ISSN
0001-5318

ACTA BIOLOGICA ET MEDICA GERMANICA

Zeitschrift für funktionelle Biowissenschaften

Symposium
acellular Protein
abolism

Band 36
Heft 11/12 · 1977
Seite 1503 – 1968

'P 48,- M

MGA J 36 (11/12) 1503—1968 (1977)

002

AKADEMIE-VERLAG
BERLIN

Aufnahmebedingungen

1. Die ACTA BIOLOGICA ET MEDICA GERMANICA, Zeitschrift für funktionelle Biowissenschaften, publiziert Arbeiten aus den Fachgebieten Biochemie, Molekular- und Zellbiologie, Physiologie (einschließlich Pathophysiologie), Pharmakologie und Immunbiologie. Es werden nur Arbeiten angenommen, die nicht an anderer Stelle mit demselben Inhalt veröffentlicht oder zur Veröffentlichung angeboten werden. Der Autor verpflichtet sich nach Annahme, die Arbeiten an keiner anderen Stelle zu veröffentlichen.

2. Die Arbeit muß wissenschaftlich wertvoll sein. Bestätigungen bekannter Tatsachen, Versuche und Beobachtungen ohne positives Ergebnis werden, wenn überhaupt, nur in kürzester Form aufgenommen. Nicht aufgenommen werden Polemiken und spekulative Arbeiten, falls sie nicht wesentlich neue Gesichtspunkte enthalten.
Die Arbeiten sollen den Charakter wissenschaftlicher Originalarbeiten haben. Als solche gelten alle Mitteilungen, die zur vorwärtsführenden Erweiterung des Erkenntnisstandes auf den genannten Fachgebieten führen. Originalarbeiten sollen 20 Manuskriptseiten nicht überschreiten. Kurzmitteilungen werden bei der Drucklegung zeitlich bevorzugt; sie dürfen 5 Manuskriptseiten nicht überschreiten. Als Kurzmitteilung gelten solche Arbeiten, in denen über neue Ergebnisse berichtet wird, ohne Details einer Originalarbeit zu enthalten.
Besonders aktuelle Untersuchungsergebnisse können in kurzer Form (bis 4 Seiten) im Offsetverfahren publiziert werden, wofür reproduktionsreife Manuskripte erforderlich sind. In Form von Übersichtsarbeiten (Reviews) werden Artikel entgegengenommen, die zu aktuellen Gebieten einen Überblick geben, in dem Fakten dargestellt, besprochen und kritisch bewertet werden.

3. Die Arbeiten müssen so kurz als möglich abgefaßt werden und in einem druckreifen Zustand geschrieben sein. Einleitung (Problematik), Methodik, Befunde und Diskussion sollen deutlich in Erscheinung treten. Der Arbeit ist eine Zusammenfassung der wesentlichsten Ergebnisse voranzustellen, wobei bei deutschsprachigen Manuskripten auch eine englische Übersetzung notwendig ist.
Arbeiten werden in Deutsch, Englisch und Russisch angenommen. Die Manuskripte sind in zweifacher Ausfertigung einzureichen. Bei Manuskripten in deutscher Sprache ist die Schreibweise des „Duden" verbindlich; bei eingedeutschten Wörtern ist die „K-Z"-Schreibweise anzuwenden.
Von den Abbildungen sind 2 Kopien sowie 1 Satz reproduktionsreife Vorlagen beizufügen. Genaue Hinweise zur Manuskriptgestaltung sind von der Redaktion der Zeitschrift anzufordern und unbedingt einzuhalten. Manuskripte, die diesen Bedingungen nicht entsprechen, gehen unbearbeitet zur Revision an den Autor zurück.

4. Die Arbeiten werden im Sofortumbruch gesetzt; Korrekturen in Form von Streichungen bzw. Zusätzen sind daher in der Umbruchkorrektur nicht zulässig.

5. Manuskripte sind an die Redaktion der ACTA BIOLOGICA ET MEDICA GERMANICA, DDR-1115 Berlin-Buch, Lindenberger Weg 70, zu senden.

6. Von jeder Originalarbeit werden kostenlos 80 Sonderdrucke geliefert.

Chefredaktion/Herausgeber

Zeitschrift ACTA BIOLOGICA ET MEDICA GERMANICA

Herausgeber: Prof. Dr. R. Baumann, Prof. Dr. H. Dutz, Prof. Dr. A. Graffi, Prof. Dr. F. Jung, Prof. Dr. O. Prokop, Prof. Dr. S. M. Rapoport.

Verlag: Akademie-Verlag, DDR-108 Berlin, Leipziger Straße 3—4; Fernruf 2236221 oder 2236229; Telex-Nr. 114420; Bank: Staatsbank der DDR, Berlin, Kto.-Nr.: 6836-26-20712.

Chefredaktion: Prof. Dr. Heinz Bielka, Prof. Dr. Werner Scheler.

Anschrift der Redaktion: DDR-1115 Berlin-Buch, Lindenberger Weg 70. Fernruf: 5697851, App. 222.

Veröffentlicht unter der Lizenznummer 1318 des Presseamtes beim Vorsitzenden des Ministerrates der Deutschen Demokratischen Republik.

Gesamtherstellung: VEB Druckerei „Thomas Müntzer", DDR-582 Bad Langensalza.

Erscheinungsweise: Die Zeitschrift erscheint monatlich. Die 12 Hefte eines Jahrganges bilden einen Band. Bezugspreis je Heft 35,— M (Preis für die DDR: 24,— M); Bandpreis 420,— M zuzüglich Versandspesen (Preis für die DDR 288,— M).

Bestellnummer dieses Heftes: 1053/XXXVI/11/12.

AN (EDV) 50117

ISSN 0001-5318

ACTA BIOLOGICA ET MEDICA GERMANICA

Herausgeber:

R. Baumann, H. Dutz, A. Graffi, F. Jung, O. Prokop, S. M. Rapoport

Chefredaktion:

H. Bielka, W. Scheler

Zeitschrift für funktionelle Biowissenschaften **Band** 36 1977 **Heft** 11—12

Intracellular Protein Catabolism III

Proceedings of the 3rd Symposium Intracellular Protein Catabolism

30 May — 4 June 1977
Schloß Reinhardsbrunn, DDR

in Honour of the 100th Birthday of Emil Abderhalden

Edited by

Horst Hanson

Siegfried Ansorge

Peter Bohley

Physiologisch-chemisches Institut,
Martin-Luther-Universität Halle-Wittenberg,
402 Halle (Saale), DDR

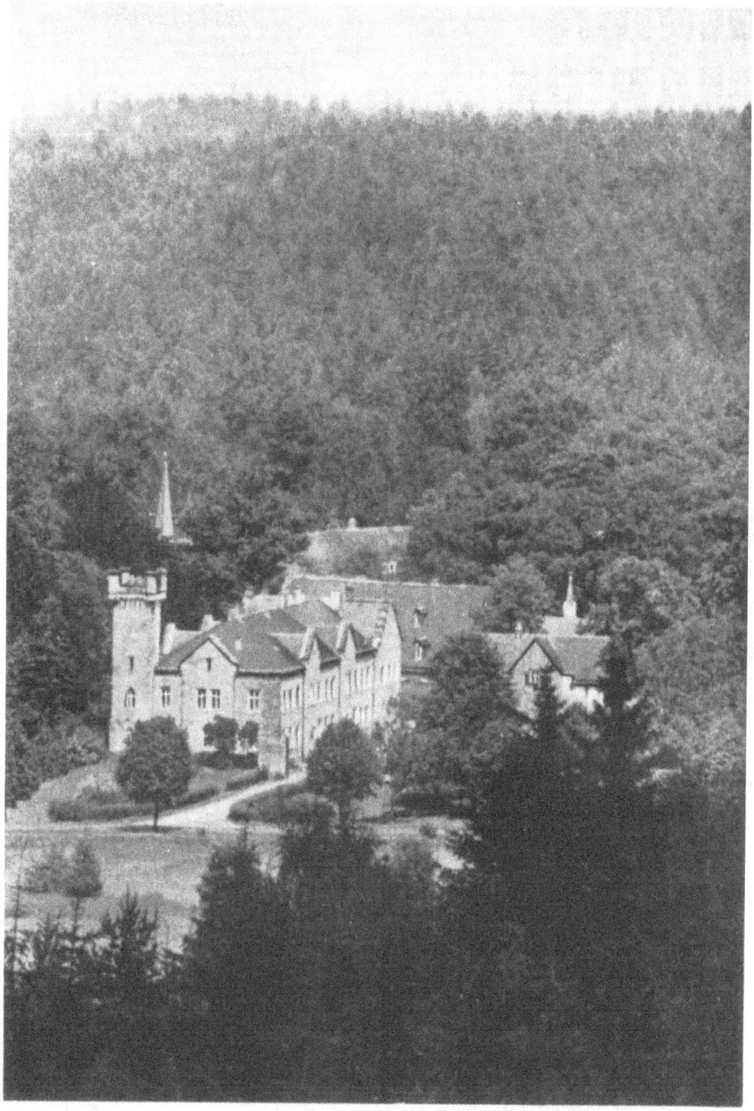

Schloß Reinhardsbrunn

Preface

This volume contains the proceedings of the 3rd Symposium on Intracellular Protein Catabolism which was held from May 30 to June 4, 1977, in Schloß Reinhardsbrunn, GDR, in honour of the 100th birthday of EMIL ABDERHALDEN *(1877—1950). The meeting was organized by the "Biochemische Gesellschaft der Deutschen Demokratischen Republik" in conjunction with the "Deutsche Akademie der Naturforscher LEOPOLDINA". It was supported by the "Martin-Luther-Universität Halle-Wittenberg". The meeting was attended by about 160 scientists, among them 60 from European Countries, Japan, USA, Australia, Sudan and Lebanon.*

This meeting has been the logical consequence of the increasing interest in the wide field of intracellular protein catabolism. After the first symposium on tissue proteinases organized by A. J. BARRETT *and* J. T. DINGLE *in 1970, a meeting dealing with the connexion of both, proteinases and turnover in vivo, was held in Schloß Reinhardsbrunn in 1973. The papers presented there were published in the book "Intracellular Protein Catabolism", edited by* H. HANSON *and* P. BOHLEY. *Two years later, the 2nd International Symposium again covering both fields was organized by our Jugoslavian friends from the J. Stefan Institute in Ljubljana and the papers were published in the book "Intracellular Protein Catabolism II", edited by* V. TURK *and* N. MARKS.

Summarizing the experiences of all these meetings we feel that our work would be unthinkable without them. We hope to find possibilities to continue this approved tradition also in the future.

This volume contains most of the papers presented at the symposium. They are arranged chronologically, largely in the form as submitted by the authors. Unfortunately, the fascinating discussions — in particular those in the night sessions — could not be included. The editors and the other members of the organizing committee (HEIDRUN KIRSCHKE, JÜRGEN LANGNER *and* BERND WIEDERANDERS) *again wish to express their thanks to all the old and new friends, who took a lively interest in the successful realization of this meeting.*

The symposium was essentially sponsored by the "Generalsekretariat der Medizinisch-wissenschaftlichen Gesellschaften beim Ministerium für Gesundheitswesen der DDR", by the "Deutsche Akademie der Naturforscher LEOPOLDINA" and by the "Martin-Luther-Universität Halle-Wittenberg". Finally, it is a pleasure to acknowledge the cooperation of the "Acta biologica et medica germanica", particularly the efforts of Prof. H. BIELKA *and Mrs.* G. GROTHE *towards rapid publication of the proceedings.*

The editors

Opening Address

by Professor H. HANSON
Chairman of the Organizing Committee,
Secretary General of the LEOPOLDINA

Dear Colleagues:

It is a great honour and pleasure for the proteolysis group of the Institute of Physiological Chemistry of the Halle-University and for myself to welcome you at the third symposium on "Intracellular Protein Catabolism". We thank you all for coming, especially our colleagues from USSR, Australia, Japan and USA. Our special welcome and thanks are devoted to the presidency and the president of the Biochemical Society of the GDR, Prof. RAPOPORT *and the Secretary General of the Medical Scientific Societies of the GDR for their aid and financial support. We are also indebted to the President of the Deutsche Akademie der Naturforscher Leopoldina, Prof.* BETHGE *and the Rector magnificus of the Martin-Luther-University in Halle, Prof.* POPPE *for their generous help in preparing our symposium. It would not have been possible to hold this symposium without the great understanding of the personalities mentioned above. The president of the Leopoldina and the rector of the university have asked me to welcome you and to wish a successful course of the symposium. President* RAPOPORT *will speak to us following my introductory words. Perhaps you will wonder why especially those three scientific institutions took part in the preparation of this symposium; this is to commemorate the centenary of the birth of* EMIL ABDERHALDEN, *a biochemist known all over the world. As one of the first scientists in the field of protein biochemistry research he was especially successful in this field. He was one of the most famous researchers and teachers of physiology and physiological chemistry at the Institute of Physiology and Physiological Chemistry of the Medical Faculty of the University of Halle from 1911—1945. Besides, from 1932 to 1950, he was the president of one of the oldest scientific academies of the world, the Deutsche Akademie der Naturforscher Leopoldina, which was founded in 1652 and has had its seat in Halle since 1878. He was my teacher from 1929—1939 and with intervals to 1945. During my work in his laboratory I learned that there must be close relations between protein turnover of the cells and the proteolytic enzyme systems existing in the cells. These problems have also been the subject of our present symposium as well as of those at Reinhardsbrunn in 1973 and in Ljubljana in 1975. We think that we could not better recall* EMIL ABDERHALDEN *to our minds than by holding this year's symposium on the occasion of his one hundredth birthday. From 1897 to 1945 he worked first in Basle in the laboratory of* GUSTAV VON BUNGE, *then from 1902—1911 in Berlin, six years of which in the laboratory of* EMIL FISCHER. *From 1911—1945, in his Halle-Institute he worked on the liberation of amino acids from proteins and peptides during the digestion in the intestine and during the intracellular degradation of cell proteins. The enzymes, which performed the digestion and degradation of proteins in the intestine and the tissues, were also a subject of his research. For he assumed that there must be correlations between the presence of proteolytic enzymes in the cells and the regulation of their activity in dependence on the processes of protein biosynthesis. The lack of appropriate methods and the poor knowledge of the structure of cells and their organelles are the reasons why the interactions between intracellular proteolytic enzyme systems, intracellular protein degradation and protein biosynthesis could not be demonstrated and proved by him. We think that it is possible now to overcome these difficulties due to advances in the field of cell particle fractionation, enzymatic micromethods and radioactive labelling of cell-own proteins. Thus we had decided to inaugurate these symposiums, the first one 4 years ago, the second in Ljubljana and now the third, to close the gap between investigations of protein turnover in vivo and the studies of intracellular proteinases in vitro and in vivo.*

I dare say that we have been successful in this respect at the two preceding symposiums and we hope that this symposium will continue the process of integrating the protein turnover studies in vivo and the molecular mechanisms of the intracellular proteolytic enzymes involved in these turnover processes.

I think we should try to perform the investigations on the field of protein turnover, intracellular protein degradation and intracellular proteolytic enzyme systems in a concerted way. In order to win clearer ideas of the regulation of the protein turnover and of the intracellular proteolytic enzymes concerned, some crucial facts would be necessary, which, however, are still missing. In case of a more detailed knowledge about the intracellular proteolytic enzyme systems and their regulation and cooperation in the living cell, we should undoubtedly be able to understand the feed back, which is almost unknown yet, between protein biosynthesis and protein degradation. Also the other regulation factors, such as intracellular enzyme activation and inhibition, limited proteolysis and intracellular enzyme synthesis and enzyme degradation could be better interpreted. Therefore criteria are necessary whose requirements must be fulfilled in the environment of the cell and their organelles and also in the structure of the cell proteins themselves, so that the intracellular proteases may initiate and finish the degradation of certain proteins in a selective manner.

We do hope that the amenities of this lovely place will create the atmosphere adequate for a scientific meeting like this.

At the end of my introductory words I should like to express my gratitude to all coworkers, named and unnamed. A special thank is due to the members of the organizing committee, all belonging to the proteolysis group in Halle. First Dr. PETER BOHLEY *and also the others: Dr.* SIEGFRIED ANSORGE, *Dr.* JÜRGEN LANGNER, *Dr.* HEIDRUN KIRSCHKE, *Dr.* BERND WIEDERANDERS.

Before we shall start our scientific programme, I should like to ask the President of the Biochemical Society of the GDR, Prof. RAPOPORT, *to take the floor.*

H. HANSON

Opening Address

by Prof. S. M. RAPOPORT
President of the Biochemische Gesellschaft der DDR

Dear Colleagues:

I am happy to express on behalf of the Biochemische Gesellschaft der DDR thanks to Prof. HANSON *and his coworkers for their fine work in organizing this symposium. I convey the best wishes for its success to all participants. Our society sponsors specialized symposia as an important element of its scientific life and as a valuable means to develop international contacts. Recurrent symposia which establish a scientific tradition we consider to be particularly useful. Even though this one is only the third of a series, the preceding ones have established a fine tradition which the present symposium is certain to continue.*

It has, however, an additional historical significance. The present symposium is devoted to the memory of the 100th birthday of EMIL ABDERHALDEN. *We honor not only a great scientist who has contributed prolificly to biochemistry and who has been a pioneer in the field of proteolysis, but also a great humanitarian. The life of* EMIL ABDERHALDEN *is an example of devotion to many aspects of human welfare, which*

should be hold up to all scientists even today. It was a tragic fate that both the beginning and the end of his life time work in Halle were overshadowed by the world wars.
Our symposium has yet another accent. We honor with it the life time work of H. HANSON, *a pupil of* ABDERHALDEN. HANSON *served in Halle nearly as long as his teacher. After the terrible catastrophe brought on by Hitler he was able to build up a fine department and a scientific school which well deserves international recognition. The preconditions for this steady development were the stability and security in all levels of life, including the individual scientist, the department, the university and the GDR as a whole. The most important precondition for the undisturbed development of science is the maintenance of peace. I feel that we owe a tribute to the untiring world-wide efforts for distension to which the USSR contributes in such an outstanding manner. We remember that one of the first decrees after the October Revolution sixty years ago was that for peace. The USSR has remained faithful to its spirit.*

S. M. RAPOPORT

Acta biol. med. germ., Band 36, Seite 1509—1514 (1977)

Institute of Genetics and Selection of Industrial Microorganisms, Moscow, USSR

Intracellular proteinase of Bacillus subtilis

V. M. STEPANOV, A. Ya. STRONGIN, L. S. ISOTOVA, and Z. T. ABRAMOV

Summary

An intracellular serine proteinase was isolated from Bacillus subtilis, strain A—50. The molecular weight of the enzyme is 30000 ± 1000, its amino acid composition is enriched in glutamic acid residues, the isoelectric point is 4.3, the N-terminal sequence Glu-Leu-Pro-Glu-Gly-Ile-Gln-Val-Ile-Lys-Ala-Pro-Glu-Leu-Xxx-Ala-Gln-Gly-Phe-Lys Gly-Ser-Asx-Ile-Lys-Ile-Ala-Val-Leu-Asx. The enzyme is structuraly homologous with secretory subtilisins.

Introduction

Although the intracellular proteinases play an important role in protein catabolism and eventually in the regulation of biological processes, our knowledge of these enzymes is rather limited. E. g., the chemical properties of bacterial intracellular proteinases are scarcely known and information on their structure is completely lacking. Recently we studied the multiple forms of the serine proteinase subtilisin secreted by Bacillus subtilis A-50 strain [1]. This proteinase of subtilisin BPN type [2] appears in the cultural filtrate as a mixture of multiple forms whose pattern changes under the influence of certain mutations not hitting the structural gene of subtilisin. The most effective were the mutations changing the surface structures of the cell. It seems that the molecule of subtilisin which is coded in a given Bacillus subtilis strain by one structural gene becomes modified in the course of its secretion presumably by limited proteolysis. The intensity of this process strongly depends on the state of the cell membrane, cell wall and periplasmic space.

We have shown that the same strain of Bacillus subtilis in addition to subtilisin of BPN type produces an intracellular serine proteinase, a structural homolog of secreted enzyme. This enzyme, which will be further abbreviated as ISP (intracellular serine proteinase), under certain conditions — presumably as a result of cell lysis or major changes in cell membrane permeability might appear in the cultural medium.

Material and methods

Cells of Bacillus subtilis A-50 (strain supplied by Dr. L. KAY, Monsanto Co., St. Louis, USA) were grown on Spizizen medium and harvested at the stationary phase (20hrs, 35 °C). The washed cells were sonicated and the cell debris separated by centrifugation. After precipitation of nucleic acids with 1 mg/ml of streptomycin sulfate and centrifugation the supernatant was fractionated with ammonium sulfate precipitation. The fraction precipitated between 0.55 and 0.80 of ammonium sulfate saturation was dialyzed and applied on Whatman DE-52 column at *p*H 8.5. After elution with a linear 50—500 mM Tris buffer gradient, *p*H 8.5, the fractions containing active proteinase (benzyloxycarbonyl-L-alanyl-L-alanyl-L-leucyl-p-nitroanilide was used as a substrate for proteinase assay throughout the procedure [3]) were collected, concentrated by ultrafiltration through a Diaflo UM-2 membrane and chromatographed on Ultragel AcA column at *p*H 8.5. Active fractions were collected, concentrated by ultrafiltration and treated by 1 mM phenylmethylsulfonylfluoride, a specific inhibitor of serine proteinases, to prevent ISP autolysis. As a final purification step disc-electrophoresis in 10 per cent polyacrylamide gels was used. After protein staining the zone corresponding to the active enzyme (run separately on the control gel) was cut off and the inactivated enzyme was extracted from the gel slices. The preparation obtained was used for amino acid assay and sequence determination. Disc-electrophoresis of the active enzyme gave another preparation which was used for preliminary enzymological tests although its specific activity was diminished obviously as a result of autolysis.

All operations were performed at 4 °C. Ca^{++}-ions were added to all solutions to 1 mM concentration which was necessary to prevent enzyme inactivation. The isolation procedure is summarized in Table 1. 100 g of wet cells gave 20—30 mg of pure protein.

In Fig. 1 discelectrophoretic patterns are shown for ISP and the secretory subtilisin BPN.

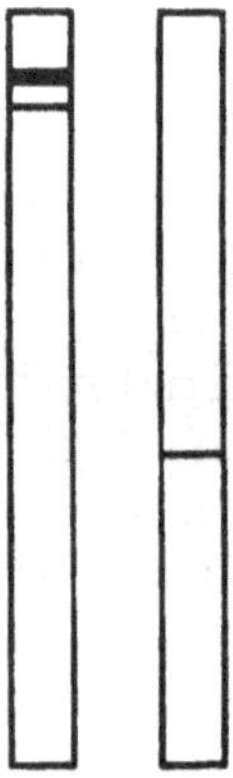

a b Fig. 1

Table 1
Purification of the intacellular serine proteinase

Purification step	Protein (mg)	Activity (units)	Specific activity (units/mg)
Cell extract	—	135	—
Streptomycin sulfate precipitation	10000	150	0.015
$(NH_4)_2SO_4$ precipitation	400	180	0.45
DEAE-cellulose chromatography	36	90	2.5
Ultragel AcA34 chromatography	15	79	5.3

Fig. 1. Polyacrylamide gel electrophoresis in 7.5% gels.
Migration was from top to bottom.
a) Subtilisin BPN; b) Intracellular serine proteinase. The faint band in a) corresponds to minor component of subtilisin. The bands were localized by Coomassie Brilliant Blue R250 staining or by substrate hydrolysis [3]

Results and discussion

The purification scheme described above allows to obtain homogenous preparation of individual specifically inhibited enzyme with satisfactory yield. The active enzyme preparation appears to be free from proteinic impurities but substantial decrease in activity level did not allow to estimate ISP catalytic constant. Polyacrylamide electrophoresis in the presence of sodium dodecyl sulfate showed that ISP has a molecular weight of 31000 ± 1000. This value is slightly higher than the molecular weight of secretory subtilisins. One may suspect that the difference is caused by eventual anomaly in SDS complexing with rather acidic ISP, but the existence of some polypeptide chain extensions in ISP cannot be excluded.

The enzyme appears to be a dimer when studied by gel filtration in non-denaturing solvents. An I. P. equal to 4.3 was found by isoelectrofocussing. Hence, ISP is clearly an acidic protein in contrast to the secretory subtilisins showing an I. P. of 7—8. This difference reflects substantial increase in the content of glutamic acid residues (Table 2). Among other amino acids whose share in ISP differs markedly from that in subtilisins lysine, phenylalanine and valine deserve to be mentioned. These differences in amino acid composition are large enough to indicate that ISP is coded by specific structural gene and cannot be considered as a precursor of secretory subtilisin. This conclusion was confirmed by comparison of cyanogen bromide fragments of ISP and subtilisin BPN. The separation of CNBr cleavage products by discelectrophoresis gave four peptide zones for subtilisin BPN whereas five peptide zones were found in the case of ISP. The fragments obtained from these proteins showed different electrophoretic mobilities.

N-Terminal sequence of ISP was determined by automated Edman degradation (Tab. 3). ISP is clearly homologous to secretory subtilisins including one produced by the same strain of Bacillus subtilis. Special run of sequencing confirmed that secretory subtilisin of Bacillus subtilis strain A-50 has exactly the same N-terminal sequence as subtilisin BPN. Among the first 30 residues of ISP at least 16 coincide with respective residues of subtilisin BPN, 18 with subtilisin „Carlsberg“. The N-terminal sequence of ISP is two amino acids shorter than that of the secretory subtilisins. The minimal amino acid substitution number is 13 for the ISP-BPN' pair, and 11 for ISP-Carlsberg (one residue is not identified in ISP sequence). These numbers are very close to 13 substitutions for the same stretch of BPN and Carlsberg sequences.

Table 2

Amino acid composition of ISP and secretory subtilisins

Amino acid	ISP	BPN	221	Carls-berg	Amylosaccha-riticus	Pfizer
Lys	20	11	6	9	8	11
His	6	6	8	5	6	4
Arg	6	2	8	4	4	4
Asp	36	28	29	28	25	28
Thr	13	13	18	19	17	17
Ser	25	37	23	32	41	31
Glu	33	15	16	12	15	15
Pro	13	14	16	9	13	14
Gly	36	33	39	35	33	29
Ala	32	37	45	41	35	32
Val	19	30	27	31	25	22
Met	5–6	5	4	5	4	5
Ile	13	13	9	10	16	9
Leu	25	15	22	16	15	13
Tyr	7	10	9	13	12	9
Phe	7	3	4	4	4	4
Trp	—	3	3	1	3	—
Sum:	296	275	283	274	275	247

Hence, the extent of N-terminal sequence divergence is of the same order of magnitude for intracellular as well as secreted subtilisins. Nevertheless, a very specific shift in amino acid composition — the enrichment in glutamic acid content — allows to consider ISP as a new type of subtilisin-like proteinases rather than just an additional member of the known family of secretory subtilisins.

ISP is fully inactivated by standard inhibitors of serine proteinases such as diisopropylfluorophosphate and phenylmethylsulfonylfluoride (Table 4). EDTA inactivates the enzyme rapidly and irreversibly owing to destabilization caused by the removal of calcium ions. p-Chloromercuribenzoate diminished the activity of ISP by 20 per cent. ISP cleaves effectively the chromogenic peptide substrates of subtilisin, benzyloxycarbonyl-L-alanyl-L-alanyl-L-leucyl-p-nitroanilide being the best from the tested ones. The specific activity against Z-Ala-Ala-Leu-pNA is 5.3 units per mg, against Z-Gly-Gly-Phe-pNA 0.13 units per mg, and against Z-Gly-Gly-Leu-pNA 0.21 units per mg. The specific activity of subtilisin BPN is 0.45 units per mg against the first substrate. ISP has a rather broad *p*H optimum at 7—10, and an optimal temperature of peptide hydrolysis at 40 °C. The enzyme shows a stability optimum at *p*H 6—7 and retains its stability up to 60 °C. The intracellular localization of ISP awaits a more careful study. Preliminary

Table 3
The alignment of N-terminal sequences of subtilisin BPN (BPN), intracellular serine proteinase (ISP) and subtilisin Carlsberg (CAR)

BPN	Ala	Gln	Ser	Val	*Pro*	Tyr	*Gly*	Val	Ser	Gln	*Ile*	*Lys*
ISP			Glu	Leu	Pro	Glu	Gly	Ile	Gln	Val	Ile	Lys
CAR	Ala	Gln	Thr	Val	*Pro*	Tyr	*Gly*	*Ile*	Pro	Leu	*Ile*	*Lys*
BPN			*Ala*	*Pro*	Ala	*Leu*	His	Ser	*Gln*	*Gly*	Tyr	Thr
ISP			Ala	Pro	Glu	Leu	Xxx	Ala	Gln	Gly	Phe	Lys
CAR			*Ala*	Asp	Lys	Val	Gln	*Ala*	*Gln*	*Gly*	*Phe*	*Lys*
BPN			*Gly*	*Ser*	*Asn*	Val	*Lys*	Val	*Ala*	*Val*	Ile	*Asp*
ISP			Gly	Ser	Asx	Ile	Lys	Ile	Ala	Val	Leu	Asx
CAR			*Gly*	Ala	*Asn*	Val	*Lys*	Val	*Ala*	*Val*	*Leu*	*Asp*

Residue Nr. 15 in ISP was not identified; identification of residues Nrs. 22 and 25 is preliminary and awaits confirmation. For calculation of coinciding residues in aligned sequences Asx-23 considered as Asn, Asx-30 as Asp. It has to be mentioned that Asx-30 corresponds to Asp-32 in secretory subtilisins which belongs to the active site of these enzymes. Symbbols in italics in the sequences of BPN and CAR represent residues identical to those in ISP.

Table 4
Some properties of intracellular serine proteinase

Molecular weight	31000 ± 1000
Isoelectric point	4.3
*p*H-optimum of activity	7—10
*p*H-optimum of stability	6—7
Temperature optimum of activity	40°
Stable to heating up to	60°
Activity retained after treatment with:	
Diisopropylfluorophosphate	0%
Phenylmethylsulphonylfluoride	0%
Ethylenediaminetetraacetate	0%
p-Hydroxymercurybenzoate	80%

tests showed that at least a part of this enzyme is bound to the cell membrane and might be solubilized only by non-ionic detergent treatment.

ISP studied in our laboratory possesses common traits with acidic intracellular proteinase found in Bacillus subtilis by REYSSERT and MILLET [4]. Unfortunately the latter enzyme had been only loosely characterized from the chemical point of view which handicaped the strict comparison. It seems that the enzyme described by these authors might be identical with ISP. One might also suspect that the unusual form of subtilisin described by SHOER and RAPPAPORT [5] as extracellular enzyme under designation W-I and possessing rather close amino acid composition to that of ISP is identical with the latter. We observed that under certain conditions ISP appears outside the cell presumably as a result of cell lysis or heavy changes in cell permeability.

The precise functional role of intracellular serine proteinase is not yet clear. The enzyme appears within the cell in noticeable quantities immediately before the sporulation concurrently with the increase in proteolytic intensity. In any case it seems to be more reasonable candidate for the role of protein catabolizing enzyme and/or modifying agent than the secretory subtilisins. Its activity is lower than that of secretory subtilisins when tested against the standard protein substrates, e. g. bovine serum albumin and hemoglobin, although ISP is much more active against peptide p-nitroanilides. It cannot be excluded that the low proteolytic activity of ISP might be explained by a disadvantageous shift in enzyme net charge at the *p*H-optimum of hydrolysis.

All data discussed above show that the genome of Bacillus subtilis contains at least two homologous structural genes for two serine proteinases — an intracellular serine proteinase and subtilisin — that arose obviously as a result of ancestor gene duplication. The presence of two homologous genes in the cell might eventually accelerate the evolution of this particular type of enzyme not only by the loosening of selection constraints but also by creation of numerous sequence variants by means of intragenic recombination. It is tempting to assume that the acceleration of this kind might be the reason of surprisingly high rate of subtilisin evolution.

Acknowledgement

We wish to thank Dr. E. A. TIMOKHINA for amino acid analysis, Drs L. P. BELYANOVA and L. P. BARATOVA for the sequenator experiments, Dr. D. I. GORODETSKY for the CNBr cleavage experiments, and Mrs. V. V. JANONIS for skillful assistance.

References

[1] STRONGIN, A. Ya., Z. T. ABRAMOV, E. D. LEVIN, and V. M. STEPANOV: Bioorgan. Khim. 1, 1441 (1975)
[2] MARKLAND, F. S., and E. L. SMITH in: The Enzymes. 3rd Ed., Vol. 3, 564. P. BOYER (Ed). Academic Press, New York, London, 1971
[3] LYUBLINSKAYA, L. A., S. V. BELYAEV, A. Ya. STRONGIN, L. F. MATYASH, E. D. LEVIN, and V. M. STEPANOV; Analyt. Biochem. 62, 371 (1974)
[4] REYSSERT, G., and J. MILLET: Biochem. biophys. Res. Commun. 49, 328 (1972)
[5] SHOER, R., and H. P. RAPPAPORT: J. Bact. 109, 575 (1972)

Acta biol. med. germ., Band 36, Seite 1515—1522 (1977)

Institute of Microbiology, Czechoslovak Academy of Sciences, Prague, Czechoslovakia

Relationships between intracellular proteolytic activity and protein turnover in Bacillus megaterium

J. Chaloupka, L. Philippová, J. Čechová, and M. Strnadová

Summary

When incubated in a sporulation medium, the sporogenous strains of Bacillus megaterium degrade proteins at a rate of 4—10% × h^{-1}. The maximal rate of protein turnover is reached after 3—4 hrs at the time of development of forespores and then decreases again. The rate of protein turnover in the asporogenous strain decreases steadily under similar conditions from 3—8% × h^{-1} at the beginning of incubation to 1% × h^{-1} after 5—6 hrs in the sporulation medium. The rate of degradation of proteins in vitro in protoplast lysates is similar or higher than the rate of protein turnover.

The exocellular, as well as periplasmic proteolytic activity, is suppressed by amino acids more severely than the activity in protoplasts. Mutants devoid of the exocellular proteolytic enzyme contain also less proteolytic activity in the periplasm than in the protoplasts, in contrast to the wild strain. However, their rate of protein turnover, as well as the degradation of abnormal proteins is similar to that in the wild strain. This supports a view that the proteolytic system in protoplasts is involved in intracellular protein catabolism. The periplasmic enzyme can be considered as a kind of the exocellular proteinase.

Introduction

During protein turnover intracellular proteolytic enzymes, together with peptidases, catalyze the hydrolysis of proteins to amino acids. They probably also play an important role in degradation of abnormal proteins, which may occur as a consequence of an incorrect translation [1, 2]. The important role of proteolytic enzymes in the sporogenesis of bacilli and in other types of cellular differentation in microorganisms is also assumed [3]. Turnover of proteins may include either activation or increased synthesis of the intracellular proteolytic system, the basic level of which is present even in a growing population. However, certain data indicate that a new specific proteinase is synthesized in nongrowing cells of bacilli which is involved in first steps of sporulation [4].

The course of intracellular proteolytic activity determined in vitro usually generally corresponds to the course of protein turnover. However, the proteolytic activity measured in cell homogenates often exceeds several times the rate of protein catabolism in vivo [5] indicating that only a part of the intracellular proteolytic system might be involved in protein turnover. The role of different cellular compartments (periplasm, protoplast) in protein degradation is not clear either.

It was the aim of the present work to study the relationships between the intracellular proteolytic activity and protein turnover in sporogenous and asporogenous strains of Bacillus megaterium. This organism was chosen as a model as it synthesizes only a single exocellular proteinase the regulation of which has already been studied [6]. It is also very sensitive to lysozyme which makes it possible to study separately proteolytic systems in the periplasm and protoplasts.

Material and methods

The sporogenous strains of Bacillus megaterium (KM-gift of Prof. ARONSON and 27 (J)-gift of Prof. TAUBENECK) were used. The strains KM 1, highly proteolytic, and its spontaneous derivative KM 7, slightly proteolytic, were used as representatives of asporogenous variants. Two mutants (KM 12 and 13) devoid of exocellular proteolytic activity were prepared from strain KM 7 by treatment with monochromatic ultraviolet light (to be published). Cultivation in a shaken water bath (35 °C) as well as media – mineral (C) and complex (C/CAA and BET) – were described in previous communications [7, 8]. The sporulation medium was a modification [8] of the medium of GREENE and SLEPECKY [9]. Ca^{2+}-ions were omitted from the sporulation medium, in order to decrease contamination of cells with the exocellular proteinase. Preparation of protoplasts, as well as lysis of cells with lysozyme were performed as described [8]. When determining β-galactosidase, toluene (50 μl) was added to 2.5 ml of the cell suspension (about 1 mg dry weight/ml) and the suspension was shaken 6 min with a Wortex mixer. Occasional changes of this procedure are mentioned in the text.

Determination of proteolytic activity using ^{14}C or ^{3}H labelled denatured bacterial proteins as substrates as well as degradation of labelled "native" proteins in vitro in the protoplast or cell lysates were described earlier [7, 8]. The rate of degradation of "native" proteins in the cell or protoplast lysates was determined after three hours incubation of the respective samples at 35 °C. As lysozyme decreased the proteolytic activity in the cell lysates, due probably to competition for the substrate with the enzyme, the values measured were corrected. The activity of β-galactosidase was assayed according to JANEČEK and RICKENBERG [10].

The measurement of protein turnover during incubation in the sporulation medium was based on the determination of the release of [^{14}C] leucine from the proteins of the overnight prelabelled culture into the TCA supernatant [8]. Protein determinations in the course of the assay of specific radioactivity of proteins was performed according to LOWRY et al. [11].

The measurement of the turnover of abnormal proteins was performed as follows: The culture was incubated in the mineral salts + glucose medium (C/G). Ethionine (5 mM) was added for 45 min to the growing population. During the last 15 min the incubation proceeded in the presence of [^{14}C] leucine (3.7 kBq/ml. 50 μM).

The labelled cells were then harvested by means of centrifugation and resuspended in the fresh C/G medium with [^{12}C]L-leucine (2 mM). The incubation proceeded for 1 h and samples were precipitated at time intervals with the same volume of 10% TCA with [^{12}C] leucine. The release of ^{14}C into the TCA supernatant was then determined.

Results

The asporogenous variant of Bacillus megaterium KM as well as the sporogenous strain 27(J) synthesize and excrete an exocellular proteinase that belongs to the group of neutral metaloproteinases and also contain a distinct intracellular proteolytic activity. The synthesis of the exocellular proteinase in both organisms is controlled by repression, in which amino acids and glucose are involved. However, the course of protein turnover during incubation in the sporulation medium is different in the asporogenous and sporogenous strains. In the sporogenous organism an increase of the rate of degradation of proteins during first 3—4 hrs was found. The rate was found to decrease again since the visible forespores were formed. The rate of the intracellular protein degradation in the asporogenous variant steadily decreases beginning with the first hour (Fig. 1). The rate of degradation of proteins, when plotted in a semilogarithmic scale, decreases with the half-life of 2—3 hrs (Fig. 2). A higher rate of protein turnover was found in the asporogenous strain

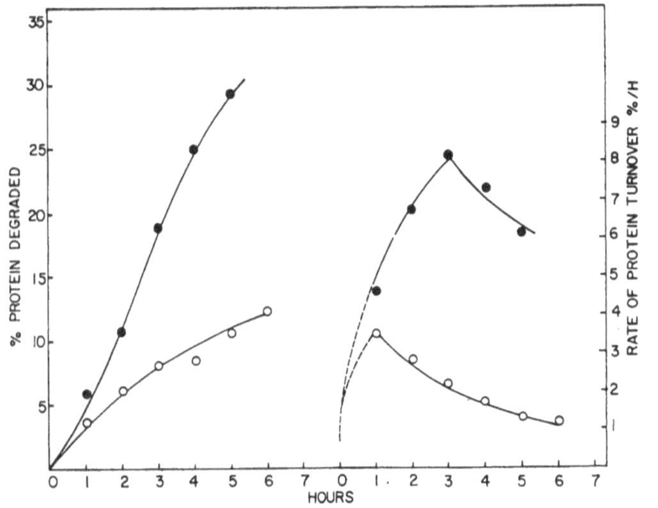

Fig. 1. Course of intracellular protein catabolism in the sporogenous and asporogenous B. megaterium.

The organisms grown and labelled in a complex medium with lactose (BET/L) were transferred at the end of growth phase (0 h) to the sporulation medium. ● sporogenous strain 27 (J); ○ asporogenous strain KM 1. Left site: course of degradation of proteins; right site: rate of degradation of proteins

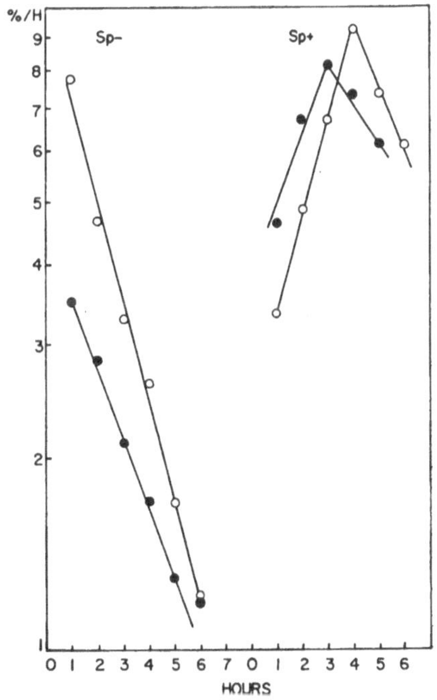

Fig. 2. Rate of intracellular protein catabolism plotted in the semilogarithmic scale.

The procedure was similar to that in Fig. 1. Sp^-: asporogenous strain KM 1, Sp^+: sporogenous strain 27 (J). ● culture was pregrown and labelled in BET/L medium; ○ culture was pregrown in the complex medium with glucose in the case of the asporogenous strain or in the complex medium with glycerol and galactose in the case of the sporogenous organism grown and labelled in the complex medium with glucose, in comparison with that grown in the same medium with lactose. The reason for this difference is not clear; it seems, however, that the growth curve of this organism in lactose media has a biphasic character. It is not excluded that during the second, slower growth phase some turnover of proteins can take place leading to the decrease of the fraction of proteins more susceptible to turnover. When the incubation of the asporogenous strain in the sporulation medium proceeds for 20 hrs or more, no substantial increase of degradation of proteins above the value 20—30% could be found (Fig. 3). The asporogenous variant seems to be similar in this respect to Escherichia coli, where also only up to 30% protein can undergo protein turnover during starvation [12]. Protein turnover in the sporulating strains is probably more extensive.

Another difference in the course of intracellular protein catabolism between the sporogenous and asporogenous strain was also observed. The inactivation of β-galactosidase in the former strain proceeded at a higher rate than the protein turnover, especially during later stages of sporogenesis. In the asporogenous strain only a negligible decrease of activity of β-galactosidase was observed at the beginning and some residual synthesis of the enzyme was found during the prolonged incubation (Fig. 4). Inactivation of β-galactosidase took place also in the sporogenous KM strain, where, however, the rate of protein turnover, as well as the extent of sporulation were lower than in the strain 27(J) under similar conditions (Table 1). In the sporogenous strain 27(J) up to 90% of sporangia were observed at t5, i. e. after 5 hrs of incubation in the sporulation medium. However, we have no evidence

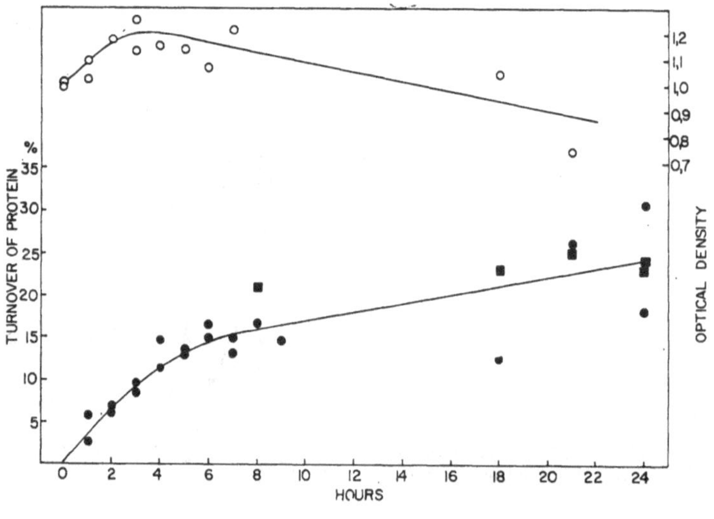

Fig. 3. Course of degradation of proteins in the asporogenous strain KM 1 in a long-term experiment.

The organism was pregrown and labelled in BET/L medium and at the end of the growth phase transferred to the sporulation medium. ○ optical density (650 nm); ● decrease of TCA precipitable radioactivity; ■ decrease of specific radioactivity of proteins.

The results of two independent experiments are given

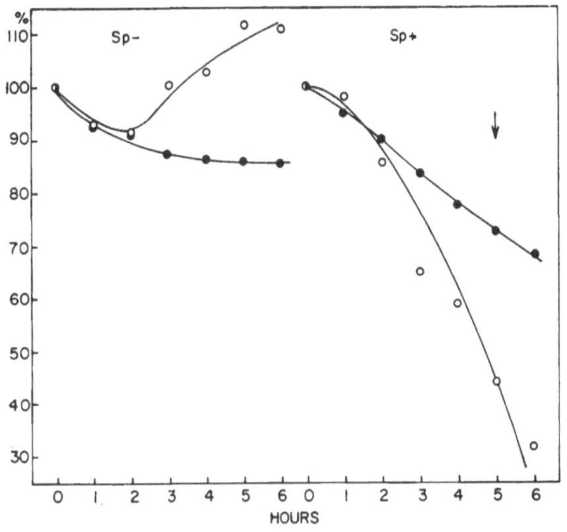

Fig. 4. Relationship between the degradation of proteins and inactivation of β-galactosidase. The asporogenous strain KM 1 (Sp^-) and sporogenous strain 27 (J) (Sp^+) were pregrown and labelled in a complex medium with glycerol and galactose and at the end of the growth phase they were transferred to the sporulation medium. ● TCA precipitable radioactivity, ○ activity of β-galactosidase.

Table 1
Intracellular protein catabolism in the sporogenous strain KM

Degradation of labelled proteins	t4 (a)	14.9%
	t5 (a)	20.0%
Inactivation of β-galactosidase	t4 (a)	27.0%
	t5 (b)	35.5%

The grown culture was transferred at the beginning of the stationary phase (t0) to the sporulation medium. The incubation proceeded for 4 (t4) or 5 (t5) hrs and the extent of degradation of proteins labelled with [^{14}C]leucine, as well as that of inactivation of β-galactosidase were determined. The activity of β-galactosidase was estimated in lysozyme cell lysates. At t7 only 20–40% cells formed sporangia. The mean values from four or more (a) or three (b) experiments are given.

that the inactivation of β-galactosidase is due to the activity of a proteolytic system.

There are two compartments in cells of bacilli and probably also in other types of bacteria, which can be considered as places where the degradation of intracellular proteins proceeds: the periplasmic space and the protoplast. In order to establish whether the proteolytic system in the protoplast fraction can display sufficient activity to hydrolyse "native" proteins, the rates of proteolysis in vitro in lysates of protoplasts and cells were determined and compared with the rate of protein turnover. The data obtained in the experiments in which glucose as well as lactose grown cells were used indicate that the proteolytic activity in protoplasts is probably sufficiently high to be responsible for the catabolism of proteins during protein turnover (Fig. 5). The course of activity in the cell lysates shows a sharp peak during the first hours, which is apparently due to the increase of the proteolytic activity in the periplasm. This peak roughly coincides with the highest capacity to synthesize the exocellular proteinase (data not shown).

Another indirect evidence also supports the view that the periplasmic proteinase is probably an enzyme of the exocellular type not involved in protein turnover. Repression of exocellular proteinase by amino acids and glucose suppresses the periplasmic proteinase to a similar extent as the exocellular enzyme (Table 2). The proteolytic activity in protoplasts is suppressed substantially less. It appears likely that most of the repressible intracellular proteolytic activity (periplasmic and protoplast activities) might represent rather an exocellular proteinase synthesized de novo, than a true intracellular enzyme involved in protein catabolism. This assumption is also supported by the experiments with nonproteolytic mutants. These mutants derived from the asporogenous strain that are devoid of the exocellular proteinase have decreased considerably their periplasmic proteolytic activity. Their activity in the fraction of protoplasts is also reduced, however, it is not further substantially decreased under conditions of repression (Table 2).

All these strains are capable of protein turnover in the sporulation medium at a rate similar to that found in the proteolytic asporogenous strain KM 1 (Table 3). They retain also the capacity to degrade the abnormal proteins formed during growth in the presence of ethionine.

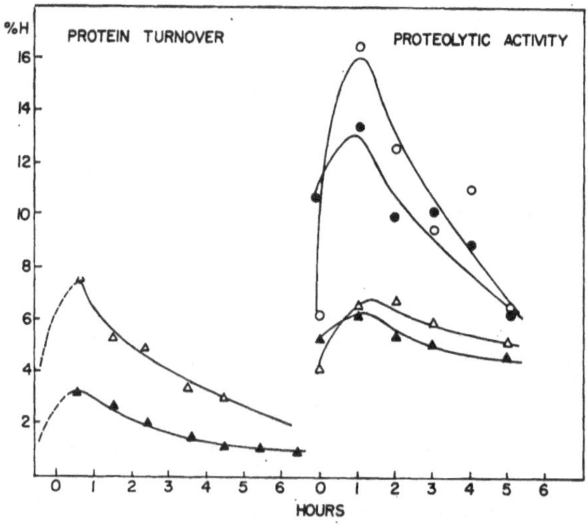

Fig. 5. Relationship between the rate of protein turnover and intracellular proteolytic activity

The asporogenous strain KM 1 was pregrown and labelled in the complex medium with either lactose (full symbols) or glucose (open symbols) and transferred at the end of the growth phase to the sporulation medium. Left site: ▲, △ rate of protein turnover; right site: ▲, △ proteolytic activity im lysates of protoplasts or: ●, ○ lysozyme lysates of cells. The rate of degradation of "native" proteins in cell or protoplasts lysates was determined.

Table 2

Suppression of proteolytic activity by 10 mg/ml of caseine hydrolysate

Strain KM	Exocellular enzyme[a]	Periplasm[a]	Protoplasts[a]	Specific activity[b] in protoplasts
1	18.1%	17.1%	33.5%	90.5 µg S × mg P^{-1} × h^{-1}
7	(4.5%)/	N	73.3%	15.8 µg S × mg P^{-1} × h^{-1}
12	N	N	59.3%	22.5 µg S × mg P^{-1} × h^{-1}
13	N	N	71.5%	26.3 µg S × mg P^{-1} × h^{-1}

The culture was grown in the mineral salts + glucose medium (C/G). To a portion of the population acid caseine hydrolysate (10 mg/ml) was added and the cultivation proceeded for 2 hrs. The activities in the medium (exocellular enzyme), in the supernatant released after protoplasting the cells ("periplasm") and in the lysate of protoplasts ("protoplasts") were then determined. The mean values of three experiments are given.

[a] Activity of the culture grown in the absence of caseine hydrolysate is taken as 100%.

[b] Specific activity in protoplasts prepared from the culture grown in the absence of caseine hydrolysate is presented.

[c] Result of a single experiment only.

S = substrate; P = protein; N = negligible even in the control grown without caseine hydrolysate. The suppression by amino acids could not be determined.

Table 3

Characteristics of non-proteolytic mutants

Strain KM	Exocellular enzyme %	Intracellular enzyme[a] %	Ratio of activity protoplasts: cells	Turnover of proteins	
				starvation[b]	abnormal protein[c]
1	100	100	0.40	6.8% × h^{-1}	20.9% × h^{-1}
7	<30	30.3	0.64	6.4% × h^{-1}	14.7% × h^{-1}
12	<0.2	15.1	0.60	5.7% × h^{-1}	21.0% × h^{-1}
13	<1	30.8	0.79	5.6% × h^{-1}	15.9% × h^{-1}

[a] Specific activity with radioactive denatured proteins determined after $2^1/_2$ hrs in the sporulation medium.

[b] Determined after 3 hrs in the sporulation medium; the culture was labelled with [^{14}C]leucine in the C/CAA/G medium.

[c] Abnormal proteins labelled with [^{14}C]leucine were synthesized during 15 min in C/G medium in the presence of 5 mM ethionine. Their degradation was determined during 1 h of growth in C/G medium

Discussion

Protein turnover can be considered as a necessary prerequisite for any kind of cellular differentiation in microorganisms. The loss of the sporulation capacity usually results in a considerable decrease of the rate of protein turnover [13]. However, the asporogenous variant of B. megaterium KM retains its capability to exert turnover of proteins under conditions where the sporogenous strains develop spores. The rates of protein turnover at the beginning of incubation on both sporogenous and asporogenous variants in a sporulation medium do not differ substantially (Fig. 1 und 2) and the characters of the respective proteolytic systems in the lysates of protoplasts seem to be also similar [8]. However, the rate of protein turnover in the asporogenous strain decreases rapidly unlike that in the sporogenous organism. The reason for the rapid decrease of the rate of protein catabolism in vivo is not clear. Progressive exhaustion of proteins primarily susceptible to the proteolytic enzymes, a decrease of proteolytic activity, or inactivation of a hypothetical system which makes proteins more sensitive to the proteolytic attack can be considered as possible causes.

The proteolytic system present in protoplasts is probably sufficiently active to be responsible for the first hydrolytic attack of protein molecules during protein turnover. Its capacity to hydrolyse denatured proteins seems to be even higher than its actual activity against "native" proteins in protoplast lysates [8].

Also the results of the experiments with non-proteolytic mutants (Tables 2 and 3) support the idea that the protoplast is the compartment where protein catabolism takes place and that the periplasmic proteolytic activity does not play any substantial role in protein turnover. It cannot be excluded either that at least a portion of proteolytc activity in the protoplast might be due to a "precursor" form of the exocellular enzyme, as it is sensitive to the repression and is decreased in mutants devoid of the exocellular proteinase.

References

[1] MANDELSTAM, J.: Ann. N.Y. Acad. Sci. **102**, 621 (1963)
[2] GOLDBERG, A. L.: Proc. natn. Acad. Sci. U.S.A. **69**, 422 (1972)
[3] SCHAEFFER, P.: Bact. Rev. **33**, 48 (1969)
[4] MILLET, J.: C. r. Acad. Sci., Paris **272**, 1806 (1971)
[5] BERNLOHR, R. W., and V. CLARK: J. Bact. **105**, 276 (1971)
[6] CHALOUPKA, J.: Ann. Inst. Pasteur **117**, 631 (1969)
[7] CHALOUPKA, J., V. OBDRŽÁLEK, P. KŘEČKOVA, M. NESMEYANOVA, and V. ZALABÁK: Folia Microbiol. **20**, 277 (1975)
[8] CHALOUPKA, J., M. STRNADOVA, and V. ZALABÁK: Folia Microbiol. **22**, 1 (1977)
[9] GREENE, R. A., and R. A. SLEPECKY: J. Bact. **111**, 537 (1972)
[10] JANEČEK, J., and H. V. RICKENBERG: Biochim. biophys. Acta **81**, 108 (1964)
[11] LOWRY, O. H., N. J. ROSEBROUGH, A. L. FARR, and R. J. RANDALL: J. biol. Chem. **193**, 265 (1951)
[12] PINE, M. J.: A. Rev. Microbiol. **26**, 103 (1972)
[13] MANDELSTAM, J. in: Microbial growth. 19th Symposium of the Society of General Microbiology. University Press, Cambridge 1969, p. 377

Acta biol. med. germ., Band 36, Seite 1523—1524 (1977)

Biochemisches Institut der Universität Freiburg im Breisgau
und Abteilung für Enzymchemie der Gesellschaft für Strahlen- und Umweltforschung, Hermann-Herder-Straße 7, D-7800 Freiburg im Breisgau, Bundesrepublik Deutschland

Characterization and function of intracellular proteinases and proteinase inhibitors from yeast

H. Holzer

Summary

Data on the proteinase inhibitors I^A, I^B and I^C from yeast and their possible intracellular interaction with the proteinases A and B and carboxypeptidase Y are presented. A role of proteolysis in "catabolite inactivation" is discussed.

Results

Proteinases A and B, carboxypeptidase Y and aminopeptidase I are the well characterized proteinases from yeast [1]. Specific inhibitors for the proteinases A [2] and B [3], and carboxypeptidase Y [4], respectively, have been isolated and characterized as proteins with molecular weights of about 7000, 9000 and 23 000, respectively. The inhibitors are localized in the cytosol, whereas the proteinases are concentrated in the vacuoles [5]. For the two "isoinhibitors" of proteinase B, I_2^A and I_2^B, a specific occurrence in Saccharomyces carlsbergensis and Saccharomyces cerevisiae, respectively, is demonstrated [6]. Furthermore experiments on nitration of I_2^B with tetranitromethane and the use of the modified inhibitor for affinity chromatography of proteinase B have been described [6].
Based on results of Cabib et al. (for a recent review see [7]) demonstrating activation of chitin synthase by limited proteolysis (cf. [8]) and our observation of a specific hydrolysis, i. e. inactivation, of I^A by proteinase B [2] and I^A by proteinase A [3], a cascade mechanism for the proteolytic control of chitin synthesis in bud scars of yeast was proposed [9]. This cascade is discussed in the lights of new findings on the interaction of proteinase A with I^B [10].
Addition of glucose to yeast cells growing on a non-sugar carbon source causes not only repression of synthesis of a group of enzymes ("catabolite repression") but also inactivation of certain enzymes. This "catabolite inactivation" (for a summary see [11]) has till now been demonstrated for 5 enzymes (maltose permease, cytoplasmic malate dehydrogenase, fructose bisphosphatase, phosphoenolpyruvate carboxykinase, α-isopropylmalate synthase) and the galactose fermenting system ("galactozymase"). Matern and Holzer (unpublished experiments) have shown, that glucose affects the galactose uptake system by increasing the apparent K_m for galactose from 3,6 to 11 mM without change in v_{max}, whereas the 4 enzymes necessary in addition for channeling galactose in the glucose degradation pathway (galactose kinase, galactose 1-phosphate uridyltransferase, UDP-galactose 4-epimerase and phosphoglucomutase) are not impaired. The possibility that "catabolite inactivation" is affected by selective proteolysis was discussed [12].

At transition from exponential to stationary growth the activities of the proteinases and their specific inhibitors increase manyfold. According to HANSEN et al. [13] release from catabolite repression after exhaustion of glucose is responsible for these changes. A role of the cytoplasmic inhibitors as "safety guard" against unwanted proteolysis caused by proteinases which leave lysed or leaky vacuoles was discussed [12].
At the transition from resting to sporulating yeast a decrease of the activites of several metabolic enzymes parallel to an increase in proteolytic activities was observed by BELZ and WEISER [14, 15]. This is discussed as evidence for proteolytic degradation of certain proteins to make amino acids available for synthesis of enzymes necessary for spore formation [15].

Conclusions

The following 3 mechanisms of intracellular proteolysis participating in metabolic regulation may be considered: 1) degradation of enzymes selected by unknown mechanisms inside vacuoles (possible physiological examples: catabolite inactivation, starvation, sporulation), 2) activation of inactive proenzymes by limited proteolysis outside the vacuoles catalyzed by proteinases released from lysed vacuoles (example: activation of chitin synthase localized in the outer plasma membrane), 3) formation of subunits from precursor proteins by limited proteolysis (example: assembly of cytochrome oxidase from cytosolic precursor protein and mitochondrial subunits according to POYTON [16]).

References

[1] HOLZER, H., H. BETZ, and E. EBNER: Curr. Top. cell. Reg. **9**, 103–156 (1975)
[2] SAHEKI, T., Y. MATSUDA, and H. HOLZER: Eur. J. Biochem. **47**, 325–332 (1974)
[3] BETZ, H., H. HINZE, and H. HOLZER: J. biol. Chem. **249**, 4515–4521 (1974)
[4] MATERN, H., M. HOFFMANN, and H. HOLZER: Proc. natn. Acad. Sci. U.S.A. **71**, 4874 to 4878 (1974)
[5] MATERN, H., H. BETZ, and H. HOLZER: Biochem. biophys. Res. Commun. **60**, 1051 to 1057 (1974)
[6] BÜNNING, P., and H. HOLZER: J. biol. Chem. (in press)
[7] CABIB, E.: Trends biochem. Sci. **1**, 275–277 (1976)
[8] HASILIK, A., and H. HOLZER: Biochem. biophys. Res. Commun. **53**, 552–559 (1973)
[9] HOLZER, H., and T. SAHEKI: Tokai J. expl. clin. Med. **1**, 115–125 (1976)
[10] HOLZER, H., P. BÜNNING, and F. MEUSSDOERFFER in: Proceedings of the Conference on Acid Proteases. Oklahoma, Nov. 1976. Plenum Publishing Corporation, New York. (in press)
[11] HOLZER, H.: Trends biochem. Sci. **1**, 178–181 (1976)
[12] HOLZER, H. in: Metabolic Interconversion of Enzymes. S. SHALTIEL (Ed.) Springer, Berlin, Heidelberg 1976, pp. 168–174
[13] HANSEN, R. J., R. L. SWITZER, H. HINZE, and H. HOLZER: Biochim. biophys. Acta **496**, 103–114 (1977)
[14] BETZ, H., and U. WEISER: Eur. J. Biochem. **62**, 65–76 (1976)
[15] BETZ, H., and U. WEISER: Eur. J. Biochem. **70**, 385–395 (1976)
[16] POYTON, R. O. in: Genetics and Biogenesis of Mitochondria and Chloroplasts. North-Holland/Elsevier, Amsterdam (in press)

Acta biol. med. germ., Band 36, Seite 1525—1530 (1977)

Biochemisches Institut der Universität Freiburg D-7800 Freiburg, BRD
and Neurobiologie Moléculaire, Institut Pasteur, 25 Rue du Docteur Roux, F-75724 Paris Cedex 15, France*

Protein degradation during the differentiation of eukaryotic cells: Studies on the sporulation of Saccharomyces cerevisiae and on the formation of the neuromuscular junction in the chick embryo

H. Betz

Summary

The role of protein degradation in cell and tissue differentiation has been investigated during the sporulation of Saccharomyces cerevisiae and during endplate formation in developing avian muscle. The results suggest that a variety of proteolytic processes as enzyme inactivation, degradation of mitochondrial membrane constituents and removal of embryonic cell surface proteins exert stringent controls over the sequence of differentiation in eukaryotic cells.

Most cellular differentiation processes occur after the cells have reached the end of proliferative growth. Thus the construction of a differentiated cellular architecture requires not only the expression of new specific functions, but simultaneously the removal of vegetative metabolic pathways which are redundant or incompatible with differentiation. Intracellular protein degradation therefore can be presumed to play a key role in cellular differentiation and morphogenetic development. In this communication, the various functions of protein degradation during the intracellular (histiotypic) differentiation of eucaryotic cells have been studied with two different systems:

I. Diploid cells of the simple unicellular eucaryote *Saccharomyces cerevisiae* can be induced to undergo meiosis and sporulation by starvation on nitrogen-free acetate medium [1]. The result of both processes is a modified cell, the ascus, which contains four haploid ascospores. Since ascus formation occurs in the absence of an exogeneous nitrogen source, protein degradation is the only means to provide the sporulating cell with amino acids for the synthesis of proteins and nucleotides required for differentiation. In fact, yeast diploids homozygous for an amino acid auxotrophy sporulate normally even in the absense of the required amino acid [2].

In previous studies, the major part of the vegetative cell proteins and also of the proteins synthesized during sporulation has been shown to be degraded during ascospore formation [3, 4]. This degradation process concerns soluble and membran-bound proteins to a similar extent and is reflected by striking increases in the activities of the different yeast proteinases [3—5]. In the case of proteinase A, the increase in activity appears to be essential for sporulation since diploid cells homozygous for a nuclear mutation resulting in constitutively low proteinase A levels are unable to sporulate [6].

* Author's present adress

Which individual functions can now be attributed to the extensive degradation of cell proteins during ascus formation? When the levels of different enzymes are followed in extracts from sporulating cells, at least four types of enzyme patterns can be distinguished [5]:

a) Enzymes and proteins remaining at fairly constant specific activity throughout the entire sporulation process, as for example the specific proteinase B inhibitor [7]. Radioimmunochemical assays reveal this latter protein to be completely stable during sporulation [5], as it is in resting cells [8];

b) enzymes mainly of RNA and protein catabolism, which increase severalfold during sporulation;

c) enzymes, which are inactivated from the onset of sporulation, as NAD-dependent glutamate dehydrogenase and enzymes of glyoxylate cycle metabolism;

d) enzymes, which are inactivated during the period of ascus maturation, as for example hexokinase.

Experiments with various metabolic inhibitors suggest that the inactivations observed under c) and d) may indeed be proteolytically mediated. Also, spectroscopic and enzymatic analysis of whole cells and isolated submitochondrial particles reveals an almost complete degradation of mitochondrial cytochromes and other inner mitochondrial membrane proteins as F_1—ATPase during sporulation, a process believed to be intimately connected to the akquisition of metabolic dormancy by the mature ascospores [5]. Since mitochondrial DNA is doubled during sporulation [9], a 5 to 10fold reduction of the mitochondrial unit size, i. e. membrane surface area per DNA copy, has to take place in the sporulating cell [5]. In Fig. 1, the temporal relationship between the different proteolytic events occuring during sporulation is depicted.

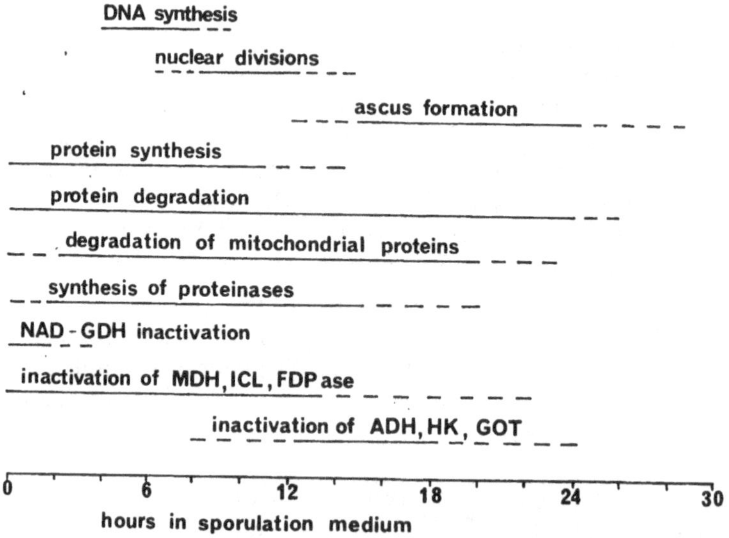

Fig. 1. Temporal relationship of proteolytic events during yeast sporulation

The central question raising from this scheme is how the temporal order of proteolytic events is achieved in the differentiating cell. The immediate stimulation of proteolysis after shift of the cells to sporulation medium is presumably mediated both by release from nitrogen catabolite repression and by cessation of protein accumulation. Experiments with various inhibitors of macromolecular synthesis and with temperature-sensitive mutants defective at different steps of RNA and protein synthesis have shown that in growing cells the stimulation of protein degradation is directly dependent on the inhibition of protein synthesis per se [10]. The factors which trigger the initiation of enzyme inactivation and cytochrome degradation are much more obscure. As a rule, it appears that inactivation begins when the intracellular substrate concentration for a given enzyme falls under a critical treshold level. The biochemical mechanisms which render the respective enzyme susceptible to degradation (as conformational changes, covalent modification etc.) are, however, unknown.

In summary, from our studies on yeast sporulation we can deduce that protein degradation exerts controls over differentiation at the level of protein synthesis by amino acid production, at that of intermediary metabolism by selective enzyme inactivation and at that of cell respiration and acquisition of dormancy by the degradation of inner mitochondrial membrane proteins. During the morphogenesis of complex tissues, protein degradation may exert regulatory functions in addition at the level of cell surface differentiation and cell-cell interaction. This type of control is demonstrated with the second system studied in this communication, the developing neuromuscular junction in the chick embryo.

II. The development of *muscle fibers* is initiated by the fusion of mononucleated myoblasts into multinucleated myotubes. Immediately after fusion, the synthesis of acetylcholine receptors (AChR) increases severalfolds, the newly synthesised receptors being randomly incorporated in the myotube membrane [11]. Upon further development, and contact formation with ingrowing motor axons, some of these "extrasynaptic" AChR molecules become concentrated at discrete spots of the myotube membrane which underly the nerve terminals. In the adult innervated myofiber, chemosensitivity and receptor sites are almost completely restricted to the subsynaptic part of the plasma membrane [12, 13].

Different electrophysiological and autoradiographical studies indicate that receptor molecules disappear from extrasynaptic membrane areas during motor endplate formation [13, 14]. Also, a decrease in the total number of receptor sites has been observed in differentiating muscle cultures [15]. When the total contents of acetylcholineesterase (AChE) and AChR are followed during breast muscle development in the avian embryo, both proteins increase continuously and in a parallel manner up to the 14th day of incubation [16]. Thereafter, however, the evolution of these postsynaptic proteins differs considerably: the total number of cholinergic receptor sites decreases with an apparent half-life of approximately 3 days until the 20th day, whereas the total activity of AChE stays more or less constant [16]. Obviously, the majority of AChR molecules synthesized during myotube differentiation is not required for the formation of the mature endplate. A comparison of the decay on total receptor number after the 14th day with the autoradiographically determined developmental profile of extrasynaptic receptor site density reveals that the reduction in total receptor number must be due to the

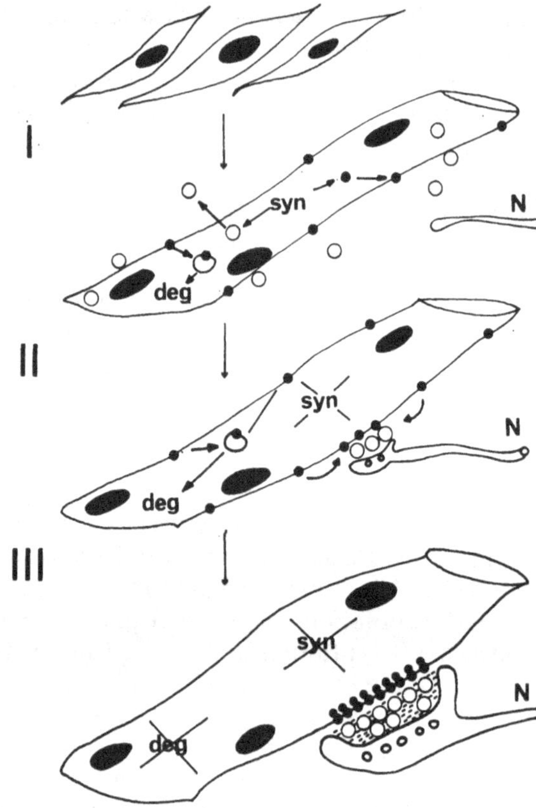

Fig. 2. Hypothetical scheme on the biochemical steps involved in vertebrate endplate formation.

The sequence of events is explained in the text. Symbols used: ● AChR; ○ AChE; ⁏ covalently modified (phosphorylated?) AChR; N motor axon; === basal membrane; syn synthesis; deg degradation

degradation of extrasynaptic sites, since the latter disappear after the 11th day with the same apparent half-live of 3 days as determined for the decay of the total receptor population [16]. In fact, different groups have demonstrated a rapid turnover of extrasynaptic AChR (half-life 15—30 hrs), whereas, in the adult endplate, subsynaptic receptors seem to be metabolically stable (half-life ≥ 5 days) [14, 17, 18]. Labelling of the cholinergic receptor sites in the developing chick embryo by injection of the specific probe α-bungarotoxin also yields a half-life of around 28 hrs (unpublished experiments).

These and the other currently available data can be combined in a hypothetical scheme on the different steps of vertebrate endplate formation as shown in Fig. 2:

Step 1: *Fusion of myoblasts into myotubes* induces the accumulation and incorporation into the membrane of AChR and the synthesis and secretion of AChE (evidence for secretion of AChE and other high molecular weight substances inducing choline acetyltransferase synthesis in cultivated motor neurons has been reported

[19, 20]; such secreted substances may in addition be responsible for chemoattraction of the nerve growth cone). The AChR in the membrane is degraded after internalisation of the protein [17] with a $t_{1/2}$ of about 20 hrs.

Step 2: Contact formation with the motor axon leads to clustering of AChR under the nerve terminal and to trapping of secreted AChE in the synaptic cleft. Acetylcholine release from the motor axon initiates muscle activity; the latter inhibits the further synthesis of AChR and AChE [21]. Continuing degradation removes the extrasynaptic receptors from the fiber surface.

Step 3: Stabilisation of the synapse [13, 22]: Covalent modification of the subsynaptic AChR renders the receptor protein resistant to degradation ($t_{1/2} \geq 5$ days) (biochemical and pharmacological differences between extra- and subsynaptic AChR species as well as a phosphorylation of the receptor protein have recently been reported [14, 23, 24]); AChE is fixed in the synaptic cleft by basal membrane formation and cross-linking to collageneous proteins.

Whether future experiments will establish this scheme to be correct or not, in any case it is evident that the degradation of extrasynaptic AChR is essential for the localization of the receptor molecules in the subsynaptic area of the muscle fiber membrane. It is tempting to speculate that similar mechanisms of plasma membrane protein degradation are also involved in other developmental processes requiring cell surface polarisation, as for example organogenesis of the central nervous system.

Acknowledgements

I am greatly indebted to Profs. H. Holzer and J.-P. Changeux for their generous support during the different parts of this work and for many of the ideas discussed in this communication. It is a pleasure to thank Mrs. U. Weiser for excellent assistance and Dr. J.-P. Bourgeois for his collaboration.

Currently, the author is supported by a fellowship from the Deutsche Forschungsgemeinschaft.

References

[1] Tingle, M., A. J. Singh Klar, S. A. Henry, and H. O. Halvorson in: Microbial Differentiation. Symposium of the Society of General Microbiology. J. M. Ashworth and J. E. Smith (Eds.). Vol. 23, pp. 209–243. University Press, Cambridge 1973
[2] Esposito, M. S., R. E. Esposito, M. Arnaud, and H. O. Halvorson: J. Bact. **100**, 180–186 (1969)
[3] Betz, H., and U. Weiser: Eur. J. Biochem. **62**, 65–76 (1976)
[4] Klar, A. J. S., and H. O. Halvorson: J. Bact. **124**, 863–869 (1975)
[5] Betz, H., and U. Weiser: Eur. J. Biochem. **70**, 385–395 (1976)
[6] Betz, H.: Proceedings of the Symposium Cellular Differentiation in Microorganisms, Animals and Plants, Reinhardsbrunn 1977. K. Mothes (Ed.). Academic Press, New York (in press)
[7] Betz, H., H. Hinze, and H. Holzer: J. biol. Chem. **249**, 4515–4521 (1974)
[8] Betz, H.: Biochim. biophys. Acta **404**, 142–151 (1975)
[9] Kuenzi, M. T., and R. Roth: Expl Cell Res. **85**, 377–382 (1974)
[10] Betz, H.: Biochem. biophys. Res. Commun. **72**, 121–130 (1976)
[11] Vogel, Z., A. J. Szytkowski, and M. W. Nirenberg: Proc. natn. Acad. Sci. U.S.A. **69**, 3180–3184 (1972).

[12] Fambrough, D. in: Biology of Cholinergic Function. A. M. Goldberg and I. Hanin (Eds.). Raven Press, New York 1976, p. 101–160
[13] Changeux, J.-P., and A. Danchin: Nature, Lond. **264**, 705–712 (1976)
[14] Brockes, P. J., D. K. Berg, and Z. W. Hall: Cold Spring Harb. Symp. quant. Biol. **40**, 235–262 (1976)
[15] Prives, J., I. Silman, and A. Amsterdam: Cell **7**, 543–550 (1976)
[16] Betz, H., J.-P. Bourgeois, and J.-P. Changeux: FEBS Lett. **77**, 219–224 (1977)
[17] Devreotes, P. N., and D. M. Fambrough: Cold Spring Harb. Symp. quant. Biol. **40**, 237–251 (1976)
[18] Chang, C., and M. Huang: Nature, Lond. **253**, 643–644 (1975)
[19] Wilson, B. W., P. S. Nieberg, C. R. Walker, T. A. Linkhart, and D. M. Fry: Develop. Biol. **33**, 285–299 (1973)
[20] Nelson, P. G.: Cold Spring Harb. Symp. quant. Biol. **40**, 359–371 (1976)
[21] Drachman, D. B., and F. Witzke: Science, N.Y. **176**, 514–516 (1972)
[22] Changeux, J.-P., P. Courrége, and A. Danchin: Proc. natn. Acad. Sci. U.S.A. **70**, 2974–2978 (1973)
[23] Gordon, A. S., C. G. Davis, and I. Diamond: Proc. natn. Acad. Sci. U.S.A. **74**, 263–267 (1977)
[24] Teichberg, V. I., A. Sobel, and J.-P. Changeux: Nature, Lond. **267**, 540–542 (1977)

Acta biol. med. germ., Band 36, Seite 1531—1535 (1977)

Department of Biochemistry, J. Stefan Institute, University of Ljubljana, Ljubljana, Yugoslavia

Studies on bovine spleen cathepsin D

V. Turk, I. Kregar, F. Gubenšek, S. Lapanje, I. Urh, and M. Kovačič

Summary

The purification procedure of cathepsin D which includes autolysis results in the destruction of the molecule to smaller polypeptide chains. Pure catepsin D obtained by the method which includes affinity chromatography, contains single polypeptide chain of 42000 daltons. The N-terminal amino acid is glycine. The specificity was studied using synthetic substrates. CD measurement of cathepsin D shows mainly unordered structure, about 26% of β-structure and only 5% of α-helix. Binding of pepstatin shows pronounced changes in the CD spectrum between 250 and 300 nm; above 7.5 no interaction was observed.

Introduction

Acid proteinases are biologically very important enzymes. They are used in widespread areas of food and pharmaceutical industry (acid proteinase from calf stomach and from microorganisms). Mammalian acid proteinases not only control processes of digestion (pepsin) and blood pressure (renin) but also play an important role in the processes of intracellular protein catabolism (cathepsins). In spite of this fact the study of the structure of acid proteases has been slow until the complete amino acid sequence of porcine pepsin was determined [1, 2] and finally very recently three new high resolution crystal structures of microbial acid proteases were reported [3, 4].

Contrary to the progress in the knowledge of microbial acid proteases and porcine pepsin, advances in the knowledge of intracellular proteinases, particularly cathepsins, are rather slow. Many laboratories are still improving purification procedures and doing basic characterization. In the cathepsin family is the most investigated cathepsin D. In our laboratory cathepsin D has been isolated for the first time using affinity chromatography on hemoglobin-agarose resin [5], pepstatin-agarose resin [6] and immobilized synthetic octapeptide inhibitor on agarose-resin [7]. All these purification procedures lead to the isolation of two pure multiple forms of cathepsin D with single polypeptide chain of 42000 daltons, whereas the third one still contains the additional polypeptide chain of 28000 daltons. Most authors using classical procedures obtained also smaller polypeptides [5, 8, 9].

In this communication we present some enzymatic properties of cathepsin D, studies on secondary structure and binding of the inhibitor pepstatin.

Materials and methods

Fresh bovine spleen was used as enzyme source. Deionized water containing 1 mM sodium azide was used in all experiments. AH-sepharose 4B was purchased from Pharmacia Fine Chemicals. The generous gifts of pepstatin from Prof. H. Umezawa (Institute of Microbial

Chemistry, Tokyo, Japan) and synthetic peptide substrates from Dr. L. BARSTOW (Vega Fox Biochem., Tucson, Az., USA) are gratefully acknowledged. All other chemicals used in this study were reagent grades from different commercial sources.

Cathepsin D was isolated using affinity chromatography method [5, 6]. Proteolytic activity was measured by the modified Anson's method [10]. Analytical polyacrylamide gel electrophoresis was done at *p*H 8.5 according to the procedures of DAVIS [11]. Electrophoresis in the presence of sodium dodecyl sulphate was performed by the procedure of WEBER and OSBORN [12]. Circular dichroism (CD) was measured with a Jobin Yvon dichrographe III in the far and near UV region from 200–320 nm. The narrowest band-pass was used when ever possible in order to achieve the highest resolution of the bands.

Results and discussion

For the isolation of enzymes the initial steps in the purification procedure are very important. Many cathepsin D purification procedures still use autolysis at the beginning of the purification [9]. Our experiments clearly show that the autolysis of homogenate or supernatant from several hours to 24 hrs at 37 °C at acid or neutral *p*H leads to the destruction of the native molecule. Similar results were obtained when the tissue extract was adjusted to *p*H 3.5 and remained for 24 hrs at 4 °C. The appearance of several additional polypeptide chains with dominant chains of 28000 and 14000 daltons was found in all experiments where incubation was included. From these results we can conclude that the method of autolysis has to be excluded from the purification procedure of cathepsin D.

Cathepsin D was isolated by short purification procedure which includes preparation of homogenate and supernatant, affinity chromatography, gel filtration and separation of three multiple forms of the enzyme by DEAE cellulose, as described previously [5, 6].

Table 1
Cathepsin D cleavage of synthetic substrates

N-a-CBZ-L-Phe↓-L-Phe
N-a-CBZ-L-Phe-↓L-Tyr
N-a-CBZ-L-Tyr-↓L-Phe
N-a-CBZ-L-Thre-↓L-Phe-Me-ester
N-a-L-Phe-↓L-Tyr-amide
Gly-L-Phe-↓L-Phe

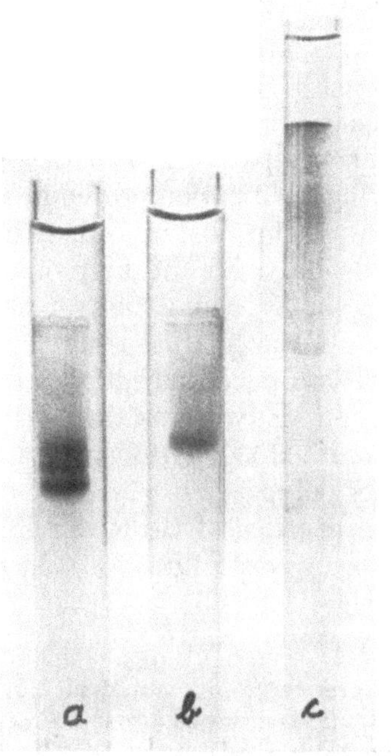

Fig. 1. Polyacrylamide gel electrophoresis of cathepsin D. (a) three multiple forms; (b) first form after separation on DEAE cellulose; (c) SDS electrophoresis of first form

Fig. 1 shows the purity of enzyme as judged by gel electrophoresis in sodium dodecyl sulphate. In all further investigations we used only the first multiple form of cathepsin D which contains a single polypeptide chain of 42000. The second multiple form contains also one polypeptide chain, whereas the third one contains an additional chain of 28000 [13].

N- terminal analysis shows that glycine is the only terminal amino acid. The method of ZANETTA et al. [14] and micro polyamide foils were used. The specificity of cathepsin D was studied using different synthetic substrates (Table 1.) As we expected Phe-Phe, Tyr-Phe and Phe-Tyr bonds were cleaved.

The CD spectrum between 200 and 250 nm (Fig. 2) in 0.1 M phosphate buffer, *p*H 6.9, was essentially the same as recorded earlier using a sample prepared by classical procedure [8]. It reveals that cathepsin D contains mainly unordered structure, about 26% of β-structure and only about 5% of α-helix, as estimated by the method of CHEN et al. [15]. It is interesting to note that similar spectra were recorded recently for pepsinogen [16] which is also mainly nonhelical and has a significant portion of its main chain in the pleated sheet conformation.

Binding of pepstatin causes pronounced changes in the near UV CD-spectrum between 250 and 300 nm (Fig. 3). It is apparent that aromatic side chains have been

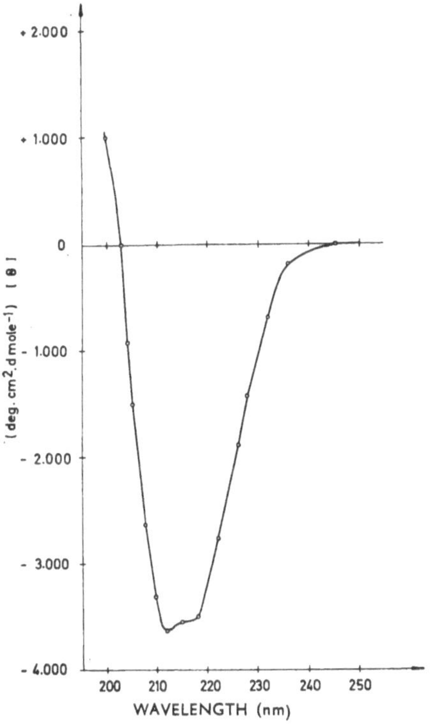

Fig. 2

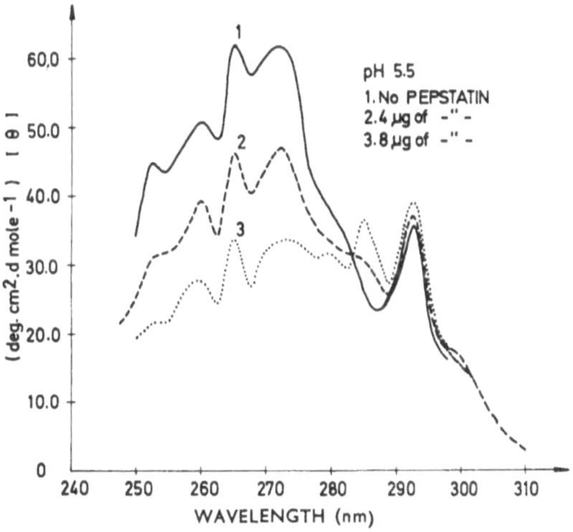

Fig. 3

Fig. 2. The far UV CD spectrum of cathepsin D

Fig. 3. Effect of pepstatin binding to cathepsin D on the near UV CD spectrum of cathepsin D perturbed upon binding, although further experiments will be needed in order to asign particular bands. From the reported CD-spectra of other proteins [17] it could be assumed that a newly formed peak at 285 nm probably belongs to a tryptophan residue.

In our previous studies with immobilized pepstatin we have shown that cathepsin D binds effectively to immobilized pepstatin also far away from the *p*H optimum of its activity [6]. The same was demonstrated by CD spectra. At *p*H 7.2 practically no interaction was observed (Fig. 4). The titration curve (Fig. 5) shows that the inflection point lies at *p*H 7.2. The only amino acid that could be titrated in this region is histidine. Thus, it seems that pepstatin could be bound to cathepsin D only when one of the histidine side chains is positively charged. Unfortunately the structure of cathepsin D is not yet known. However, three similar acid proteinases have been extensively studied by crystallographers. These are penicillopepsin [4] and acid proteases from Rhisopus chinensis and Endothia parasitica [3]. In the known sequences [4] there is only one common histidine. It does not belong to highly homologous part of the molecules but apparently lies on the surface next to the enzymatic cleft.

The mean residue ellipticity of the sharp peak at 265 nm was plotted against concentration of added pepstatin and a clear end point of such a titration could be determined (Fig. 6). It is evident that no further change of ellipticity occurs upon further addition of pepstatin.

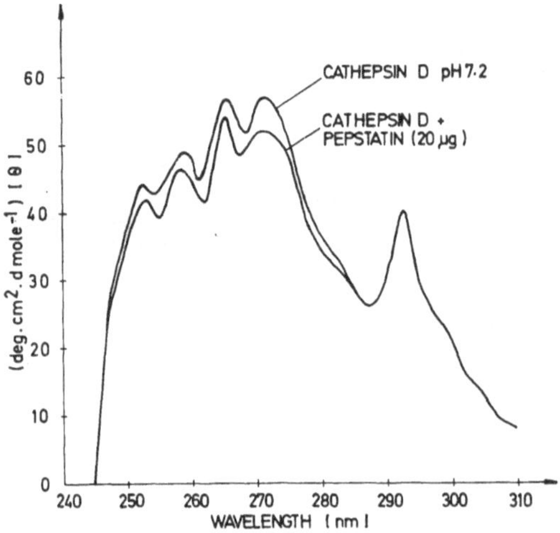

Fig. 4

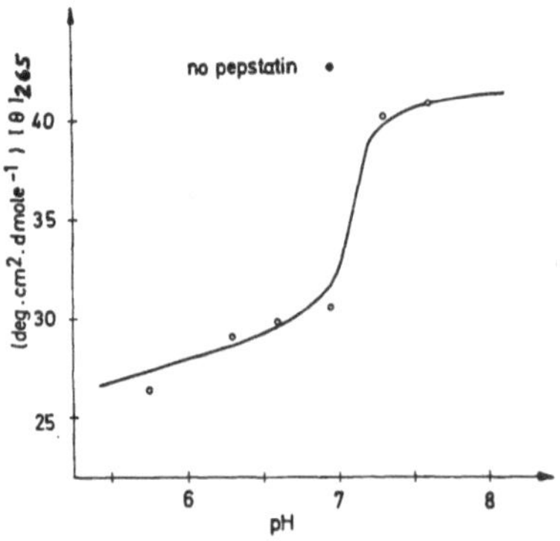

Fig. 5

Fig. 4. CD spectra of cathepsin D and cathepsin D + 3fold molar excess of pepstatin at *p*H 7.2

Fig. 5. Binding of pepstatin to cathepsin D as could be observed by CD at 265 nm. Cathepsin D concentration was 0.177 g/100 ml and pepstatin was added in two-fold molar excess

Fig. 6. Titration of cathepsin D with pepstatin. The molar ellipticity was measured at 265 nm

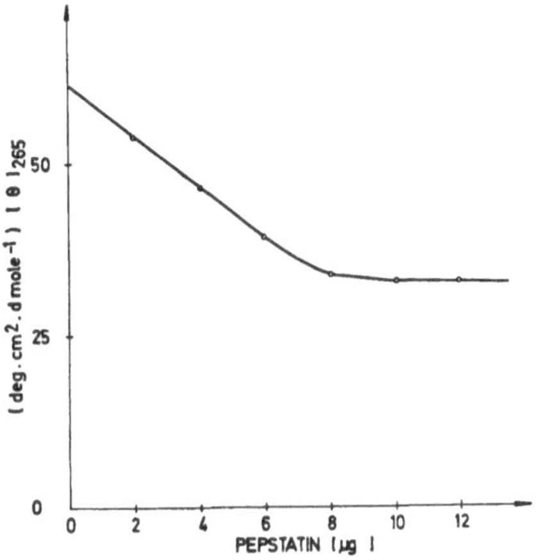

We can expect that in the near future also crystallographic data will contribute to the final elucidation of the structure of cathepsin D.

This work was supported in part by the Research Council of Slovenia and National Science Foundation Grant, F 7 FO3DY, USA. We are grateful to Mrs. M. PREGELJ, Mrs. N. PELICON and Mr. K. LINDIČ for their excellent technical assistance.

References

[1] TANG, J., P. SEPULVEDA, J. MARCINISZYN, K. CHEN, W. Y. HUANG, N. TAO, D. LIU, and J. P. LANIER: Proc. natn. Acad. Sci. U.S.A. **70**, 3437 (1973)
[2] SEPULVEDA, P., J. MARCINISZYN, D. LIU, and J. TANG: J. biol. Chem. **250**, 5082 (1975)
[3] SUBRAMANIAN, E., I. D. A. SWAN, M. LIU, D. R. DAVIS, J. A. JENKINS, I. J. TICKLE, and T. L. BLUNDELL: Proc. natn. Acad. Sci. U.S.A. **74**, 556 (1977)
[4] NAN HSU, I., L. T. J. DELBARE, and M. N. G. JAMES: Nature, Lond. **266**, 140 (1977)
[5] SMITH, R., and V. TURK: Eur. J. Biochem. **48**, 245 (1974)
[6] KREGAR, I., I. URH, R. SMITH, H. UMEZAWA, and V. TURK in: Intracellular protein catabolism II. V. TURK and N. MARKS (Eds). Plenum Press, New York and London 1977, p. 250
[7] GUBENŠEK, F., L. BARSTOW, I. KREGAR, and V. TURK: FEBS Lett. **71**, 42 (1976)
[8] TURK, V., I. KREGAR, F. GUBENŠEK, R. SMITH, and S. LAPANJE in: Intracellular protein catabolism. H. HANSON and P. BOHLEY (Eds). Barth, Leipzig 1974/6, p. 260
[9] BARRETT, A. J. in: Proteases and biological control. E. REICH, D. RIFKIN and E. SHAW (Eds). Cold Spring Harbour Laboratory, Cold Spring Harbour, Long Island, New York 1975, p. 467
[10] ANSON, M. L.: J. gen. Physiol. **22**, 79 (1939)
[11] DAVIS, B. J.: Ann. N.Y. Acad. Sci. **121**, 404 (1964)
[12] WEBER, K., and M. OSBORN: J. biol. Chem. **244**, 4406 (1969)
[13] TURK, V., I. URH, I. KREGAR, J. BABNIK, F. GUBENŠEK, and R. SMITH in: Intracellular protein catabolism II. V. TURK and N. MARKS (Eds.). Plenum Press, New York and London 1977, p. 240
[14] ZANETTA, J. P., G. VINCENDON, P. MANDEL, and G. GOMBOS: J. Chromat. **51**, 441 (1970)
[15] CHEN, Y. H., J. T. YANG, and K. H. CHAU: Biochemistry **13**, 3350 (1974)
[16] JIRGENSONS, B.: Biochim. biophys. Acta **434**, 58 (1976)
[17] PUETT, D., A. NUREDDIN, and L. A. HOLLADAY: Int. J. Pept. Prot. Res. **8**, 183 (1976)

Acta biol. med. germ., Band 36, Seite 1537—1546 (1977)

Department of Enzyme Chemistry, Institute for Enzyme Research, School of Medicine, Tokushima University, Tokushima 770, Japan

Intracellular protein catabolism and new serine proteases

Nobuhiko Katunuma, Yukihiro Sanada, Eiki Kominami, Keiko Kobayashi, and Yoshiko Banno

The strategy to success in the study of intracellular protein catabolism should consider the following items: (1) Proteases which possess certain properties required for participating on intracellular protein degradation must be found in the required subcellular location of the relevant organs. (2) In order to know the participation of a certain protease which degrades a particularintracellular protein group, the relationship between alteration of the protease activity in physiological or pathological conditions and the relevant substrate protein level in the cell should be studied. (3) Alteration in the conformation of the substrate protein renders it more susceptible to the action of our proteases, so that such a change in conformation is considered to be the initial step in intracellular protein degradation. (4) Of particular interest is the identification of the rate-limiting steps in the degradation pathway and the nature of the factors which regulate them. For the purposes of discussion, we can represent the elemental items of intracellular protein degradation in a cell by the following series of steps [1—2]

Non-susceptible form (Holoenzyme) → Susceptible form (Apoenzyme) → Limited proteolytic products ----→ Amino acids

Limited proteolytic products ⇢ (Lysosome) ⇢ Amino acids

Outline of properties of serine proteases in various organs

Several diffrent kinds of new serine proteases from skeletal muscle, liver, muscle layer of intestine and bone-marrow cells were isolated in our laboratory. These new proteases have been purified to homogeneity and proteases from muscle layer of intestine and from bone-marrow cells have been crystallized [3—6]. The molecular weights of the proteases from skeletal muscle, liver, intestinal muscle and bone-marrow cells are 24,000, 24,000, 25,000 and 18,000, respectively. Their immunochemical properties distinguish them from each other. The active sites of all of the proteases are serine and histidine and they react in the alkaline *p*H range. The proteases from skeletal muscle, liver and intestinal muscle hydrolyze N-acetyl-L-tyrosine ethyl ester (ATEE) and are inhibited specifically by chymostatin. The protease from bone-marrow cells cleaves acetyl-$(ala)_3$-methyl-ester and is inhibited specifically by elastinal [10]. The proteases show a common attack of the apo-form of several pyridoxal enzymes and also specifically attack a certain protein which is located in the same location as that of the protease. The susceptible enzyme proteins for our proteases are as follows; ornithine aminotransferase, serine dehydratase, cystathionase, β-aminolevulinate synthetase and phosphorylase etc., but malate dehydrogenase (DH), glutamate DH, glyceraldehyde-3-phosphate DH, glucose-6-phosphate DH, aspartate aminotransferase, tyrosine aminotransferase, xanthine oxidase, D-amino acid oxidase, arginase, glutaminase, pyruvate kinase, and ornithine transcarbamylase are non-susceptible.

Serine protease from skeletal muscle

The amount of the protease in various types of muscle differs greatly, the activity being higher in red muscle than in white, whereas none could be detected in heart. A significant increase in the level of the protease during atrophy of the gastrocnemius muscle was demonstrated by an experiment in which the ischiadicus nerve was amputated only on one side. The level of the protease in the amputated side was about three times higher thant that in the normal side. The level of phosphorylase on the amputated side decreased to 20% of that on the normal side [5, 6]. As shown in Table 1, the serine protease in atrophy muscle of patients with myogenic muscular dystrophy such as Duchenne type dystrophy (DMD) and Becker type dystrophy (BMD) showed 20—50 times higher activity than that in the normal muscle. On the other hand, a patient with amyotrophic lateral sclerosis (ALS) which is a neurogenic muscular atrophy showed a similar level to that of normal muscle.
The electrophoretic pattern of structural proteins of muscle of patients with muscular dystrophy shows a characteristically destroyed pattern of myofibrillar protein. When a large amount of purified serine protease was added and incubated at *p*H 8.5 and 37 °C with myofibrillar protein extracted from normal muscle, the same kind of the destroyed pattern as that from dystrophic muscle could be demonstrated. Addition of chymostatin to the incubation system prevented this degradation. Therefore, this abnormally high activity of the protease in dystrophic muscle might participate in the production of the special pattern of degradation of myofibrilar protein in this disease [7, 8].

Serine protease from liver

Hepatoma 8999 showed extremely high activity of the serine protease, but similar activities of other lysosomal proteases compared to normal liver. The distribution of the serine protease activities in the subcellular fractions of liver and hepatomas 8999 are illustrated in Table 2. The highest specific activity of the serine protease was detected in the mitochondrial fraction in both preparations. Furthermore, the serine proteases in liver and hepatoma 8999 were restricted to the inner membranes of the mitochondrial fraction as shown in Table 3 [1, 9].
The liver protease activities were altered under various physiological or pathological conditions. The liver protease activity remained very low until 3 weeks after birth and reached an adult level at 6 weeks. On the other hand, twelve hours after partial hepatectomy the protease activity began to decrease and after about 48—72 hrs reached a minimum, which was less than 20% of that in sham-operated rats [5, 6]. Also when rats were treated with clofibrate and newly synthesized liver mitochondria were much increased, the mitochondrial protease activity decreased as expressed in terms of mitochondrial protein as shown in Fig. 1 [9].
Under these conditions, in which the synthesis rate of mitochondrial proteins is accelerated, activity of the serine protease is maintained at a low level to depress the rate of degradation.

Table 1
Enzyme activities in dystrophic muscle

Case	Type	Age	Position	Total protein (mg/100 mg wet wt.)	Serum creatine phosphokinase (Units/mg/min)	Muscle	
						Lactate dehydrogenase (µmoles/mg/min)	New serine protease (Units/mg/hr)
1	DMD[1]	12	M. vastus lateralis	7.5	570	1.02	24.0
2	DMD	4	M. vastus lateralis	6.3	1,400	2.14	11.0
3	BMD[2]	20	M. vastus lateralis	18.9	200	3.50	15.4
4	BMD	25	M. vastus lateralis	19.0	140	2.15	16.0
5	ALS[3]	52	M. deltoideus	21.6	12	1.66	1.7
6	Normal	69	M. rectus femoris	21.4	<25	—	3.5
7	Normal	56	M. deltoideus	22.3	<25	1.26	<0.5
8	Normal	78	M. iliopsoas	19.6	<25	0.72	<0.5

[1] Duchenne type muscular dystrophy; [2] Becker type muscular dystrophy; [3] Amyotrophic lateral sclerosis

Table 2

Distributions of the serine protease and various marker enzymes in rat liver and hepatoma 8999.
Rat liver and hepatoma 8999 were fractionated by differential centrifugation as described by DE DUVE et al.
Values are means of those in five separate experiments. The specific activities of various marker enzymes are expressed as nmoles of product formed per min per mg protein

Fraction	Succinate dehydrogenase		Acid phosphatase		Glucose-6-phosphatase		Serine protease	
	Normal liver	Hepatoma 8999	Normal liver	Hepatoma 8999	Normal liver	Hepatoma 8999	Normal liver	Hepatoma 8999
Homogenate	43	59	61	66	57	13	—	2.700
Nuclei	10	9	17	14	59	12	21	4.200
Mitochondria	71	79	30	28	28	7	205	53.500
Lysosomes	10	30	198	151	98	24	4	7.300
Microsomes	6	25	98	109	149	35	≑0	30
Supernatant	5	7	31	47	41	12	≑0	≑0

Table 3

Intramitochondrial location of serine protease.

Values are the means of those in four separate experiments. The activities of kynurenine 3-hydroxylase and malate dehydrogenase are expressed as nmoles of porduct formed/min per mg of protein. Cytochrome oxidase activity is expressed as moles of product formed/min per mg protein. Serine protease activity of rat liver was measured using apo-OTA as substrate. Total recoveries of various fractions are expressed as percentages of the values for whole mitochondria

Fraction	Protein (mg)	Kynurenine 3-hydroxylase		Cytochrome oxidase		Malate dehydrogenase		Serine protease			
								Normal liver		Hepatoma 8999	
		Spec. act.	(%)	Spec. act.	(%)	Spec. act.	(%)	Spec. act.	(%)	Spec. act.	(%)
Whole mitochondria	339	4.3	100	38	100	1,800	100	41	100	53,500	100
Inner membrane	55	1.0	14.2	191	89.7	545	5.0	962	161	183,800	143
Matrix	150			0.6	1.0	2,186	53.8	≑0	≑0	640	0.5
Outer membrane	31	24.3	51.4	44	2.6	960	4.9	59	8.6	12,100	2.3
Intermembrane space	94	5.3	18.8	—	—	1,900	39.8	—	—	170	1.2

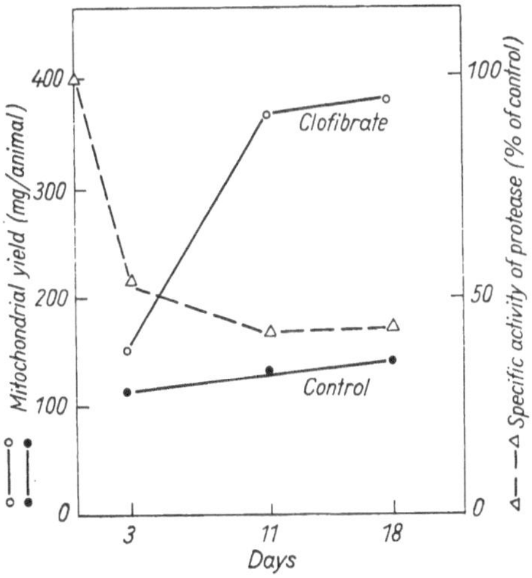

Fig. 1. The influence of clofibrate on the mitochondrial content and serine protease activity

δ-Aminolevulinate synthetase in mitochondria, which has a short half-life, is a good substrate for the liver serine protease. When the isolated mitochondria were incubated at 37 °C and *p*H 8.0, activity of the synthetase decreased to 30% of the initial activity within 60 min, while the addition of chymostatin, a specific inhibitor of the serine protease, showed protection against the inactivation up to 70—80%.

We examined whether the large difference in the protease activities of liver and hepatomas 8999 resulted in changes in the subunit composition of mitochondrial proteins by subjecting the isolated mitochondria from both tissues to polyacrylamide gel electrophoresis with sodium dodecylsulfate. These were no qualitative differences but hepatoma mitochondria contained less of the slowest moving protein subunit, estimated to have a molecular weight of 155,000 (Fig. 2). Incu-

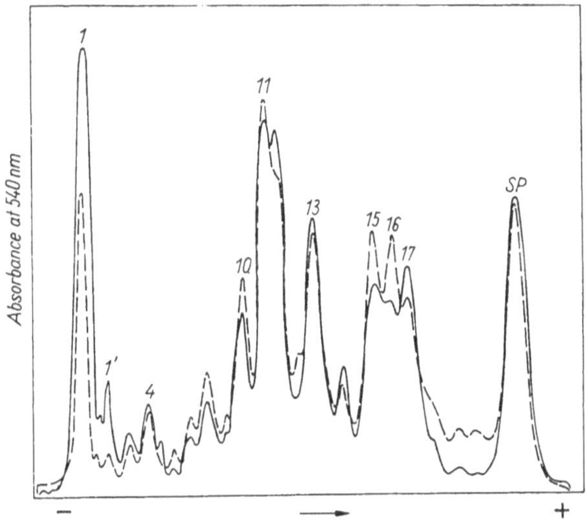

Fig. 2. Densitometer tracing electrophoretograms of mitochondrial protein from rat liver (———) and hepatoma 8999 (— — —) on dodecylsulfate-polyacrylamide gel

bation of isolated liver mitochondria and hepatoma 8999 mitochondria at 37 °C resulted in progressive decrease of the slowest moving protein subunit with appearance of another band of slower mobility. The amount of other protein components did not change on the incubation. In the case of hepatoma 8999, the slowest moving protein subunit decreased much faster than that in liver mitochondria (Fig. 3). The presence of chymostatin or PMSF completely prevented the loss of this slowest component. These results show that this major component of the matrix is a good substrate for the serine protease of mitochondria [9].

Serine protease from bone-marrow cells

The protease activity in erythroblasts of patients suffering from rheumatoid arthritis associated with anemia was markedly elevated and a clear inverse relationship (correlation coefficient = —0.82) was observed between the synthetase and the protease activities as illustrated in Fig. 4. It is possible that the decrease of the synthetase in mitochondria is due to acceleration of degradation of the enzyme by this protease [1, 10].

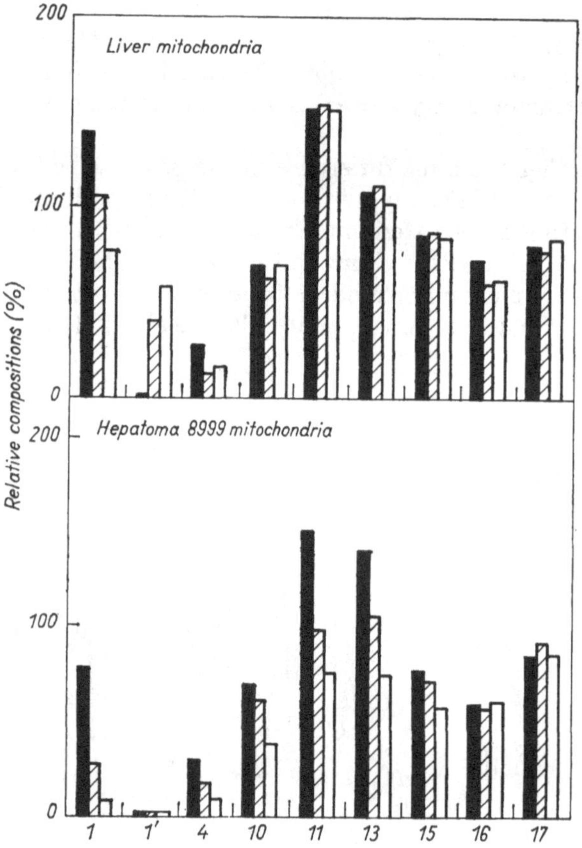

Fig. 3. Relative compositions of the major mitochondrial polypeptides of rat liver and hepatoma 8999 and their changes during incubation.
■ = 0 hr; ▨ = 1 hr; □ = 2 hrs. The numbers correspond to those in Fig. 2

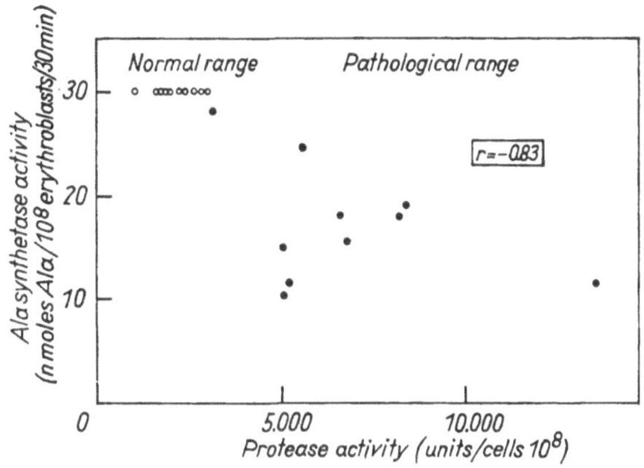

Fig. 4. Inverse relation of protease activity and δ-aminolevulinic acid synthetase activity in erythroblasts. of bone marrow

Serine protease from muscle layer of intestine

The primary structure of the serine protease from muscle layer of intestine was decided by cowork with the Neurath group (Seattle, Washington) [11]. The sequences around the active-site histidine or serine and at the amino terminal are compared with those of chymotrypsin A and trypsin in Table 4. We have also established the position of the three disulfide bonds within the protein molecule.

Table 4

Primary structure of the serine protease from muscle layer of intestine

Amino terminal sequence	
New serine protease (NSP)	*Ile-Ile-Gly-Gly-Val-Glu-Ser-Ile-Pro-His-Ser-Arg-Pro-Tyr*
Bovine chymotrypsin A (BCA)	*Ile-Val-Asn-Gly-Glu-Glu-Ala-Val-Pro-Gly-Ser-Trp-Pro-Trp*
Bovine trypsin (BTr)	*Ile-Val-Gly-Gly-Tyr-Thr-Cys-Gly-Ala-Asn-Thr-Val-Pro-Tyr*
Sequence around active-site histidine	
NSP	*Phe-Val-Leu-Thr-Ala-Ala-His-Cys-Lys-Gly*
BCA	*Trp-Val-Val-Thr-Ala-Ala-His-Cys-Gly-Val*
BTr	*Trp-Val-Val-Ser-Ala-Ala-His-Cys-Tyr-Lys*
Sequence around active-site serine	
NSP	*(Ala)-Met-Gly-Asp-Ser-Gly-Gly-Pro-Leu-Leu-Cys-Ala*
BCA	*Cys-Met-Gly-Asp-Ser-Gly-Gly-Pro-Leu-Val-Cys-Lys*
BTr	*Cys-Gln-Gly-Asp-Ser-Gly-Gly-Pro-Val-Val-Cys-Ser*

All trypsin related serine proteases previously described contain a disulfide bond at the carboxyl terminal, around the active-site serine area which contains the sequence corresponding to the primary substrate binding pocket. But our new serine protease is unique in that the disulfide bond between 191 and 221 in the area of the active-site serine and the substrate binding pocket is not present. These differences may well be related to the different specificities of action of the new protease and chymotrypsin.

The rate of decay of ornithine aminotransferase in intestine in vivo was faster in cases of vitamin B_6-deficiency, in wich the intracellular apoenzyme level was greatly increased over that of the normal animal. The half-life ($t_{1/2}$) of the enzyme in the muscle layer of the intestine in B_6-deficient rats was estimated as 4—5 hrs, whereas that in normal rats was 9—10 hrs. These results suggest that the conversion of holo- into apo-form is the rate limiting and initiating step in the degradation of these B_6 enzymes in vivo [1, 12].

Rate limiting step in degradation of intracellular protein

To identify the initial step and the rate limiting step in the protein degradation pathway in the cell, the following series of experiments were designed [1, 12, 13]. Incubation of the homogenates of muscle layer of small intestine resulted in rapid inactivation of endogenous ornithine aminotransferase. The half-life of the enzyme inactivation was 60 to 70 min. The formation of the apoenzyme in the homogenate occurs prior to the proteolytic inactivation. Addition of coenzymes or various keto acids which act as substrates inhibited conversion of the holoenzyme to the apoenzyme and its subsequent inactivation. These observations suggest that the rate of inactivation depends on the rate of conversion of holoenzyme to apoenzyme. It seems likely that the inactivation is initiated by formation of the apoenzyme.

Addition of phenylmethyl sulfonyl fluoride or chymostatin to the homogenates completely prevented the inactivation of the enzymes. This shows that the inactivation is due to proteolysis by a serine protease.

If the proteolytic inactivation of ornithine aminotransferase in the homogenates is due to limited proteolysis by the serine protease and is not rate-limiting in the degradation, the same breakdown products as those from the purified enzyme system should accumulate in the homogenate. Proteolysis of the aminotransferase by the purified protease produced breakdown intermediates which showed no catalytic activity but which retained immunological activity.

The relationship between the rate of loss of enzyme activity and the rate of change in concentration of the material cross-reactable with the antibody was studied. The enzyme activity was lost approximately 10 times faster than the losses of the immunological activity (activity $t_{1/2} = 1$ hr, and immunological activity $t_{1/2} = 10$ hrs). Antigen-antibody precipitates from homogenates containing inactivated enzyme were separated by sodium dodecyl sulfate gel electrophoresis. A solution of the antigen-antibody complex gave three major bands which corresponded in position to light and heavy chains of rabbit γ-globulin and ornithine aminotransferase as shown in Fig. 5. The band which coincided in position with the pure aminotransferase used as standard split into two bands during enzyme inactivation, and addition of 2-oxoglutarate to the homogenates prevented both enzyme

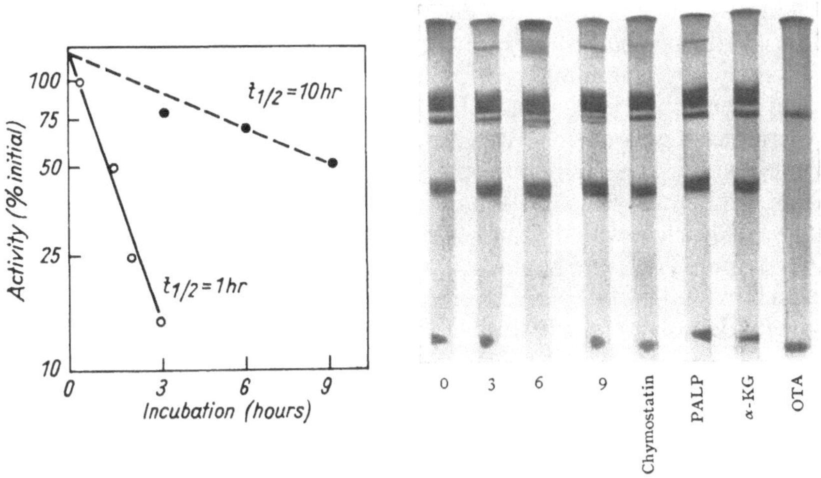

Fig. 5. Comparison of losses of catalytic (○) and immunological (●) activities of ornithine ATase during incubation of homogenate of muscle layer of intestine (left panel) and SDS electrophoresis of antigen-antibody precipitates of the inactivated enzyme (right panel)

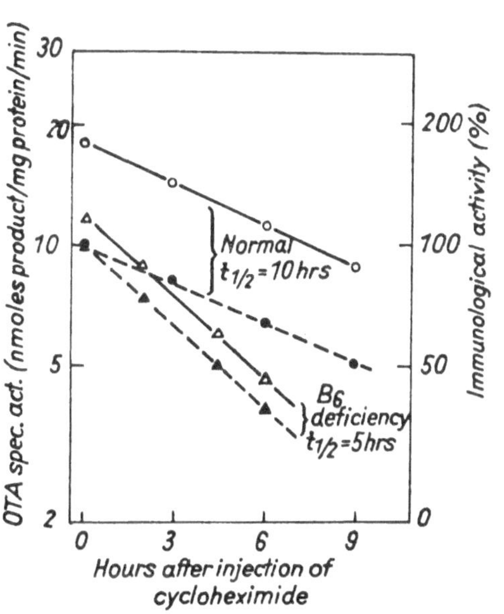

Fig. 6. Comparison of losses of catalytic and immunological activities during degradation of ornithine aminotransferase under control and pyridoxine deficient conditions. ○——○ Enzyme activity, ●– – –● immunological activity under control conditions; △——△ enzyme activity, ▲– – –▲ immunological activity under pyridoxine deficient conditions.

inactivation and splitting of the band of the aminotransferase. The protein band which showed slightly increased electrophoretic mobility is a breakdown product. The degradation products in the homogenate system of the aminotransferase were identical to those in the purified enzyme system and inactivation of the enzyme in homogenates was due to limited proteolysis as well.

However, this does not mean that the results obtained in vitro reflect actual reactions in vivo. The rate of inactivation of the enzyme observed in vitro was extremely rapid, compared with the apparent half-life of the enzyme in vivo (10 hrs). Results in vivo were different from those in vitro. As shown in Fig. 6, there is no difference between the rates of decrease of enzyme activity and of immunological activity during the decrease of the aminotransferase when protein synthesis is inhibited by cycloheximide. An analysis of immunoprecipitates by the same method of electrophoresis revealed no degradation products. But the rate of decay of the aminotransferase was faster in B_6-deficiency, in which the cellular apoenzyme level was much increased, than under normal conditions. The apparent half-life of both catalytic and immunological activity in B_6-deficient rats was estimated as 5 hrs whereas that in normal rats was 9 to 10 hrs as mentioned in the previous chapter. The same kind of data on the other B enzymes has been accumulated, which indicates that the half lives are prolonged by administration of their coenzyme in vivo, particularly in the case of B_6 deficient animals. In a comparison of B_6 treated and nontreated rats, the total amounts of serine dehydratase were increased and its half-life prolonged in the treated group [14]. These results suggest that a step in the conversion of the holoenzyme to the apoenzyme is rate limiting in the degradation of this B_6 enzyme in vivo.

References

[1] KATUNUMA, N., E. KOMINAMI, Y. BANNO, K. KITO, Y. AOKI, and G. URATA: Adv. Enzyme Reg. **14**, 325–345 (1976)
[2] KATUNUMA, N., E. KOMINAMI, K. KOBAYASHI, Y. HAMAGUCHI, Y. BANNO, K. CHICHIBU, T. KATSUNUMA, and T. SHIOTANI: Intracellular Protein Turnover, R. T. SHIMKE and N. KATUNUMA (Eds). Academic Press, New York 1975, p. 187–204
[3] KATUNUMA, N., E. KOMINAMI, K. KOBAYASHI, Y. BANNO, K. SUZUKI, K. CHICHBIU, Y. HAMAGUCHI, and T. KATSUNUMA: Eur. J. Biochem. **52**, 37–50 (1975)
[4] KOMINAMI, E., Y. BANNO, K. CHICHIBU, T. SHIOTANI, Y. HAMAGUCHI, and N. KATUNUMA: Eur. J. Biochem. **52**, 51–57 (1975)
[5] BANNO, Y., T. SHIOTANI, T. TOWATARI, D. YOSIKAWA, T. KATSUNUMA, E.-G. AFTING, and N. KATUNUMA: Eur. J. Biochem. **52**, 59–63 (1975)
[6] KATUNUMA, N.: Rev. Physiol. Biochem. Pharmac. **72**, 83–104 (1975)
[7] SANADA, Y., N. YASOGAWA, and N. KATUNUMA: J. Biochem. **83**, 27–33 (1978)
[8] KATUNUMA, N., N. YASOGAWA, K. KITO, Y. SANADA, H. KAWAI, and K. MIYOSHI: J. Biochem. **83**, 625–628 (1978)
[9] BANNO, Y., H. P. MORRIS, and N. KATUNUMA: J. Biochem. (in press.)
[10] AOKI, Y., F. TAKAKU, G. URATA, and N. KATUNUMA: Biochem. biophys. Res Commun. **65**, 567–574 (1975)
[11] WOODBURY, R., N. KATUNUMA, L. ERIESSON, H. NEURATH, and K. TITANI: ASBC Meeting, San Francisco 1976
[12] KOMINAMI, E. and N. KATUNUMA: Eur. J. Biochem. **62**, 425–430 (1976)
[13] KATUNUMA, N. and E. KOMINAMI: Proteinases of Mammalian Cells and Tissues. Biological and Medical Press, Amsterdam 1977, p. 151–180.
[14] KHAIRALLAH, E. A., and H. C. PITOT in: Symposium on Pyridoxal Enzymes. Maruzen Press, Tokyo 1968, p. 159–164

Acta biol. med. germ., Band 36, Seite 1547—1548 (1977)

Institute of Physiological Chemistry Martin Luther University of Halle,
402 Halle (Saale), GDR

Cathepsin H: An endoaminopeptidase

H. KIRSCHKE

Two years ago we reported on two proteinases from rat liver lysosomes: cathepsin L and cathepsin B_3. In the meantime the purification and properties of both enzymes have been described [1, 2]. Cathepsin L proved to be a usual proteinase whereas cathepsin B_3 has been found to be a proteolytic enzyme with rather unusual catalytic properties. This enzyme has to be designated as an endoaminopeptidase because it catalyzes the hydrolysis of proteins, N-terminal substituted proteins and amino acid derivatives, respectively, as well as peptides of various chain lengths and N-terminal free amino acid derivatives.
Because of its similarities to cathepsin B, the endoaminopeptidase from rat liver lysosomes was named first cathepsin B_3. But there are also striking differences, and therefore this enzyme was given a letter of its own, which is now named cathepsin H.
An extension of the so far known two classes of proteolytic enzymes, endo- and exopeptidases, has now proved to be necessary by adding a further class: the endoexopeptidases, which are enzymes showing both endopeptidase activity as well as exopeptidase activity. It is well known that some endopeptidases hydrollyze also exopeptidase substrates (papain [3]) and that some exopeptidases have slight endopeptidase avtivity (carboxypeptidase A [4]). These enzymes were given the name according to their main catalytic property. Endoaminopeptidases have endo- and aminopeptidase activity in the same order of magnitude. It is impossible to decide whether these enzymes are endopeptidases or exopeptidases and therefore we propose the new class of endoexopeptidases.
Up to now only three or four endoaminopeptidases have been described: an enzyme from the fruiting body of a mushroom [5], an enzyme from E. coli [6] and the enzyme from rat liver lysosomes, cathepsin H [2]. JÄRVINEN and HOPSU-HAVU [7, 8] have described an enzyme from rat skin, which they called BANA-hydrolase. DAVIDSON [9] has described a similar enzyme. These enzymes seem also to be endoaminopeptidases and show close similarities to cathepsin H. The other endoaminopeptidases are different from each other with regard to their molecular weight, specifity, stability and *p*H activity optimum — but one of their common properties is their endopeptidase activity connected with an aminopeptidase activity. Endocarboxypeptidases are unknown yet.
The designation of an enzyme as an endoaminopeptidase requires definite proofs. Here are some points which are evident enough to show the endoaminopeptidase nature of cathepsin H.
1. The first point is the purity of the enzyme. The purity of cathepsin H has been revealed by disc electrophoresis at various *p*H and SDS-gel electrophoresis. The molecular weight of cathepsin H is 28000.

2. The enzyme hydrolyzes endo- as well as aminopeptidase substrates in the same order of magnitude [2].
3. A strong evidence for the endoaminopeptidase nature of cathepsin H is the competitive inhibition of the enzyme activity by aminopeptidase and endopeptidase substrates between one another.
4. Another evidence is the identical inactivation pattern by heat of the endopeptidase activity as well as of the aminopeptidase activity. In contrast to most of the proteinases, cathepsin H is relatively heat resistant. The enzyme maintained 80% of its activity after 30 min at 60 °C.
5. Maximum hydrolysis of all substrates by cathepsin H was measured nearly at the same *p*H (*p*H 6.5). But this requirement does not afford in all cases a proof of an endoaminopeptidase, because the *p*H activity optimum is also dependent on the conformation of the substrate, which also depends on the *p*H.
6. Inhibitors have the same effect both on endopeptidase and aminopeptidase activity. Cathepsin H has to be regarded as a thiol enzyme. SH-reagents inhibit the hydrolysis of proteins and synthetic endopeptidase substrates as well as aminopeptidase substrates [2]. Leucine chloromethyl ketone has been found to be the strongest irreversible inhibitor ($K_i = 8 \cdot 10^{-8}$M). Leupeptin acts as a reversible competitive inhibitor of cathepsin H ($K_i = 5 \cdot 10^{-6}$M). Puromycin inhibits the enzyme only weakly [2].

These six points may in general serve as proofs of the endoaminopeptidase nature of an enzyme. From our results we can conclude that these enzymes are wide spread. By an immunological technique cathepsin H has been detected in extracts of homogenates from all organs of the rat as lung, spleen, kidney, skin, muscle and heart. We used an antiserum from chicken against cathepsin H from rat liver.

References

[1] KIRSCHKE, H., J. LANGNER, B. WIEDERANDERS, S. ANSORGE, and P. BOHLEY: Eur. J. Biochem. **74**, 293 (1977)
[2] KIRSCHKE, H., J. LANGNER, B. WIEDERANDERS, S. ANSORGE, P. BOHLEY, and H. HANSON: Acta biol. med. germ. **36**, 185 (1977)
[3] KIMMEL, J. T., and L. SMITH: J. biol. Chem. **207**, 515 (1954)
[4] LOGUNOV, A. J., and V. N. OREKHOVICH: Biochem. biophys. Res. Commun. **46**, 1161 (1972)
[5] DOONAN, S., H. DOONAN, R. HANFORD, C. A. VERNON, J. M. WALKER, L. P. AIROLDI, F. BOSSA, D. BARRA, M. CARLONI, P. PASELLA, and F. RIVA: Biochem. J. **149**, 497 (1975)
[6] LAZDUNSKI, C., J. BUSUTTIL, and A. LAZDUNSKI: Eur. J. Biochem. **60**, 363 (1975)
[7] JÄRVINEN, M., and V. K. HOPSU-HAVU: Acta chem. scand. **B 29**, 671, 772 (1975)
[8] JÄRVINEN, M.: Acta chem. scand. **B 36**, 53 (1976)
[9] DAVIDSON, E.: Thesis, The Rockefeller University, New York and the University Catholic Louvain 1976

Acta biol. med. germ., Band 36, Seite 1549—1554 (1977)

Molecular Pathology Department, Strangeways Research Laboratory, Cambridge CB1 4RN, England

The effect of human neutrophil elastase and cathepsin G on the collagen of cartilage, tendon, and cornea

PHYLLIS M. STARKEY

Summary

The degradation of collagen in a number of inflammatory diseases is associated with infiltration of the tissues by neutrophil leucocytes.

The neutrophil serine proteinases, elastase and cathepsin G, solubilize type II collagen from articular cartilage by an attack on the terminal peptides, destroying the inter- and intra-molecular crosslinks. Both enzymes also solubilize type IV collagen from kidney basement membrane.

Elastase attacks the terminal peptides of type I collagen of tendon, cornea and skin, and also attacks the helical region of type I skin collagen.

It seems probable that the neutrophil proteinases play an important role in collagen degradation in vivo in a variety of pathological conditions.

Introduction

The destruction of collagen by proteolytic attack is an important feature of several inflammatory conditions, including inflammatory joint diseases and gout, inflammations of the cornea, and damage to the kidney basement membrane in glomerulonephritis. The degradation of the collagen is often associated with a massive infiltration of the tissues by neutrophil leucocytes. These cells carry with them in their granules large amounts of proteolytic enzymes which are known to be released when the cells encounter the immune complexes or activated complement factors often present in rheumatoid arthritis and glomerulonephritis, the bacteria present in septic arthritis and corneal ulceration, or the urate crystals present in gout [1].

The major neutral-acting proteinases of human neutrophil leucocytes are the specific collagenase [2] and the serine proteinases, elastase and cathepsin G [3, 4]. Neutrophil collagenase has very little activity against collagen fibres [2]. It therefore appeared of interest to investigate the action of neutrophil elastase and cathepsin G on the collagen of articular cartilage, tendon, and cornea.

Results

Human neutrophil elastase and cathepsin G were prepared as described previously [5, 6]. Other enzymes were obtained commercially.

Degradation of type II collagen of cartilage

Slices of pig articular cartilage (about 0.5 mm thick) were incubated with buffer alone, neutrophil elastase or cathepsin G, or porcine trypsin at about 1.3 μg of enzyme/mg of cartilage (wet. wt.) at *p*H 7.5 and 37 °C for 18 hrs. The percentage solubilization of collagen (as hydroxyproline) during 18 hrs was 0.5 (control), 4.5 (trypsin), 21.5 (elastase) and 17.9 (cathepsin G). Trypsin, like the neutrophil proteinases, produced almost complete release of proteoglycan under these conditions showing that solubilization of the collagen does not automatically follow from removal of the proteoglycan. All of the hydroxyproline in the material solubilized by the neutrophil enzymes was precipitable by 15% (w/v) trichloroacetic acid, and therefore was of molecular weight > 5000 [7].

To discover whether part of the collagen not solubilized during the enzyme treatments had been degraded in any way, samples of the residues were treated either with 1 M NaCl at 4 °C overnight, or with 1% sodium dodecyl sulphate (SDS) and 0.5% mercaptoethanol at 100 °C for 10 min. After the action of the neutrophil enzymes, a further 10% of the collagen was solubilized by the NaCl, whereas 50% became soluble in SDS. After treatment with trypsin or buffer alone, less than 5% was solubilized by either treatment. Clearly, the collagen remaining insoluble after treatment with the neutrophil enzymes had been degraded in some way.

A dose-response experiment in which cartilage slices were incubated with increasing amounts of the neutrophil proteinases showed that both elastase and cathepsin G caused essentially complete release of the proteoglycan from the cartilage at 0.1 μg of enzyme/mg of cartilage. The solubilisation of collagen required larger amounts of the enzymes.

To investigate the mechanism by which the neutrophil enzymes solubilize collagen from cartilage a further experiment was made with pig laryngeal cartilage that had been extracted with 1 M NaCl to remove part of the proteoglycan (given by Dr. D. EYRE). The collagen solubilized directly by the neutrophil proteinases or extracted subsequently in 1 M NaCl formed a highly viscous solution at concentrations of a few mg/ml, and readily formed a gel at low ionic strength. These properties are suggestive of tropocollagen not extensively degraded in the helical region. Samples of the soluble materials were run in SDS gel electrophoresis (Fig. 1) alongside standards of type I collagen and type II collagen extracted from the same cartilage by use of pepsin [8]. Almost all of the collagen solubilized by elastase or cathepsin G ran as α chains of mobility indistinguishable from that of the modified $\alpha 1$(II) chains obtained with pepsin. There was no evidence of further degradation of the α chains, but there were traces of β components in the elastase digests.

Experiments have also been made with both young and adult human articular cartilage. Qualitatively, the results were similar to those with porcine cartilage, but the rate of solubilization of collagen from the older tissues was slower.

Degradation of type I collagen of tendon and cornea

To compare the susceptibilities to the neutrophil proteinases of achilles tendon collagen (type I) and articular cartilage collagen (type II), samples of porcine tissue were incubated at 37 °C and *p*H 7.5 for 18 hrs with neutrophil elastase and cathepsin G. For a given wet weight of tissue, the tendon collagen was about five-fold more resistant to degradation by elastase than was the cartilage collagen. Cathepsin G had almost no activity against the tendon collagen. In a similar

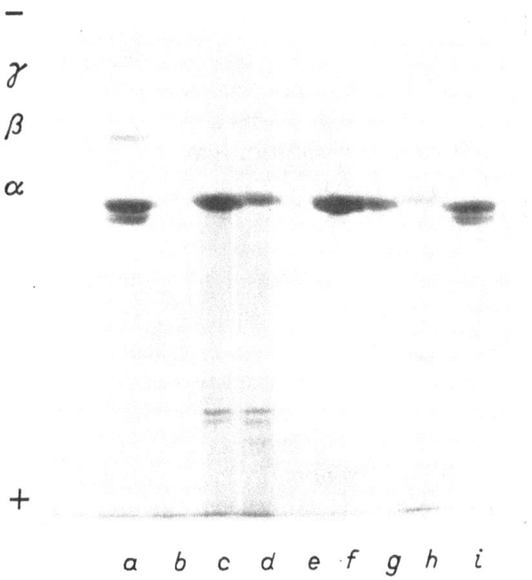

Fig. 1. Solubilization of collagen from cartilage as seen in SDS gel electrophoresis. The samples were a reference sample of type I rabbit skin collagen (a,i), collagen solubilized from pig laryngeal cartilage in buffer (0.05 M Tris HCl), *p*H 7,5, 0.15 M NaCl) alone (b), by neutrophil elastase (c), and by cathepsin G (d), material subsequently extracted in 1 M NaCl from the residues of (b–d), (e–g) and a reference sample of type II collagen pepsin solubilized from the pig cartilage (h)

experiment with rabbit cornea, elastase also was shown to solubilize the collagen of this tissue, the susceptibility to degradation of corneal collagen being similar to that of tendon collagen.

Degradation of isolated collagen

Acid-soluble rabbit skin collagen (type I) in solution was incubated with each of the neutrophil serine proteinases overnight at *p*H 7.5. Experiments were made at 28, 32 and 37 °C. The enzymes were inactivated with phenylmethane sulphonylfluoride before the samples were treated with SDS at 100 °C prior to electrophoresis. The enzymes were used at up to 50 µg/mg of collagen. Examination of the stained gels revealed that at each temperature the neutrophil elastase had almost completely eliminated β and γ components. This showed that the enzyme is capable of cleaving the amino terminal peptides that contain the inter-chain crosslinks. Several-fold higher concentrations of the pancreatic serine proteinases, elastase, trypsin and chymotrypsin had little or no effect under the same conditions. That the neutrophil elastase also attacked the helical region of the type I collagen was shown by the appearance of multiple sub-α components in some experiments. The variable intensity of these bands between experiments was attributable to the fact that they appeared only transiently during the course of the incubation. Cathepsin G had little or no effect on the skin collagen.

Discussion

Degradation of collagen in vivo may well occur in two stages; a phase of lysosomal intracellular digestion probably by acid proteinases, following preliminary extracellular degradation at neutral *p*H. Human neutrophil leucocytes contain little cathepsin D [9], though they may contain cathepsin B [10]. This latter enzyme degrades collagen [11] and may well be involved in the degradation of the banded collagen fibres observed in cells at the pannus-cartilage junction in rheumatoid arthritis [12].

In cartilage the collagen is protected by the proteoglycan matrix, and the first stage in the extracellular degradation of cartilage in vivo is the loss of proteoglycan. This occurs readily because of the sensitivity of proteoglycans to proteolysis, and neutrophil leucocytes exposed to aggregated IgG have been shown to secrete a proteoglycan-degrading activity which is at least in part attributable to elastase and cathepsin G [13, 14]. The depletion of proteoglycan is reversible, but until this component is replaced the collagenous framework of the tissue lacks its normal protection against mechanical stresses and enzymic attack, and can then be damaged irreversibly [15].

Human neutrophil collagenase has very little activity against collagen fibres, though it is reported to act synergistically with the serine proteinases on skin collagen [2]. The collagenase of human rheumatoid synovium has some activity against insoluble tendon collagen, but it is very much less active against mature cartilage collagen [16, 17].

The release of collagen from cartilage and tendon by the neutrophil serine proteinases was first demonstrated in our laboratory [18]. We have recently shown that elastase also attacks type I collagen of cornea, and that both elastase and cathepsin G solubilize type IV collagen from human kidney basement membrane [19].

Since we have found no evidence for fragmentation of the helical region of the type II α chains of cartilage collagen (as opposed to skin collagen) by elastase or cathepsin G it appears that the solubilization of collagen from this tissue is attributable solely to an attack on the terminal peptides of the collagen molecules which are essential for the integrity of the inter- and intra-molecular crosslinks. Cleavage of the crosslinks is almost certainly the most important mechanism by which the neutrophil enzymes solubilize the type IV collagen of kidney basement membrane, and the elastase solubilizes type I collagen of tendon and cornea. The further action of elastase on the helical region of type I collagen is reminiscent of the greater sensitivity of this collagen to the action of collagenase [20].

It is known that the amino acid sequences of the terminal peptides of $\alpha1$(I), $\alpha2$, and $\alpha1$(II) chains differ, although it is being found that the regions proximal to the crosslinks always contain hydrophobic amino acid residues. The various specificities of pepsin [21], neutrophil elastase [22] and cathepsin G [23] with polypeptide substrates are broad, but show clear preferences for hydrophobic residues. It is therefore not surprising that the two neutral proteinases have an action similar to that of pepsin on cartilage collagen. The sequence differences in the terminal peptides of $\alpha1$(I) and $\alpha1$(II) chains are presumably responsible for the greater susceptibility to the neutrophil proteinases of the type II collagen.

We found that after treatment of cartilage with the neutrophil proteinases a further 10—50% of the collagen of the tissue could be extracted with M-NaCl or SDS. This was to be expected as collagen fibres are stabilized by non-covalent interactions between helical regions of individual molecules as well as covalent crosslinks. Under the conditions of digestion by the neutrophil proteinases the non-covalent interactions would not have been disturbed, and some of the partially degraded collagen molecules would have remained insoluble until extracted in high salt or SDS.

Under physiological conditions many collagen molecules might persist for some time in the cartilage despite cleavage of the terminal peptides by the neutrophil proteinases. However, these molecules would make little contribution to the mechanical strength of the tissue. Furthermore, this loosening of the structure of the fibres would predispose them to further enzymic degradation in which collagenase might participate. The loss of crosslinks would tend to bring the cartilage to the state seen in osteolathyrism, in which the formation of crosslinks is chemically blocked. Such cartilage has a high degree of hydration and low mechanical strength.

It is clear then that neutrophil elastase and cathepsin G have the capacity to degrade the collagen as well as the proteoglycan of articular cartilage, and the collagen of kidney basement membrane, and that elastase can also attack type I collagen of tendon, cornea and skin. Whether they act similarly in disease processes in vivo depends on a variety of complex factors, including their interaction with naturally occurring inhibitors. It seems quite probable however that the neutrophil proteinases do play a role in cartilage and tendon breakdown in rheumatoid and septic arthritis and in gout, in the destruction of cornea in ulceration, and in the breakdown of the kidney basement membrane in certain forms of glomerulonephritis.

Acknowledgement

Elastase and cathepsin G from blood leucocytes were kindly prepared by Professor James Travis. Financial support was from the Arthritis and Rheumatism Council.

References

[1] Henson, P. M.: J. exp. Med. **134**, 114s—135s (1971)
[2] Lazarus, G. S., J. R. Daniels, J. Lian, and M. C. Burleigh: Am. J. Path. **68**, 565—576 (1972)
[3] Starkey, P. M., and A. J. Barrett: Biochem. J. **155**, 265—271 (1976)
[4] Starkey, P. M., and A. J. Barrett: Biochem. J. **155**, 273—278 (1976)
[5] Starkey, P. M., and A. J. Barrett: Biochem. J. **155**, 255—263 (1976)
[6] Baugh, R., and J. Travis: Biochemistry **15**, 836—841 (1976)
[7] Harris, E. D. Jr., and S. M. Krane: Biochim. biophys. Acta **258**, 566—576 (1972)
[8] Miller, E. J.: Biochemistry **11**, 4903—4909 (1972)
[9] Folds, J. D., I. R. H. Welsh, and J. K. Spitznagel: Proc. Soc. exp. Biol. Med. **139**, 461—463 (1972)
[10] Davies, P., A. C. Allison, and W. J. Hylton: Biochem. Soc. Trans. **2**, 432—434 (1974)
[11] Burleigh, M. C., A. J. Barrett, and G. S. Lazarus: Biochem. J. **137**, 387—398 (1974)
[12] Harris, E. D. Jr., A. M. Glauert, and A. H. G. Murley: Arth. Rheum. (in press)
[13] Oronsky, A. L., and R. J. Perper: Ann. N.Y. Acad. Sci. **256**, 233—253 (1975)
[14] Malemud, C. J., and A. Janoff: Arth. Rheum. **18**, 361—368 (1975)

[15] Harris, E. D. Jr. in: Rheumatoid Arthritis. E. D. Harris Jr. (Ed.). Medcom Press, New York 1974, pp. 72–98
[16] Leibovich, S. J., and J. B. Weiss: Biochim. biophys. Acta **251**, 109–118 (1971)
[17] Wooley, D. E., R. W. Glanville, M. J. Crossley, and J. M. Evanson: Eur. J. Biochem. **54**, 611–622 (1975)
[18] Starkey, P. M., A. J. Barrett, and M. C. Burleigh: Biochim. biophys. Acta, **483**, 386–397 (1977) (in press)
[19] Davies, M., A. J. Barrett J. Travis, E. Sanders, and G. A. Coles: Clin. Sci. molec. Med. (in press)
[20] Woolley, D. E., K. A. Lindberg, R. W. Glanville, and J. M. Evanson: Eur. J. Biochem. **50**, 437–444 (1975)
[21] Sanger, F., and H. Tuppy: Biochem. J. **49** 481–490 (1951)
[22] Blow, A. M. J.: Biochem. J. **161**, 13–16 (1977)
[23] Blow, A. M. J., and A. J. Barrett: Biochem. J. **161**, 17–19 (1977)

Acta biol. med. germ., Band 36, Seite 1555—1563 (1977)

Agricultural Research Council Meat Research Institute and Bristol University Department of Comparative Pathology, Langford, Bristol, BS18 7DY. UK

The action of cathepsin B and collagenolytic cathepsin in the degradation of collagen

D. J. Etherington and P. J. Evans

Summary

Cathepsin B and collagenolytic cathepsin were obtained from bovine spleen and human placenta and identified as thiol proteinases. Both enzymes degraded insoluble fibrous collagen maximally at *p*H 3.5 and soluble monomeric collagen near *p*H 4.5. The response to activators and inhibitors was similar for both enzymes. Collagenolytic cathepsin was unable to degrade the synthetic substrates of cathepsin B and was also shown to differ in its physico-chemical properties. Minor differences were noted in the action of these cathepsins on insoluble fibrous collagen from different tissues. It was concluded that the rate and extent of the dissolution of fibrous collagen was determined by the number and location of the interchain cross-links, the amount of the associated non-collagenous components and the type of solvent ions, but not by the collagen phenotype.

The major organic structural elements in higher animals are formed from collagen. This protein is secreted by fibroblasts as long, thin, rod-like molecules which align themselves in parallel to form the individual fibres in the connective tissues. These fibres may be randomly orientated or ordered in one or more directions depending upon the tissue and the specific mechanical stresses to which it is normaly subjected. The individual molecules became stabilized within each fibre by the formation of interchain cross-links. The type and number of these cross-links are again dependant upon the particular tissue [1].

The cross-linked fibre is resistant to non-specific proteolytic action and estimates of collagen catabolism have revealed that the normal turnover rate for this protein is exceedingly low. However under specific circumstances collagen degradation can proceed in an efficient and controlled manner. The stimuli to initiate collagen resorption have been defined as (1) normal, (2) induced, or (3) pathological [2].

From electron-microscope studies fragments of collagen fibres, with an otherwise normal ultrastructure, have been observed within cytoplasmic vacuoles of uterine macrophages in the early phase of resorption during post-partum involution. These phagosomes and phagolysosomes then appear to digest this collagenous material quite rapidly [3]. Similar vacuolar processes containing collagen fibres have now been identified in macrophages in several pathological disorders where there is an abnormally high rate of catabolism of the connective tissues [4, 5]. In the periodontal ligament the fibroblasts appear to function in the normal turnover of the collagen fibres by an analogous process [6, 7]. Although there is some evidence that cathepsins may act extracellularly on bone collagen during remodelling of the skeletal structures [8] it is now generally believed that the initial stage in the resorption of collagen occurs with the secretion of collagenase and other neutral proteinases, which can fragment or dissolve the fibre at neutrality in the extracellular space. A collagenase has been identified in each tissue examined [9], but its action is closely regulated by serum inhibitors [10] and it remains uncertain how efficient these enzymes are in degrading the fibre at this stage. In the second stage the digestion is continued intracellularly with the lysosomal cathepsins completing the dissolution of the collagenous debris. In the now acidic environment monomeric subunits and oligomers are rapidly denatured and become exposed to the action of the full range of lysosomal peptide hydrolases [9, 11]. A simplified scheme to illustrate these events is presented in Fig. 1.

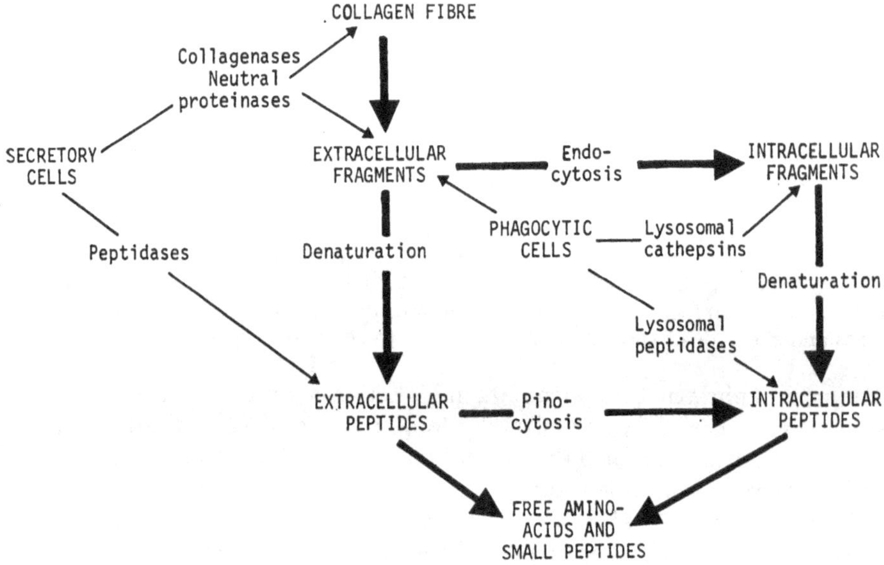

Fig. 1. Possible pathways in the metabolism of collagen.

Identification and fractionation of collagen-degrading cathepsins

The in vitro testing for collagenolytic activity of these lysosomal cathepsins was made with insoluble cross-linked fibrous collagen. The standard assay consisted of a fine dispersion of fibres incubated at 37 °C in 0.1 M sodium formate fuffer, *p*H 3.4, containing 1 mM-EDTA and 0.5 mM-dithiothreitol. The soluble hydroxyproline released from the substrate was then estimated [12].

Extracts of various tissues have been shown to solubilize fibrous collagen in the *p*H range 2.5—4.5 [11]. Bovine spleen contained a high level of activity and autolysed extracts were therefore fractionated to isolate the collagen-degrading enzymes. Two enzymes were separated by chromatography on Amberlite CG-50. One was cathepsin B and this was subsequently purified to yield two homogenous isoenzyme forms. The other was different from all the other described cathepsins and has been provisionally called "collagenolytic cathepsin" [13]. The best preparations obtained so far of this latter enzyme were still slightly impure. Cathepsin B and collagenolytic cathepsin have recently been isolated from human placental tissue using a modified procedure [14]. Flow diagrams of the separation techniques are given in Fig. 2. Collagenolytic cathepsin was slightly unstable to

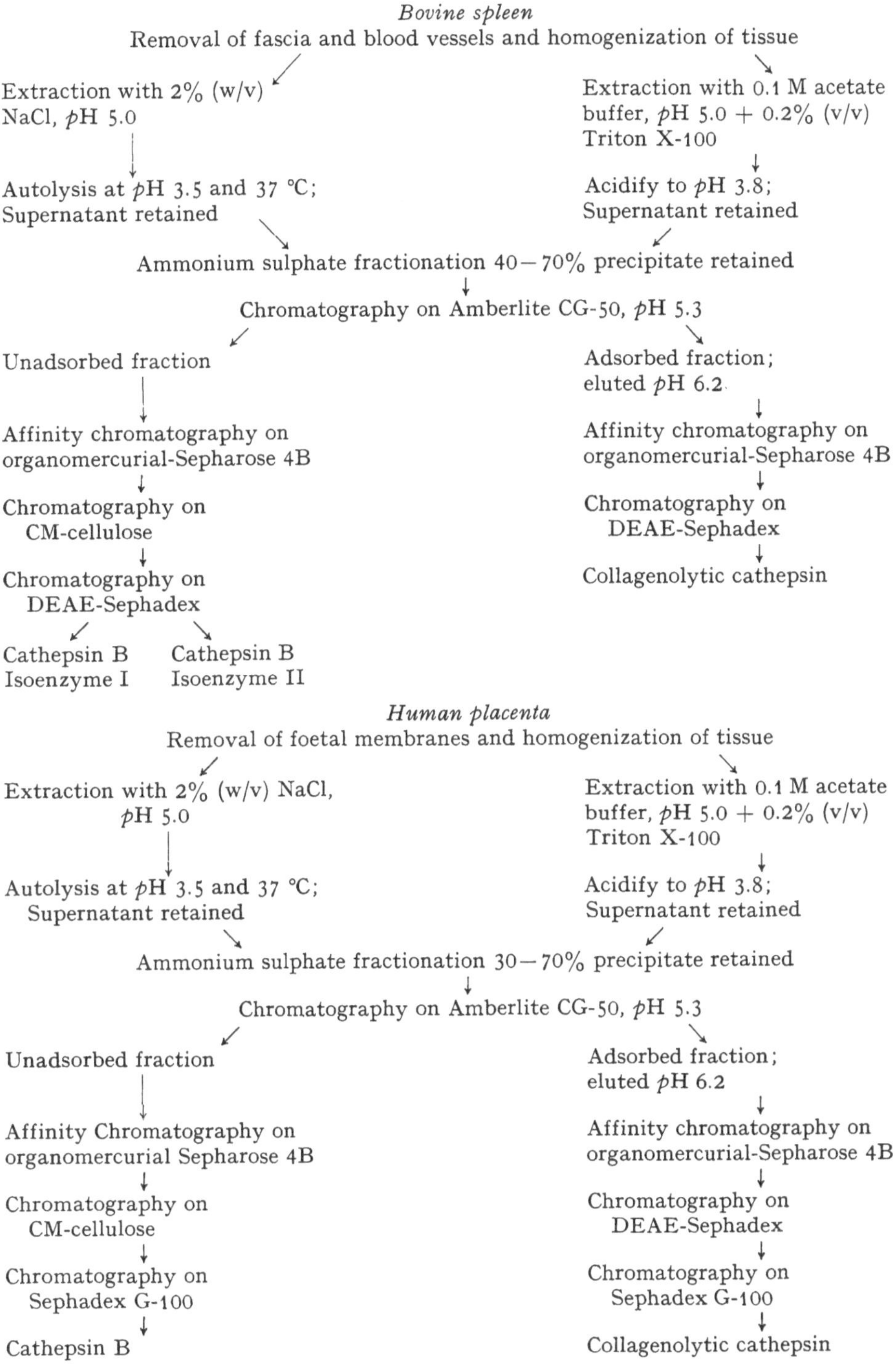

Fig. 2. Flow diagrams summarising the procedures for the purification of cathepsin B and collagenolytic cathepsin from bovine spleen and human placenta.

the autolytic treatment at *p*H 3.5 and acid precipitation at *p*H 3.8 and 4 °C was preferred in the preparation of this enzyme. Purified or partially-purified enzymes were dialysed finally against 1 mM-EDTA and were then safely stored at —25 °C in 33% (v/v) glycerol.

Properties of cathepsin B and collagenolytic cathepsin

Both cathepsins degraded fibrous collagen optimally at *p*H 3.4—3.5 and with negligible activity above *p*H 4.5. When cathepsin B and collagenolytic cathepsin were recombined the collagenolytic activity was enhanced [15]. This apparent synergism indicated that the two enzymes were not acting in an identical manner. Since these two enzymes exist together in the lysosome then their combined action in vivo must be more effective than has been indicated from previous studies on the isolated cathepsins.

Soluble monomeric collagen was tested at temperatures below 30 °C in order to prevent thermal denaturation of this substrate. Both cathepsins were shown to cleave off the short, non-helical telopeptides which carry the intramolecular cross-links and the helical region was totally resistant. This action was demonstrated in the *p*H range 3—6 [13, 15]. Using purified isoenzymes of bovine cathepsin B, these cleavage sites in calf skin, type 1 collagen have been investigated by end-group analysis and located between the lysine-derived cross-links and the first triplet sequence in the helical region [13].

At 37 °C monomeric collagen is spontaneously denatured and was shown to be further cleaved by pure cathepsin B to smaller peptide fragments [16]. From viscometric analysis we demonstrated that cathepsin B acted optimally on the denatured substrate near *p*H 4.6 [13].

The lower *p*H range observed for the degradation of the native fibre is believed to arise from conformational changes in the substrate that could influence the ease of formation of the enzyme-substrate complex [13]. Collagen fibres swell markedly in acid and this is normally apparent below *p*H 4. Hence this collagen was much less accessible to penetration by the cathepsins in the *p*H range 4—6, which spans the intralysosomal level of acidity.

Cathepsin B has been shown to cleave a variety of proteins near *p*H 5 [17] and synthetic chromogenic peptide substrates near *p*H 6 [18, 19] and aryl-arginyl peptides were used routinely for the assay of this enzyme. Collagenolytic cathepsin has been similarly tested against the chromogenic substrates at *p*H 3.5 and 6.5. The human enzyme was totally inactive against these peptides, but the bovine enzyme exhibited a very weak activity against α-N-benzoyl-DL-arginine-β-naphthylamide at *p*H 6.5. These data are recorded in Table 1. Although most protein substrates other than collagen remained apparently undegraded by collagenolytic cathepsin, we have recently found that the human enzyme will release TCA-soluble peptides from basic proteins such as lysine-rich histone.

Both cathepsin B and collagenolytic cathepsin possess a thiol group that is essential for acitivity. Heavy metals and a variety of alkylating agents were inhibitory to both enzymes in the collagen assay. Cathepsin B was assayed also against the synthetic substrate Bz-DL-Arg-4-nitroanilide at *p*H 6.5 and minor differences were noted in the effect of some compounds. These data are presented in Table 2. The activity of both enzymes was blocked by chicken-egg-white inhibitor and by

Table 1
Hydrolytic activity of cathepsin B and collagenolytic cathepsin against peptide substrates

	Bovine spleen		Human placenta	
	Cathepsin B	Collagenolytic cathepsin	Cathepsin B	Collagenolytic cathepsin
	(Percent activity relative to cathepsin B in the standard assay)			
Bz-L-Arg-2-naphthylamide[1]	100	0.2	100	0
Bz-DL-Arg-4-nitroanilide[2]	2.7	0	12	0
Cbz-L-Lys-4-nitrophenyl ester[3]	1076	0	n. d.	n. d.
Cbz-Gly-4-nitrophenyl ester[3]	176	0	n. d.	n. d.
L-Arg-2-naphthylamide[1]	13	0	47	0
L-Arg methyl ester[3]	n. d.	n. d.	0	0
L-Lys methyl ester[3]	n. d.	n. d.	0	0
Ac-L-Lys methyl ester[3]	n. d.	n. d.	0	0
Bz-L-Tyr-4-nitroanilide[2]	n. d.	n. d.	0	0

n. d. = not determined.
Peptide substrates were tested according to published methods: [1] [20]; [2] [17]; [3] [21]. Activity values were calculated as μmoles/min/mg and converted to percent of the respective activity value for cathepsin B against Bz-L-Arg-2-naphthylamide. The activity of the collagenolytic cathepsin in the table was calculated relative to the equivalent collagenolytic activity of the cathepsin B preparation.

the Actinomycete inhibitors antipain, chymostaton and leupeptin. The latter compound is a structural analogue of the arginine-containing peptide substrates for cathepsin B. Since it was equally effective as an inhibitor of both enzymes in the collagen assay it is suggested that the substrate requirement for collagenolytic cathepsin may be similar to cathepsin B. However all attempts so far to identify a synthetic substrate for collagenolytic cathepsin have been unsuccessful.

The physico-chemical properties of cathepsin B and collagenolytic cathepsin are recorded in Table 3. Bovine and human cathepsin B were very similar, although for the latter preparation no minor isoenzyme forms were observed. The two collagenolytic cathepsins exhibited a substantial difference in both size and in isoelectric point. However, both enzymes appeared to be stable at physiological *p*H, in contrast to cathepsin B.

During these studies of the collagen-degrading cathepsins it had become apparent that in the dissolution of insoluble fibrous collagen, the integrity of the original substrate was of paramount importance to the ultimate effectiveness of these enzymes. The potential factors which may contribute to the inherent resistance to collagenolysis were tentatively identified as: (1) number and location of the interchain cross-links, (2) extent of association with proteoglycans and/or glycosaminoglycans, (3) collagen phenotype, and (4) lyotropic properties of the solvent. In order to examine these factors, insoluble bovine collagens were prepared from various tissues of mature animals and included the four known pheotypes. Collagens from foetal, young and old animals were also prepared. Each collagen preparation was analysed chemically for contaminants and then tested for its susceptibility to

Table 2

Activators and inhibitors of cathepsin B and collagenolytic cathepsin

	Bovine spleen			Human placenta		
	Cathepsin B		Collagenolytic cathepsin	Cathepsin B		Collagenolytic cathepsin
	BAPNA (pH 6.5)	Collagen (pH 3.5)	Collagen (pH 3.5)	BAPNA (pH 6.5)	Collagen (pH 3.5)	Collagen (pH 3.5)
Cysteine	+	+	+	+	+	+
Dithiothreitol	+	+	+	+	+	+
EDTA	+	+	+	+	+	+
$HgCl_2$	−	−	−	−	−	−
$ZnSO_4$	−	N. E.	N. E.	n. d.	n. d.	n. d.
2,2′-Dipyridyl-disulphide	−	−	−	−	−	−
Iodoacetamide	−	−	−	−	−	−
p-Hydroxymer-curibenzoate	−	−	−	−	−	−
Chymostatin	−	−	−	−	−	−
Leupeptin	−	−	−	−	−	−
Antipain	n. d.	n. d.	n. d.	−	−	−
Tos-Lys-CH_2Cl	−	−	−	n. d.	n. d.	n. d.
Ac-$(Ala)_3$-Ala-CH_2-Cl	−	−	−	n. d.	n. d.	n. d.
Phenylpyruvic acid	N. E.	−	−	n. d.	n. d.	n. d.
Chicken's-egg-white inhibitor	−	−	−	n. d.	n. d.	n. d.

BAPNA, Bz-DL-Arg-4-nitroanilide; +, activation; −, inhibition; N. E., no effect; n. d., not determined. Each test compound was pre-incubated with enzyme at pH 6. The activity was then determined against insoluble collagen at pH 3.5 or BAPNA at pH 6.5 [15].

Table 3

Physico-chemical properties of cathepsin B and collagenolytic cathepsin

	Bovine spleen		Human placenta	
	Cathepsin B	Collagenolytic cathepsin	Cathepsin B	Collagenolytic cathepsin
M. W. (exclusion chromatography)	26,000	20,000	24,5000	34,600
pI (isoelectric focusing)	4.9	6.4	5.4	5.1
Minor isoenzyme forms	2−4	−	? NIL	−
Stability at pH 7.4	unstable	stable	unstable	stable

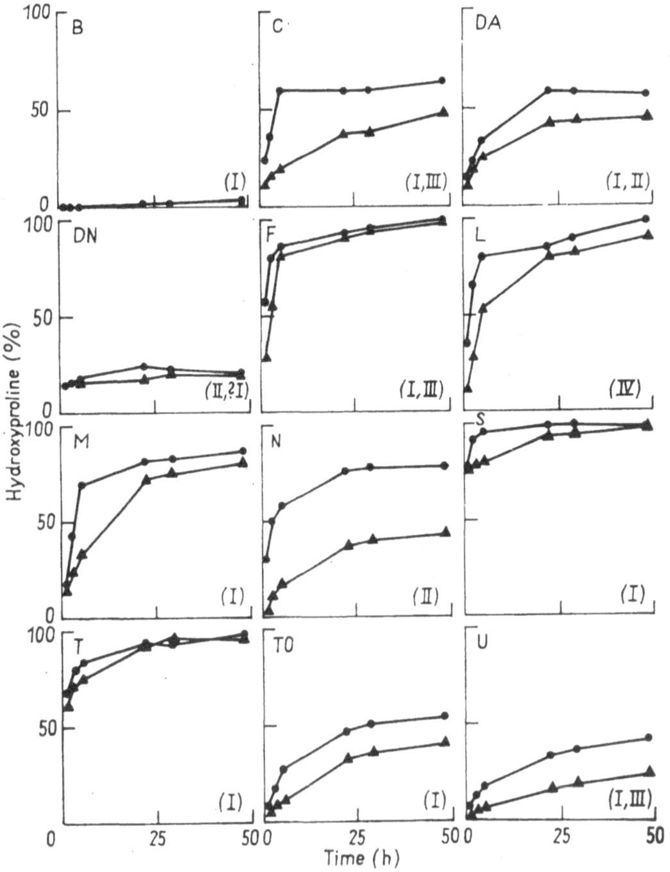

Fig. 3. Dissolution of insoluble bovine collagens by bovine spleen cathepsin B and collagenolytic cathepsin at *p*H 3.4 and 37 °C.

Collagens, which were prepared by extraction with neutral salt and acetic acid, were freeze-dried and then chemically analysed for hydroxyproline. Insoluble collagens were obtained from the following tissues and the percent of hydroxyproline in each preparation is shown in parenthesis:

B, bone (12.6); C, calf skin (4.8); DA, disc annulus (12.3); DN, disc nucleus (10.8); F, foetal calf skin (6.2); L, anteria lens capsule (12.1); M, meniscus cartilage (12.6); N, nasal cartilage (6.7); S, skin (11.4); T, tendon (12.2); TO, old tendon (11.6); U, umbilicus fascia (10.0). The collagen phenotypes (I, II, III or IV) present in each preparation are shown in the figure. Cathepsin B (●) and collagenolytic cathepsin (▲) were each incubated with collagen at the rate of 0.005 unit of collagenolytic activity/mg hydroxyproline in 0.13 M sodium formate buffer, *p*H 3.4, containing 1.3 mM EDTA and 0.7 mM dithiothreitol. Samples were removed at intervals and the extent of dissolution calculated from the percent solubilization of the collagen hydroxyproline

dissolution by each of the bovine cathepsins. Full details of this investigation have been published elsewhere [20].

Progress curves for the dissolution of twelve insoluble collagen preparations over 48 hrs at 37 °C are shown in Fig. 3. Foetal skin, adult skin and anterior lens capsule were almost completely degraded. In contrast to these, disc nucleus and bone collagens were very resistant. Collagens from the remaining tissues exhibited an intermediate range of susceptibilities and for several preparations a resistant collagenous residue was obtained. Additional studies on collagens in which the acid labile cross-links had been stabilized by prior reduction with potassium borohydride reduced the susceptibility and made the preparation more like the equivalent collagens from old animals.

Nasal cartilage collagen was more susceptible to cathepsin B than to collagenolytic cathepsin. Smaller differences were also noted for some of the other preparations, but these could not be correlated with collagen phenotypes and in studies of mixed-type-fibre preparations no differences in susceptibility were revealed for either collagen in the respective preparations.

Several collagen preparations remained heavily contaminated by non-collagen components. Nasal cartilage collagen was additionally treated with chondroitinase ABC. This removed much of the associated proteoglycan and the substrate was more susceptible to degradation. Both cathepsins solubilized twice as much material in a 48 h period at 25 °C, but at 37 °C the improvement was less marked. In a parallel study with pepsin, the increase in susceptibility after this chondroitinase ABC treatment was very much greater and supported the concept of these components acting as a blockade to the enzyme-sensitive telopeptides.

The effect of the solvent ions on the activity of the collagen-degrading cathepsins has not been examined in detail. However, we have studied the lyotopic effect of different ions, ionic strength and *p*H on peptic activity and this enzyme was shown to be influenced greatly by changes in any of these parameters. It is clear from this study that the more highly swollen the fibre, the more rapidly it is degraded. Buffer cations restrict fibre swelling and it was noted in earlier studies that collagenolysis by the cathepsins was enhanced in buffers of low ionic-strength [12].

The action of these cathepsins in vivo is to complete the dissolution of the fibrous fragments that have entered the phagosomal-lysosomal system. The collagen has already been partially degraded extracellularly and it may be anticipated therefore that it can swell more readily in the less acidic environment of the digestive vacuole. The preparation of fibrous collagen used for the assay substrate in these in vitro studies had not been fragmented or weakened by any such enzymatic pretreatment and it was therefore probably not a true physiological substrate for these lysosomal cathepsins. Associated non-collagenous components that may provide a blockade of the cleavage sites in the collagen molecule would be removed through the action of lysosomal glycosidases. The action of the specific collagen-degrading cathepsins therefore may be assisted by these enzymes to complete the dissolution of this ingested collagen.

Acknowledgements

We are grateful to the Arthritis and Rheumatism Council for a grant to support part of this investigation. We also thank Professor SILVER for providing laboratory facilities to P. J. EVANS.

References

[1] Bailey, A. J., S. P. Robins, and G. Balian: Nature, Lond. **251**, 105 (1974)
[2] Woessner, J. F., jr. in: Treatise on Collagen. B. S. Gould (Ed.). **2B**, 253. Academic Press, London, New York 1968
[3] Parakkal, P. F.: J. Ultrastruct. Res. **29**, 210 (1969)
[4] Sambe, K., K. Kamagaya, M. Oda, and I. Okasaki in: Biochemistry and Pathology of Connective Tissue. Y. Ohtaka (Ed.). Igakushoin, Tokyo 1974, p. 249
[5] Renteria, V. G., V. J. Ferrans, H. Jones, and W. C. Roberts: Lab. Invest. **35**, 439 (1976)
[6] Tencate, A. R., and D. A. Deporter,: Anat. Rec. **182**, 1 (1975)
[7] Garant, P. R.: J. Periodont. **47**, 380 (1976)
[8] Vaes, G. in: Lysosomes in Biology and Pathology. J. T. Dingle and H. B. Fell (Eds.). **1**, 217. North-Holland Publishing Co., Amsterdam 1969
[9] Harris, E. D., jr., and S. M. Krane: New Engl. J. Med. **291**, 557 (1974)
[10] Ohlsson, K., and M. Delshammar in: Dynamics of Connective Tissue Macromolecules. P. M. C. Burleigh and A. R. Poole (Eds.). North-Holland Publishing Co., Amsterdam 1975
[11] Etherington, D. J.: Ann. rheum. Dis. **36**, Suppl. 2, 14 (1977)
[12] Etherington, D. J.: Biochem. J. **127**, 685 (1972)
[13] Etherington, D. J.: Biochem. J. **137**, 547 (1974)
[14] Evans, P. J., and D. J. Etherington: Archs Int. Physiol. Biochim. **84**, R9 (1976)
[15] Etherington, D. J.: Biochem. J. **153**, 199 (1976)
[16] Burleigh, P. M. C., A. J. Barrett, and G. S. Lazarus: Biochem. J. **137**, 387 (1974)
[17] Otto, K. in: Tissue Proteinases. A. J. Barrett and J. T. Dingle (Eds.). North-Holland Publishing Co., Amsterdam 1917, p. 1
[18] McDonald, J. K., and S. Ellis: Life Sci. **17**, 1269 (1975)
[19] Bajkowski, A. S., and A. Frankfater: Anal. Biochem. **68**, 119 (1975)
[20] Etherington, D. J.: Connect. Tissue Res. **5**, 135 (1977)
[21] Barrett, A. J.: Anal. Biochem. **76**, 374 (1976)

Acta biol. med. germ., Band 36, Seite 1565–1573 (1977)

Central Research and Development Department
E. I. du Pont de Nemours and Company
Wilmington, Delaware 19898 U.S.A.

Protein cleavage in virus-infected cells

B. D. KORANT

Summary

A variety of proteins, including viral precursor polypeptides, were bound to a solid support and used in a sensitive assay for proteolytic enzymes in HeLa cells. A trypsin-like endoprotease, present on ribosomes of HeLa cells, loses activity after picornavirus infection. The decline follows synthesis and processing of a viral protein. Inhibition of cellfree activity of HeLa protease occurs when protein trypsin inhibitors or double-stranded RNA are added. After the mid-point of infection, protease activity with enhanced specificity for viral substrates is detected. The new protease has a *p*H optimum and heat stability different from endogenous host enzymes, and is synthesized following infection. A viral mutant was isolated which produces a temperature-sensitive protease. The results indicate that a poliovirus gene product participates enzymatically in the final cleavages of some polioviral proteins. A model for the regulation of poliovirus replication based on specific proteolysis is presented.

Introduction

Many animal and bacterial viruses utilize protein cleavages to produce their capsid polypeptides. The picornaviruses (e. g., poliovirus and rhinovirus) rely on cleavage to an exaggerated degree; all stable viral proteins are produced from precursors. Most of the information describing steps in the cleavage process has relied on pulse-chase experiments, protease inhibitors, or amino acid analogs. Once inhibitors are available, viral precursors can be accumulated and used as substrates in vitro, permitting comparisons of proteolytic activities between control and virus-infected tissue culture cells. The published data collectively indicate that the primary cleavages occurring in nascent viral polypeptides are mediated by cellular proteases, while the ultimate conversion of intermediates to stable proteins, e. g., the capsid polypeptides, is carried on by proteases which are induced after infection (reviewed in [1, 2]).

Materials and methods

Tissue culture cells, media and viruses. The "0" strain of HeLa cells was used throughout. Cells were grown in McCoy 5A medium (monolayer) or in Joklik-modified Eagle's medium, with 7% horse serum. Poliovirus type 2 (atten.), rhinovirus type 1A and the P2r variant were grown and assayed as in prior reports [1, 3].
Gel electrophoresis was in 0.1% dodecyl sulfate on polyacrylamide slab gels, as was previously described [1, 4].
Zonal sedimentation was performed in 5–25% or 8–56% sucrose (w/v) gradients, containing 0.01 M NaCl, 0.01 M Tris *p*H 7.2 and 1 mM Mg^{2+} (RSB). Centrifugation was in a Beckman SW27 rotor, or in DuPont-Sorvall SS-90 and TV850 vertical rotors, in Sorvall OTD-2 or

RC-2B centrifuges, at 4 °C. Cell samples were swelled in RSB, mechanically broken and, after removal of nuclei, treated with deoxycholate and Triton X-100 prior to centrifugation.
Protease assays were done in slab gels [1] or with solid-phase substrates, as described in the text.
Labeling of cellular or viral proteins was done with [^{35}S]-methionine, [^{3}H]-uridine or mixtures of [^{3}H]-amino acids (10—50 μCi/ml) in vivo, or with [^{125}]iodine, using chloramine T or the Bolton-Hunter reagent, in vitro. Trasylol was the generous gift of Professor E. Wecker, University of Würzburg.
Amino acid analogs were purchased from Sigma Chemical Company.

Results

The scheme for poliovirus protein cleavage is indicated in the diagram of Fig. 1. The reactions will occur in vitro, if suitable precursors are added to homogenates of poliovirus-infected cells [3—6]. In order to easily quantitate the proteolytic reactions, precursors are attached covalently to sepharose beads [7, 8]. Protease activity is then conveniently assayed by the release of radioactive precursors from the beads (Fig. 2).
Exposure in vitro of poliovirus precursors to extracts of HeLa cells infected with poliovirus indicates that the endogenous protease activity in the uninfected cells

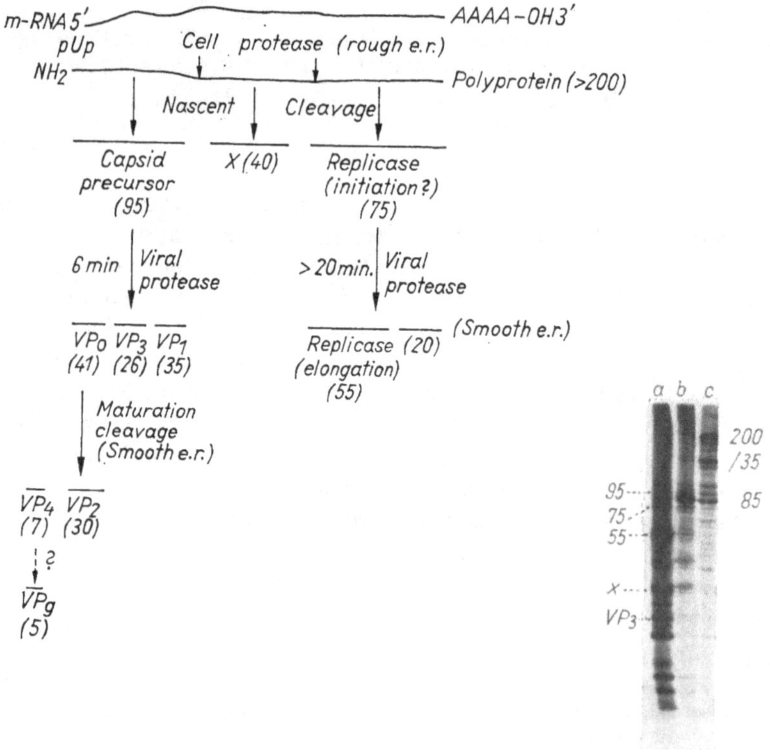

Fig. 1. Proteolytic processing of viral precursor polypeptides in poliovirus-infected cells. Insert: Gel electrophoresis of ^{35}S-labelled poliovirus polypeptides.
a) Untreated cells; b) cells treated with $5 \cdot 10^{-4}$ M iodoacetamide [3]; c) cells treated with $1 \cdot 10^{-4}$ M TLCK [4]. Larger proteins are at the top of the gel

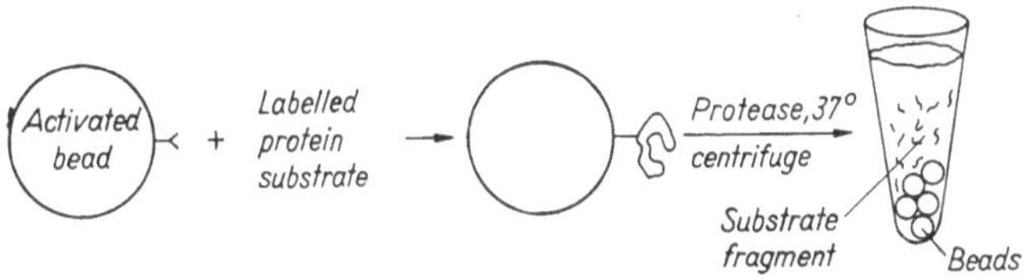

Fig. 2. Assay for protease using a solid-phase protein substrate.
The substrate may be labelled isotopically [7, 8] or with a fluorescent marker. The supernate is counted after incubation of the beads with a protease. Best results have been obtained by treating the beads in 0.1% dodecyl sulfate prior to centrifugation [8]

declines by 50% or more following infection, so that a minimum is reached at 2.5 hrs post infection. An increase in protease activity within the infected cells begins by 3 hrs after infection and continues as infection proceeds (Fig. 3).

Inactivation of HeLa cell protease

Viral inactivation of HeLa protease occurs with kinetics resembling the viral inhibition of cellular protein synthesis, and the inhibition of cellular protease proceeds in the presence of guanidine.

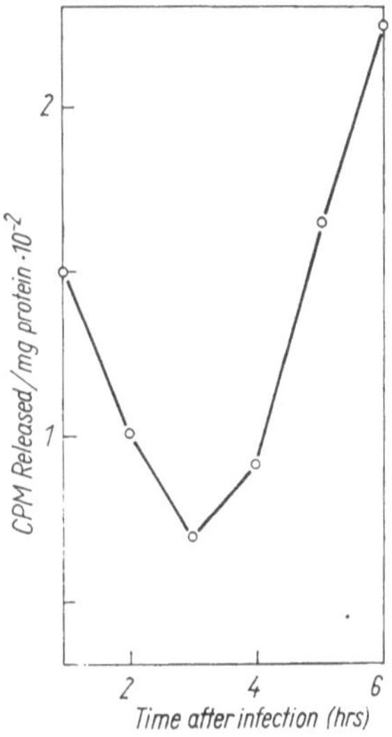

Fig. 3

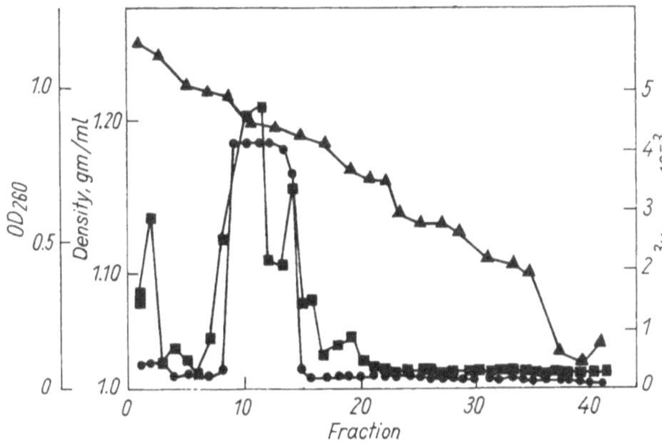

Fig. 4

Fig. 3. Protease activites in poliovirus-infected HeLa cells at various times after infection
Substrate was solid phase-linked poliovirus precursor polypeptides

Fig. 4. Polyribosomal protease activity.
Polyribosomes were prepared from uninfected HeLa cells ($3 \cdot 10^7$ cells) and rebanded in a discontinuous sucrose gradient for 17 hrs at 25.000 rpm. The polysomes were initially adjusted to 25% sucrose (w/v), but banded in approximately 45% sucrose. Protease activity was assayed on ^3H labeled HeLa cell protein extracts (shown) and on ^{127}I-labelled hemoglobin (not shown), with similar results

An interesting feature of the HeLa protease is that a part of the activity sediments as a particulate in sucrose gradients, coinciding with cellular ribosomes [8]. A higher degree of purification was achieved by isopycnic banding of HeLa cell polyribosomes in a discontinuous sucrose gradient (Fig. 4). Protease activity still remained associated with the polyribosomal fraction under these conditions. Freeze-thaw, high concentrations of KCl, and EDTA treatments reduced the protease activity considerably [8].

Because the decline in host protease activity is kinetically similar to the viral inhibition of cellular translation, we surveyed some chemical inhibitors of translation initiation, and found that double-stranded RNA is able to inhibit HeLa cell protease in a dose-dependent manner (Fig. 5). The ribosomal protease in HeLa cells detected under these conditions appears to be trypsin-like, as indicated by the inhibitory effects of α_1A trypsin inhibitor, basic pancreatic trypsin inhibitor (Trasylol), and TLCK (Fig. 6).

The inhibitory effect of poliovirus infection on ribosomal protease activity was studied using iodine-labeled Trasylol. As shown in Fig. 7, Trasylol is a homogeneous protein of molecular weight approx. 6,500. The protein was labeled with ^{125}iodine, using both the Bolton-Hunter and chloramine T methods, and dialyzed to remove unbound iodine. Ribosomes were prepared from uninfected HeLa cell cultures, and from cells infected for 3 hrs with poliovirus in the presence of 2 mM guanidine.

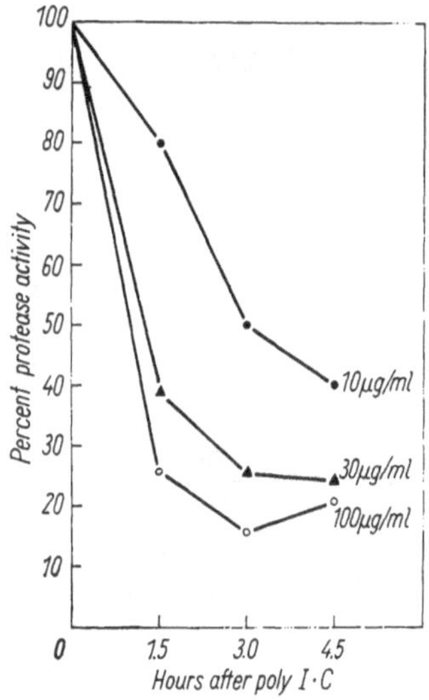

Fig. 5

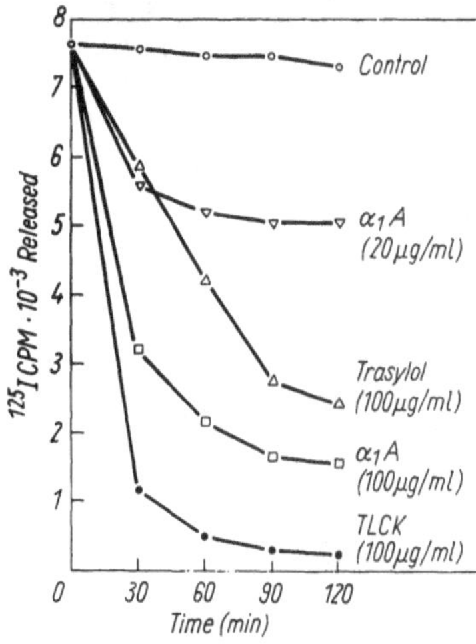

Fig. 6

Fig. 5. Effect of double-stranded RNA (poly rI · poly rC) at three concentrations on ribosomal protease.
The RNA is inhibitory at $10^{-6}-10^{-7}$ M, a level somewhat higher than is necessary to inhibit protein synthesis [9]

Fig. 6. Effects of trypsin inhibitors on HeLa cell ribosomal protease activity.
Substrate was ^{125}I-labeled hemoglobin. Inhibitors were human α_1A trypsin inhibitor, bovine pancreatic trypsin inhibitor (Trasylol) and tosyl lysyl chloromethyl ketone (TLCK)

The purified monosomes were incubated with the labelled Trasylol and chromatographed to separate unbound Trasylol from the ribosomes. As shown in Fig. 7, much less of the protease inhibitor is bound to the ribosomes from infected cells, which correlates with their reduced proteolytic activity. It is not clear whether the lack of binding is due to specific loss of the protease polypeptide, or to a more general effect of the infection on ribosome structure. Neither is the function of ribosomal protease yet understood, but it may participate in processing of nascent cellular polypeptides [8, 10].

Production of virus-specific protease in poliovirus-infected cells

I will now discuss some properties of the proteases which participate in the later stages of poliovirus infection. The increase in protease activity later in infection does not occur if cycloheximide or guanidine is added at 2 hrs after infection, therefore production of the protease is dependent on a functional viral genome

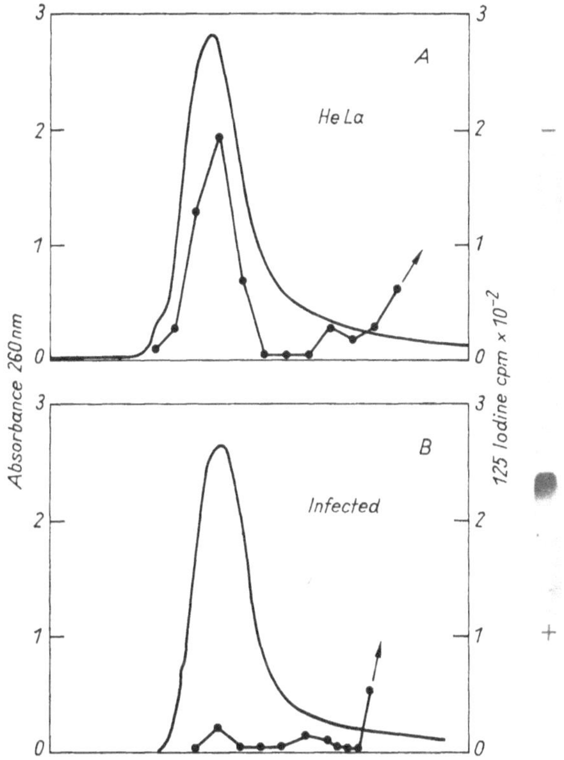

Fig. 7. Binding of ^{125}I Trasylol to ribosomes.
Ribosomes were purified by zonal sedimentation, following detergent treatment of uninfected or polio-infected HeLa cells. The ribosomes were incubated for 30 min at 25 °C with Trasylol labeled by the Bolton-Hunter reagent. The mixture was then passed through a Biogel P150 column, buffered at *p*H 7.2 and containing 1 mM $MgCl_2$ and 0.01 M NaCl. The monosomes were recovered in the void volume, and unbound Trasylol was retained. ^{125}I was determined by liquid scintillation counting.
Panel A: Uninfected cells; Panel B: Poliovirus-infected. Insert: SDS gel of Trasylol. Autoradiography showed only one radioactive species

and viral protein synthesis. The specificity of the polio protease is directed toward its homologous substrate. Infections by unrelated, but cytopathic viruses including rhinovirus 1A and VSV do not induce proteases active on polio substrate.

In Fig. 8 is shown the production of protease activity in HeLa cells infected with a human rhinovirus, type 1A. There is an initial decline in endogenous cellular protease in the cytoplasm, as with poliovirus infection. After a 3 h latency, there is induced a new activity, which is able to cleave a rhinovirus substrate, but has much lower activity on poliovirus substrate, or on hemoglobin or gelatin.

A major question remaining is whether the proteases which produce stable viral polypeptides are themselves viral proteins, or cellular enzymes, activated by infection. To study this problem, HeLa cells were infected with a high multiplicity of poliovirus, in the presence of actinomycin D, in order to insure thorough inhibition of cellular protein synthesis. At 3 hrs after infection, that is the time point when intracellular protease activity begins to rise, amino acid analogs were added to the medium. Cells were harvested at 6 hrs after infection, and the cell extracts were heated at 55 °C for up to 1 h, then assayed on polio substrate.

There was little effect of the analogs on the production of the protease. Up to 0.3 mM of each of azatryptophan, fluorophenylalanine and azaleucine did not reduce the yield of enzyme more than 20% (Figure 9).

By comparison, the yield of infectious virus is greatly reduced following a similar level of treatment. This result implies the protease activity is not a function of a native virus coat protein. However, the enzyme from analog-treated cells was more heat sensitive than that from control cultures, which demonstrates that it was synthesized in the presence of the analogs, that is, after 3 hrs of infection. This is a time of virus replication after which no cellular proteins are synthesized (Fig. 10).

If the induced protease is viral in origin, then a viral polypeptide should be associated with it. In order to examine for a viral contribution, cytoplasmic extracts from infected HeLa cells containing radioactive viral proteins were chromatographed, as follows: Homogenates of the infected cells, with nuclei removed, were

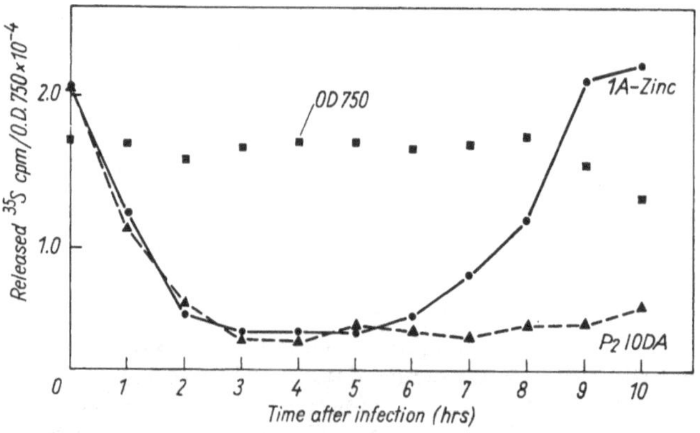

Fig. 8. Cleavage of viral substrates by rhinovirus-infected cell extracts.
HeLa cells were infected with rhinovirus type 1A, and samples were removed at the indicated times, and homogenized. Protease activity in the extracts was measured on either poliovirus (P2 IODA ref. [3]) or rhinovirus (1A Zinc, ref. [11]) substrates

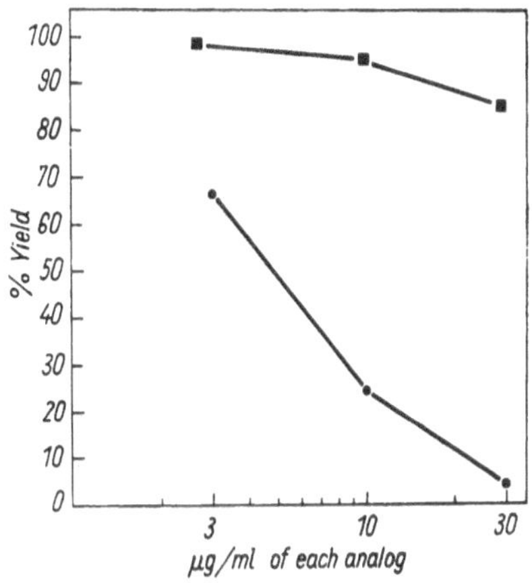

Fig. 9

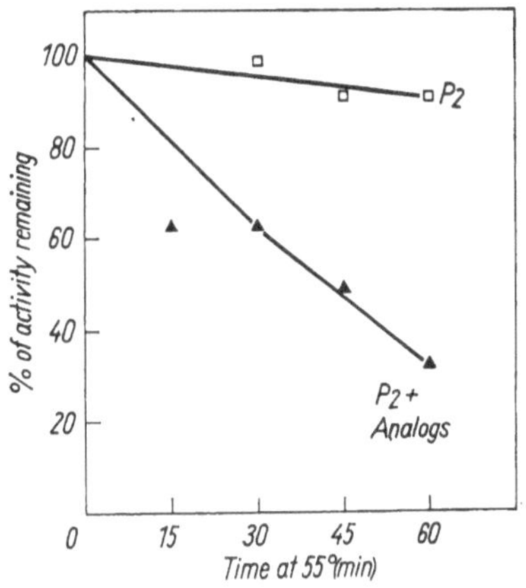

Fig. 10

Fig. 9. Effect of amino acid analogs on production of poliovirus and activity of virus-induced protease.

At 3 hrs after infection with poliovirus, the culture was divided in four aliquots. One was not treated, the others received various levels of azaleucine, azatryptophan and parafluorophenylalanine. After an additional 3 hrs the cultures were harvested, and homogenates assayed for protease (■) and infectious virus (●)

Fig. 10. Stability of poliovirus protease in heated cell extracts.

Protease extracted from amino acid analog treated cells or from control cultures was heated at 55 °C for up to 1 h, then chilled to 0°, and assayed at 35 °C. Untreated (□); plus 30 μg/ml of each analog (▲)

detergent-treated and resolved by ion-exchange and hydroxylapatite chromatography, the latter in SDS. Protease-containing fractions from the DEAE-Sephadex contain many cell proteins. These are greatly reduced following hydroxylapatite chromatography. The viral protein contribution was established by autoradiography. Present in the peak of protease activity is only the cytoplasmic polypeptide X of the virus. However, following radioiodine labeling of the "purified" protease-containing fraction, many host protein contaminants were detected (not shown). It must be concluded that presently there is insufficient purity of the best preparations to permit assignment of the enzymatic activity to a specific viral polypeptide.

A virus mutant was selected which is able to maintain for an extended time the maximal rate of RNA synthesis, and which also displays greater stability of certain cytoplasmic proteins [1]. The levels of protease in cells infected by the parent virus or the mutant were assayed. The unregulated virus mutant is deficient in production of active protease, compared to the parent virus (Fig. 11). A possible explanation for the low protease activity of the mutant virus is that it codes for a missence protease polypeptide. To test this, protease was extracted at 6 hr after infection, and the stability of the parental or mutant protease to heat was measured (Fig. 12). The results indicate that the mutant induces an altered, temperature-sensitive protease. This is further support for the proposal that the enzyme is a viral gene product.

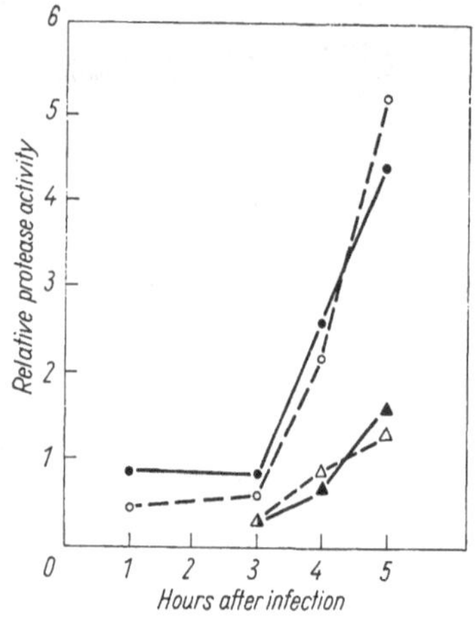

Fig. 11

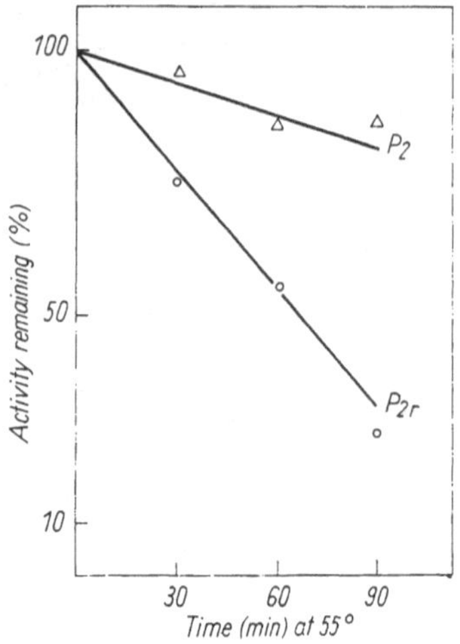

Fig. 12

Fig. 11. Protease activities in cells infected by parental or mutant polioviruses. Infected HeLa cells were extracted at the indicated times after infection, and assayed on substrates of either the parental of mutant virus. Parent virus enzyme, parental substrate (○ – – – ○); parent virus enzyme, mutant substrate (● ——— ●); mutant virus enzyme, parental substrate (▲ ——— ▲); mutant virus enzyme, mutant substrate (△ – – – △).

Fig. 12. Heat inactivation of parental and mutant viral proteases. After 6 hrs of infection, extracts were made of cells infected with parental virus (P2) or mutant (P2r) and these were heated at 55 °C for up to 90 min, chilled to 0°, and assayed at 35 °C

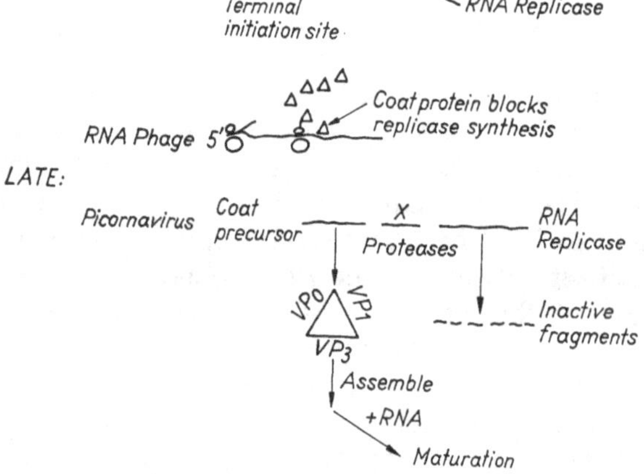

Fig. 13. Comparison of the regulation of RNA metabolism by phages (translational control) and by picornaviruses (posttranslational cleavage)

Acta biol. med. germ., Band 36, Seite 1575–1585 (1977)

Department of Biochemistry, University of Leeds, Leeds LS2 9LS, U. K.

Peptidases of the kidney microvillus membrane

A. J. KENNY, A. G. BOOTH, and R. D. C. MACNAIR

Summary

The microvillus membrane of the kidney is highly differentiated in its complement of enzymes and other proteins. In addition to the five well documented peptidases that are present in the membrane, recent work suggests that aminopeptidase P, carboxypeptidase P and an enzyme tentatively referred to as "leucine hydrazidase" are also microvillus enzymes. Microvillus serine peptidase (dipeptidyl peptidase IV) has been purified after detergent solubilization. The catalytic and molecular properties of this form and the form released by autolysis have been compared in an attempt to gain understanding of the intramembranous domain of this protein. Current views on the molecular organization of the microvillus are discussed.

Introduction

The cells that line the renal proximal tubule exhibit polarization and possess highly differentiated plasma membranes. The luminal pole is specialized into microvilli and these structures contain a battery of hydrolases capable of cleaving glycosidic, ester and peptide bonds. The group of peptidases is the most studied (Table 1) and three of these, aminopeptidase M, serine peptidase and neutral

Table 1
Kidney microvillus membrane peptidases

Enzyme	EC Number	Active site	Assay substrate	Specific activity in microvilli (nmol/mg/min)	References
Neutral endopeptidase	3.4.24.-	Zn^{2+}	[^{125}I]iodo-insulin B chain	28	[3, 4]
Serine peptidase (dipeptidyl peptidase IV)	3.4.21.- (3.4.14.-)	Serine	Gly-Pro-2-NNap	1590	[5, 6, 7]
Aminopeptidase M	3.4.11.2	Zn^{2+}	Leu-2-NNap	2350	[8, 9, 10]
Aminopeptidase A	3.4.11.7	Me^{2+}	α-Glu-2-NNap	950*	[11, 12]
γ-Glutamyl transferase	2.3.2.2.	—	γ-Glu-2-NNap + acceptor	810*	[13, 14, 15, 16]
Aminopeptidase P	3.4.11.9	—	Gly-Pro-Hyp	128	[17]
Carboxypeptidase P (prolyl carboxypeptidase)	3.4.12.-	—	Z-Pro-Met	125	[18]
"Leucine hydrazidase"	—	—	Leu-$NHNH_2$	120	[19]

* Rabbit; other values are for pig. NNapt: 2-naphthylamide

endopeptidase are major proteins in the membrane, each constituting about 4% of the microvillus protein [1]. Five of the enzymes listed in Table 1 are well documented [2] and their general properties need not be expanded here (for references see Table 1). However the last three are peptidases not previously reported to be microvillus enzymes and they merit some explanation for their inclusion in this group. Additionally, we are reporting some preliminary conclusions on the intramembranous domain of microvillus serine peptidase. This enzyme may be solubilized by autolysis or by detergents. A comparison of the two forms of the purified enzyme indicates that the hydrophobic foot is a relatively small peptide which forms part of the N-terminal sequence of the protein. Current views on the organization of the proteins in the microvillus are discussed.

Material and methods

Unless otherwise stated, enzyme assays were those previously described [2]. Aminopeptidase P was assayed as described by DEHM and NORDWIG [17] on dialysed samples, preincubated with 2 mM $MnCl_2$, carboxypeptidase P was determined in early experiments by the same authors' method [18] but in later experiments by a modification in which Z-Pro-Met was the substrate and methionine released was determined enzymically by L-amino acid oxidase [20]. All samples were dialysed before assay and 1 mM Mn^{2+} was present in the incubation mixture. Leucine hydrazidase was assayed by the Fermognost LAP-Test (VEB Arzneimittelwerk, Dresden, DDR). Microvilli were prepared from frozen pig kidneys as described [21]. Other methods were those described in previous papers [1, 7].

Results and discussion

Carboxypeptidase P, aminopeptidase P and "leucine hydrazidase" as microvillus enzymes

The first two enzymes were previously reported as kidney microsomal peptidases by DEHM and NORDWIG [17, 18]. The existence of the third peptidase was suggested to us by Dr. H. J. HÜTTER (personal communication). The substrate, L-leucine hydrazide is part of a clinical enzyme assay kit for the determination of serum leucine aminopeptidase. HÜTTER had noted that crude human kidney brush border membranes hydrolysed this substrate, but that there were differences in properties, paricularly the reponses to Mn^{2+} ions, that distinguished the brush border activity from leucine aminopeptidase. Furthermore the substrate was not hydrolysed by a purified preparation of aminopeptidase M.

Table 2
Enrichment of aminopeptidase P and carboxypeptidase P in pig microvillus preparations

Enzyme	No. of preparations	Specific activities (nmol/min/mg, mean ± S. E.) Homogenate	Microvilli	Enrichment
Aminopeptidase P	6	20.7 ± 1.5	128 ± 17.2	6.2
Carboxypeptidase P	11	8.17 ± 0.97	125 ± 14.3	15.3

Marker enzymes (microvillus serine peptidase and aminopeptidase M, 4 and 2 preparations respectively), showed a mean enrichment of 7.0

In our preparations of pig kidney microvilli both aminopeptidase P and carboxypeptidase P were consistently enriched (Table 2). The former to a degree comparable with two marker enzymes (serine peptidase and aminopeptidase M). These enrichment values are lower than previously reported for the rabbit [21], but pig microvillus preparations seldom exceed a value of 10. The value for carboxypeptidase P is, however, unexpectedly high. The reasons for this are not yet clear, but we have some evidence that the homogenate activity is depressed by the presence of an inhibitor. When portions of homogenate and microvillus fractions were mixed before assay some experiments showed the resulting activity to be about two-thirds of the sum of the two separate activities. When boiled homogenate was added to a microvillus fraction the latter's activity was again reduced by the same fraction. The inhibitor is heat-stable and non-diffusible, but we have not attempted to characterize it further. The presence of such a factor in the homogenate, and its absence from the microvillus fraction, would tend to magnify the apparent enrichment values. Any contribution to the hydrolysis of these substrates by other microvillus peptidases must also be considered. Microvillus serine peptidase might be capable of cleaving the Pro-X bond in the assay substrates, Gly-Pro-Hyp and Z-Pro-Met [7]. It is also possible that neutral peptidase might attack Z-Pro-Met, though the presence of a free α-carboxyl group makes it very unlikely [3]. Both these possibilities have been excluded by inhibition experiments. The addition of 1 mM Dip-F and 20 μM phosphoramidon [2] to homogenate and microvilli did not reduce the activity of either aminopeptidase P or carboxypeptidase P.

The enrichment values for leucine hydrazidase in microvillus preparations have been invariably less than unity. This is not surprising bearing in mind the high activity of leucine aminopeptidase (EC 3.4.11.1) in the kidney cytosol. Indeed, the microvillus activity towards leucine hydrazide might be no more than a loose and nonspecifically bound form of the cytosol enzyme. Although this is a possibility that has not been completely excluded, it is clear that the leucine hydrazidase could not be displaced by repeated washing of the mirovillus fraction with 0.15 M NaCl. Another possibility, that the activity might be attributable to aminopeptidase M, was unequivocally excluded by several experiments in confirmation of HÜTTER's observations. Thus, EDTA in the range 0.1 mM to 50 mM inhibited aminopeptidase M to a maximum of 50% but did not affect leucine hydrazidase. Secondly, $MnCl_2$ in the range 0.1 mM to 100 mM activated leucine hydrazidase three-fold but had no effect on aminopeptidase M. Thirdly, heat treatment for various periods at 60 °C revealed that leucine hydrazidase was consistently the more labile of the two.

The effect of incubation of microvillus fractions with papain is one criterion for classifying the membrane-bound enzymes [1]. Four of the five "established" peptidases are released; only neutral endopeptidase remains bound to the membrane. The effect of papain on the release of the three putative microvillus enzymes is shown in Fig. 1. Carboxypeptidase P is rapidly and virtually completely released from the membrane in a manner comparable to aminopeptidase M. Aminopeptidase P is more slowly released and approaches a maximum of only 50%. The curve for leucine hydrazidase is quite atypical: 40% of the membrane-bound enzyme is rapidly released in 5 min and the rest stays firmly bound during the

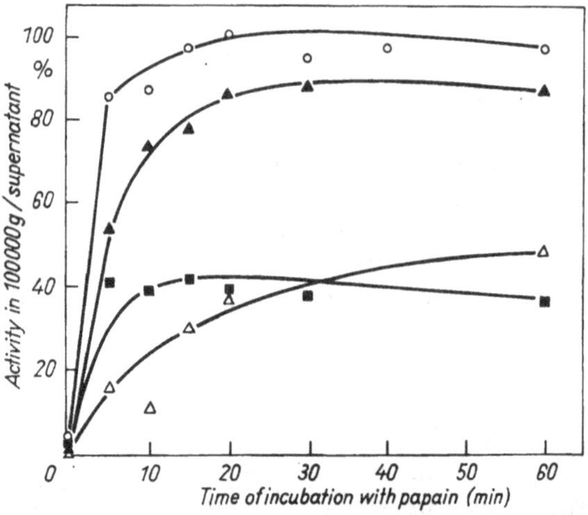

Fig. 1. Solubilization of enzymes by incubation of microvillus preparations with papain. Solubilization implies % activity in 100000 × *g* supernatant. Papain: microvillus protein ratio was 1 : 10.
○ aminopeptidase M; ▲ carboxypeptidase P; △ aminopeptidase P; ■ leucine hydrazidase

subsequent 55 minutes incubation. This is difficult to interpret: it might imply that there are two enzymes in this preparation, one accessible and the other inaccessible to papain. The latter might be an intrinsic membrane protein, but could conceivably be due to (cytosol) leucine aminopeptidase trapped within vesiculated microvilli at the time of homogenization. At present we have not resolved these alternatives. However our conclusions, at this preliminary stage, are that there are two and possibly three additional peptidases in the microvillus membrane. They further add to the complexity of this already enzymically complex membrane.

Serine peptidase (dipeptidyl peptidase IV) — the intramembranous domain

This enzyme is readily solubilized by autolysis at *p*H 3.8, without significant losses in activity [7]. The properties and specificity of this form of the enzyme have been described in detail [6, 7] and need only be summarized here. The enzyme attacks substrates with N-terminal sequences, X-Pro-Y and X-Ala-Y to release dipeptides, X-Pro and X-Ala. Substrates of the latter type are hydrolysed at rates 3—5% of those of the former type. A free α-amino group is not obligatory: Z-Gly-Pro-Leu-Gly-Pro is also cleaved at the Pro-Leu bond. The active site contains a serine residue that is exquisitely sensitive to diisopropylphosphorofluoridate (Dip-F) and very insensitive to phenylmethanesulphonyl fluoride. The subunit molecular weight determined by SDS-gel electrophoresis of the enzyme released by autolysis is 130000 and its mobility hardly distinguishable from that of the [^{32}P] Dip-labelled band in SDS-gel electrophoresis of the microvillus membrane. This observation suggests that the intramembranous portion that remains associated with the membrane when the enzyme is released by autolysis is relatively small, probably less than 5000 daltons. Some further information about this fragment has been sought by comparing the autolysed form of the enzyme with that released by a non-ionic detergent.

The solubilization of the serine peptidase, together with other enzymes, may be efficiently accomplished by Triton X-100. The scheme of preparation is shown in Fig. 2 and the results of one such purification in Table 3. It is noteworthy that, once the proteins substantially purified, it is possible to omit detergent from the buffers. In contrast, omission of detergent at earlier stages encouraged aggregation of proteins and produced anomalous behaviour on ion-exchange columns. We have now compared the two forms of the enzyme in regard to catalytic and molecular properties.

The values for K_m and V_{max} for each of the two substrates, Gly-Pro-2-NNap and Ala-Ala-2-NNap, are shown in Table 4. In no case are the values significantly different for the two forms of the enzyme and we conclude that the "hydrophobic tail" has no effect on the catalytic site. The reaction of each form of the enzyme with Dip-F was also similar: the inhibition curves being superimposable. Sedimentation-velocity experiments are shown in Table 5. The uncorrected sedimentation coefficients are generally similar — in some comparisons the detergent form had a slightly lower coefficient and in one (in which the protein concentrations were carefully matched) the values were identical. Our view is that any expected increase

Fig. 2. Purification scheme for microvillus serine peptidase (detergent form). Triton-X100 was present in all buffers except where noted otherwise

Kidney cortex homogenized in 0.25 M sucrose
↓
Microsomal pellet
↓ Triton-X 100
Solubilized fraction
↓ *p*H 4.2
CM-Cellulose
↓ *p*H 7.9
DEAE-Cellulose
↓
Sepharose 6B
↓
DEAE-Cellulose (Triton omitted)

Table 3
Purification of microvillus serine peptidase (detergent form)

Fraction	Protein (mg)	Total units (μmol of Gly-Pro/min)	Recovery (%)	Specific activity (units/mg of protein)	Purification (fold)
Kidney cortex (900 g) homogenate	145000	3950	100	0.028	1
Microsomal fraction	20360	1468	37	0.072	2.57
Triton supernatant	8890	1150	29	0.129	4.6
CM-cellulose	558	772	20	1.38	49.2
DEAE-cellulose	157	506	13	3.21	114
Sepharose 6B	70.2	500	12.6	7.12	253
DEAE-cellulose	44.2	490	12.4	11.1	394

Table 4

Kinetic constants for detergent and autolysis-solubilized forms of microvillus serine peptidase (MSP-Det and MSP-Aut)

	Substrate			
	Gly-Pro-2-NNap		Ala-Ala-2-NNap	
	V_{max}	K_m	V_{max}	K_m
MSP-Det	52	493	2.88	1057
MSP-Aut	59	578	2.74	977

Values are means of 4 or 5 experiments (V_{max}: µmol/min/mg; K_m: µM)

Table 5

Sedimentation-velocity determinations (21 °C, 0.1 M Tris/HCl, *p*H 7.9) on the detergent and autolysis solubilized forms of microvillus serine peptidase

Run	MSP-Det		MSP-Aut	
	Protein (mg/ml)	*S*	Protein (mg/ml)	*S*
1	1.54	9.3 ±0.1	—	—
2	1.54	9.6 ±0.03	1.54	10.25±0.1
3	1.54	9.75±0.02	1.54	10.45±0.01
4	1.91	10.25±0.01	1.97	10.25±0.002

in molecular size of the detergent form, attributable to the additional length of the polypeptide chain, may well be countered by a buoyancy effect due to bound detergent. In SDS-gel electrophoresis the two forms show a consistent, but very slight difference in mobility. The difference was not sufficient to resolve the two forms when run together, but in parallel tracks, the detergent form exhibited a slightly lower mobility. Electron micrographs of the two forms showed that each form is a dimer, the subunits of both forms are about 7 nm in diameter.

Nevertheless, in spite of these general similarities in the two forms, some clear differences in molecular properties have now been demonstrated. Gel filtration by Sepharose 6B has shown that the detergent form has a smaller elution volume than the autolysis form (Table 6). In these experiments the two forms were run concurrently, the autolysis form being detected as the [^{32}P]Dip-enzyme and the detergent form as the active enzyme. In each of five runs the two forms were always partially resolved, a result that was independent of the presence of Triton-X 100 in the elution buffer. The probable difference in molecular size of the two forms is about 20000 daltons in some runs the difference seemed larger and in others smaller. The size of a Triton-X100 micelle is reported to be 5 nm in diameter and about 90000 mol. wt [22]. None of our results seems consistent with the detergent form being larger than the autolysis form by this amount and our present view is that the enzyme-associated detergent must be in a non-micellar form. Incubation of the two enzyme forms with papain abolished the difference in elution volume, the detergent form now behaved like the untreated autolysis form.

Table 6

Gel-filtration on Sepharose 6B of the detergent (MSP-Det) and autolysis (MSP-Aut) forms of microvillus serine peptidase.
Papain treated samples were incubated for 60 min at 37 °C with papain (0.1 mg/0.3 mg MSP-Det). The number of experiments is shown in parentheses.

Enzyme form	Elution buffer	
	5 mM Tris/HCl *p*H 7.9	5 mM Tris/HCl *p*H 7.9 0.15% Triton-X 100
MSP-Det	1.71 (2)	1.72 (3)
MSP-Aut	1.81 (2)	1.79 (3)
MSP-Det (Papain treated)	1.79 (1)	—
MSP-Aut (Papain treated)	1.79 (1)	—

End group determinations have revealed differences in the N-terminal amino acid residues of the two enzymes. The dansyl chloride method [23] has been applied to three preparations of the autolysis form, each with serine as the N-terminal amino acid, and to two preparations of the detergent form in which leucine was identified as the N-terminus. Incubation of each form with papain (two preparations of each) resulted in two end groups being identified in the detergent form (serine and leucine) and no change in end group in the autolysis form.
The simplest, though not necessarily the only interpretation of this result is that the intramembranous domain (the hydrophobic foot) is located at the N-terminal sequence of the protein. This is in line with the work of MAROUX's group in Marseille on the intestinal microvillus aminopeptidase M [24, 25]. The postulated structures of the two enzymes are compared in Fig. 3. The size of the intramem-

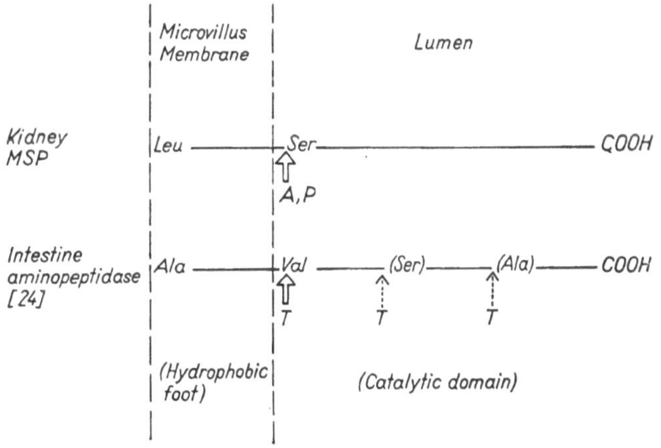

Fig. 3. Comparision of the postulated orientation of the kidney microvillus serine peptidase and intestine aminopeptidase M in the membrane
A, P: autolysis and papain-sensitive sites; T: trypsin-sensitive sites. The dashed arrows indicate that other sites in the catalytic portion of the aminopeptidase are sensitive to trypsin; these result in the artifactual "subunits" reported for the intestinal enzyme and the kidney enzyme prepared by toluene-trypsin extraction

brane portion of the serine peptidase is probably considerably less than 5000 daltons; that of the intestinal aminopeptidase is reported to be about 9000 daltons and to be rich in hydrophobic residues [24]. However the final confirmation of this postulated organization of these two microvillus enzymes will depend on establising that the sequence of the hydrophobic foot is identical to that of the N-terminal portion of the detergent form of each enzyme.

Molecular organization of the microvillus proteins

A feature of the microvillus surface, both in kidney and intestine, is that proteins project from the membrane and are visible as knobs in the electron microscope (see for example [26]). Most such proteins are 'intrinsic' in the sense that a portion, often minor and not including the catalytic site, is intimately associated with the lipid bilayer. This hydrophobic foot may serve simply as an anchor, or it may penetrate the membrane and have some additional function at the cytoplasmic or core face. The transmembrane domain of such a protein might be concerned with the maintenance of structure by interaction with core cross-bridges or might have a function in transport. We have attempted to identify kidney microvillus transmembrane proteins by radio-iodine labelling using the lactoperoxidase method [27]. The experimental approach is shown in Fig. 4. It depends on the accessibility of the interior space of the microvilli to the labelling reagents (glucose oxidase and lactoperoxidase) when brush borders are fragmented by homogenization. Subsequent incubation of the preparation permits fusion of the membrane, thus

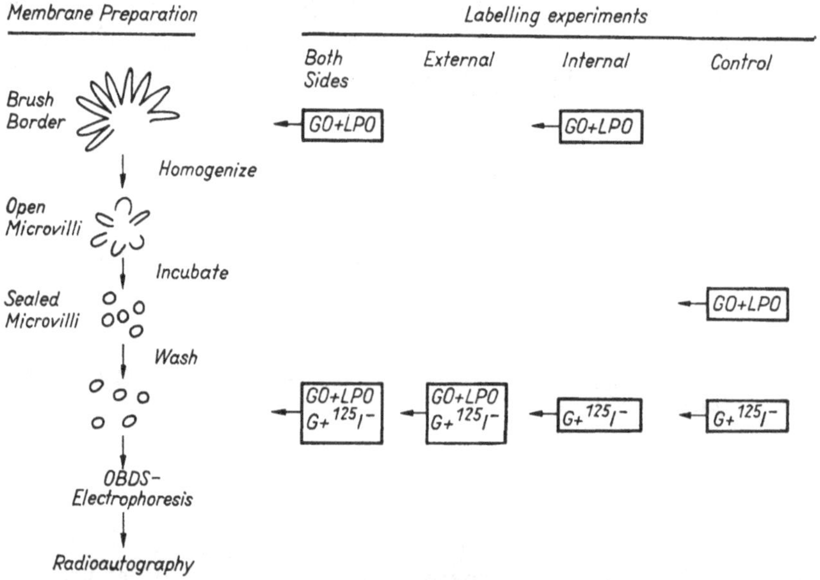

Fig. 4. Experimental design for ^{125}I-labelling of microvillus proteins at internal and external faces of the membrane.

GO, glucose oxidase; LPO, lactoperoxidase; G, glucose; OBDS, organic base dodecyl sulphate [28] producing sealed microvillus vesicles. When the washed vesicles are incubated with glucose and $Na^{125}I$, it is possible to preferentially label core proteins together with those proteins at the inner face of the membrane. External labelling is achieved by adding all the reagents (i. e. enzymes and substrates) after the vesicles are sealed. Both surfaces are labelled by a combination of the two treatments. A con-

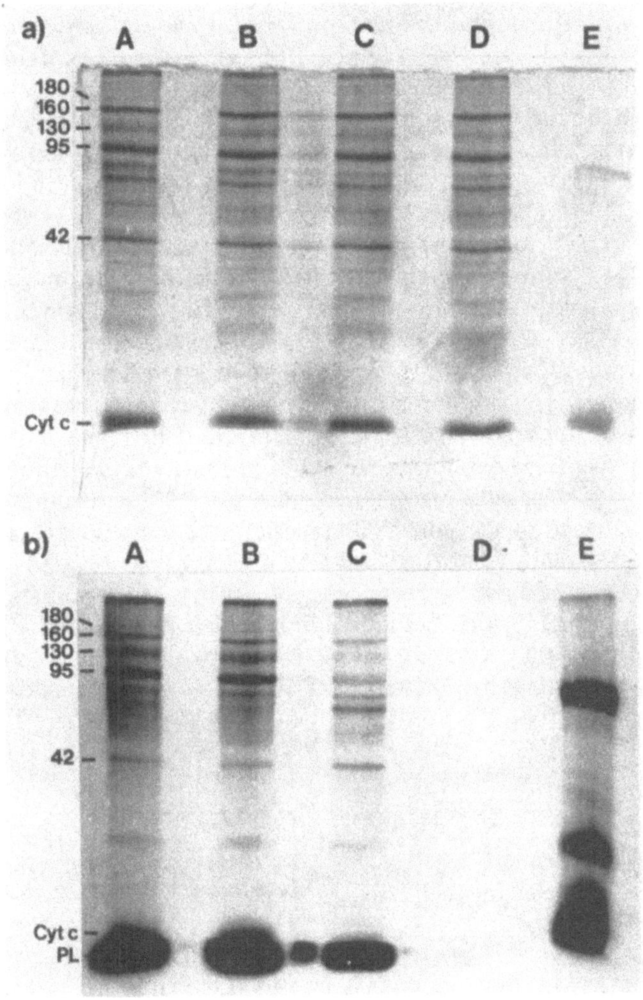

Fig. 5. Electrophoretic separation of radio-iodinated kidney microvillus proteins. See Fig. 4 for the design of the experiment. The proteins were separated by organic base dodecyl sulphate-polyacrylamide gel electrophoresis [28]; 50 μg protein was loaded in each track. Fig. 5a shows pattern after staining with Coomassie Brilliant Blue R250 and Fig. 5b is a radio-autograph of the same dried gel.

A, internal + external iodination; B, external iodination; C, internal iodination; D, microvillus control; E, control iodination, without microvilli. Cytochrome c (Cyt c) was added as an external marker protein to all samples (A–E) after the incubation designed to seal the microvillus vesicles. The radioactivity designated PL is attributed to labelled phospholipids trol, to demonstrate that washing removed any adsorbed glucose oxidase and lactoperoxidase, was also included in these experiments. The labelled vesicles were analysed by a new electrophoretic system that allows stacking of the proteins from samples containing high concentrations of salt [28]. The results are shown in Fig. 5. The pattern of stained polypeptide bands seen in this electrophoretic system is similar to that we have reported with a conventional SDS system [1] and the identities then established hold for the new system. The pattern of radioactive bands is complex and we will confine the interpretation to the major bands that can be confidently identified: bands 180 (glycovillin, an extrinsic protein), 160 (aminopeptidase M), 130 (serine peptidase) and 95 (neutral endopeptidase) are membrane proteins. Another band 95 of slightly lower mobility than neutral endopeptidase is attributed to α-actinin and band 42 is actin. Glycovillin is labelled only externally, but the three peptidases identified with bands 160, 130 and 95 are iodinated internally and externally. This supports the view that these enzymes are transmembrane proteins. α-Actinin is resolved from neutral endopeptidase: it is iodinated only by the internal label. Actin is strongly labelled internally, but some radioactivity is also detectable, albeit weakly, by the external labelling. Both are core proteins and predictably labelled by the internal reagents. However the anomalous external labelling of actin is unexpected. It is not due to leaky vesicles permitting access to external reagents, since some proteins, which are very clearly resolved by a two-dimensional electrophoretic system [28], are uniquely labelled by the internal reagents. The most likely explanation for the external actin labelling is that a small amount of actin is released during homogenization [25] and some of this actin is bound on the surface of the microvillus vesicles. Glycovillin, previously designated an extrinsic protein, is labelled only by the external reagents. These iodination experiments should not be regarded as definitive in establishing which proteins traverse the membrane. Some free iodine may be liberated and its diffusion across a membrane may produce spurious results. But the results so far obtained are consistent with information obtained by independent means for

Table 7
Principal proteins in kidney microvilli

Type and name	Band (=Mol.Wt. × 10^{-3})	Trans-membrane domain	Gly-cosylation	Papain release	Proportion of micro-villus protein (%)	Copies per micro-villus
Extrinsic membrane protein		0				
Glycovillin	180		+	+	?	?
Intrinsic membrane protein						
Aminopeptidase M	160	+	+	+	4.1	450
Serine peptidase	130	+	+	+	3.9	530
Neutral endopeptidase	95	+	+	0	4.1	760
Core proteins						
α-Actinin	95	0	0	0	~2.5	~470
Actin	42	0	0	0	9.0	3800

some of the proteins. These include the elegant experiments by LOUVARD et al. [25] in which a macromolecular photolabel was used to show that the aminopeptidase in intestinal microvilli is a transmembrane protein. Our view of the organization of the principal proteins of the microvilli [29] may now be extended to indicate the presence of a transmembrane domain in the three peptidases (Table 7). All three are glycoproteins, aminopeptidase M being the major glycoprotein in the membrane. Papain releases aminopeptidase M and serine peptidase, suggesting that the main part of each protein projects as a knob; but neutral endopeptidase is unaffected by such treatment indicating that it either lacks a susceptible bond, or more likely that it is more deeply embedded in the membrane.

Acknowledgement

We thank Mrs. JEAN INGRAM for expert technical assistance and the Medical Research Council for financial support.

References

[1] BOOTH, A. G., and A. J. KENNY: Biochem. J. **159**, 395 (1976)
[2] KENNY, A. J. in: Proteinases of Mammalian Cells and Tissues. A. J. BARRETT (ed.). North Holland, Amsterdam 1977 p. 393
[3] KERR, M. A., and A. J. KENNY: Biochem. J. **137**, 477 (1974)
[4] KERR, M. A., and A. J. KENNY: Biochem. J. **137**, 489 (1974)
[5] HOPSU-HAVU, V. K., and G. G. GLENNER: Histochemie **7**, 197 (1966)
[6] BARTH, A., H. SCHULZ, and K. NEUBERT: Acta biol. med. germ. **32**, 157 (1974)
[7] KENNY, A. J., A. G. BOOTH, S. G. GEORGE, J. INGRAM, D. KERSHAW, E. J. WOOD, and A. R. YOUNG: Biochem. J. **157** 169 (1976)
[8] HANSON, H., H. J. HÜTTER, H. G. MANNSFELDT, K. KRETSCHMER, and C. SOHR: Hoppe-Seyler's Z. physiol. Chem. **348**, 680 (1967)
[9] WACKER, H., P. LEHKY, E. H. FISCHER, and E. A. STEIN: Helv. chim. Acta **54**, 473 (1971)
[10] WACKER, H., P. LEHKY, F. VANDERHAEGHE, and E. A. STEIN: Biochim. biophys. Acta **429**, 546 (1976)
[11] GLENNER, G. G., and J. E. FOLK: Nature, Lond. **192**, 338 (1961)
[12] GLENNER, G. G., P. J. MCMILLAN, and J. E. FOLK: Nature, Lond. **194**, 867 (1962)
[13] SZEWCZUK, A., and T. BARANOWSKI: Biochem. Z. **338**, 317 (1963)
[14] TATE, S. S., and A. MEISTER: J. biol. Chem. **249**, 7593 (1974)
[15] TATE, S. S., and A. MEISTER: Proc. natn. Acad. Sci. U.S.A. **73**, 2599 (1976)
[16] ZELAZO, P., and M. ORLOWSKI: Eur. J. Biochem. **61**, 147 (1976)
[17] DEHM, P., and A. NORDWIG: Eur. J. Biochem. **17**, 364 (1970)
[18] DEHM, P., and A. NORDWIG: Eur. J. Biochem. **17**, 372 (1970)
[19] HÜTTER, H. J.: Personal communication
[20] NICHOLSON, J. A., and Y. S. KIM: Anal. Biochem. **63**, 110, (1975)
[21] BOOTH, A. G., and A. J. KENNY: Biochem. J. **142**, 575 (1974)
[22] YEDGAR, S., Y. BARENHOLZ, and V. G. COOPER: Biochim. biophys. Acta **363**, 98 (1974)
[23] GROS, C., and B. LABOUESSE: Eur. J. Biochem. **7**, 463 (1969)
[24] MAROUX, S., and D. LOUVARD: Biochim. biophys. Acta **419**, 189, (1976)
[25] LOUVARD, D., M. SEMERIVA, and S. MAROUX: J. molec. Biol. **106**, 1023 (1976)
[26] ROSTGAARD, J., and L. THUNEBERG: Z. Zellforsch. mikrosk. Anat. **132**, 473, (1972)
[27] HUBBARD, A. L., and Z. A. COHN: J. Cell Biol. **64**, 438 (1975)
[28] BOOTH, A. G.: Biochem. J. **163**, 165 (1977)
[29] KENNY, A. J., and A. G. BOOTH: Biochem. Soc. Trans. **4**, 1011 (1976)

Acta biol. med. germ., Band 36, Seite 1587—1604 (1977)

Bureau of Biological and Department of Physiology Rutgers University
New Brunswick, N. J. 08903, U.S.A.

Degradation of myofibrillar proteins by cathepsins B and D

J. W. C. Bird, W. N. Schwartz, and A. M. Spanier

Summary

Cathepsin B and cathepsin D were purified from rat liver and skeletal muscle. Electrophoretic analyses revealed that the enzymes were highly purified, and isoelectric focusing demonstrated multiple forms of both enzymes. Purified actin and myosin, as well as actin and myosin in myofilaments and myofibrils, were degraded by the purified cathepsins B and D. Degradation of myosin was completely blocked by the cathepsin B and D inhibitors, leupeptin and pepstatin, respectively. Cathepsins B and D were visualized by electron microscopy, using CBZ-Ala-Arg-Arg-4-methoxy-β-naphthylamine and BZ-Arg-Gly-Phe-Phe-Leu-4-methoxy-β-naphthylamine as substrates.

Introduction

Biochemical studies have established the existence of lysosomal proteinases in skeletal muscle [1, 2]. Morphological evidence suggests that in normal muscle the lysosomes exist primarily as part of the longitudinal sarcotubular system as well as golgi vesicles, and become clearly recognizable as distinct, sub-cellular particles during conditions of accelerated protein turnover [2—4].

It has long been known that myofibrillar proteins undergo a continual process of turnover, and that the degradation of these proteins is accelerated in physiological stress or pathological insult. There is no known single proteinase that can affect the total breakdown of any particular protein, let alone all proteins of cells. Thus it seems clear that a system of many different proteinases must participate in normal or accelerated protein turnover [5]. The only known intracellular system of proteinases are those found in the lysosomal apparatus.

There are two well known endopeptidases in cells with the potential of initiating the degradation of myofibrillar proteins. These are the lysosomal cathepsins B and D. At the previous meeting in Yugoslavia we reported that cathepsin B, when released from strong inhibition in the cytoplasm, was capable of limited degradation of purified myosin [6]. The experiments we would like to report today demonstrate that purified cathepsins B and D will degrade purified native or denatured myosin and actin, as well as the actin and myosin in preparations of myofilaments and myofibrils. We will also show that the enzymes can be visualized intracellularly by electron microscopy techniques.

Materials and methods

Cathepsins B and D were purified by the method of Barrett [7, 8] with modifications for use with rat liver and skeletal muscle [9, 10]. Cathepsin B activity during purification was monitored using BZ-DL-Arg-$NHC_{10}H_7$ as substrate, where one unit of activity released 1 µmole of 2-naphthylamide per min at 40 °C [11]. Cathepsin D activities were measured using denatured bovine hemoglobin as substrate, where one unit of activity released 1 µmole of tyrosine equivalents, soluble in trichloroacetic acid, per min at 40 °C [10]. Protein concentrations were determined using bovine serum albumin as standard [12], or by measurement of absorbance at 280 nm with the $A^{1\%}_{1\,cm}$ assumed to be equal to 10.0.

Myosin and actin were purified from rabbit and rat skeletal muscle [13, 14] and myofilaments and myofibrils were prepared from guinea pig gastrocnemius muscles [15]. Disc electrophoresis in polyacrylamide slab gels containing sodium dodecyl sulfate was performed in the buffer system of LAEMMLI and FAVRE [16]. Gels were electrophoretically fixed, stained with Coomassie Brilliant Blue R-250, and then destained in a Pharmacia GD-4 gel destainer with a Pharmacia DPS destainer power supply [10].

Tissue samples for electron microscopy, all from guinea pigs, were either a "total mitochondrial fraction" separated from gastrocnemius homogenates by differential centrifugation [17]; or, ultrathin sections from the medial head of the gastrocnemius. Tissues were fixed in 1.5% glutaraldehyde, containing 2% sucrose and 0.05 M cacodylate buffer at *p*H 6.8. Tissues were postfixed in 1% osmium tetroxide (0.05 M cacodylate buffer, *p*H 7.8), dehydrated in a series of ethanols followed by acetone, embedded in Epon, and sectioned by standard methods. The sections were stained with lead citrate and uranylacetate, and viewed on a Seimans Elmiskop-1 A electron microscope at 80 kV. Substrates for cytochemistry of cathepsins B and D were CBZ-Ala-Arg-Arg-4-methoxy-β-naphthylamine and BZ-Arg-Gly-Phe-Phe-Leu-4-methoxy-β-naphthylamine, respectively, using the technique of SMITH and VAN FRANK [18].

Results

Purification of enzymes and degradation of proteins

The results of the purification of cathepsin B and D, and their subsequent degradation of myosin and actin can be summarized as follows (see [9, 10, 17] for details):

(a) Cathepsin B and D were completely separated from each other during the chromatography step using Sephadex G-75 (superfine).

(b) The final purification step of cathepsin B was by gradient elution from a column of CM-cellulose, and the enzyme was optimally active against BZ-DL-Arg-$NHC_{10}H_7$ at about *p*H 6.0, and only in the presence of a reducing agent. The specific activity increased 13,300fold. The BZ-DL-Arg-$NH_{10}H_7$-hydrolyzing activities could be inhibited by typical inhibitors of thiol enzymes. The enzyme was also completely inhibited by leupeptin (10 μM), but not by pepstatin. Molecular weights, as determined by gel filtration, were within the range of 24,000—27,000; on slab gels in the presence of SDS a polypeptide molecular weight of 27,000 was obtained. Disc electrophoresis at *p*H 9 [20] yielded two closely migrating zones of protein; at *p*H 4.3 [21] there was one diffuse band of protein which corresponded to a zone of BZ-DL-Arg-$NHC_{10}H_7$-hydrolyzing activity. Gel isoelectric focusing of purified cathepsin B resolved 4 major bands of protein, each corresponding to a band of BZ-DL-Arg-$NHC_{10}H_7$-hydrolyzing activity. The isoelectric points of the enzyme forms were 6.9, 6.7, 6.2 and 5.3.

(c) The final purification step of cathepsin D was by preparative isoelectric focusing and three major peaks of cathepsin D activity were resolved, corresponding to isoelectric points of 5.7, 6.1 and 6.5. The latter peak (6.5) had a 5300fold increase in specific activity over the original homogenate. Purified cathepsin D demonstrated proteolytic activity against hemoglobin with an optimum *p*H of 3.5. Molecular weights, as determined by gel filtration were withing the range of 42,000—45,000 for the 3 major isoenzymes; on slab gels in the presence of SDS a polypeptide molecular weight of 41,000 was obtained. Disc gel electrophoresis at *p*H 9 or *p*H 4.3 yielded one protein band with cathepsin activity.

(d) The degradation of purified myofibrillar proteins by purified lysosomal proteases was clearly demonstrated with the application of SDS-PAG electrophoresis. Following incubation with enzyme, the polypeptide band representing the substrate decrease in intensity and lower molecular weight products appeared.

(e) Cathepsins B and D, purified from either rat liver or skeletal muscle, were shown to degrade myosin, purified from rabbit or rat muscle. Soluble denatured myosin was degraded more extensively than insoluble native myosin. Degradation by cathepsin B was inhibited by lack of reducing agent, myoglobin, iodoacetic acid, and leupeptin, but not by pepstatin. The same potential modifiers were applied to cathepsin D, and only pepstatin produced inhibition.

(f) Rat liver cathepsin B had a *p*H optimum of 5.2 on native myosin. The *p*H optimum of cathepsin D was 4.0 on myosin.

(g) Purified rat muscle cathepsin B had greater myosin degradative activity, on the basis of its naphthylamidase activity, than did a corresponding preparation from liver. The difference appeared to be quantitative rather than qualitative.

(h) Cathepsin D purified from muscle and the three major cathepsin D isoenzymes from rat liver had the same activities on native rabbit myosin.

(i) Rat liver cathepsins B and D were demonstrated to degrade rabbit F-actin at *p*H 5.0, and were inhibited by leupeptin and pepstatin, respectively.

(j) The degradation of myosin and actin by cathepsin D was more extensive than that by cathepsin B.

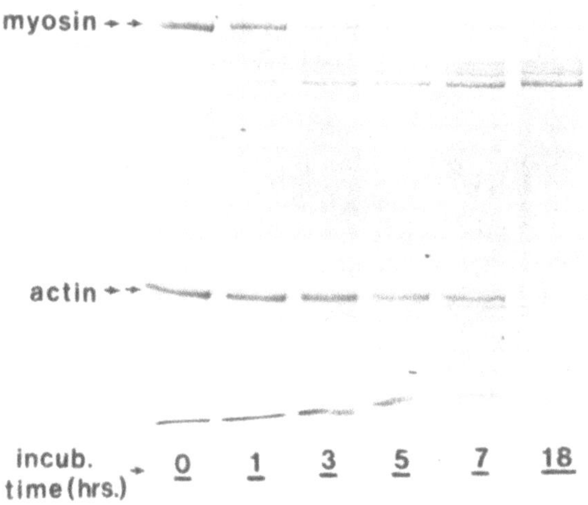

Fig. 1. Degradation of myofilaments by a lysosome-rich fraction (TMF) as a function of time. The final concentration of the myofilament (Mf) preparation in the reaction mixture was 0.325 mg protein/ml. Treatment with TMF (0.186 mg protein/ml) was carried out at 37 °C in 50 mM sodium acetate buffer, *p*H 5.0, containing 1.0 mM Na_2 EDTA and 1.0 mM DTT. Assays were terminated at appropriate time intervals by treatment with an equal volume of solubilization solution. Samples of 100 µl (16.25 µg of substrate protein) were subjected to SDS-PAGE in a 7.5% gel stained with Coomassie Brilliant Blue R-250

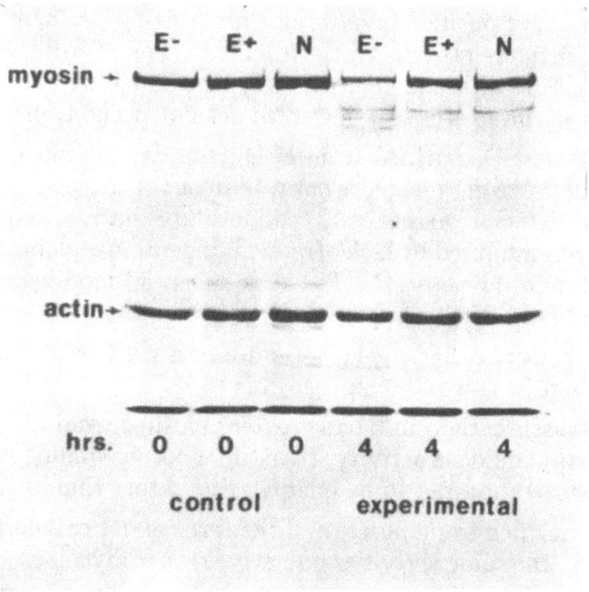

Fig. 2. Myofilament degradation by lysosome-rich fractions from 15 day vitamin E-deficient, (E−); vitamin E-supplemented, (E+); and normal, (N) guinea pig gastrocnemius muscle. Assay conditions were the same as those described for Fig. 1 with the following exceptions: (1), only one time interval was chosen (4 hrs); (2), the substrate's final concentration was 0.281 mg protein/ml; and (3), the TMF was prepared from 3 cources (E−, E+, and N), and applied separately to the substrate at a final concentration of 0.200 mg protein/ml. 100 μl samples, equivalent to 14.05 μg of substrate protein, were applied to the 7.5% gel. Solubilization, SDS-PAGE, and staining were identical to that described in Fig. 1.

We then tested our experimental procedure further by measuring myosin and actin degradation in an experimental muscular dystrophy induced in guinea pigs by feeding them vitamin E-deficient diets (E—) for 15 to 21 days [17, 23]. Controls were animals fed a normal diet (N) or a vitamin E-deficient diet supplemented with dl-alpha-tocopherol (E+). Myofilaments and myofibrils, from normal animals, isolated and purified by the method of Etlinger et al. [15], were solubilized by addition of an equal volume of solubilization media [1] followed by incubation in a boiling water bath for 5 min. The preparations were then incubated with lysosome-rich fractions isolated from skeletal muscles of the (N), (E+) and (E—) animals by differential centrifugation [17].

First, let us consider the degradation of actin and myosin in myofilament preparations at *p*H 5.0 as a function of time. Lysosomal extract was prepared from the medial head of the gastrocnemius muscle and served as enzyme source. There was apparent degradation of myosin, with the concomitant appearance of lower molecular weight end-products, after one hour of incubation at 37 °C (Fig. 1). Actin was visually degraded after 3 hrs of incubation, and there was extensive degradation of both actin and myosin for the remaining incubation times. No degradation of myosin or actin was observed in a control gel containing only the incubated myofilaments.

Myofilaments were then incubated with lysosomal extract from the gastrocnemii of the three dietary groups of animals (N; E+; E—) (Fig. 2). In that the amount of enzyme protein in each reaction mixture was the same, the increased degradation of protein in the (E—) preparation represents the increased specific activity of the enzymes involved. Fig. 3 represents a densitometric scan of the gels, and shows

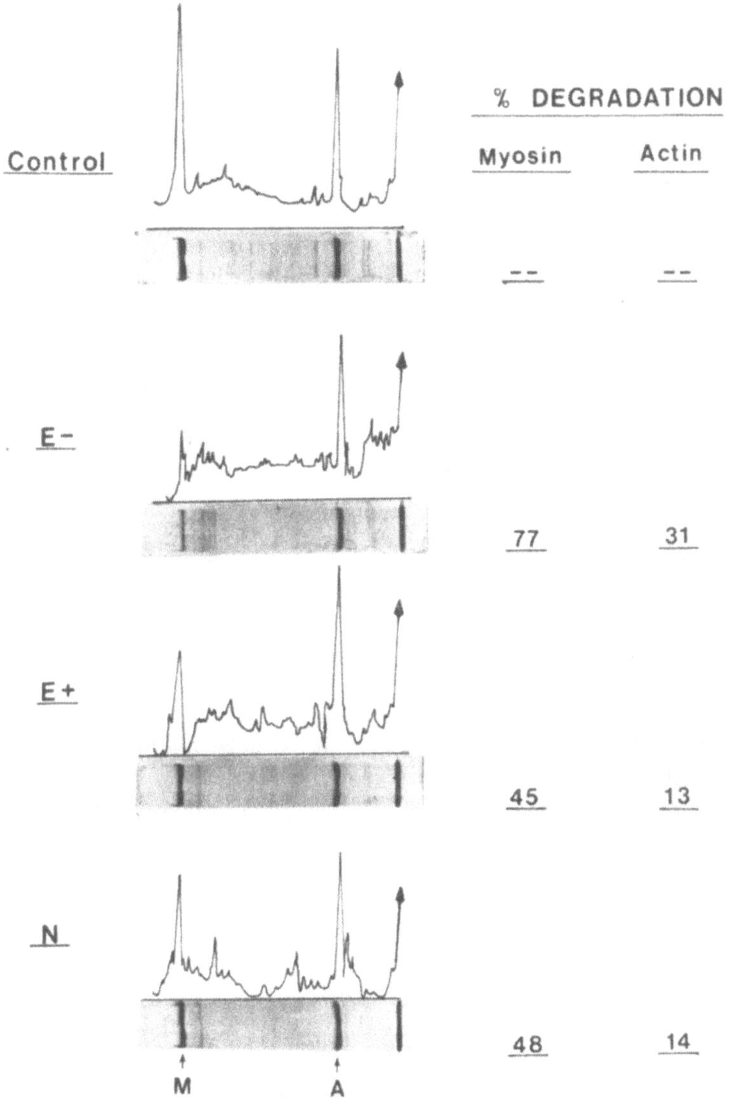

Fig. 3. Densitometric tracing and quantification of myofilament degradation by lysosome-rich fractions.
Densitometric tracings were made of the gels in Fig. 2 on a Canalco D scanning densitometer gel scanner which was coupled with a Canalco 8G recorder. The wavelength was set at 530 nm using a green Wratten # 55 filter.

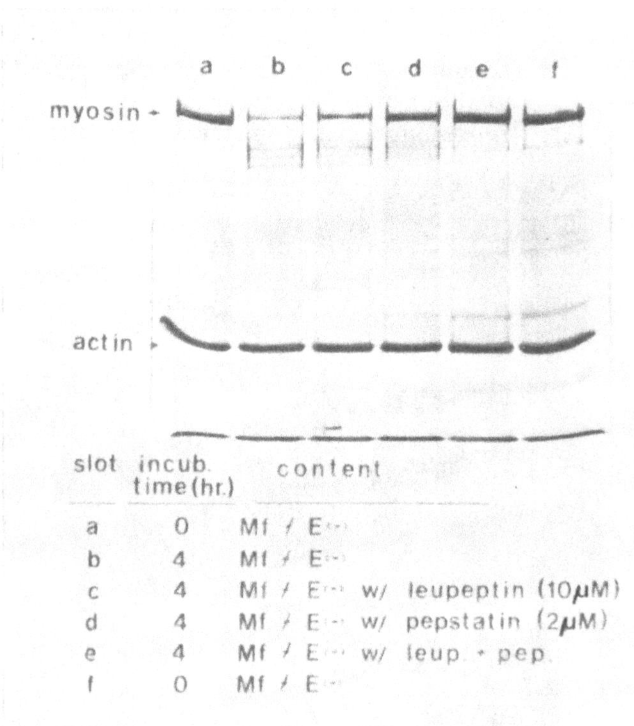

Fig. 4. Effect of two potential modifiers of enzyme activity on the degradation of myofilaments.

Assay conditions were exactly as described for Fig. 2, except that only the TMF of the E-animals were used, and potential modifiers of enzyme activity were also present.

that there is a significantly greater decrease in actin and myosin in the (E—) group, as compared to the (N) and (E+) groups, with no significant differences between the degradation in the (E+) and (N) groups [19].

In that the lysosomal extract is a mixture of many lysosomal enzymes and possible contaminent proteases, we tested the effects of leupeptin and pepstatin in our system, as these are known specific inhibitors of cathepsin B and cathepsin D, respectively [24, 25] (Fig. 4). The addition of leupeptin (10 μM) and pepstatin (2 μM) individually to the reaction mixtures both partially inhibited the breakdown of protein (principally myosin), pepstatin more than leupeptin; and, both of the inhibitors in the same reaction mixture appeared to completely inhibit the degradation of myosin. Therefore, the conditions of this experiment suggest that cathepsin B and cathepsin D are the only endopeptidases involved.

When the substrate is increased an order of magnitude in structure, i. e. using a myofibrillar preparation, there is also degradation of the myosin and actin. As a function of *p*H, the degradation of the polypeptide band patterns was most extensive at *p*H 5, and continued as high as *p*H 7 (Fig. 5). The polypeptide band pattern at *p*H 7.0 resembled that seen when purified myosin was incubated with purified cathepsin B. Control reactions, without the addition of a lysosomal

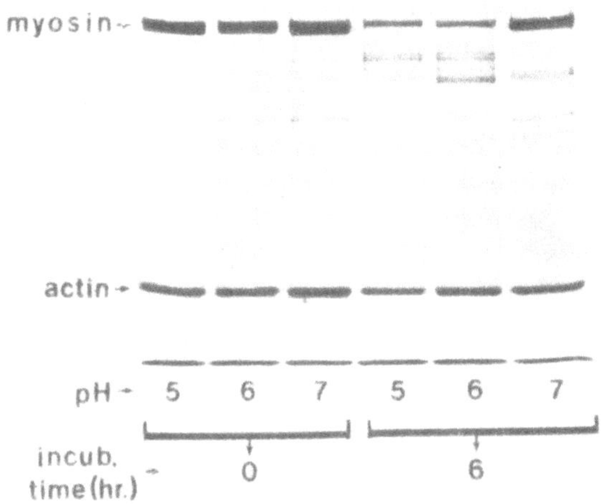

Fig. 5. Degradation of myofibrils (MF) by a lysosome-rich fraction as a function of *p*H. The final concentration of myofibrils (MF), (prepared as described in the text) in the reaction mixture was 0.358 mg protein/ml. Treatment with TMF (0.221 mg protein/ml prepared by pooling 15 and 21 day E−, E+, and N gastrocnemius TMF) was carried out at 37 °C for 6 hrs in 50 mM sodium acetate buffer, *p*H 5.0, 6.0 or 7.0, containing 1.0 mM Na_2 EDTA and 1.0 mM DTT. 125 μl samples, equivalent to 17.9 μg of substrate protein, were applied to the 7.5% gel. Solubilization, SDS-PAGE, and staining were identical to that described in Fig. 1.

extract and incubated for 6 hrs, did not indicate degradation of the polypeptides, suggesting that the degradation at *p*H 7.0 was not due to a contaminant enzyme in the myofibrillar preparation.

Cytochemical visualization of cathepsins B and D

SMITH and VAN FRANK [18] have recently published detailed methods for the ultrastructural localization of some known proteolytic enzymes, including cathepsins B and D. The enzymes are identified in their subcellular sites of proteolytic activity by deposition of an insoluble azo-dye metal chelate. The enzymes cathepsin B and D hydrolyze amino acid derivatives of 4-methoxy-β-naphthylamine, i. e. CBZ-Ala-Arg-Arg-4-methoxy-β-naphthylamine and BZ-Arg-Gly-Phe-Phe-Leu-4-methoxy-β-naphthylamine, respectively. The released 4-methoxy-β-naphthylamine is coupled with hexazotized pararosaniline (3:1) resulting in a dye product with a high degree of osmiophilia, with no appreciable diffusion of dye product before metal chelation. By using pararosaniline, as long as reducing conditions are maintained, osmium is linked directly to the dye via the amino and azo groups. The result is an electron dense product which can be visualized by electron microscopy.

For those of us interested in intracellular mechanisms of protein turnover, we now have a technique with which we may visualize the intracellular proteases during compartmentalization and intracellular transport.

Fig. 6 represents a low magnification of the lysosome-rich "total mitochondrial fraction", isolated by differential centrifugation [17] from homogenates of the medial head of guinea pig gastrocnemius muscles. In addition to the large numbers of mitochondria, which one would expect to find in this fraction, there are numerous lysosomes with the dense reaction product from the action of cathepsin B.

A high magnification of a lysosome from a "total mitochondrial fraction" (Fig. 7) demonstrates that the reaction product to cathepsin B activity is usually found concentrated at the periphery of the organelle. Note that there is also reaction product on the mitochondria, but in a random type of distribution. The reaction product on the mitochondria in this image is more than is usually seen, but we show it to emphasize the necessity of doing good baseline controls for reaction product.

A type of experimental muscular dystrophy can be induced in young guinea pigs by placing them in a vitamin E-deficient diet for 15 days or more [22, 23].

Fig. 8 demonstrates a typical section of gastrocnemius muscle from one of these animals, reacted for cathepsin B. Again, the reaction product for cathepsin B activity is localized mainly on the periphery of the lysosomes and on associated membranes. Fig. 9 is a higher magnification, showing intense reaction product on the lysosome as well as on a profile of sarcoplasmic reticulum.

For reasons that are still not clear to us, we have had better success with the cytochemical localization of cathepsin D. Controls rarely show artifactual reaction product, and experimental sections indicate reaction product only on lysosomes and profiles resembling sarcoplasmic reticulum.

Fig. 10 demonstrates two types of lysosomes reacting for cathepsin D. One type is found in the perinuclear region in the vicinity of golgi stacks, with very intense reaction product, and the other type is found in the interior of the myofibril. A high magnification of a lysosome in the interior of the cell demonstrates a fairly common image, and the reaction product on the periphery appears to have a laminar arrangement (Fig. 11).

To keep the morphologists happy, and of course to strengthen our argument, we would also like to examine these samples in cross-section. Fig. 12 demonstrates a cross-section cut through the A-band of a muscle fiber. Several mitochondria are present, as well as a lysosome with intense reaction product for cathepsin D. On higher magnification in Fig. 13 the reaction product appears to be concentrated on the periphery of the lysosome, as well as on associated membranous structures. We believe the associated structures are elements of the sarcoplasmic reticulum.

The in vitro degradation of purified myosin and actin, as well as the actin and myosin contained in myofilaments and myofibrils, was clearly demonstrated in these experiments with SDS polyacrylamide gel electrophoresis. This type of analysis permitted detection of proteolysis regardless of the sizes of the hydrolysis products.

Discussion

SCHWARTZ and BIRD have made calculations on the in vivo significance of the concentrations of cathepsins B and D in skeletal muscle [10, 19]. At *p*H 5.0, cathepsins B and D could degrade all of the myosin, in the native state, in 6—9 days.

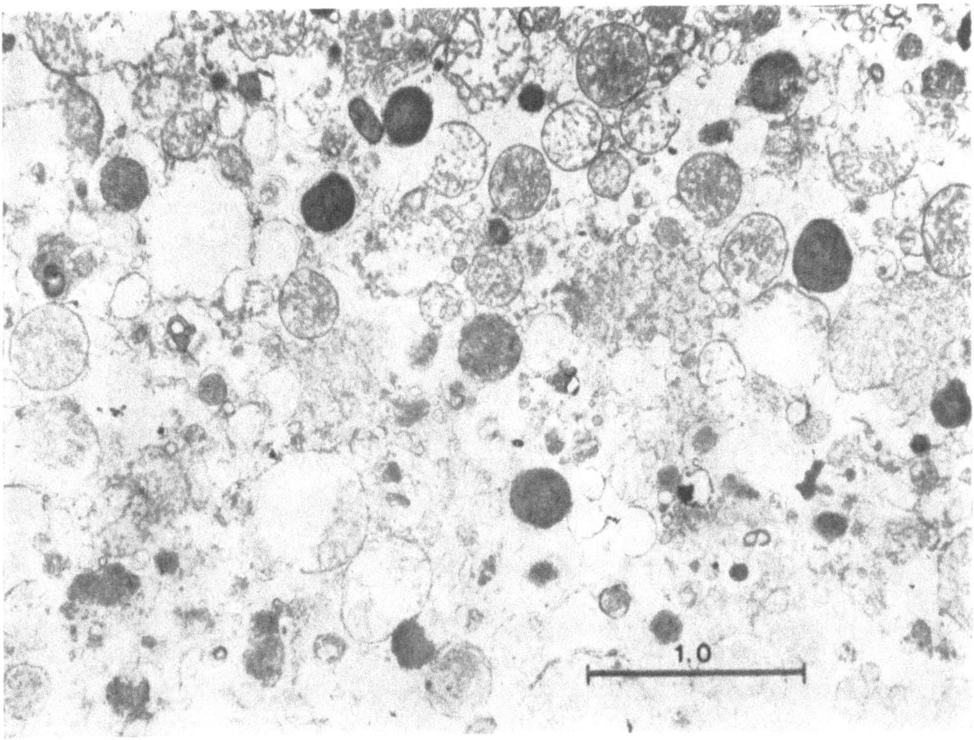

Fig. 6. Lysosome-rich "total mitochondrial fraction", isolated by differential centrifugation from homogenates of the media head of guinea pig gastrocnemius muscles. Dense reaction product from cathepsin B activity. Stained with uranyl acetate and lead citrate.

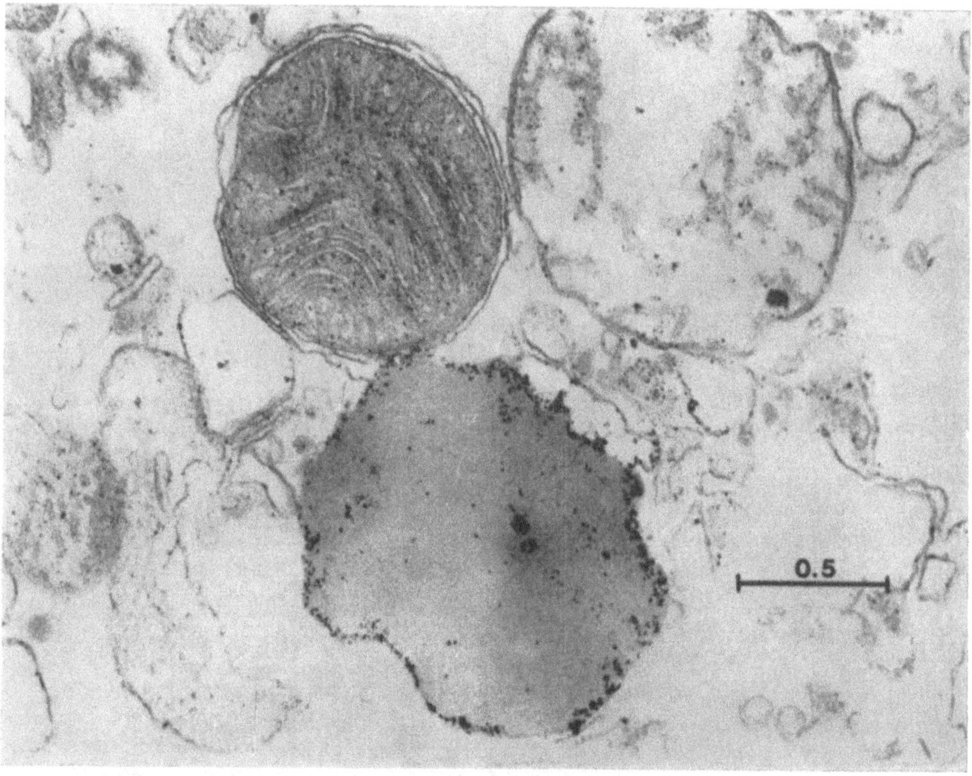

Fig. 7. High magnification of TMF, prepared as described in Fig. 6. Reaction product from cathepsin B activity is seen on periphery of lysosome. Stained as in Fig. 6.

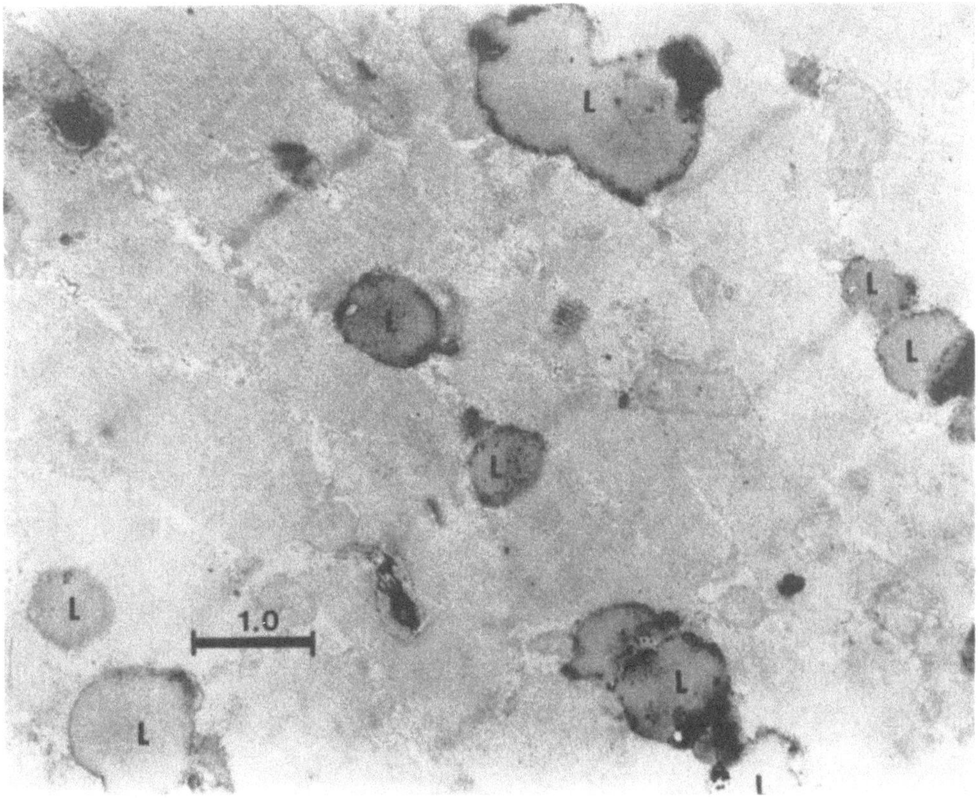

Fig. 8. Ultra-thin section from medial head of vitamin E-deficient gastrocnemius muscle. The numerous lysosomes (L) contain reaction product from cathepsin B activity. Stained as in Fig. 6.

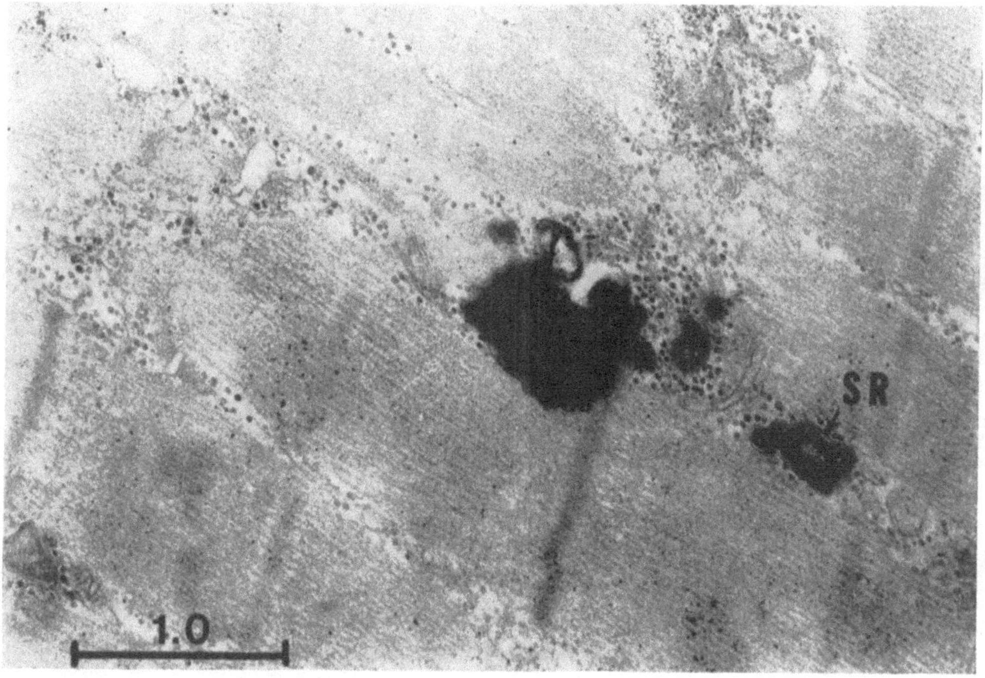

Fig. 9. High magnification showing intense reaction product from cathepsin B activity in a lysosome (L) and profile of sarcoplasmic reticulum (SR). Stained as in Fig. 6.

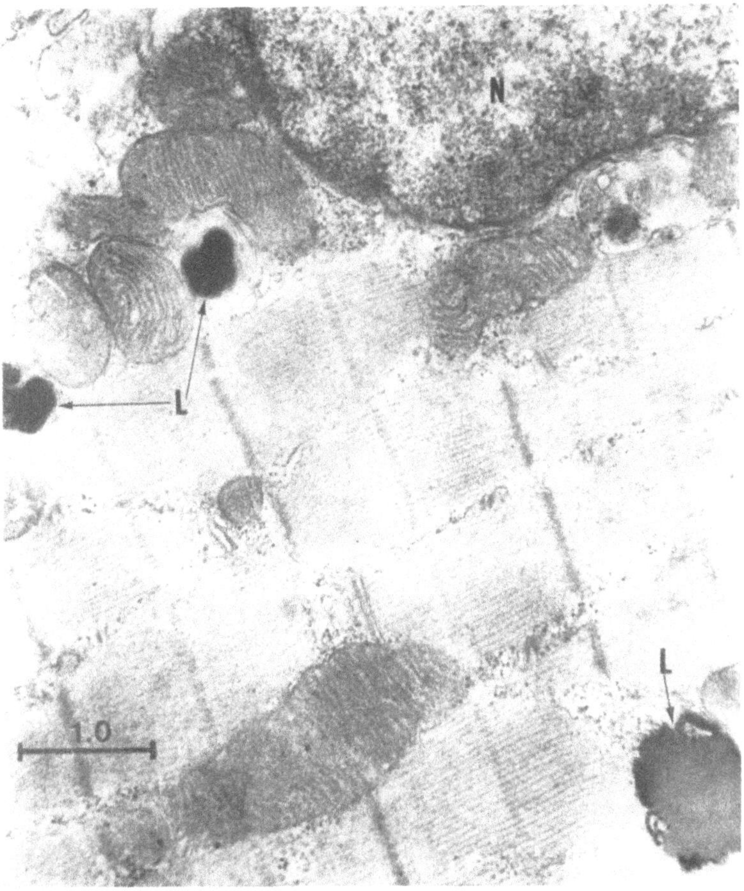

Fig. 10. Two "types" of lysosomes found in skeletal muscle. Note intense reaction product in lysosomes (L) in perinuclear region (in close approximation to golgi stacks); and the lysosome in the myofibrillar interior. Reaction product represents cathepsin D activity. Stained as in Fig. 6.

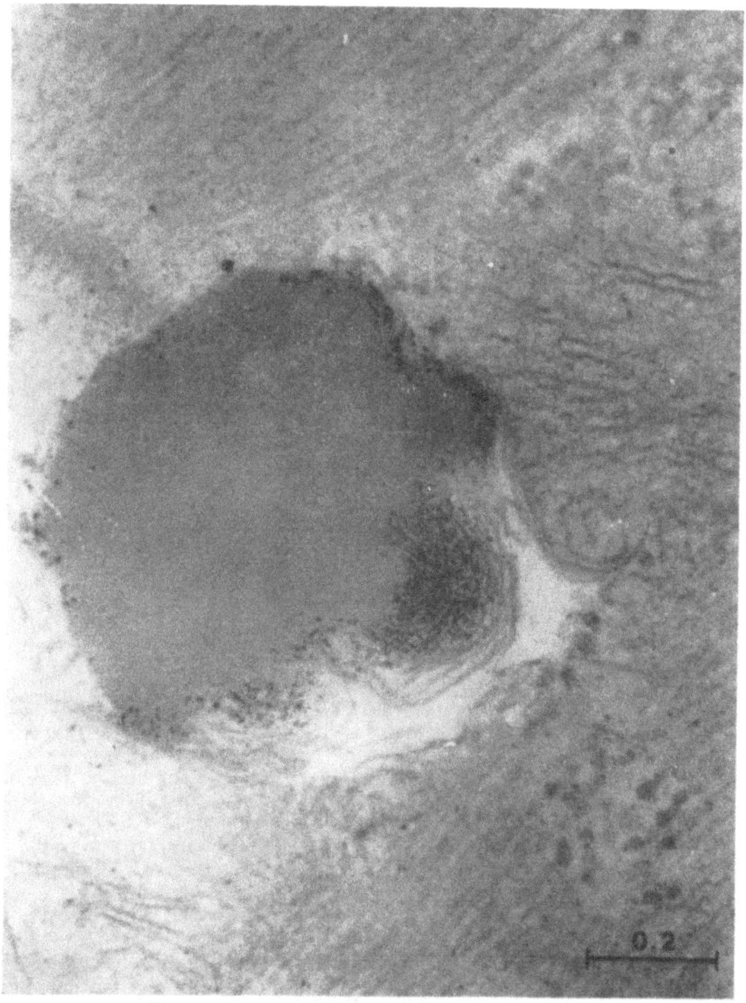

Fig. 11. A high magnification of a lysosome in muscle cell, reacted for cathepsin D. Reaction product on periphery of lysosome appears to have laminar arrangement. Stained as in Fig. 6.

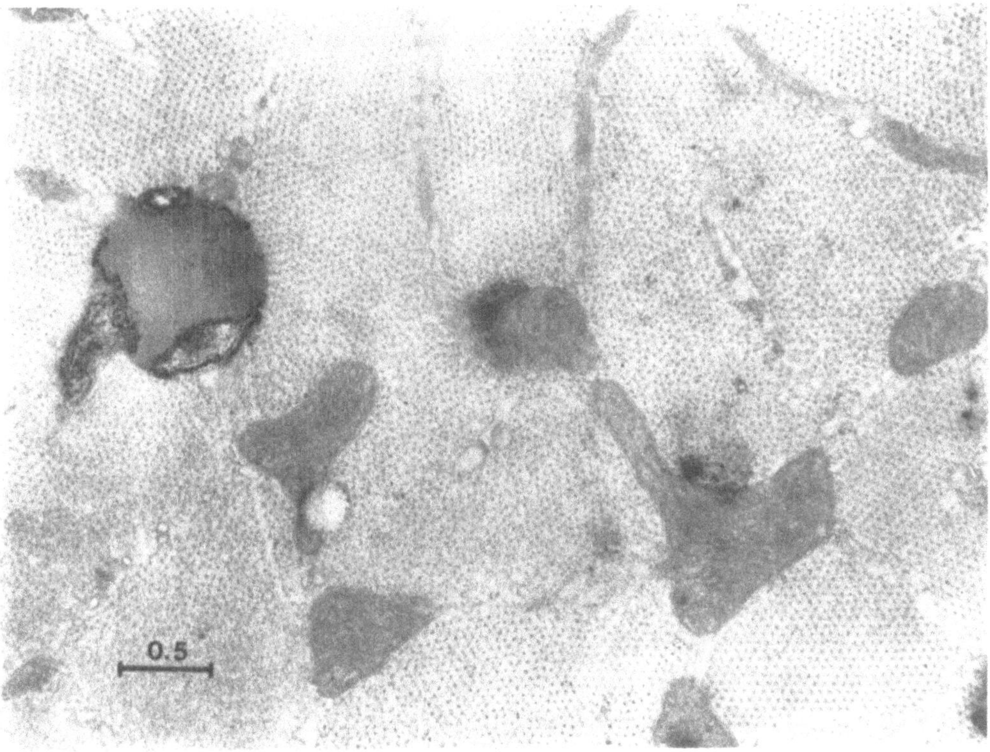

Fig. 12. Low magnification of cross-section of gastrocnemius, cut through A-band. Reaction product represents cathepsin D activity. Stained as in Fig. 6.

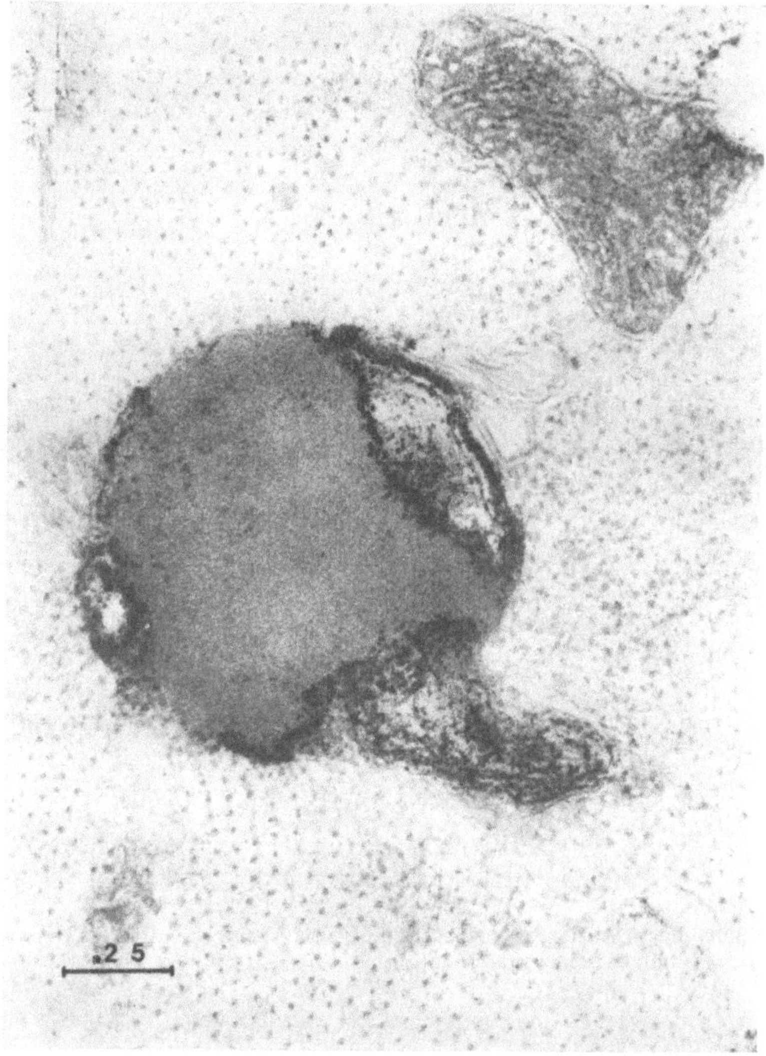

Fig. 13. High magnification of lysosome in Plate 7. Reaction product from cathepsin D activity is concentrated on periphery of lysosome, as well as on associated membranous structures. Stained as in Fig. 6.

When one considers the possible enhancement of degradation by denaturation and the additional contribution of the lysosomal exopeptidase, the physiological significance of these enzymes in protein turnover becomes quite apparent. There is presently no agreement on the half-lives of actin and myosin. However, MILLWARD and GARLICK [26] have estimated the half-life of actomyosin to be 26 days in quadriceps muscle.

The visualization of cathpesins B and D in muscle cells by electron microscopy adds another dimension to our understanding of protein catabolism. We are now able to observe the intracellular compartmentalization and transport of these enzymes.

Acknowledgements

The authors wish to thank Dr. RICHARD TRIEMER for his valuable contributions to the electron microscopy studies, Ms. LAURA WOOD for her superb technical assistance, the Charles and Johanna Busch Memorial Fund, Muscular Dystrophy Association, National Institutes of Health (NS-07180), and the Rutgers University Research Council and Biomedical Research Support Grant for partial support of these studies.

References

[1] CANONICO, P. G., and J. W. C. BIRD: J. Cell Biol. **45**, 321 (1970)
[2] BIRD, J. W. C.: Skeletal Muscle Lysosomes. In: Lysosomes in Biology and Pathology. Vol. **4**., pp. 75–109. J. TINGLE, and R. T. DEAN (Eds.). American Elsevier Pub. Co., New York, 1975
[3] PEARCE, G. W.: Ann. N.Y. Acad Sci. **138**, 138 (1966)
[4] HOFFSTEIN, S., D. E. GENNARO, G. WEISSMAN, J. HIRSCH, F. STREULI, and A. C. FOX: Am. J. Path. **79**, 193 (1975)
[5] POOLE, B., and C. DEDUVE in: Intracellular Protein Catabolism. H. HANSON and P. BOHLEY (Eds.). Wissenschaftliche Beiträge der Martin-Luther-Universität Halle-Wittenberg **1974**/6, pp. 13–30
[6] BIRD, J. W. C., and W. N. SCHWARTZ in: Intracellular Protein Catabolism. II. V. TURK and N. MARKS (Eds.). Plenum Press, New York, London 1977, pp. 167–182
[7] BARRETT, A. J.: Biochem. J. **131**, 809 (1973)
[8] BARRETT, A. J.: Biochem. J. **117**, 601 (1970)
[9] SCHWARTZ, W. N., and J. W. C. BIRD: Biochem. J. **167**, 811 (1977)
[10] SCHWARTZ, W. N.: Cathepsins B and D; Purification and Degradation of Myofibrillar Proteins. Ph. D. Dissertation, Rutgers University, New Brunswick, New Jersey 1977
[11] BARRETT, A. J.: Anal. Biochem. **47**, 280 (1972)
[12] LOWRY, O. H., N. J. ROSEBROUGH, A. L. FARR, and R. J. RANDALL: J. biol. Chem. **193**, 265 (1951)
[13] OFFER, G., C. MOOS, and R. STARR: J. molec. Biol. **74**, 653 (1973)
[14] SARAYDARIAN, K., E. J. BRISKEY, and W. F. H. M. MOMMAERTS: Biochim. biophys. Acta. **133**, 399 (1967)
[15] ETLINGER, J. D., R. ZAK, and D. A. FISCHMANN: J. Cell Biol. **68**, 123 (1976)
[16] LAEMMLI, U. K., and M. FAVRE: J. molec. Biol. **80**, 575 (1973)
[17] SPANIER, A. M.: Studies of the Lysosomal Apparatus in Progressive Muscle Degeneration Induced by Vitamin E-deficiency. Ph. D. Dissertation, Rutgers University, New Brunswick, New Jersey 1977
[18] SMITH, R. E., and R. M. VAN FRANK in: Lysosomes in Biology and Pathology. Vol. **4**, pp. 193–249. J. T. DINGLE and R. T. DEAN (Eds). American Elsevier Pub. Co., New York 1975
[19] SPANIER, A. M., J. W. C. BIRD, and R. E. TRIEMER: Fedn Proc. Fedn. Am. Socs exp. Biol. **36**, 1497 (1977)
[20] REISFIELD, R. A., V. J. LEWIS, and D. E. WILLIAMS: Nature, Lond. **195**, 281 (1962)

[21] DAVIS, B. J.: Ann. N.Y. Acad. Sci. **121**, 404 (1964)
[22] BENDER, A. D., D. D. SCHOTTELIUS, and B. A. SCHOTTELIUS: Proc. Soc. exp. Biol. Med. **102**, 362 (1959)
[23] BOND, J., and J. W. C. BIRD: Proc. Soc. exp. Biol. Med. **146**, 608 (1974)
[24] WINGENDER, W. in: Bayer-Symposium V. "Proteinase Inhibitors" Springer, Berlin 1974, pp. 548–559
[25] BARRETT, A. J. in: Proteases and Biological Control. E. REICH, D. B. RIFKIN, and E. SHAW (Eds.). Cold Spring Harbor Laboratory, Cold Spring Harbor, Long Island, New York 1975, pp. 467–482
[26] MILLWARD, D. J., and P. J. GARLICK in: Intracellular Protein Catabolism. H. HANSON, and P. BOHLEY (Eds.). Wissenschaftliche Beiträge der Martin-Luther-Universität Halle-Wittenberg 1974/6, pp. 158–164

Acta biol. med. germ., Band 36, Seite 1605—1619 (1977)

Institut of Biochemistry, University of Medical Sciences Szeged, Hungary

Degradation of myones as a consequence of disuse and denervation

F. Guba, Magda G. Mészáros, and Ö. Takács

Summary

After denervation or immobilization in both slow an fast muscles of rabbits a rapid decrease in weight and protein content and a focal degeneration of cell ultrastructure were observed. As a consequence marked changes in the ratio of soluble to myofibrillar protein and in regulatory proteins of myofibrillar system occurred.

Introduction

The close correlation between the function of the various organs and their morphological and biochemical structure have long been known in biology. The consequences of use and disuse are particularly striking in the skeletal muscles, in which systematic and enhanced functioning leads to a relatively rapid, well-visible and measurable mass increase and metabolic modification [1, 2]. In contrast, the disuse of muscle of pathological or experimental origin results in marked atrophy of the musculature, and appreciable changes in the chemical constituents [3].
Inactivation of muscles can be brought about in various ways under experimental conditions. It may be achieved, for example, by transsection of the medulla [4] by tenotomy [5], and by different forms of immobilization, with a plaster cast, and with articular fixation [6].
In the experimental series reported in the present paper, biochemical and morphological methods were used to study the tonic and tetanic muscles in rabbit hind limbs immobilized with a plaster cast or denervated, it was hoped to acquire new data on the pathogenesis of the disuse and neurogenic atrophy of skeletal muscles.

Material and methods

4-month-old New Zealand rabbits of both sexes, originating from one strain, and each weighing about 3 kg were used. The right hind leg was immobilized in full extension with a plaster cast. The animals were decapitated and bled to death on the 5th, 10th, 14th, 28th day following immobilization; in a few cases they were killed on the 7th day, rather than on the 5th or 10th day. Two functionally different muscles, the tetanic m. gastrocnemius and the tonic m. soleus, were then isolated and excised. They were weighed, and compared with the corresponding muscle from the contralateral nonimmobilized limb of the same animal as control. The muscle in atrophia was also compared with that of a non-immobilized, intact animal. In an another experimental series the motor nerve of the hind limb was exposed and excised between two ligatures. The processing of muscles was identical with previous experiments.
For electron microscopic processing samples with an average weight of 30 mg, fastened out to their normal length, were prepared from the central parts of the muscles in question. They were next double-fixed in glutaraldehyde-osmium tetroxide and embedded in Durcupan. Semithin and ultrathin sections were cut with an LKB ultramicrotome.
To increase the contrast of the electron microscopic images, both a uranyl acetate (in 70% alcohol) and a final uranyl acetate — lead citrate double-staining were performed.
A JEOL 100-B type microscope was used in this work.

We developed a method for quantitative separation and analysis of the protein compartments of the muscle tissue and muscle cells. The results for the intact animals are in good agreement with the relevant literature data, which were generally obtained by selective extraction methods.

The myofibrillar fraction obtained by the procedure described was further resolved by fractionation using SDS-polyacrylamide gel electrophoresis [7]. Staining was performed by 0.025% Coomassie brilliant blue. 50 or 100 μg of protein were run from each sample, and a Kipp and Zonen densitometer was employed for evaluation.

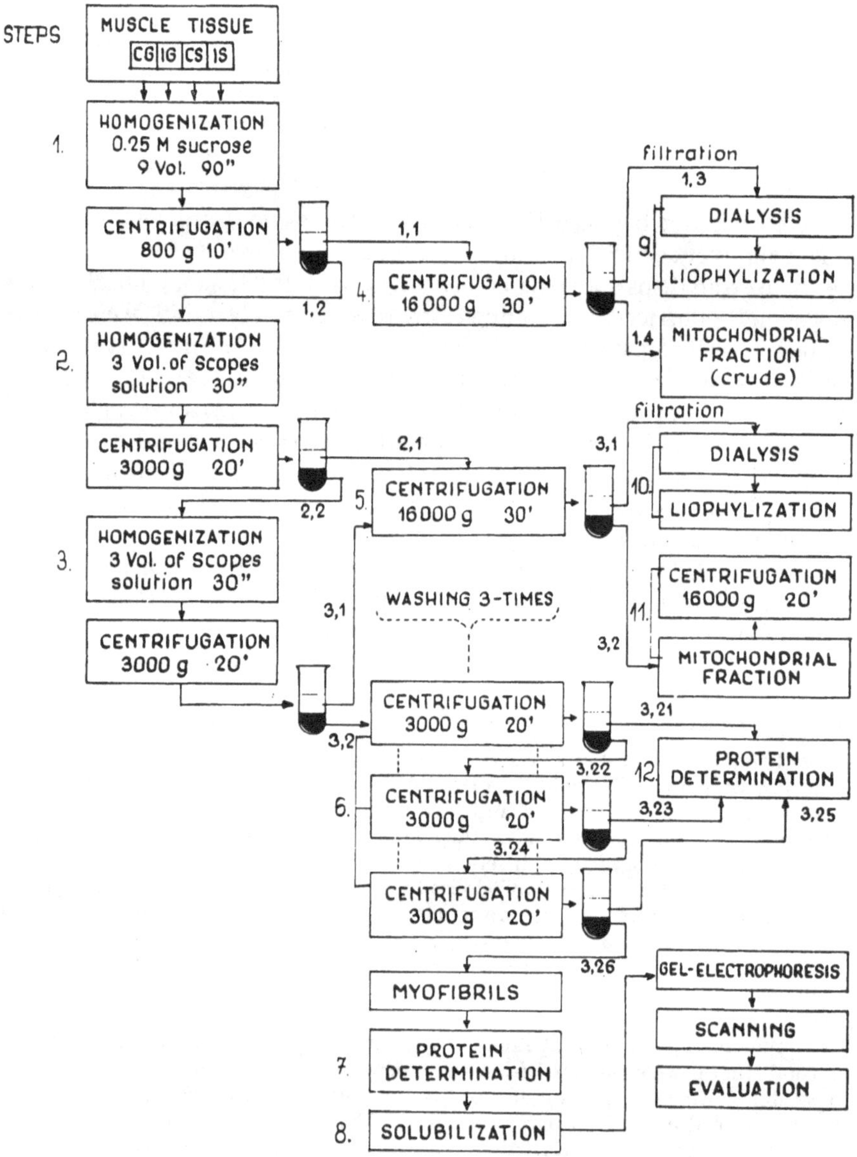

Fig. 1. Scheme for separation of protein compartments of muscle tissue and muscle cells

Results

In Fig. 2a and 2b one can see cross-sectional and longitudinal pictures of the normal m. soleus at the same magnification. The longitudinal picture clearly reveals the retention of the characteristics of the intact muscle: e. g. the sarcomeres lie in register, and the myofibrillar compartment is very compact. The micrograph also depicts the average diameter of the myofibrils. An average of 30 myosin filaments can be counted per myofibril. The cross-sectional picture similarly corresponds to the normal muscle. Fig. 3 shows the initial stage of disintegration of the myofibrillar system. The first splitting appears in the "A" band. This is followed by splitting of the ,,Z" membrane, and then by the slipping-apart of the myofibrillar fragments parallel to the longitudinal axis of the cell.

The most striking evidence deriving from our micrographs is that a multitude of very slightly altered myofibrils are to be found in the immidiate vicinity of a very severely damaged area (Fig. 4). This is the phenomenon known as focal atrophy in the literature. An even greater degree of disintegration can be seen in the Fig. 5a and 5b. There are almost no thick filaments, this being more clearly visible in the cross-sectional part of micrograph. The number of myosin filaments may be counted along a straight line. Fig. 6 illustrates a very characteristic final stage of the degeneration. The muscle cell even loses its typical spindle shape, the cell is shrunk and a highly invaginated plasma membrane is obvious.

In atrophy after denervation the destruction of myones is also marked but somewhat different from that in atrophy after disuse of muscle.

The changes start in the Z region and inside the myofibrils. The compact appearence of myofibrillar structure diminishes and spaces filled with vesicles of 3—500 Å in diameter are clearly visible (Fig. 7, 8). In this case in spite of the fact that at the cell membrane an accumulation of pinocytotic vesicles can be seen there is no such marked invagination of cell boundary as was observed by the atrophy after disuse of muscle.

The musculus gastrocnemius shows similar but less enhanced changes as described for the m. soleus.

Fig. 9 shows changes in weight of m. gastrocnemius and m. soleus after immobilization and denervation.

Table 1 gives the changes in the protein fractions of normal, disused and denervated rabbit muscles. One can see that during 4 weeks of immobilization, the total

Table 1
Changes in the protein fractions of the gastrocnemius (G) and soleus (S) muscles after 4 weeks of denervation or disuse

Protein fractions	Normal (mg/g)	Denervated G (mg/g)	Denervated S (mg/g)	Immobilized G (mg/g)	Immobilized S (mg/g)
Total	195.4±8.3	171.5±15.5	170.9±13.6	168.5±6.7	168.7±5.1
Myofibrillar (M)	113.6±7.0	81.3± 8.6	85.6± 7.1	84.3±6.6	79.4±4.6
Sarcoplasmic (S)	51.5±6.2	39.6± 4.1	42.5± 5.4	63.7±7.1	67.3±3.4
Particulate + connective tissue	20.3±4.4	45.4± 9.6	43.2± 8.8	20.5±3.1	21.9±2.5
S/M ratio	0.47	0.49	0.49	0.75	0.84

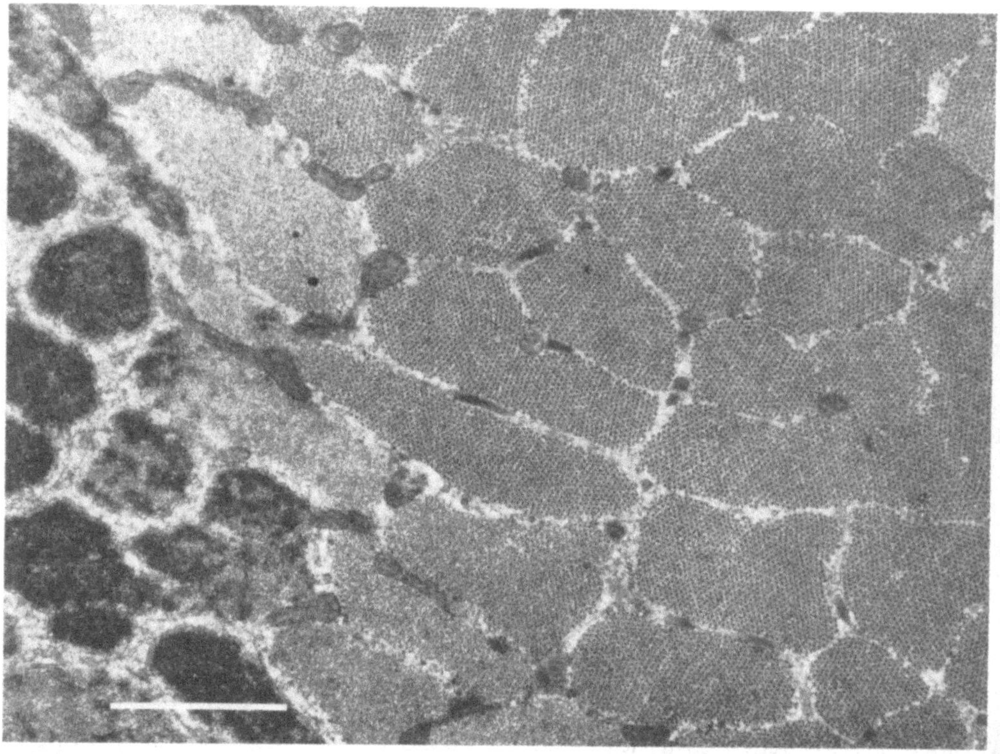

Fig. 2a. Cross-sectional electronmicrograph of the normal m. soleus of rabbit

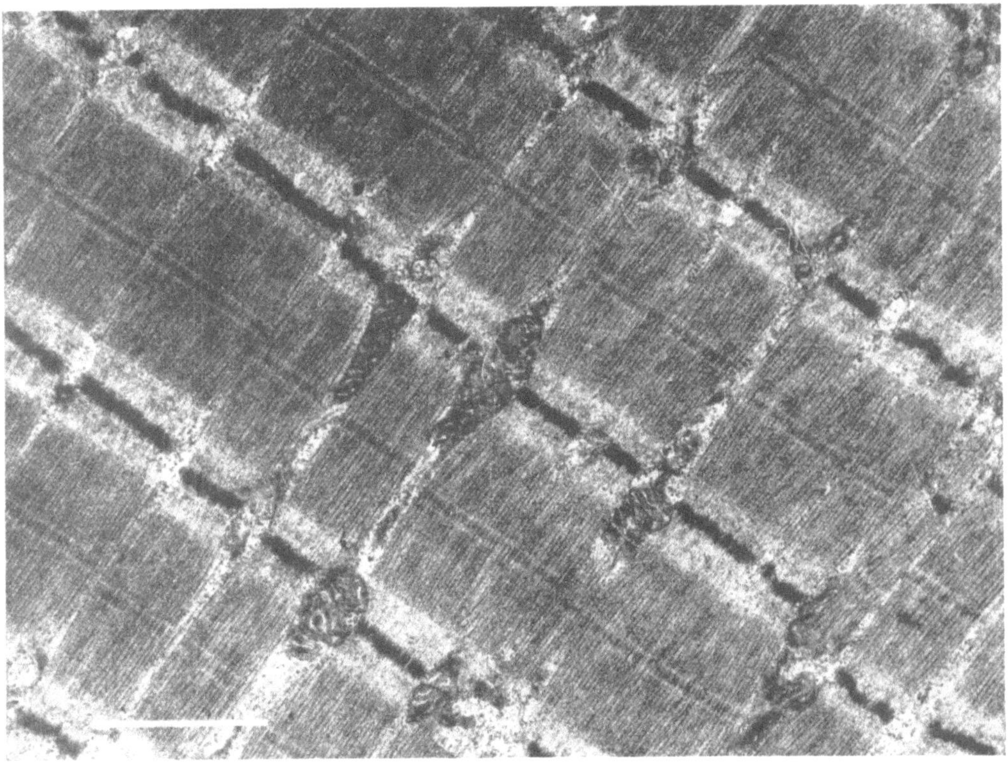

Fig. 2b. Longitudinal section of the normal m. soleus of rabbit

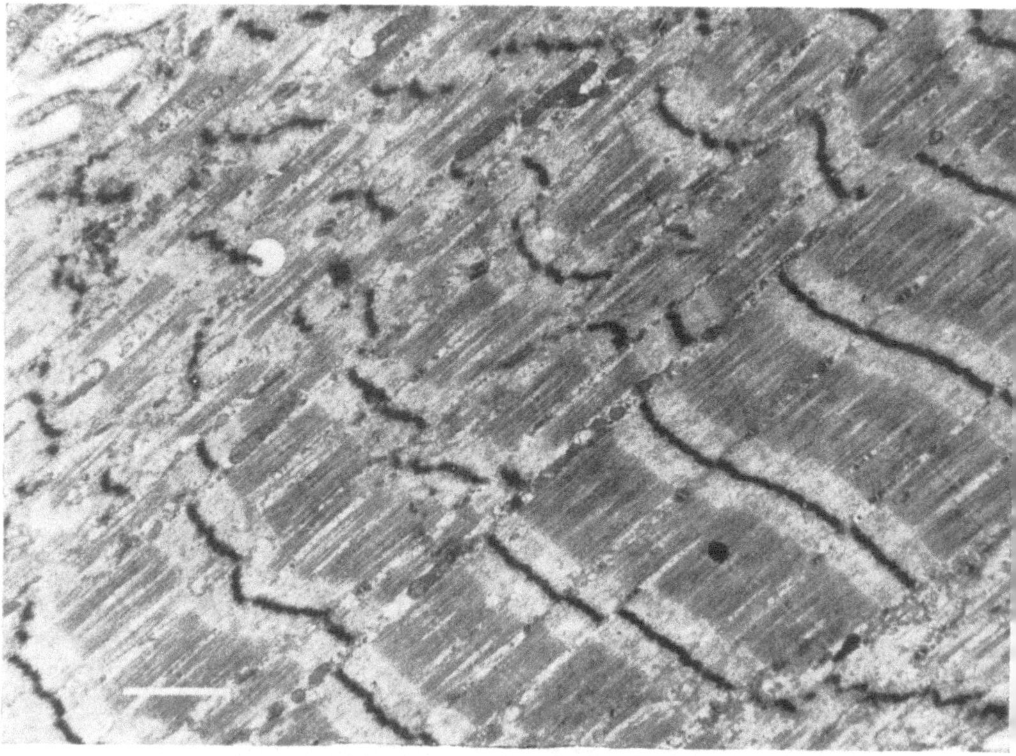

Fig. 3. Initial stage of disintegration of the myofibrillar system after immobilisation of the m. soleus

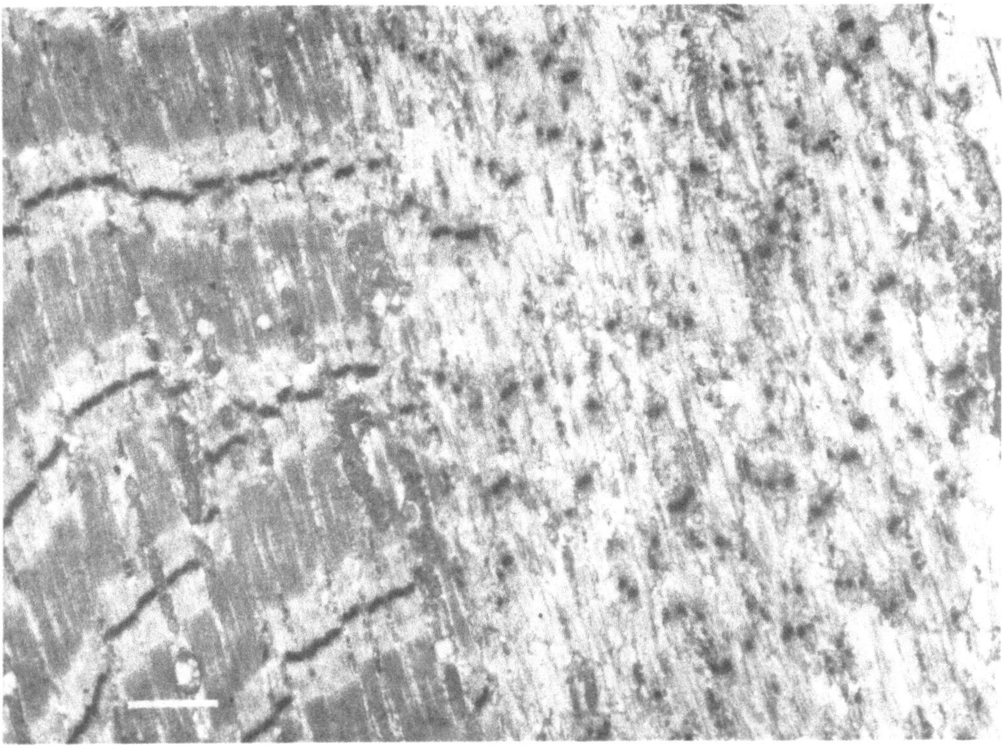

Fig. 4. "Focal atrophy" of a muscle cell after immobilisation

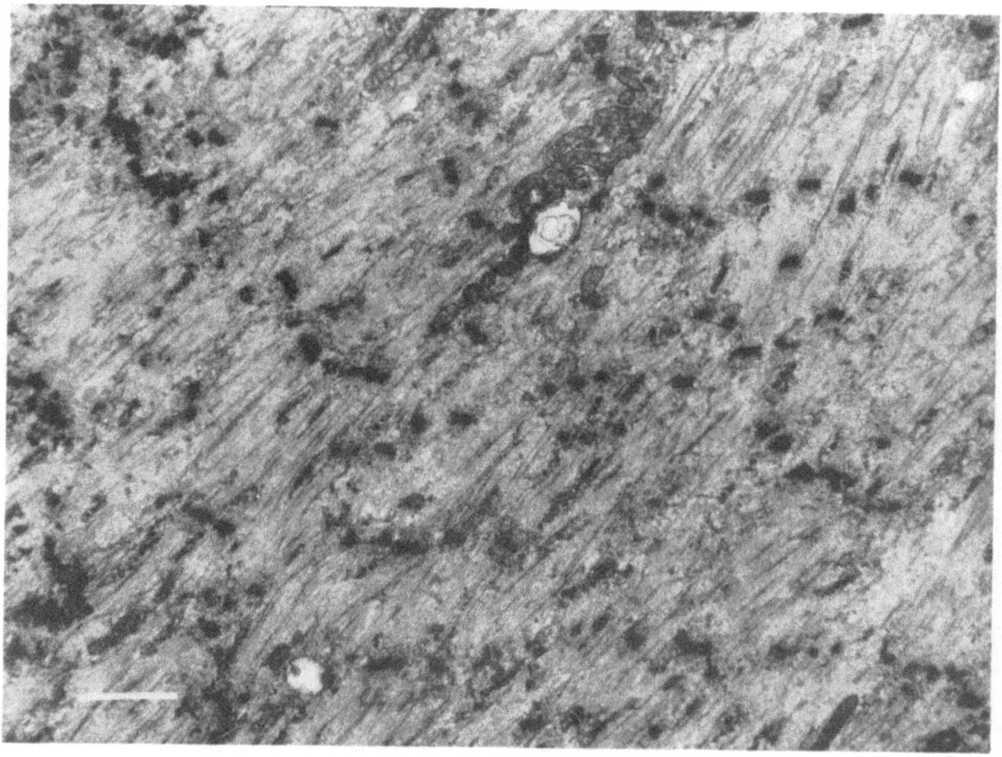

Fig. 5a. Longitudinal section of the immobilized m. soleus muscle cell. Enhanced disintegration of myofibrillar structure is appearent

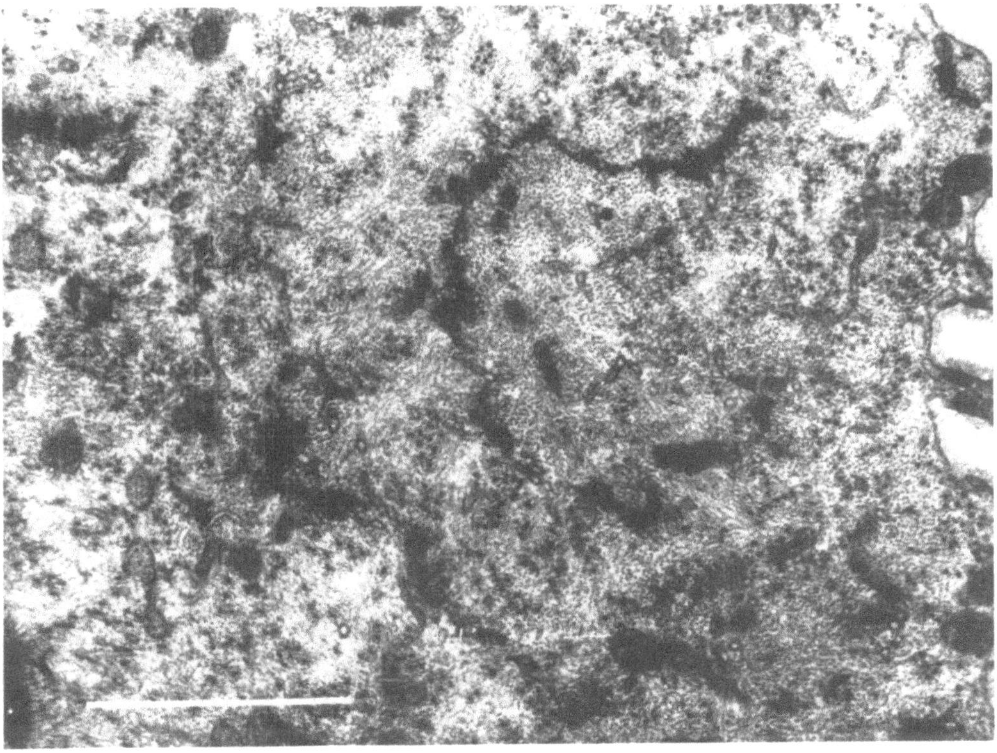

Fig. 5b. Cross section of the same muscle as in Fig. 5a. The marked loss in the number of thick filaments is obvious

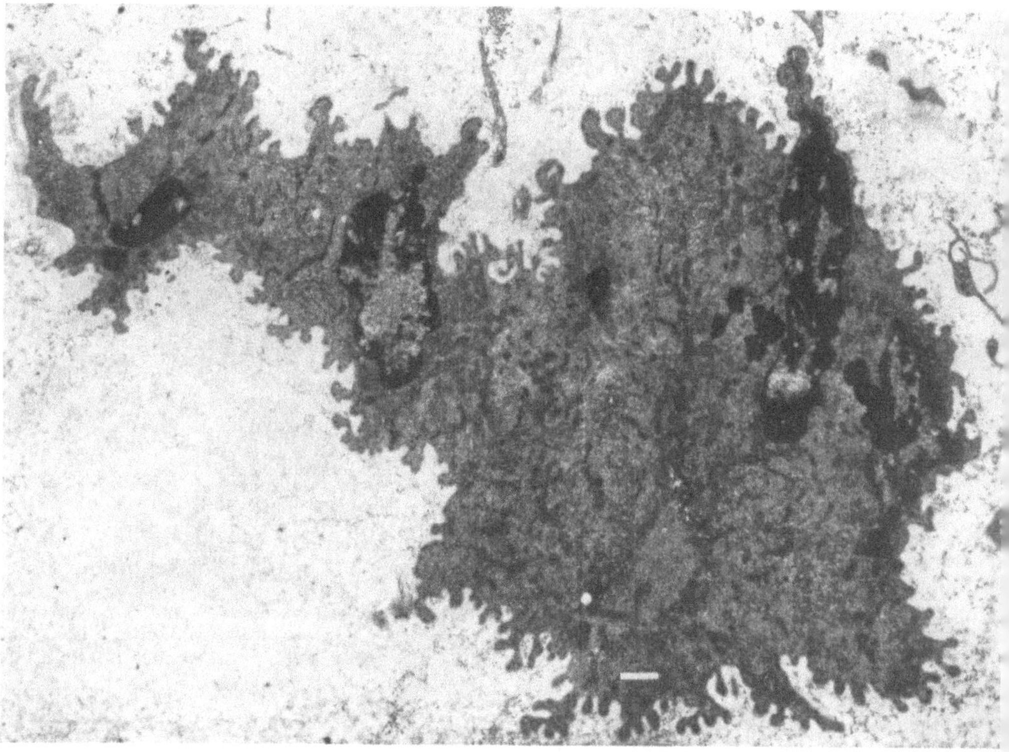

Fig. 6. Highly degenerated muscle cell in disuse atrophy of the m. soleus. A marked invagination of the cell membrane can be noticed

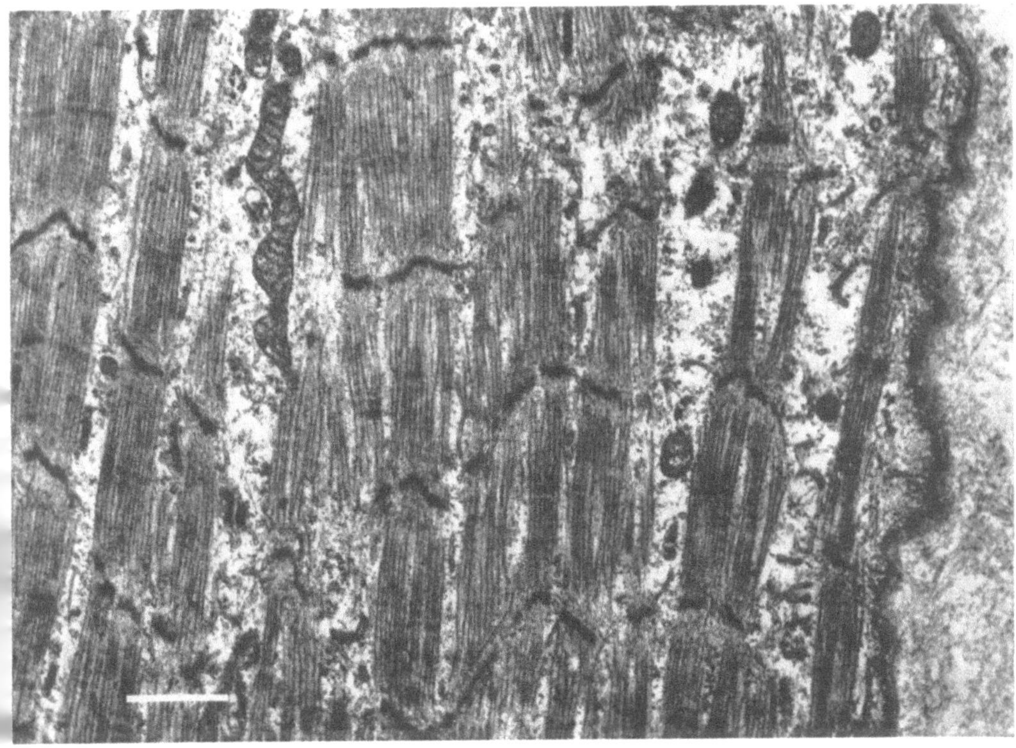

Fig. 7. Characteristic feature of disintegration of the myofibrillar system in the m. soleus after denervation

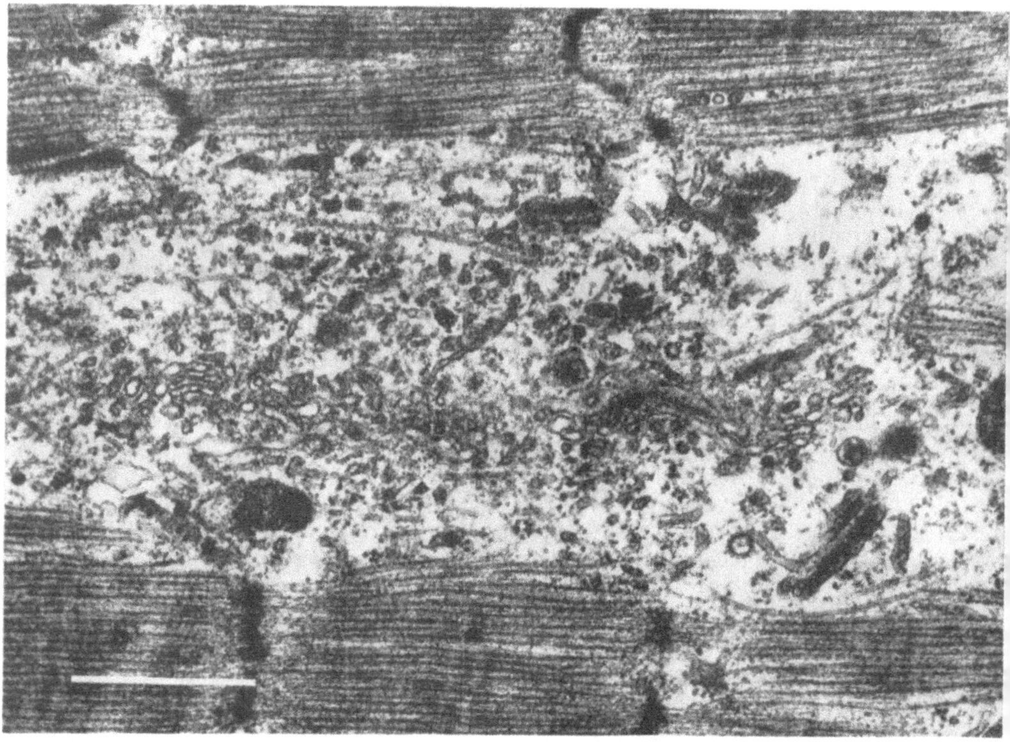

Fig. 8. Disintegrated myofibrillar system of the m. soleus in denervation atrophy. Spaces filled with vesicles of 3 – 500 Å in diameter are observed

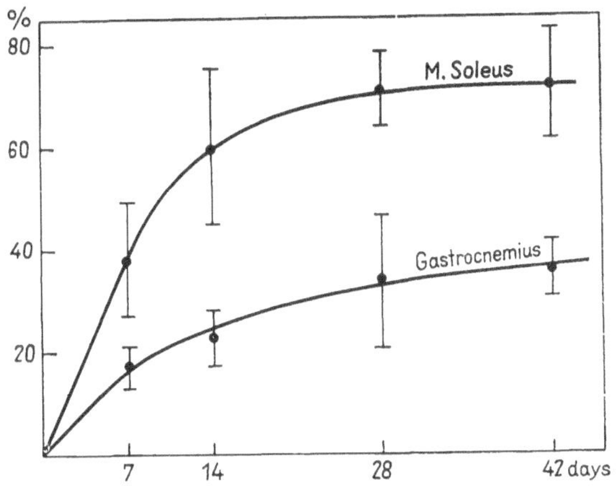

Fig. 9. Changes in weight of the m. soleus and m. gastrocnemius after immobilisation and denervation

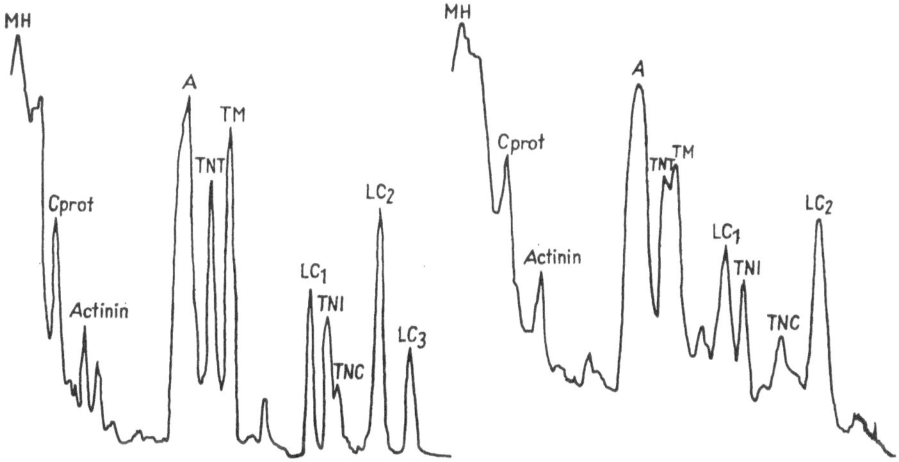

Fig. 10. The SDS-gel electrophoresis pattern of myofibrillar proteins of normal m. soleus and m. gastrocnemius

protein content of muscles decreases. The situation is the same in the case of denervation. The differences in the two forms of atrophy appear to be in the ratios of sarcoplasmic to myofibrillar protein fractions. In the denervation atrophy this ratio is 0.49 while in disuse atrophy it proved to be 0.75 for m. gastrocnemius. Fig. 10 gives the composition of myofibrillar proteins in the normal m. soleus and m. gastrocnemius.

The Fig. 11 shows the composition of disused gastrocnemius muscle compared to the normal. As a consequence of four weeks disuse a very high degree of decrease in the relative amount of LC_3 and TN-I, while that of the TN-T increased. The tropomyosin content also decreases.

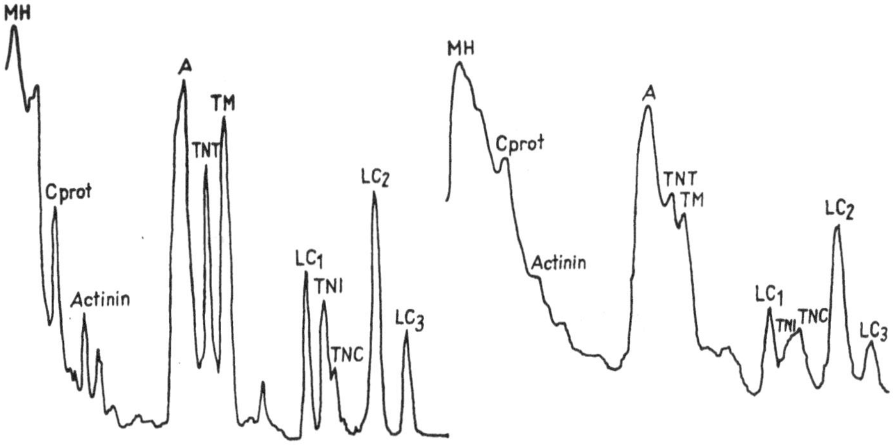

Fig. 11. The protein pattern of normal and disused m. gastrocnemius

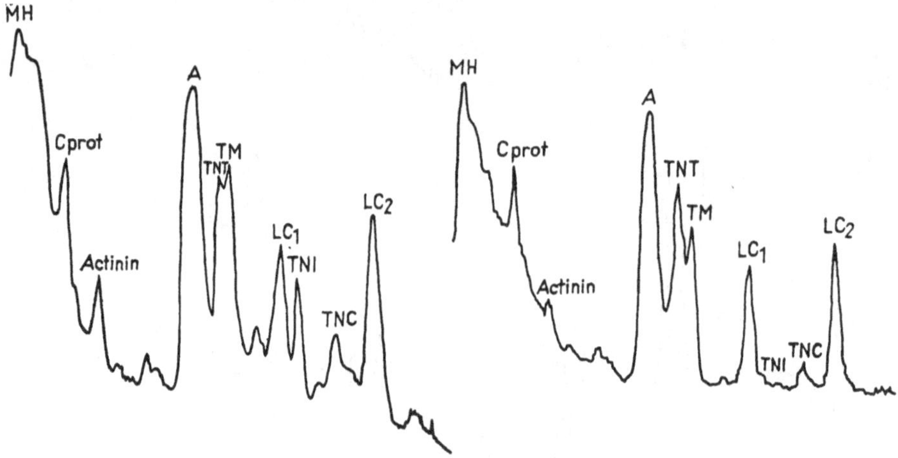

Fig. 12. The protein pattern of normal and disused m. soleus

In the m. soleus the changes are more marked than in the gastrocnemius (Fig. 12). Here, too, mainly the relative amounts of tropomyosin, LC_1-LC_2 and TN-C are reduced.

Following denervation the main changes in the m. gastrocnemius are the decrease of the components LC_3, tropomyosin and TN-I (Fig. 13). In contrast to disuse atrophy, from the troponin subunits the relative quantity of TN-C increases and that of the TN-T decreases. It is noteworthy to consider that the quantity of the myosin relatively to actin decreases.

Discussion

It was found that the differences in the effects of disuse and denervation on the myones appear to be in the alteration of the sarcoplasmic to myofibrillar protein quotient. In denervation the decrease of the cell compartments is proportional, while in disuse the decrease of the myofibrillar fraction is a higher order of degree.

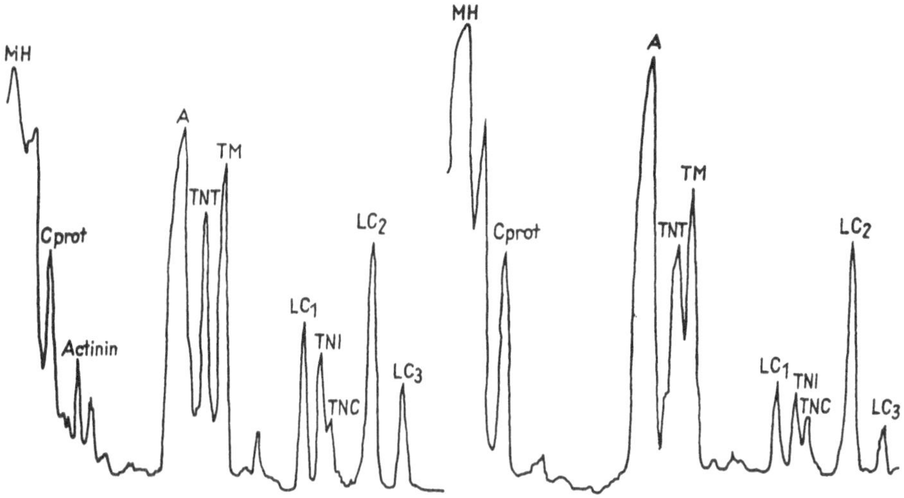

Fig. 13. The protein pattern of normal and denervated m. gastrocnemius

There is an essential difference in the alteration of the structural proteins. In denervation the calcium binding component of the troponin (TN-C) shows a relative increase, and the TN-T decreases. In disuse atrophy the TN-T increases while the TN-C decreases.

The ratio of myosin to actin and the quantity of tropomyosin shows a continuous fall in both types of atrophy. Most probably the differences found are in close correlation with the influence of innervation of myones or that of the disuse.

In conclusion: The neurogen and disuse atrophy differ in their effects on the turnover of the protein compartments of myones, and that of the single components.

References

[1] GUTMANN, E.: J. Physiol., Lond. **203**, 46 (1969)
[2] GOLDBERG, A., L. in: Cardiac Hypertrophy. ALBERT (Ed.). Academic Press, New York 1971, p. 35—53
[3] ECCLES, J. C.: J. Physiol., Lond. **103**, 243 (1944)
[4] GOLDBERG, A. L., and H. M. GOODMAN: Am. J. Physiol. **216**, 1116 (1969)
[5] KÁRPÁTI, G., and W. K. ENGEL: Neurology **18**, 681 (1968)
[6] TAKÁCS, Ö., I. SOHÁR, I. GUBA, and T. SZILÁGYI: Acta biol. hung. **28**, 213 (1977)
[7] WEBER, K., and M. OSBORN: J. biol. Chem. **244**, 4406 (1969)

Acta biol. med. germ., Band 36, Seite 1621—1624 (1977)

Institute of Biochemistry, University of Medical Sciences, H-6701 Szeged, Hungary

The influence of immobilization on soluble proteins of muscle

I. SOHÁR, Ö. TAKÁCS, and F. GUBA

Summary

1. The right hind legs of rabbits were immobilized in full extension with a plaster cast for various periods.

2. The mainly fast, white m. gastrocnemius and the mainly slow, red m. soleus were separated, and the activities or relative amounts of the following soluble proteins were measured: fructose-1,6-diphosphate aldolase, lactic acid dehydrogenase, lactic acid dehydrogenase isoenzyme, glutamic acid pyruvic acid-transaminase, acid phosphatase, myoglobin and myokinase.

3. The quantities of the enzymes playing important roles in the metabolic processes fall as a result of disuse to a relatively greater extent than the weight decrease.

4. In m. gastrocnemius the quantity of acid phosphatase, a hydrolytic enzyme involved in catabolism, does not change during the atrophy, but in m. soleus it decreases compared to the muscle weight loss.

5. As regards the isoenzymes, the activities of LDH-1 and LDH-2, which play important roles in the oxidation processes, decrease considerably, whereas the activities of LDH-4 and LDH-5 barely change in the course of the atrophy.

6. The catabolism of myoglobin is inhibited in m. gastrocnemius, and hence an increase in its relative amount can be observed.

7. The catabolism of myokinase is inhibited in m. soleus, while in m. gastrocnemius its quantity decreases, similarly to those of the other enzymes.

Introduction

Many authors have dealt with the composition of the soluble proteins of the skeletal muscles with regard to function and metabolism [1, 2]. The composition of the soluble proteins is changed by damage or various diseases of the muscle [3—5]. The effect of disuse has mainly been examined with histochemical reactions. In a previous electrophoretic examination we described changes in the soluble protein composition [6]. Numerous authors have similarly reported on the presence and the increase in activity of the proteolytic and hydrolytic enzymes in the skeletal muscle [7—11]. At the earlier Symposium we also have described changes in proteolytic enzyme activity following denervation [12]. JAKUBIEC-PUKA et al. [13] likewise dealt with autolysis resulting from lack of movement. The effect of immobilization on the protein turnover in the skeletal muscle has been investigated recently by GOLDSPINK [14].

Our present examinations were carried out on the mainly red, slow m. soleus and the white, fast m. gastrocnemius in rabbits whose movement was inhibited. From the enzyme activity changes resulting form the immobilization, conclusions were drawn on the various protein catabolic rates of these enzymes.

Material and methods

Four-month-old New Zealand rabbits of both sexes from one breed, weighing 3000 g, were used in groups containing 10 animals each. The right hind legs of the animals were immobilized in full extension with plaster casts, and 7, 14, 28 or 42 days later the animals were decapitated and drained of blood, and the two functionally different muscles, m. gastrocnemius and m. soleus, were isolated and excised. After purification from connective tissue and fatty tissue, the muscle was homogenized twice for 30 s in a Waring blender in a 20fold volume of 50 mM phosphate buffer of *p*H 7.25, containing 5 mM EDTA and 0.1% Triton X-100. This was followed by further treatment in a teflon-glass homogenizer, with subsequent centrifugation at 16,000 × *g*. The entire procedure was carried out at 0–4 °C. Protein [15] and enzyme activities were determined on the supernatant. Activities were measured as described in [16]. Enzyme activities were calculated per unit dissolved protein. The following enzymes were measured: lactic acid dehydrogenase (LDH) (E.C.1.1.1.27); glutamic acid-pyruvic acid transaminase (GPT) (E.C.2.6.1.2); acid phosphatase (Ac.P.) (E.C.3.1.3.2); and fructose-1,6-diphosphate aldolase (ALD) (E.C.4.1.2.7). The LDH isoenzymes were separated according to Dietz and Lubrano [17].

The relative amounts of myoglobin (MG) and myokinase (MK) (E.C.2.7.4.3) within the soluble proteins were measured by electrophoresis with a Kipp and Zonen densitometer after staining with Coomassie Brilliant Blue. Hyland enzyme control was used in the activity measurements, and Boehringer standards in the electrophoresis.

Results

In our previous contribution we have described that after the fourth week of immobilization the weight of the atrophied muscle no longer decreases with in-

Table 1
Changes in the activity of various enzymes and of myoglobin and myokinase

Days	GPT (U/g)	Ac. P. (U/g)	ALD (U/g)	LDH (U/g)	Myoglobin (%)	Myokinase (%)
Musculus soleus						
0	50.0±0.8	14.5±1.7	142.8±11.5	2.9±0.5	7.5±0.5	1.4±0.2
7	32.5±5.5 yes	17.0±2.2 yes	115.8±11.5 yes	2.3±0.4 no	6.3±1.0 yes	2.9±0.4 yes
14	27.8±8 yes	19.1±3.8 yes	100.2±23.5 yes	1.7±0.2 yes	4.98±1.0 yes	3.5±0.5 yes
28	5.8±1.4 yes	12.6±1.0 yes	94.0±16.0 yes	1.1±0.3 yes	3.0±0.5 yes	3.1±0.5 yes
Musculus gastrocnemius						
0	26.2±5.5	9.4±1.9	1107±158	10.7±1.8	1.4±0.3	3.2±0.4
7	18.8±4.4 yes	11.5±1.2 yes	985±161 yes	10.1±3.7 no	7.0±0.3 yes	2.0±0.2 yes
14	12.6±2.2 yes	12.7±1.3 yes	734±118 yes	7.8±0.8 yes	7.6±0.5 yes	1.4±0.2 yes
28	9.7±2.1 yes	12.7±1.2 yes	481±35 yes	3.7±0.7 yes	7.7±0.5 yes	1.05±0.3 yes

Means ± S. D.; significance p <0,05 = yes; no: not significant compared to the controls by Students *t*-test

crease of the duration of immobilization, compared to the muscle of the contralateral leg. Accordingly, the present measurements relate to the first 4 weeks. The same muscle taken from the right hind legs of untreated, intact animals served as control. Table 1 lists the mean activities measured for m. soleus and m. gastrocnemius, together with the standard deviations. It is obvious that the greatest decrease in the m. soleus is found for GPT. After one week only the activity per unit protein decreases by 35%. The changes in LDH and ALD were lower. The Ac. P. activity increased for the first 2 weeks of immobilization on average by 32%, and then fall to the normal level after 4 weeks. Also in the case of the m. gastrocnemius the highest degrease is found for GPT, while the activities of LDH and ALD fall in almost the same way during immobilization. In this muscle the activity of the acid phosphatase attains its maximum in the fourth week.
Table 1 furthermore depicts the changes in MG and MK compared to the control. The relative increases of MG in m. gastrocnemius and of MK in m. soleus are outstanding.
In Fig. 1 the LDH isoenzyme distribution in the m. soleus and m. gastrocnemius are demonstrated. In the m. soleus the isoenzymes LDH-1 and LDH-2 display a relative decrease, and LDH-4 an increase. There is no LDH-5 in rabbit m. soleus. The variations observed in the m. gastrocnemius are of a similar nature as in the m. soleus; the maximum changes were found in the fourth week.

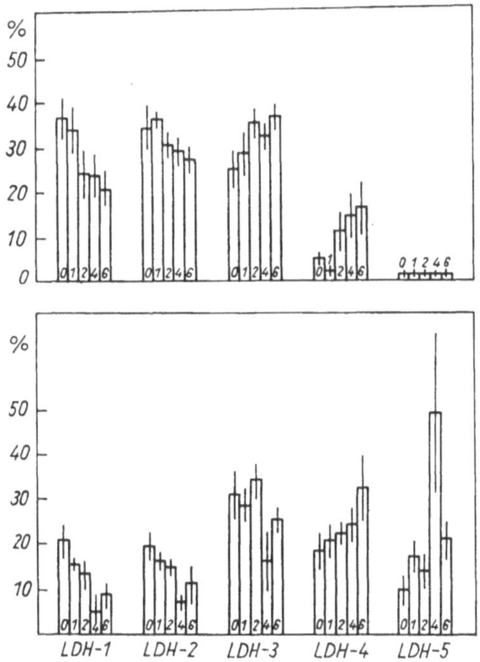

Fig. 1. Percentage distribution of LDH isoenzymes in m. soleus and m. gastrocnemius after various periods of immobilization. The numbers in the columns indicate the duration of immobilization in weeks

Discussion

The results demonstrate that the activities and quantities in the muscle of the soluble proteins examined varied in different manners with the duration of the immobilization. As a result of disuse, the muscles of the two types are forced to change their metabolisms, and hence they undergo damage. Since the changed conditions favour the catabolic processes, the hydrolytic enzymes are activated. The increasing proteolytic activity catabolizes the individual enzymes in different ways. Our experiments confirmed that in both cases the activity of GPT decreases to the highest extent, followed by LDH and ALD. The percentage degradation of the enzyme protein proved to be independent of the magnitude of the initial activities in the two muscles, which exhibit a very large difference in the case of ALD, for instance.

References

[1] PETTE, D., and G. DÖLKEN: Adv. Enzyme Reg. **13**, 355 (1975)
[2] BASS, A., P. BRDICZKA, P. EYER, S. HOFER, and D. PETTE: Eur. J. Biochem. **10**, 198 (1969)
[3] GUTMANN, E.: Ärztl. Forsch. **23**, 33 (1969)
[4] PEARSON, M.: Rev. can. Biol. **21**, 533 (1962)
[5] HOGAN, E. L., D. DAWSON, and F. ROMANUL: Archs Neurol. **13**, 274 (1965)
[6] TAKÁCS, Ö., I. SOHÁR, T. SZILÁGYI, and F. GUBA: Acta biol. hung. (in press)
[7] BIRD, J. W. C.: Frontiers of biology. Vol. **43**. Lysosomes in biology and pathology. North-Holland Publishing Co., Amsterdam 1975
[8] DRABIKOWSKI, W., A. GORECKA, and A. JAKUBIEC-PUKA: Int. J. Biochem. **8**, 1 (1976)
[9] IODICE, A. A., J. CHIN, S. PERKER, and I. M. WEINSTOCK: Archs Biochem. Biophys. **152**, 166 (1972)
[10] HÁJEK, I., E. GUTMANN, and I. SYROVY: Fiz. Bohem. **13**, 32 (1963)
[11] BERLINGUET, L., and U. SRIVASTAVA: Can. J. Biochem. **44**, 613 (1966)
[12] GUBA, F., Ö. TAKÁCS, Zs. KISS, and T. PELLE: Intracellular Protein Catabolism Symposium, Reinhardsbrunn 1973. H. HANSON and P. BOHLEY (Eds.). Barth, Leipzig 1974/76, p. 415
[13] JAKUBIEC-PUKA, A., W. DRABIKOWSKI and A. GORECKA: Intracellular Protein Catabolism Symposium, Reinhardsbrunn 1973. H. HANSON and P. BOHLEY (Eds.). Barth, Leipzig 1974/76, p. 409
[14] GOLDSPINK, D. F.: J. Physiol., Lond. **264** 267 (1977)
[15] GOA, J.: Scand. J. clin. Lab. Invest. **5**, 218 (1953)
[16] BERGMEYER, H. U. (Ed.): Methoden der enzymatischen Analyse. Akademie Verlag, Berlin 1970
[17] DIETZ, A. A., and T. LUBRANO: Anal. Biochem. **20**, 246 (1967)

Acta biol. med. germ., Band 36, Seite 1625—1635 (1977)

Department of Biochemistry, University College, Cardiff CF1 1XL, Wales, U. K.

A neutral protease from rat intestinal muscle. A possible role in the degradation of native enzymes

ROBERT J. BEYNON and JOHN KAY

Summary

A membrane-limited protease has been solubilised and partially purified from the intestinal smooth muscle of rats fed on protein free diets. This neutral protease has a mol. wt. of around 33,000 and from its susceptibility to several known modifiers of proteolytic enzymes, it appears to be trypsin-like. It is stable over a relatively narrow *p*H range and it appears to have a markedly enhanced ability over trypsin for inactivating substrate enzymes in their native conformations through limited proteolysis.
The rate of inactivation of substrate enzymes can be modulated by cofactors, allosteric ligands, or by changes in ionic strength. In addition, a specific protein inhibitor of the protease has been measured and levels of this are high in animals fed on normal diets. On administration of protein free diets, the inhibitory activity is depleted. Contamination of the muscle tissue by lumenal, mucosal or blood proteases and inhibitors has been excluded.
A role for the neutral protease in initiating the turnover of intracellular enzymes is postulated.

Introduction

The intracellular level of an enzyme is determined by the balance between its individual rates of synthesis and degradation. Extensive studies on the turnover of enzymes from rat liver have revealed a wide range of half lives, and several mechanisms have been proposed to explain the selectivity of the degradative process implicit in these observations (for review, see [1]). The relationship of subunit molecular weight to half-life, together with the observation that large proteins are proteolysed in vitro more rapidly than those of lower molecular weight [2], suggest that proteolysis itself might be involved in determining the rate limiting step of an enzyme's catabolism. The major proteolytic organelle is the lysosome, and direct evidence has been presented for lysosomal involvement in gross protein breakdown [3—5]. However, the restricted localisation and acidic *p*H optima of the cathepsins seem to prevent their introducing the selectivity which is necessary to account for each enzyme having its own characteristic rate of turnover, although two theories have been presented to allow the lysosome to function selectively [6, 7].
One alternative hypothesis would be to have proteolysis at a region distinct from the lysosome regulating the turnover of intracellular proteins. The proteases responsible for this non lysosomal proteolysis would presumably have to show optimal activity at neutral or slightly alkaline *p*H, and evidence for such intracellular neutral proteases is accumulating. The histone degrading protease [8], the insulin degrading protease [9] and the myofibril degrading Ca^{2+} activated protease [10] are three of the better characterized activities found in animal tissues. In addition,

the "group specific proteases" described by Katunuma et al. [11] were suggested to be responsible for the initiation of degradation of pyridoxal phosphate, NAD, and FAD dependent enzymes, with a different protease initiating the catabolism of each class of substrate enzyme. The protease active towards pyridoxal phosphate enzymes was subsequently purified from a variety of rat tissues and shown to be chymotrypsin-like [12]. It was proposed that the group specific proteases would catalyse a limited cleavage of a susceptible form of the substrate enzyme (such as the apoenzyme), facilitating subsequent degradation by the lysosomal system. The selectivity of this system would provide an attractive mechanism to explain the variety of enzyme half lives observed in vivo. We have therefore been looking at the neutral proteolytic activity present in the intestinal smooth muscle of rats, which is capable of inactivating native enzymes. This paper reports the nature of the proteolytic activity and possible control mechanisms to modulate its activity in vivo.

Material and methods

Materials

Azocasein, azoalbumin, oxaloacetic acid, NADH, p-hydroxymercuribenzoate, α-N-benzoyl-arginine, benzamidine, soybean trypsin inhibitor, D-tryptophan O-methyl ester, tosyl arginine methyl ester, benzoyl arginine ethyl ester, acetyl tyrosine ethyl ester, benzoyl tyrosine ethyl ester, isocitrate dehydrogenase, glucose 6-phosphate dehydrogenase and urease were all obtained from Sigma (London) Ltd. Glutamate dehydrogenase was obtained from Boehringer. Malate dehydrogenase and lactate dehydrogenase were generous gifts from Miles Research Laboratories. Lima bean trypsin inhibitor was purchased from Worthington Biochemicals Ltd. Phosphorylase *b*, proflavin, and pepstatin were the generous gifts of Drs. P. Cohen, R. McRorie, and H. Umezawa respectively. An 8% casein, niacin free diet and a protein free diet were obtained from Micro Bio Laboratories. A 2% casein, 6% gelatin diet was obtained from Cooper Nutritional Biochemicals.

Animals

Male Wistar rats (150–200 g) were maintained on normal laboratory diet until transfer to the experimental diet. All animals were starved for 24 hrs before they were sacrificed by cervical dislocation. With some animals, prior to excision of the small intestine, the vascular bed of the gut was perfused with isotonic saline through the hepatic portal vein.

Preparation of crude intracellular protease

It was necessary to remove any possibility of contamination from the intestinal lumen (i. e. pancreatic proteases) by means of a rigorous washing procedure. Whole small intestine was washed with 9 aliquots of 25 ml of isotonic KCl with agitation between washes. No activity towards azocasein, tosyl arginine methyl ester or benzoyl tyrosine ethyl ester could be detected in the washings after the sixth aliquot had been passed through. The mucosal layer was removed by slitting the intestine longitudinally and then scraping the internal surface with a glass microscope slide. The muscle layer was then rinsed with isotonic KCl to remove loosely adhering mucosal tissue and used as the source of proteolytic activity. This separation procedure gave a muscle tissue preparation which contained only 8% of the total intestinal alkaline phosphatase activity, and less than 2% of the total intestinal maltase activity (both of these enzymes are found in large amounts in the mucosal layer of small intestine).

The muscle layer was chopped into small pieces and homogenised in 3 volumes of 0.02 M phosphate buffer, *p*H 7.5, at half speed for 30 s with a Polytron PT2 homogeniser. Centrifugation at 100,000 × *g* for 20 min gave a clear supernatant (S1) and a pellet (P1) which contained the proteolytic activity. Solubilisation of the activity could be achieved by incubation at 4 °C in high (0.5 M) or low (0.02 M) concentrations of phosphate buffer, *p*H 7.5, for

20 hrs. Treatment with Triton X100 (0.5% w/v) or sonication were also effective for this purpose. Centrifugation of the extracted material at 100,000 × *g* for 1 h gave a second supernatant (S2) which contained most of the proteolytic activity. On ammonium sulphate fractionation of the solubilised protease fraction (S2), the activity precipitated between 1.2 M and 2.55 M ammonium sulphate and was accompanied by marked increases in total activity. The 2.55 M supernatant was desalted and concentrated by ultrafiltration through an Amicon UM 2 membrane.

Assays

Malate dehydrogenase was assayed by monitoring the disappearance of NADH. The assay was performed at 25 °C using 0.1 M sodium phosphate buffer, *p*H 7.5, in the presence of 0.125 mM NADH and 0.3 mM oxaloacetate.

Proteolytic activity was measured using two systems to distinguish the action of the intracellular protease from exogenous proteases such as trypsin and chymotrypsin. This comparison permits a reasonable evaluation of the extent of contamination of the preparations by these pancreatic proteases, since the intracellular protease shows a limited capacity for digesting azocasein, but readily inactivates malate dehydrogenase. The converse is true for the pancreatic proteases.

The digestion of azocasein was followed by monitoring the release of dye-containing peptides soluble in 4% trichloroacetic acid. Azocasein (11 mg) was incubated with protease (0.1 ml) in a final volume of 1.1 ml of 0.1 M phosphate buffer, *p*H 7.5, at 30 °C. At suitable time intervals (usually 0, 30, 60, and 90 min) aliquots (0.25 ml) were removed and added to 1 ml of 5% (w/v) trichloroacetic acid. After centrifugation at 800 × *g* for 5 min, the absorbances of the supernatants were determined at 340 nm. The rate of increase in absorbance was taken as a measure of proteolysis, defining one unit as that amount of activity causing a rate of increase in absorbance of 0.001/min.

Proteolysis of malate dehydrogenase was monitored by observing the time dependent loss of activity of the dehydrogenases.

Mitochondrial malate dehydrogenase (pig heart; 50 µg) was incubated at 30 °C with a suitable amount of protease in a final volume of 0.25 ml of 0.02 M phosphate, *p*H 7.5. At appropriate time intervals, aliquots were diluted into cold 0.1 M phosphate buffer, *p*H 7.5, and portions were assayed for residual malate dehydrogenase activity. One unit of proteolytic activity was defined as that amount of protease causing an initial rate of loss of activity of 1%/min.

The effect of modifiers on the proteolytic activity

Several known modifiers of proteolytic enzymes were tested for their ability to affect the rate of inactivation of malate dehydrogenase by the muscle protease. The protease and modifiers were preincubated for 5 min before the addition of malate dehydrogenase to initiate digestion under normal assay conditions. In the case of p-hydroxymercuribenzoate the excess of free reagent in the inactivation mixture would itself have modified the activity of malate dehydrogenase. The pretreated protease sample was therefore dialysed against 2,000 volumes of 0.02 M phosphate buffer, *p*H 7.5, to remove the excess of reagent. The remaining activity was compared with that of a sample which had been treated identically except for the omission of p-hydroxymercuribenzoate. In the case of benzamidine, α-N-benzoyl arginine, and proflavin, direct interaction between malate dehydrogenase and the inhibitors (which could have led to a protective effect) was excluded on the basis of lack of effect of these reagents on malate dehydrogenase activity.

The effect of pH on the stability of the protease

Samples of the intestinal muscle protease were incubated at 30 °C for 60 min in 0.1 ml of buffer at the indicated *p*H. The buffers used were: *p*H 4.5–7.5, 0.01 M succinate/NaOH; *p*H 7.5–9.5, 0.01 M glycine/NaOH. At the end of the preincubation period, 0.15 ml of 0.1 M phosphate buffer, *p*H 7.5, was added to each reaction mixture, and the *p*H was adjusted to 7.5. Residual activity towards malate dehydrogenase was then determined.

Studies on the specificity of the protease

Malate dehydrogenase was used routinely as a substrate but, in addition, the susceptibilities of phosphorylase *b*, glutamate dehydrogenase, isocitrate dehydrogenase, lactate dehydrogenase, glucose 6 phosphate dehydrogenase and urease to the protease were tested and compared to the effects produced by trypsin under identical conditions. All substrate enzymes were assayed under optimal conditions and control incubations without protease were performed in every case.

Assay of inhibitory activity towards the protease

Samples thought to contain inhibitor were preincubated with the muscle protease for 5 min at 30 °C before adding malate dehydrogenase to initiate the proteolytic inactivation. One unit of inhibitory activity is defined as that amount which inhibits one unit of protease.

Sodium dodecyl sulphate (SDS) polyacrylamide gel electrophoresis

Samples were prepared using agarose-soybean trypsin inhibitor according to the method described previously [13]. SDS polyacrylamide gel electrophoresis was performed according to the method of Weber and Osborne [14].

Results

Assay of the protease

Using malate dehydrogenase as the substrate for the intracellular protease, a linear relationship between the amount of protease and the initial rate of inactivation was observed (Fig. 1). This permitted a reasonable evaluation of the level of protease present in the preparations. First order analysis was not possible since at low protease levels the inactivation slowed considerably as it progressed. Using azocasein as a 'general' proteolytic substrate the rate of increase in absorbance at 340 nm was linear, provided that the final absorbance did not exceed 0.4.

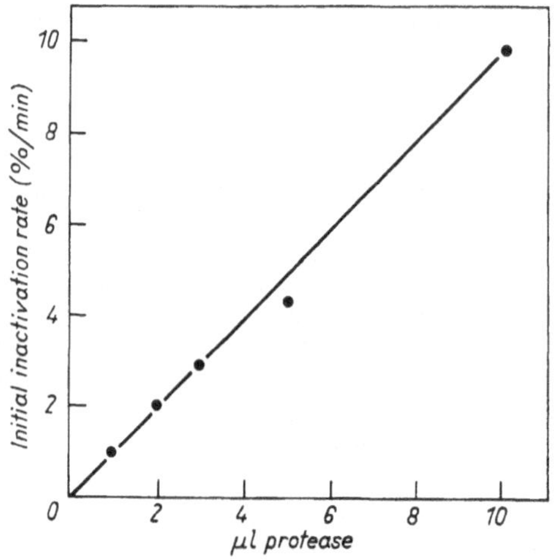

Fig. 1. Relationship between inactivation rate and amount of protease.
Malate dehydrogenase (0.2 mg/ml) was incubated with the indicated quantities of crude protease in a final volume of 0.25 ml of 0.02 M phosphate buffer, *p*H 7.5. At appropriate times, aliquots were removed and assayed for remaining dehydrogenase activity. Initial rates of inactivation were calculated from plots of percentage activity remaining against time

Purification of the protease

The initial steps in the purification of the protease permitted essentially complete solubilisation of the protease. Fractionation of the solubilized protease between 1.2 M and 2.55 M ammonium sulphate was accompanied by a variable increase in

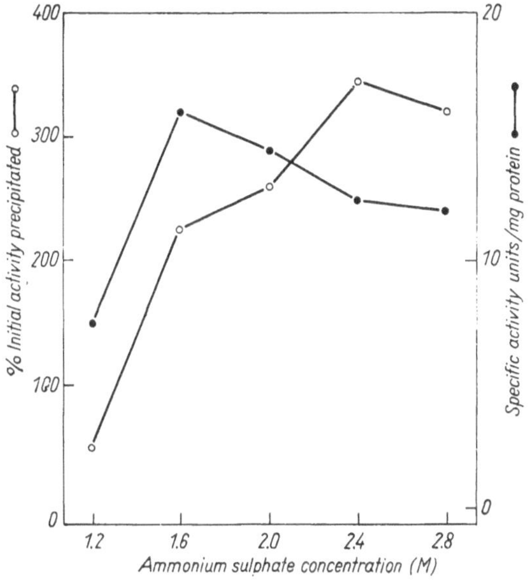

Fig. 2. Effect of ammonium sulphate on the solubility of the protease.
Solid ammonium sulphate was added to equal amounts of S2 containing proteolytic activity to give the indicated concentration. The precipitate was separated from the supernatant by centrifugation and after dialysis of the redissolved pellet, proteolytic activity and protein were determined. Total activity (O) is expressed as a percentage of the original value for the unfractionated S2 material

total activity towards malate dehydrogenase (Fig. 2). Subsequent desalting and concentration of the 2.55 M supernatant revealed the presence of an inhibitory activity towards the protease.

Nature of the protease

The effects of known modifiers of proteolytic enzymes on the intracellular protease (as purified to the ammonium sulphate stage) were investigated (Table 1). The

Table 1
The effect of modifiers on the protease

Modifier	Concentration	Percentage activity
None	—	100
Soybean trypsin inhibitor	5 μM	0
Lima bean trypsin inhibitor	10 μM	0
Benzamidine	1 mM	12
Proflavin	0.5 mM	22
α-N-benzoyl-L-arginine	1 mM	54
D-tryptophan-0-Me	1 mM	100
Pepstatin	0.36 mM	100
EDTA	10 mM	100
$CaCl_2$	1 mM	100
2-mercaptoethanol	15 mM	100
p-hydroxymercuribenzoate	0.1 mM	100

Protease (10 units) was preincubated with the indicated concentrations of modifiers for 5 min before determination of residual activity towards malate dehydrogenase. Results are expressed as the percentage of activity observed compared to the activity measured in the absence of modifiers.

trypsin-like nature of the protease suggests that it is different to the other proteases that have been reported to exist in muscle tissue.

Gel filtration of the protease preparation gave a single peak of activity towards malate dehydrogenase, corresponding to a molecular weight of 33,000.

Since malate dehydrogenase is itself sensitive to *p*H changes, a conventional *p*H/activity curve could not be determined. However, a study of the effect of *p*H on the stability of the protease (Fig. 3) indicated that the activity was stable over a narrow *p*H range centred at slightly alkaline *p*H. This contrasts with trypsin, which shows a broad range of *p*H values over which it is stable.

The protease also appeared to be different from trypsin in having a marked ability to inactivate native enzymes compared to its ability to degrade denatured protein substrates. If the azocasein degrading abilities of trypsin and the muscle protease are equated as an approximate measure of general digesting capacity, then it can be seen that the intracellular protease is one to two orders of magnitude more

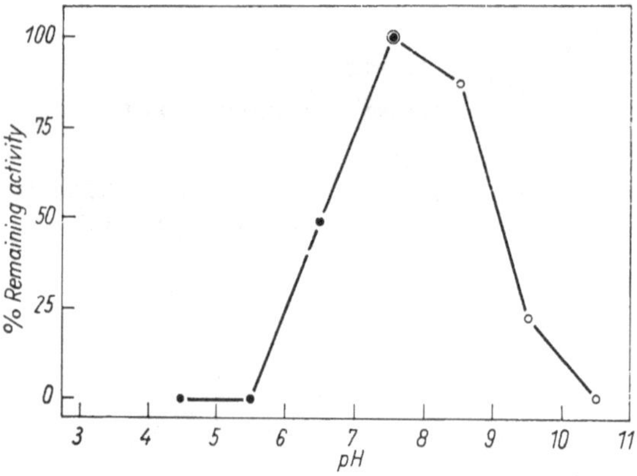

Fig. 3. Effect of *p*H on the stability of the protease.

Samples of protease were incubated at 30 °C for 60 min at the indicated *p*H, before returning the *p*H to 7.5 and assaying residual activity towards malate dehydrogenase. Results are expressed as a percentage of activity compared to a control sample kept at *p*H 7.5. (●) 0.01 M succinate/NaOH buffer, (○) 0.01 M glycine/NaOH buffer

Table 2
The inactivation of native enzymes by the intestinal protease and trypsin

Substrate	Units	
	Trypsin	Intestinal muscle protease
Azocasein	10	10
Azoalbumin	1.2	1.1
Malate dehydrogenase	0.10	5.0
Glutamate dehydrogenase	0.21	5.1
Isocitrate dehydrogenase	*	17.5
Lactate dehydrogenase	<0.01	0.4
Glucose 6-phosphate dehydrogenase	0.03	1.5
Phosphorylase *b*	2.0	200
Urease	0	0

* not determined

Units of azocasein and azoalbumin are as previously described, and units of activity towards native enzymes are the same as defined for malate dehydrogenase. The loss of activity of each enzyme was monitored during incubation with intestinal protease or trypsin, and recalculated on the basis of equal azocasein degrading activity (10 units).

efficient than trypsin at catalysing the inactivation of several native enzymes (Table 2). However, since the preparation is not homogeneous, a more exact determination is not possible at this stage.
Studies on the extent of proteolysis of glutamate dehydrogenase, phosphorylase (see [15]) and malate dehydrogenase using sodium dodecyl sulphate polyacrylamide gel electrophoresis showed that the extent of proteolysis was fairly limited in the first two cases, but that malate dehydrogenase was more extensively proteolyzed.
Saturating concentrations of the cofactors NADH (for malate dehydrogenase), and NAD^+ (for glutamate dehydrogenase) caused a reduction of 50% in the rate of inactivation of these enzymes. In addition, the rate of inactivation of malate dehydrogenase was slowed markedly at high ionic strength, but this was due to an effect on the susceptibility of the substrate to alterations in its ionic environment rather than on the protease (unpublished observations). No significant hydrolytic activity was observed towards the trypsin substrates tosyl arginine methyl ester and benzoyl arginine ethyl ester, the chymotrypsin substrates, acetyl tyrosine ethyl ester and benzoyl tyrosine ethyl ester or the elastase substrate N-tert. butyloxycarbonyl alanine p-nitrophenol ester.

Inhibitors of the protease

The intestinal muscle protease seems to fit the criteria expected of a neutral protease which might have a role in protein catabolism in that it shows a neutral *p*H optimum and has a considerable ability to inactivate native enzymes. It might be predicted that the protease would itself be controlled in some way, and the action of intracellular inhibitors would provide one possibility. As mentioned already, marked but variable increases in total protease activity were observed on ammonium sulphate fractionation of the muscle protease (Fig. 2). Desalting and concentration of the 2.55 M ammonium sulphate supernatant revealed the presence of an inhibitory activity (Fig. 4). This suggests that the protease might exist in a partially inhibited form although the possibility that homogenisation exposes the protease to an inhibitor pool, which is normally remote from it, cannot be excluded.

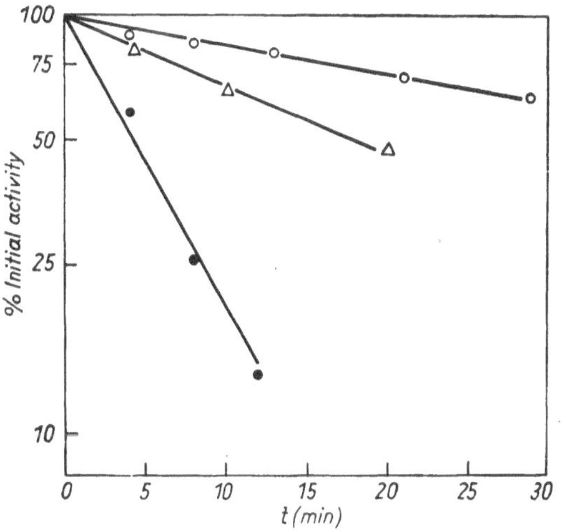

Fig. 4. Effect of endogenous inhibitors on the protease.

Samples of protease were preincubated for 5 min with 50 µl of S1 from rats fed on normal diets (Δ), 10 µl of desalted, concentrated 2.55 M ammonium sulphate supernatant (○), or without inhibitor (●). The loss of malate dehydrogenase activity was followed in an assay initiated by addition of the substrate enzyme

Table 3
The effect of various dietary manipulations on the levels of protease and inhibitor in the muscle layer of the small intestine

Diet	Period	% Weight change	Units/g small intstine muscle	
			S1 Inhibitor	S2 Protease
Normal (perfused gut)	—	~+10	550	3.5
Normal (unperfused gut)	—	~+10	581	4.1
8% Casein, Niacin Deficient diet	6 weeks	0	*	10
2% casein, 6% gelatin Niacin adequate diet	3 weeks	−10	0	140
Protein free diet (perfused gut)	3 weeks	−27	0	245
Protein free diet (unperfused gut)	3 weeks	−27	0	220
Starvation	3 days	−14	327	9

* not determined

The initial supernatant fraction (S1) also contained inhibitory activity towards the protease (Fig. 4). The levels of inhibitor in this fraction, as isolated from rats in which the gut had been perfused prior to dissection, were similar to those from unperfused tissues (Table 3) which suggests that contamination by plasma inhibitors is not a likely source of the inhibitory activity.

It has also been observed that the inactivation of malate dehydrogenase at low protease levels deviated from linear first order kinetics. This was not due to a time dependent denaturation of the protease, but resulted from a form of product inhibition, presumably by (a) peptide (s) from proteolysis of the malate dehydrogenase. Since the malate dehydrogenase was from pig heart and not from rat intestine, and since the subcellular location of the protease has not yet been determined, the precise significance of this observation to the in vivo situation remains to be elucidated.

The relationship between nutritional status and the levels of protease and inhibitor

Preliminary data have suggested that the level of the protease in vivo may be altered in response to changes in the level of dietary protein. No evidence was obtained to support a correlation with the level of niacin in the diet (Table 3), but marked increases in protease activity, accompanied by reduction in the inhibitor level in S1, occurred when animals were deprived of dietary protein. This increase in protease activity occurred rather late during protein deprivation (unpublished observation). Starvation depleted the inhibitor pool in S1 but caused only a slight increase in the protease level in S2. The situation is at present unclear and further studies are being undertaken to rationalise these findings. Perfusion of the vascular bed of the gut did not significantly alter the level of protease observed.

Discussion

The proteolytic activity which is capable of inactivating malate dehydrogenase appeared to be membrane-limited, and could be solubilized by a number of treatments. Characterisation studies performed on the protease indicate it to be a trypsin-like serine protease, in that it was inhibited by soybean and lima bean trypsin inhibitors, benzamidine, proflavin and α-N-benzoyl arginine. No inhibition was observed by the chymotrypsin inhibitor D-tryptophan 0-methyl ester, of with modifiers of thiol-, carboxyl- or metalloproteases. These results suggest that the protease is distinct from the Ca^{2+} activated protease [10] and the chymotrypsin-like histone degrading protease [8].

The intestinal protease differs from trypsin in a number of respects. The molecular weight, from gel filtration, was determined to be 33,000, and the protease was stable over a narrow *p*H range centred at slightly alkaline values. Trypsin has a molecular weight of 23,000 and is stable over a broad range of *p*H.

Since the intestinal muscle preparation was not homogeneous it is difficult to quantitate the amount of protease used in these studies and so compare the activity of this protease directly with that of trypsin. However, if the azocasein degrading activities of the two proteases are equated as an approximate measure of their general digesting abilities, then it can be seen (Table 2) that the intestinal muscle protease apparently has a greater ability than trypsin to inactivate native enzymes. Examination of the extents of digestion of phosphorylase [15], glutamate dehydrogenase and malate dehydrogenase by SDS-gel electrophoresis indicated that the proteolysis was quite limited in all cases.

If a comparison is made of the properties of the intestinal smooth muscle protease and the group specific protease of KATUNUMA et al. [12] which is active towards apo-pyridoxal enzymes, then it would appear that these are not the same. The latter protease [12] has been shown to be chymotrypsin-like with a high activity towards N-acetyl tyrosine ethyl ester whereas the intestinal muscle protease does not hydrolyse this nor any other of the esters tested. However, there is a general similarity of the intestinal muscle protease to another group-specific protease (whose preliminary description has suggested it to be "specific" towards NAD-dependent enzymes [11]). The question of "group-specificity" is by no means resolved since it can be seen (Table 4) that a similar order of susceptibility to proteolysis is obtained for native enzymes when trypsin and the intestinal muscle protease are compared, even although the intracellular protease, in quantitative terms, is about two orders of magnitude more efficient in its proteolytic capacity. Thus, it would seem that it is the susceptibility of the substrate enzyme which determines the ease of proteolysis and that this is the basis of the "specificity"

Table 4
The relative rates of inactivation of native enzymes by trypsin and intestinal muscle protease

Native enzymes ranked in order of ease of inactivation by:

Trypsin	High	*Intestinal muscle protease*
Phosphorylase *b*	↓	Phosphorylase *b*
Glutamate dehydrogenase		Glutamate dehydrogenase
Malate dehydrogenase		Malate dehydrogenase
Glucose-6-phosphate dehydrogenase		Glucose-6-phosphate dehydrogenase
Lactate dehydrogenase		Lactate dehydrogenase
Urease	Low	Urease

observed here. This is supported by the observations that proteins with short half-lives in vivo are proteolysed more readily by pancreatic, bacterial [16] and lysosomal proteases [17] in vitro.

Thus, it could be possible for the intestinal muscle protease to have a function in vivo wherein it inactivates enzymes in their native conformation. The rate at which this proteolysis occurs could be defined by the susceptibility of the substrate enzyme which could thus control its own rate of turnover. The main consequence of this would be the loss to the cell of the expression of that particular enzymic activity. The large fragments produced by limited proteolysis would be of lesser importance to the cell and so could be removed by a "general" (lysosomal?) mechanism at a rate which needs not necessarily be of direct importance (Fig. 5).

Native enzyme (non-susceptible form) ⇌ (1) Native enzyme (susceptible form)

Inactivation ↓ (2)

non functional product

↓ (3)

non selective removal

Fig. 5. A postulated scheme of removal of enzyme activity in the cell

In step 1, each enzyme could determine its particular rate of degradation, and factors such as cofactor or ligand binding, association/dissociation phenomena or covalent modification could alter the equilibrium position at this stage. As examples of this, nicotinamide coenzymes protected malate and glutamate dehydrogenases from inactivation by the intestinal muscle protease, and several allosteric ligands modified the susceptibility of phosphorylases *a* and *b* to proteolysis [15]. Step 2, leading to inactivation, could be neutral proteolysis which would then direct the protein fragments for complete degradation, perhaps by facilitating binding to the lysosomal membrane [6] or by some other process.

This initial proteolysis would, however, not necessarily have to lead to inactivation, and examples have been reported where relatively limited proteolytic cleavage has actually activated [13, 18] or modified [19] an enzymic activity. These active but nicked proteins might then more readily enter the subsequent degradative process.

It would be reasonable to suggest that a neutral protease acting in this capacity would be finely controlled, and inhibitory activity towards the intestinal protease was demonstrated in the initial supernatant (S1) of rats fed on a normal diet. The level of this inhibitor fell on administration of a protein free diet, with a concomitant rise in protease level. It is not yet known whether protein deprivation was accompanied exclusively by increase in total protease, or by a decrease in total inhibitor, or whether both events occurred simultaneously. Prior perfusion of the vascular bed of the gut of control animals was without significant effect on the levels of S1 inhibitory activity, and similarly, the level of protease in S2 was not affected by perfusion of the gut of protein depleted animals. The protease and inhibitor preparations would therefore seem to be essentially free of contamination either from plasma inhibitors or granulocyte proteases. One report has appeared [20] which describes evidence for the intracellular existence of plasma protease inhibitors, but the significance of this observation to these studies is not yet clear.

Thus, control of the proteolytic activity could be regulated directly or indirectly in several ways; 1) through the action of endogenous inhibitors; 2) by the proteolytic susceptibility of the substrate enzymes, and 3) by the alteration of this susceptibility by ligand binding or other modification. Further studies are in progress to elucidate the relationships between these processes.

Acknowledgements

Supported by MRC Grant No. G974/126/B. RJB thanks the SRC for a Studentship and the Catherine and Lady Grace James Foundation for travel assistance, We wish to thank Drs. G. M. Powell and C. G. Curtis of this Department for performing the perfusion experiments

References

[1] Goldberg, A. L., and A. C. St. John: A. Rev. Biochem. **45**, 747—803 (1976)
[2] Dice, J. F., P. J. Dehlinger, and R. T. Schimke: J. biol. Chem. **248**, 4220—4228 (1973)
[3] Dean, R. T.: Nature, Lond. **257**, 414—416 (1975)
[4] Ray, D., E. Cornell, and D. Schneider: Biochem. biophys. Res. Commun. **71**, 1246—1250 (1976)
[5] Neely, A. N., and G. E. Mortimore: Biochem. biophys. Res. Commun. **59**, 680—687 (1974)
[6] Dean, R. T.: Biochem. biophys. Res. Commun. **67**, 604—609 (1975)
[7] Segal, H. L., G. A. Dunaway, and J. R. Winkler in: Proteolysis and Physiological Regulation. D. W. Ribbons and K. Brew (Eds). Academic Press, New York 1976, pp. 287—308
[8] Jusic, M., S. Seifert, E. Weiss, R. Haas, and P. C. Heinrich: Archs Biochem. Biophys. **177**, 355—363 (1976)
[9] Duckworth, W. C., M. Heinemann, and A. E. Kitabchi: Biochim. biophys. Acta **377**, 421—425 (1975)
[10] Dayton, W. R., D. E. Goll, M. G. Zeece, R. M. Robson, and W. J. Reville: Biochemistry **15**, 2150—2158 (1976)
[11] Katunuma, N., E. Kominami, S. Kominami, K. Kito, and T. Matsuzawa in: Metabolic Interconversions of Enzymes. O. Wieland, E. Helmreich, and H. Holzer (Eds). Springer Verlag, Berlin 1972, pp. 159—174
[12] Katunuma, N., E. Kominami, K. Kobayashi, Y. Banno, K. Suzuki, K. Chichibu, and T. Katsunuma: Eur. J. Biochem. **52**, 37—50 (1975)
[13] Beynon, R. J., and J. Kay: Int. J. Biochem. **7**, 449—455 (1976)
[14] Weber, K. and M. Osborne: J. biol. Chem. **244**, 4406—4412 (1969)
[15] Kay, J., I. T. Carney and R. J. Beynon: Acta biol. med. germ. **36**, 1637 (1977)
[16] Goldberg, A. L., E. M. Howell, J. B. Li, S. B. Martel, and W. F. Prouty: Fedn Proc. Fedn Am. Socs exp. Biol. **33**, 1112—1120 (1974)
[17] Segal, H. L., J. R. Winkler, and M. P. Miyagi: J. biol. Chem. **249**, 6364—6365 (1974)
[18] Kuczenski, R.: J. biol. Chem. **248**, 2261—2265 (1973)
[19] Nakashima, K., and B. L. Horecker: Archs Biochem. Biophys. **146**, 153—160 (1971)
[20] Twining, S. S., and A. S. Brecher: Clinica chim. Acta **75**, 143—148 (1977)

Acta biol. med. germ., Band 36, Seite 1637—1644 (1977)

Department of Biochemistry, University College, Cardiff CF1 1XL, Wales, U.K.

The susceptibility of glycogen phosphorylase to inactivation by endogenous and exogenous proteases

JOHN KAY, IAN T. CARNEY, and ROBERT J. BEYNON

Summary

Phosphorylases *a* and *b* were inactivated very rapidly by a neutral, trypsin-like protease from rat intestinal muscle. With ^{32}P-phosphorylase *a* as substrate, it was shown that the initial event in the inactivation was the release of a small, phosphopeptide from the N-terminus of the enzyme, leaving the original 100,000 subunit form virtually unchanged. Subsequent proteolysis was very limited, producing 85, 70 and 65,000 mol. wt. derivatives.

The effects of several allosteric modulators of phosphorylase on the rates of inactivation of the two enzymes were studied. Removal of the pyridoxal phosphate cofactor from phosphorylase increased the susceptibility of the *b* form by three fold while the *a* form was unaffected.

By comparison of these effects with those obtained from digestion with trypsin and chymotrypsin, it is concluded that the intestinal muscle protease has a markedly enhanced ability for inactivating enzymes in their native conformation. Assuming that this property is reflected in vivo, a possible role such neutral proteases in initiating protein degradation is advanced.

Introduction

Phosphorylase fulfils a vital role in controlling the turnover of glycogen in various cells and, in skeletal muscle, in particular, it can constitute up to about 3% of the protein present. The enzyme contains pyridoxal phosphate as a prosthetic group and exists as an oligomeric protein composed of monomers, dimers or tetramers of a 100,000 subunit. Its activity is subject to precise regulation both by allosteric modulators and by a 3′,5′ cyclic AMP dependent phosphorylation-dephosphorylation of a single serine residue at position 14 in the polypeptide chain [1]. This phosphorylation converts phosphorylase *b* (which is inactive unless certain allosteric activators e. g. AMP are present) into active phosphorylase *a* and changes the response of the enzyme to various allosteric modifiers.

The turnover of such a major catalytic protein in muscle is therefore important since changes in the total amount of enzyme would have profound consequences in the cell. It has been suggested [2] that there might be extra-lysosomal proteolytic enzymes to initiate protein degradation so that it was of interest to see whether a protease such as that from intestinal muscle would be able to inactivate a muscle enzyme like phosphorylase and whether the phosphorylated and dephosphorylated forms of the enzyme might exhibit different susceptibilities. Since it has been shown [2] that the intestinal muscle protease has a trypsin-like activity, comparisons have been made with the effects of trypsin and chymotrypsin on phosphorylase. It has been known for some time [3] that phosphorylase is much more susceptible to trypsin than to chymotrypsin or other exogenous proteases.

Materials and methods

The intestinal muscle preparation was obtained as described by Beynon and Kay [2]. Rabbit skeletal muscle phosphorylase *a* was obtained from Boehringer Corp. Ltd. Phosphorylase *b* and ^{32}P-labelled phosphorylase *a* were kind gifts from Dr. P. Cohen. Trypsin, chymotrypsin, soybean trypsin inhibitor and agarose-soybean trypsin inhibitor were products of Miles Laboratories Ltd.

Samples for scintillation counting were placed in vials containing 10 ml of PCS scintillant (Amersham-Searle) and counted in a Beckman LS100 liquid scintillation counter.

Phosphorylase *b* activity was measured in the presence of 1 mM AMP whereas phosphorylase *a* was assayed without AMP [4].

Proteolytic inactivations were performed at 30 °C by dissolving 0.5 mg of phosphorylase in 0.1 ml of 0.1 M maleate buffer, *p*H 6.8 (for *b*), or 0.05 M glycerophosphate buffer, *p*H 6.8 + 1 mM EDTA (for *a*) and adding 0.2 ml of 0.05 M pyrophosphate buffer, *p*H 8.5. The final *p*H was 8.4. Reactions were started by addition of protease in a small volume (1 – 5 µl) and samples were removed for assay of the phosphorylase activity remaining at various times. For SDS-polyacrylamide gel electrophoresis [5], samples containing approximately 30 µg of protein were removed and prepared as described previously [6].

In digestions of ^{32}P-phosphorylase *a*, samples (20 µl) were removed into 0.2 ml of 20% TCA. Soybean trypsin inhibitor (0.5 mg) was added as a carrier to ensure complete precipitation of the protein. After centrifugation, the supernatants were removed for scintillation counting while the pellets were washed extensively with 4% TCA before being dissolved in 0.2 ml of 0.1 M NaOH. Samples of these (0.05 ml) were added to 10 ml of PCS scintillant and stored overnight in the dark before counting.

The SDS-polyacrylamide gels obtained from the ^{32}P-phosphorylase *a* digest were sliced into the various protein bands. These were swollen in 0.5 ml of NCS tissue solubiliser (Amersham-Searle) for 6 h at 50 °C. PCS scintillant (10 ml) was added to each extract and the samples were kept in the dark for a few days before counting.

Results

From the inactivation profiles (Fig. 1) it can be seen that 1 µl of the intestinal muscle protease preparation inactivated phosphorylase *b* with a pseudo first order rate constant (K_{app}) of 0.024 min^{-1} whereas phosphorylase *a* was more resistant since 2 µl of the preparation produced a K_{app} of 0.015 min^{-1}. However, SDS-gel electrophoresis (Figs. 2 and 3) showed that the extent of digestion in both cases was very restricted, producing fragments of approximate mol. wts. 85, 70 and 65,000. Even when virtually all of the enzymic activity had been removed, virtually all of the protein remained in the position of the original 100,000 subunit. This suggested that the inactivation was being effected by the removal of a small

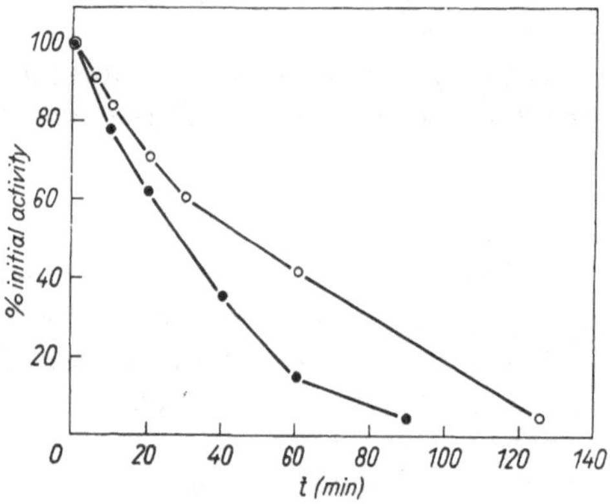

Fig. 1. Incubation of phosphorylases *a* and *b* with intestinal muscle protease.

Phosphorylase *b* (●) and phosphorylase *a* (○) were incubated (0.5 mg of each) at 30 °C in 0.3 ml of maleate/pyrophosphate buffer or glycerophosphate/pyrophosphate buffer, *p*H 8.4, with 1 and 2 µl, respectively, of the protease preparation.

Phosphorylase activity was assayed in the presence of AMP (1 mM) for phosphorylase *b* but without any ligands for phosphorylase *a*

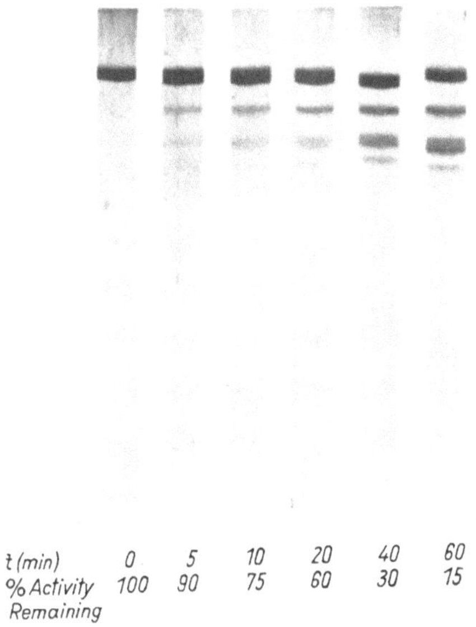

Fig. 2

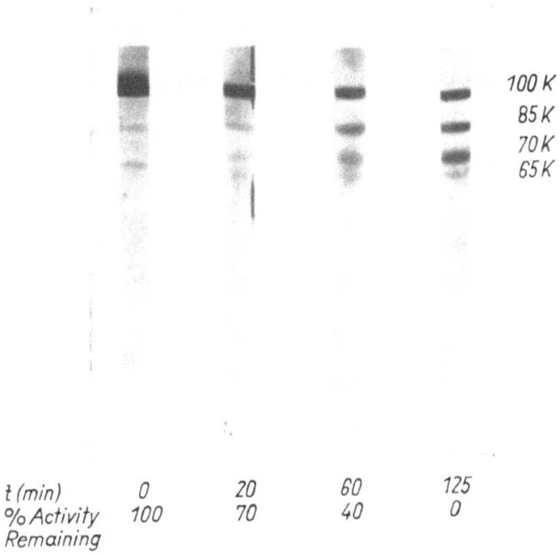

Fig. 3

Fig. 2. The extent of digestion of phosphorylase *b* by the intestinal muscle protease. Incubations were carried out as described in the legend to Fig. 1 and samples (20 μl) were removed at the indicated times and added to 0.2 ml of insolubilized soybean trypsin inhibitor. After centrifugation, the supernatants were freeze-dried before analysis by SDS-gel electrophoresis

Fig. 3. The extent of digestion of phosphorylase *a* by the intestinal muscle protease. Incubations and preparation of samples for SDS-gel electrophoresis were carried out as described in the legends to Figs. 1 and 2

peptide from one end of the polypeptide chain. Since the sole phosphoserine residue in phosphorylase *a* occurs at residue 14 in a basic region of the polypeptide chain and is believed to extend away from the main body of the subunit [7], it might therefore be exposed, thus facilitating attack by a trypsin-like protease.

Accordingly, ^{32}P-labelled phosphorylase *a* was treated with the intestinal muscle protease (Fig. 4) and the release of ^{32}P containing material from a TCA insoluble to a soluble form paralleled the loss in enzymic activity. SDS-gels showed the expected banding pattern and when the various protein bands were extracted and counted, it was found that the radioactivity was lost from the 100,000 subunit position at a similar rate to the loss of enzymic activity (Fig. 4). No radioactive label could be detected in any of the other protein bands produced by digestion.

By examination of the SDS-gel patterns, it appeared that, although the *a* form was relatively more resistant to proteolysis by the endogenous protease, the digestion patterns obtained with both forms were very similar. Thus, it was of interest to examine the effects of several known allosteric modifiers of both *a* and *b* forms on the susceptibilities of the two enzymes to proteolysis.

The effects of various ligands on the rate of inactivation of phosphorylase *b* can be grouped into three classes (Table 1) — those ligands with no effect, those which

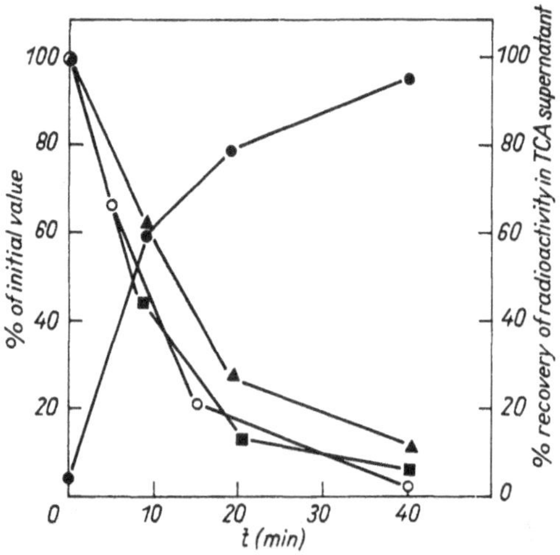

Fig. 4. Inactivation of ^{32}P- phosphorylase *a* by the intestinal muscle protease. ^{32}P-phosphorylase *a* (0.33 mg; $1.54 \cdot 10^4$ dpm) was incubated at 30 °C in 0.15 ml of 0.05 M glycerophosphate/0.05 M pyrophosphate buffer, *p*H 8.4, with 5 µl of intestinal muscle protease. Samples were removed 1) for assay of phosphorylase activity remaining (○); 2) and added to 0.2 ml of 20% trichloroacetic acid containing 0.5 mg of carrier soybean trypsin inhibitor. After centrifugation, the supernatants were counted (●) and after washing with 4% trichloroacetic acid, the insoluble material (▲) was taken up in 0.2 ml of 0.1 M NaOH for scintillation counting; 3) samples for SDS-gel electrophoresis were treated as described in the legend to Fig. 2. After staining with Coomassie Blue and destaining electrophoretically, each individual protein band was sliced out from the gel, swollen and counted. The radioactivity in the position of the 100,000 subunit is shown (■). No counts could be detected in any of the other bands

Table 1

The effect of various ligands on the rate of inactivation of phosphorylases *a* and *b* by rat intestinal muscle protease. Values for the pseudo first order rate constants (K_{app}) are given

Ligand	Phosphorylase *b*	Phosphorylase *a*
	$K_{app} \cdot 10^2$ (min^{-1})	$K_{app} \cdot 10^2$ (min^{-1})
None	2.2	0.77
UDP-glucose (10 mM)	2.3	0.26
NADH (1 mM)	2.8	n. d.
Glucose-6-P (3 mM)	1.1	0.72
IMP (3 mM)	1.3	0.17
Adenine (3 mM)	1.3	n. d.
Phosphate (10 mM)	1.5	0.19
AMP (2 mM)	0.27	0.17
CMP (2 mM)	0.25	0.38

n. d. = not determined.

reduced the rate of proteolysis by about half and those which stabilised the enzyme against inactivation. In contrast, some of these ligands had different protective effects on the inactivation of phosphorylase *a*. Glucose-6-phosphate protected the *b* form by about 50% but had no effect on the inactivation of phosphorylase *a*. In contrast, UDP-glucose had no effect in protecting phosphorylase *b* but could partially reduce the rate of inactivation of phosphorylase *a*. IMP stabilised phosphorylase *a* but only afforded partial protection to phosphorylase *b*. CMP produced precisely the opposite situation.

All of the ligands that had a protective effect on the proteolysis of the enzymes bind to the V-shaped cleft that contains the active site of phosphorylase [7]. Although recent X-ray crystallographic studies have shown that, in addition to this, the enzyme has another "dinucleotide fold" structure similar to that found in dehydrogenases, NADH had no protective effect.

The function of the pyridoxal phosphate cofactor in phosphorylase has not been elucidated but since it has been suggested that the N-terminal region of the protein is involved in interations with the cofactor [8] it was of interest to see whether removal of the cofactor from phosphorylases *a* and *b* might affect the extents of proteolysis. It has already been shown that this proteolysis takes place at the N-terminal region.

Apo-phosphorylase *b* was about three fold more susceptible to the intestinal muscle protease than its corresponding holo-form (Fig. 5) whereas, in contrast, the removal of the cofactor from the *a* form had no appreciable effect.

In order to get some sort of quantitative assessment of the susceptibility of holo-phosphorylase to the intestinal muscle protease, inactivations of the *b* form with trypsin and chymotrypsin were carried out (Fig. 6). Under these digestion conditions, trypsin (5 µg) produced inactivation with K_{app} of 0.14 min^{-1} whereas chymotrypsin (5 µg) was slightly less efficient (K_{app} = 0.09 min^{-1}). Examination of the SDS-gels (Figs. 7 and 8) showed different degradation patterns, both of which were different, in turn from that obtained with the intestinal muscle protease. Trypsin and chymotrypsin both rapidly removed the 100,000 subunit although their patterns of degradation still seemed to be relatively limited.

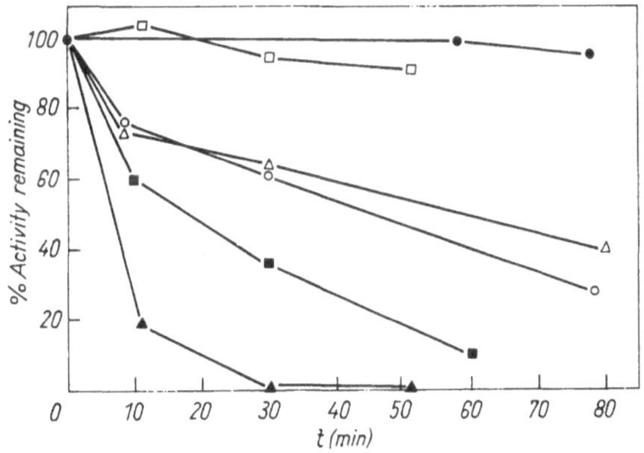

Fig. 5. Comparison of the susceptibilities of apo- and holo-phosphorylases *a* and *b* to the intestinal muscle protease.

Apophosphorylases *a* (△) and *b* (▲) were incubated with 2 µl of the intestinal muscle protease as described in the legend to Fig. 1 except that the incubation temp. was 25 °C. Samples were removed and preincubated with 0.06 mM pyridoxal phosphate for 30 min to reconstitute holoenzyme before assay of the activity remaining. Holophosphorylase *a* (○) and *b* (■) were incubated with the protease at 25 °C as described in the legend to Fig. 1. Apophosphorylases *a* (●) and *b* (△) were quite stable without protease

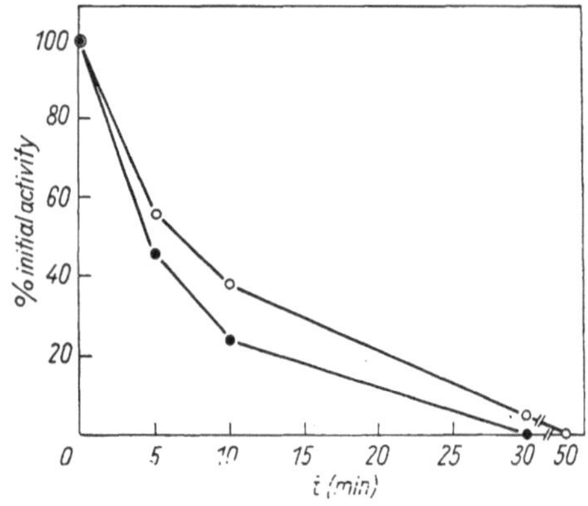

Fig. 6. Inactivation of holophosphorylase *b* by trypsin and chymotrypsin. Phosphorylase *b* (0.5 mg) was incubated at 30 °C with 5 μg of trypsin (●) or chymotrypsin (○) as described in the legend to Fig. 1

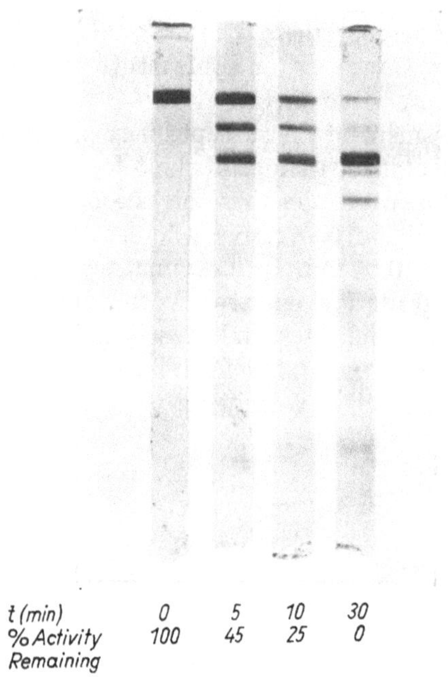

Fig. 7

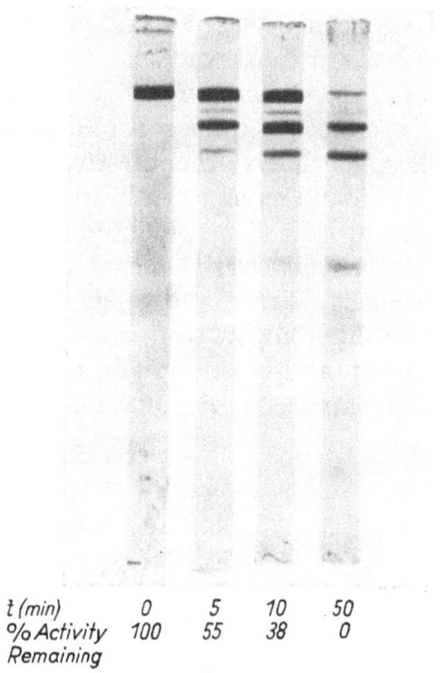

Fig. 8

Fig. 7. The extent of digestion of holophosphorylase *b* by trypsin. Incubations and preparation of samples for SDS-gel electrophoresis were carried out as described in the legends to Figs. 6 and 2

Fig. 8. The extent of digestion of holophosphorylase *b* by chymotrypsin. Conditions as for Fig. 7

Discussion

All three proteases inactivated phosphorylase *b* very rapidly while the *a* form was rather more resistant to digestion by the intestinal muscle protease (and to trypsin and chymotrypsin — see Table 2). The intestinal protease appeared to catalyse the hydrolysis of only a few peptide bonds since a virtually unchanged 100,000 subunit persisted as the major protein band throughout the course of the inactivations. Confirmation of this was obtained from the studies with ^{32}P-phosphorylase *a* where the protease released the radioactive label into a TCA soluble form at a similar rate to the loss in enzymic activity. The loss of radioactivity from both the TCA insoluble material and the original 100,000 subunit obtained on gel electrophoresis, also paralleled the loss in enzymic activity. Thus, it would appear that the initial step is a cleavage close to the N-terminus of phosphorylase resulting in loss of activity and phosphopeptide but leaving the molecular weight of the subunit essentially unchanged.

Table 2
Comparison of the abilities of several serine proteases for inactivating phosphorylases *a* and *b*

Protease	Specificity	Phosphorylase *b*	Phosphorylase *a*	
		$K_{app} \cdot 10^2$	$K_{app} \cdot 10^2$	Phosphopeptide release
Subtilisin[1]	broad	5.0	5.0	v. slow
Chymotrypsin[1]	Phe, Tyr, Trp	2.1	0.04	v. slow
Group-specific protease[2]	chymotrypsin-like	0.08	0.076	No
Trypsin[1]	Lys, Arg	3.1	0.87	Yes
Intestinal muscle protease	trypsin-like	184	57.6	Yes

Approximate pseudo first order rate constants have been calculated for each protease under roughly the following conditions (at 20° – 30 °C):
Phosphorylase *a* or *b*: approx. 0.5 – 3 mg/0.3 ml; protease 1 μg/0.3 ml

[1] Data from NOLAN et al. Biochem. **3**, 542 (1964)
[2] Data from MATSUDA and FISCHER in: Intracellular Protein Turnover, pp. 213 – 222. Academic Press, (1975)

In an attempt to compare the effects of several serine proteases on phosphorylases *a* and *b* quantitatively, Table 2 presents a very approximate summary of the pseudo first order rate constants that can be calculated from our data and from the literature [3, 9] accepting that small differences in experimental parameters such as temperature and phosphorylase concentration may introduce substantial errors. Since the intestinal muscle protease preparation was not homogeneous, it is difficult to quantitate the precise amount of protease used in our studies. However, if one equates its azocasein degrading ability with that of trypsin [2] as an approximate measure of the "general" digesting capacities of the two proteases, then 1 μl of the intestinal muscle preparation ≙ 0.013 μg of trypsin. This was the basis on which the figures (Table 2) for the intestinal muscle protease were obtained. Even allowing for this approximation to be in error by an order of magnitude, it can be seen that the intestinal muscle protease is considerably more active towards both forms of phosphorylase. In general, chymotrypsin-like enzymes do not appear to release the phosphopeptide from phosphorylase *a* and are relatively ineffective at inactivating the enzyme (apart from the microbial protease, subtilisin which "cuts" the enzyme in half [3, 10]). The "group-specific protease" of KATUNUMA et al. [11] appears to be the least efficient protease of all although the apo-form of phosphorylase *b* has been reported [9] to be 10 times more susceptible than the holo form.

Thus the intestinal muscle protease is different from trypsin, from the skeletal muscle group specific protease [9] and evidence in the previous paper [2] shows it to be different from the group-specific protease from intestinal muscle described by KATUNUMA et al. [11]. It must also be different from the myofibrillar protease [12] since it is not affected by Ca^{2+} and it was not isolated from skeletal muscle. Consequently, no attempt was made to assess its ability to digest the myofibrillar proteins of striated muscle. Instead, we have concentrated on one of the major catalytic proteins.

Thus with such a marked ability for inactivation of native enzymes, a possible role in the turnover of intracellular protein seems plausible. Inactivation of the substrate enzyme seems to be accompanied by limited proteolysis so as to generate large polypeptides. This "priming" reaction might facilitate uptake and further degradation of these polypeptide fragments by the lysosomes. However, the subcellular location of the intestinal muscle protease has not been determined so that whether it would have free access to these substrate enzymes remains to be elucidated, particularly since it seems to be membrane-limited in some way.

The existence of specific inhibitors for the protease [2] affords one method of regulation of the proteolytic activity, but, in addition, further control through changes in susceptibility of the substrate enzyme could be effective. Thus, from this data, the control of glycogen turnover not only depends on the phosphorylation-dephosphorylation cycle of the phosphorylase $b \rightarrow a$ transition but can also be affected by changes in the susceptibility ot the particular form of phosphorylase to proteolysis and regulation of this by cellular levels of important metabolites which can affect the enzyme allosterically.

Acknowledgement

Supported by the MRC (Grant No. G974/126/B). ITC acknowledges the receipt of an SRC/CASE Studentship in cooperation with Miles Laboratories. RJB thanks the SRC for a Studentship. We are very grateful to Dr. PHILIP COHEN, University of Dundee for his generosity and his constant encouragement.

References

[1] GRAVES, D. J., and J. H. WANG in: The Enzymes. P. D. BOYER (Ed.). **7**, 435–482, Academic Press, London, New York 1972
[2] BEYNON, R. J., and J. KAY: Acta biol. med. germ. **36**, 1625 (1977)
[3] NOLAN, C., W. B. NOVOA, E. G. KREBS, and E. H. FISCHER: Biochemistry **3**, 542–551 (1964)
[4] CARNEY, I. T., R. J. BEYNON, J. KAY and N. BIRKETT: Analyt. Biochem. **84** (1978) (in press)
[5] WEBER, K., and M. OSBORNE: J. biol. Chem. **244**, 4406–4412 (1969)
[6] BEYNON, R. J., and J. KAY: Int. J. Biochem. **7**, 449–453 (1976)
[7] FLETTERICK, R. J., J. SYGUSCH, H. SEMPLE, and N. B. MADSEN: J. biol. Chem. **251**, 6142–6146 (1976)
[8] GRAVES, D. J., G. CARLSON, J. SKUSLER, R. PARRISH, T. CARLY and G. TESSMER: J. biol. Chem. **250**, 2254–2258 (1975)
[9] MATSUDA, Y. and E. H. FISCHER in: Intracellular Protein Turnover. R. T. SCHIMKE, and N. KATUNUMA (Eds.). Academic Press, New York 1975, pp. 213–222
[10] RIBAUD, O., and M. E. GOLDBERG: Biochemistry **12**, 5154–5161 (1973)
[11] KATUNUMA, N., E. KOMINAMI, K. KOBAYASHI, Y. BANNO, K. SUZUKI, K. CHICHIBU, Y. HAMAGUCHI and T. KATSUNUMA: Eur. J. Biochem. **52**, 37–50 (1975)
[12] DAYTON, W. R., D. E. GOLL, M. G. ZEECE, R. M. ROBSON and W. J. REVILLE: Biochemistry **15**, 2150–2158 (1976)

Acta biol. med germ., Band 36, Seite 1645—1652 (1977)

Department of Physiology and Biophysics, University of Iowa, Iowa City, Iowa, 52242, U.S.A.

Studies on the possible physiological controls of skeletal muscle proteases

W. T. STAUBER, A. M. HEDGE, and B. A. SCHOTTELIUS[1]

Summary

This work compares the autolytic activity in homogenates from a red anterior latissimus dorsi (ALD) (tonic) and a white posterior latissimus dorsi (PLD) (phasic) avian skeletal muscle. Autolytic activity was stimulated by either calcium or magnesium ions at 10^{-3} M at *p*H 4.0, 7.0, and 8.5. At neutral *p*H (7.0), the addition of calcium at physiological concentrations (10^{-4} M) in the presence of physiological concentrations of magnesium (10^{-3} M) yielded for both muscles about 50% of the maximal activity obtained with 10^{-3} M calcium, whereas a total calcium concentration of 10^{-7} M with 10^{-3} M magnesium abolished almost all the autolytic activity. This indicates that physiological shifts of calcium ion concentrations in skeletal muscle tissues, which normally contain more than 10^{-3} M magnesium, can regulate at least one protease active at physiological *p*H values.
Other studies on skeletal muscle proteases using the artificial substrate, N-benzoyl-DL-arginine-β-naphthylamide (BANA), were begun as a result of the observation that commercial collagenase preparations used in our cell preparation techniques contained an ion-activated hydrolase (Clostripain) which was active at neutral *p*H and degraded BANA. At least two BANA hydrolase activities were assayable in skeletal muscle-H_2O extracts demonstrating acid and neutral-alkaline activities. These activities were inhibited by either homogenization of muscle in Hank's solution or by the addition of 1 mM ATP, being most pronounced for the PLD muscle.

Introduction

A variety of proteases covering the *p*H range 4—9 have been described for skeletal muscle [1—5] and most have been implicated in normal protein turnover and in muscle diseases. However, only a few have been purified and evaluated for activity on native proteins [1, 2, 5]. The paucity of information concerning the physiological control of protein degradation has left the interpretation of such data obscure. We have undertaken investigations to test the hypothesis that physiological fluctuations in calcium, and perhaps magnesium, result in increased proteolysis [6] either directly by altering protease activity or indirectly by inhibiting the production of ATP.
The chicken anterior latissimus dorsi (ALD) and posterior latissimus dorsi (PLD) skeletal muscles were chosen for study because of the homogeneity of fiber types [7] and because tonic and phasic muscles have different rates of protein turnover [8]. The tonic, ALD, muscle would be expected to have higher protein turnover rates than the phasic, PLD, muscle. The ALD contains more cathepsin D [9], cathepsin B and DAP II (unpublished observations) than the PLD muscle. This is consistent with a lysosomal role in protein turnover. However, in all muscle

[1] This work was supported in part by grants from the Muscular Dystrophy Association and the American Heart Association with local support from the Iowa Heart Association.

disease states so far investigated (denervation atrophy, starvation, and hereditary muscular dystrophy) except chloroquine-induced myopathy the PLD is preferentially affected. Therefore, it is not clear what role lysosomes actually play in normal and pathological protein degradation. Thus, we decided to measure autolysis at *p*H values where protease activity had been described [4] and to attempt to develop assay techniques for other muscle proteases.

Materials and methods

Autolysis studies

ALD and PLD muscle homogenates from young (at least 2 weeks old) Cornish-cross chickens were prepared as described elsewhere [6]. 1 ml of homogenate was added to 1 ml of buffer, covered and incubated for 3 hrs. The buffers used were 0.2 M acetate, *p*H 4.0; 0.2 M Tris-HCl, *p*H 7.0; 0.2 M Tris-HCl, *p*H 8.5. The reaction was stopped with cold TCA (10%), filtered, and tyrosine equivalents measured [10]. All determinations were made in triplicate.

BANA hydrolytic studies

Collagenase I and II (Sigma Chemical Co.) and Clostripain (Boehringer-Mannheim) were prepared (1 mg/ml) in either distilled water or Hank's solution (Table 4) and further diluted prior to use.

Extracts were prepared from the muscle homogenates, as described above (autolysis studies) by removal of a 1,000 $g \times 10$ min pellet. The supernatant contained most of the BANA hydrolytic activity and was used for these studies.

BANA hydrolytic activity was determined by the method of BLACKWOOD and MANDL [11] using N-benzoyl-DL-arginine-β-naphthylamide (BANA) as the substrate and modified as follows: 0.2 M Tris-HCl buffers were used for the entire *p*H range studied and the various reagents were added (at neutral *p*H) to these buffers. The assay mixture was incubated at 37 °C for times up to 6 hrs and each determination was made in duplicate.

BANA hydrolytic activity was tested at *p*H 6.2 and *p*H 7.0 for collagenase I and II and Clostripain. The results presented are for *p*H 7.0 but were quite similar to those found at *p*H 6.2.

Protein was determined by the method of LOWRY et al. [12] using human serum albumin as the standard.

Results

Autolysis

Autolytic activity resulting from the concerted action of many proteases and peptidases to produce TCA-soluble tyrosine equivalents from native proteins is shown in Table 1 for homogenates from ALD and PLD muscles. The tonic, ALD, muscle had more autolytic activity at *p*H 4.0 (compatible with the cathepsin D data), less at *p*H 7.0, and about the same activity at *p*H 8.5 as the phasic, PLD, muscle. Additition of 1 mM $CaCl_2$ increased the activity at least two-fold at all *p*H values for both muscles; the relative increase was greatest at *p*H 8.5. Addition of 1 mM $MgCl_2$ also increased the activity at all *p*H values, being most pronounced for the PLD at *p*H 8.5 where there was an eight-fold increase. Since these homogenates contained some calcium, calcium was removed by the action of the calcium-specific chelator [Ethylenebis(oxethylene-nitrilo)]tetraacetic acid (EGTA) to test the effect of magnesium alone (Table 2). The same pattern of increases in activity, although less pronounced, was present for the ALD at all *p*H values. But for the PLD, activity was uniquely absent at *p*H 7.0.

Table 1
Autolysis of ALD and PLD skeletal muscle homogenates

Muscle	pH	No additions	1 mM $CaCl_2$	1 mM $MgCl_2$
ALD	4.0	1.55 ± 0.11	3.12 ± 0.15[2]	7.71 ± 0.39[2]
	7.0	0.24 ± 0.04	0.49 ± 0.05[1]	0.81 ± 0.06[2]
	8.5	0.24 ± 0.04	1.00 ± 0.12[2]	1.92 ± 0.18[2]
PLD	4.0	1.11 ± 0.15	2.07 ± 0.12[2]	3.07 ± 0.36[2]
	7.0	0.43 ± 0.04	1.33 ± 0.10[2]	0.82 ± 0.07[2]
	8.5	0.29 ± 0.03	1.00 ± 0.13[2]	0.96 ± 0.07[2]

[1] $= p < 0.05$, [2] $= p < 0.01$ indicates statistical significance of value compared to corresponding "No additions" value.
TCA-soluble tyrosine (nmoles tyrosine/mg protein/h) released by autolytic digestion at pH 4.0, 7.0, and 8.5 in the presence of various reagents is expressed as mean ± standard error for at least 10 determinations, each of which was run in triplicate.
Reproduced from STAUBER et al. [6] by permission of Pergamon Press, Inc.

Table 2
Effects of magnesium in the absence of calcium on autolytic activity of ALD and PLD homogenates

Muscle	pH	1 mM EGTA	1 mM $MgCl_2$[a] + 1 mM EGTA
ALD	4.0	2.19 ± 0.17	6.31 ± 0.90[1]
	7.0	0.09 ± 0.03	0.24 ± 0.06[1]
	8.5	0.18 ± 0.04	1.10 ± 0.16[2]
PLD	4.0	1.49 ± 0.16	2.81 ± 0.39[1]
	7.0	0.02 ± 0.01	0.04 ± 0.02
	8.5	0.08 ± 0.02	0.45 ± 0.11[1]

[1] $= p < 0.05$, [2] $= p < 0.01$ indicates statistical significance of value compared to the corresponding 1 mM EGTA value.
[a] 1 mM $MgCl_2$ is assumed to be below physiological $MgCl_2$ levels.
TCA-soluble tyrosine (nmoles tyrosine/mg protein/h) released by autolytic digestion at pH 4.0, 7.0, and 8.5 in the presence of various reagents is expressed as mean ± standard error for at least 10 determinations, each of which was run in triplicate.
Reproduced from STAUBER et al. [6] by permission of Pergamon Press, Inc.

Because of the differences observed with $MgCl_2$ (Table 1) and $MgCl_2$ plus EGTA (Table 2), calcium concentrations were varied in the presence of 1 mM $MgCl_2$ (Table 3). Increased activity was noted at only neutral and alkaline pH values, being greatest at pH 7.0. Fig. 1 illustrates further the effect of calcium on ALD and PLD muscle autolysis at physiological pH in the presence of physiological magnesium concentrations. At least 50% of the maximal stimulated autolytic activity was present at a total calcium concentration of 10^{-5} M. Therefore, physiological changes in calcium concentrations that occur during contraction (10^{-5}M) and relaxation (10^{-7}M) of muscle could alternately activate and inhibit some of the proteolytic activity in skeletal muscle tissues.

Table 3
Autolysis of skeletal muscle homogenates in the presence of 1 mM $MgCl_2$[b]

Muscle	*p*H	1 mM EGTA	0.01 mM $CaCl_2$[a]	0.1 mM $CaCl_2$	1 mM $CaCl_2$
ALD	4.0	6.31 ± 0.90	5.18 ± 0.19	5.23 ± 0.16	6.09 ± 0.43
	7.0	0.24 ± 0.06	0.71 ± 0.14	1.11 ± 0.27[1]	1.17 ± 0.06[2]
	8.5	1.10 ± 0.16	1.68 ± 0.35	1.92 ± 0.38	2.31 ± 0.27[1]
PLD	4.0	2.81 ± 0.39	2.79 ± 0.27	2.67 ± 0.38	3.19 ± 0.35
	7.0	0.04 ± 0.02	1.09 ± 0.12[2]	1.91 ± 0.20[2]	2.21 ± 0.04[2]
	8.5	0.45 ± 0.11	0.97 ± 0.08[1]	1.50 ± 0.35[1]	1.81 ± 0.09[2]

[1] = $p < 0.05$; [2] = $p < 0.01$ indicates statistical significance of value compared to the corresponding 1 mM $MgCl_2$ and 1 mM EGTA value representing essentially zero calcium concentrations.
[a] 10^{-5} M $CaCl_2$ is within physiological limits. [b] 1 mM $MgCl_2$ is assumed to be below physiological $MgCl_2$ levels.
TCA-soluble tyrosine (nmoles tyrosine/mg protein/h) released by autolytic digestion at *p*H 4.0, 7.0 and 8.5 in the presence of various reagents is expressed as mean ± standard error for at least 10 determinations each of which was run in triplicate.
Reproduced from STAUBER et al. [6] by permission of Pergamon Press, Inc.

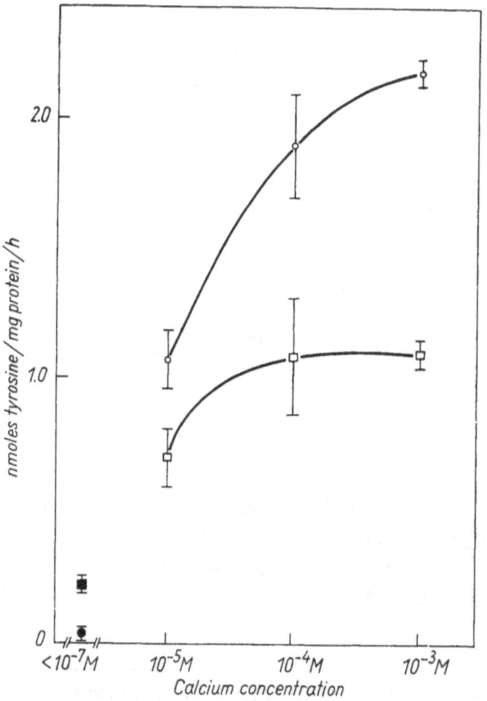

Fig. 1. Autolysis of ALD (□) and PLD (○) skeletal muscle homogenates at *p*H 7.0 as a function of calcium concentration in the presence of 1 mM $MgCl_2$.
The solid circle and square represent additions of 1 mM EGTA and, thus, calcium concentrations can be assumed to be less than 10^{-7} M.
Reproduced from STAUBER et al. [6] by permission of Pergamon Press, Inc.

BANA hydrolysis

At this time, we were about to begin zonal centrifugation studies on lysosomal proteases and to assay for cathepsin B in our enzyme-prepared tissue [9]. The collagenase preparation we used to allow more gentle homogenization of muscle was assayed for its ability to degrade N-benzol-DL-arginine-β-naphthylamide, BANA. Fig. 2 depicts an experiment using collagenase I and II (Sigma Chemical Co.) prepared in distilled water or in Hank's solution, the incubation solution for those studies [9]. Both collagenase preparations have BANA activity and were stimulated by Hank's solution. Since less activity was present in the more purified collagenase II, the presence of the trypsin-like protease, Clostripain, which had been shown to have BANA activity [11], was suspected. The BANA activity of Clostripain (Boehringer-Mannheim) was about 10 times that observed for collagenase I and also was stimulated by Hank's solution (Fig. 3).

These results (a possible ion-stimulated trypsin-like enzyme capable of degrading BANA at neutral *p*H) led us to test for such activity in muscle homogenates. First, the effect of *p*H on BANA activity was tested (Fig. 4) in Tris-HCl buffers

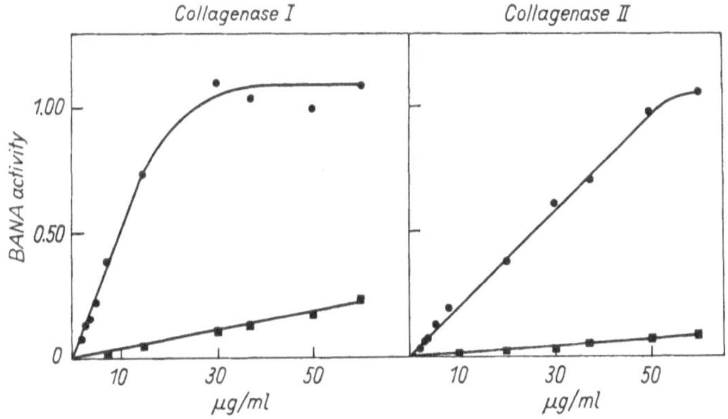

Fig. 2. BANA activity as a function of enzyme concentration for collagenase I and II (Sigma Chemical Co.).
■, water; ●, Hank's solution

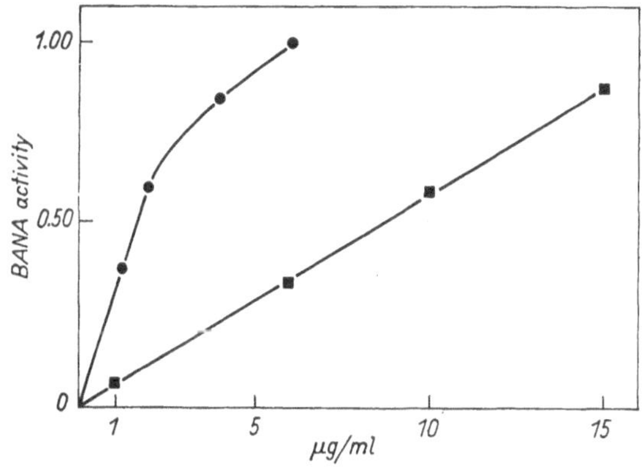

Fig. 3. BANA activity as a function of enzyme concentration for Clostripain (Boehringer, Mannheim). ■, ● cf. Fig. 2

(0.2 M). Two peaks of activity were observed for the ALD muscle extracts, at *p*H 5.0 and 8.0; whereas, only one distinct peak (*p*H 8.0) was present for the PLD muscle. The addition of 1 mM p-hydroxymercuriphenyl sulfonic acid abolished all activity. In contrast, the addition of 1 mM EDTA and 2 mM cysteine increased activity at all *p*H values and shifted the *p*H profiles (Fig. 4). Two peaks of BANA activity were again present for the ALD muscle, but now occurring at *p*H 6.0 and 7.5. In the PLD, activity peaks were present at *p*H 7.0, 5.0 and possibly 6.0.

Next, the muscles were homogenized in Hank's solution as in the Clostripain experiment and assayed for BANA activity in the presence of cysteine and EDTA (Fig. 5). There was some inhibition of activity above *p*H 7.0 (30% at *p*H 7.5 and 8.0) for the ALD muscle and marked inhibition of the PLD muscle activity at all *p*H values. It appears that some component(s) in the Hank's solution, probably calcium, inhibited BANA hydrolytic activity.

Finally, ATP (1 mM) was added to the assay mixture. Relatively no effect was seen for the ALD muscle while inhibition of activity was noted at all *p*H values

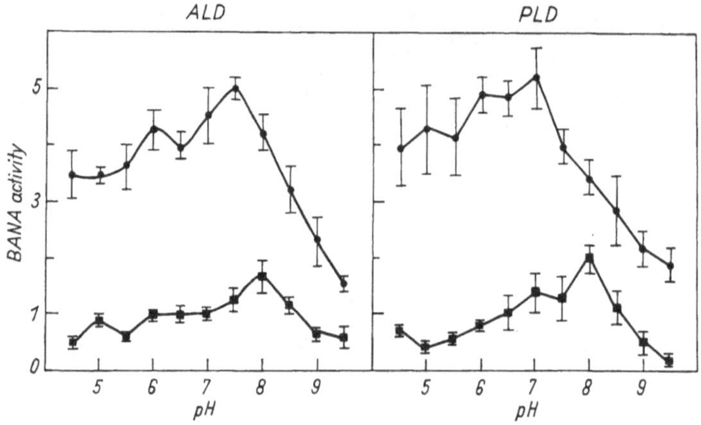

Fig. 4. BANA activity as a function of *p*H for ALD and PLD muscle extracts. Values represent the means ± standard errors of at least five experiments each run in duplicate. ●, 1 mM EDTA + 2 mM cysteine; ■, no additions

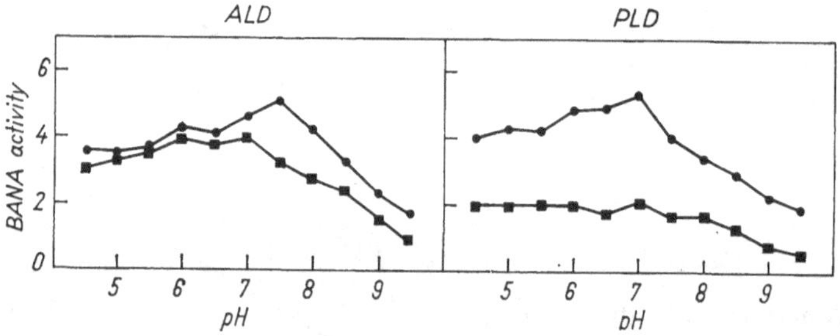

Fig. 5. BANA activity as a function of *p*H for ALD and PLD muscle extracts. Control was homogenized in distilled water and experimental in Hank's solution. Points represent the means of at least 3 experiments. ●, control; ■, homogenized in Hank's solution

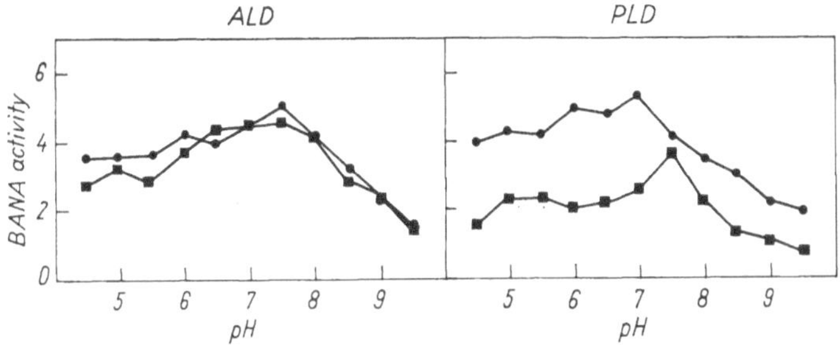

Fig. 6. BANA activity as a function of *p*H for ALD and PLD muscle extracts. The control assay mixture contained 1 mM EDTA plus 2 mM cysteine and the experimental, an additional 1 mM Na-ATP. Points represent the means of at least 3 experiments. ●, control; ■, 1 mM ATP

except *p*H 7.5 for PLD muscle extracts (Fig. 6). At no time during these experiments was the hydrolysis of ATP greater than 50% as calculated at the end of the experiment from the phosphate liberated.

Discussion

Two basic problems arose from the autolysis studies: 1) they could not be used to assay for protease activity in tissue fractionation or cytochemical localization studies, and 2) the results of similar studies on diseased muscles were difficult to interpret because it was not possible to determine if the numerator (enzyme activity), the denominator (cellular protein content) or substrate concentration (specific proteins) was the dependent variable of the disease process. Therefore, other assay techniques need to be developed to better understand the role of these ion stimulated proteases in normal and disease processes.

Calcium overload is a phenomenon that has been hypothesized as the general mechanism for muscle necrosis (atrophy) in most disease states [13]. Our results help explain this phenomenon in terms of ion control of muscle proteolytic activity. However, these studies do not indicate why ATP should inhibit BANA hydrolysis for the PLD muscle in an organelle and cell free system. ATP has been shown to inhibit a myofibrillar protease [14] but this enzyme is apparently absent in chickens ([15] and our own unpublished results). Also, since EDTA was present, the possibility of ATP acting as a chelator and removing an activating ion must be ruled out.

The markedly different autolytic and BANA activity responses in the tonic, ALD, and phasic, PLD, muscles might help account for the selective and preferential degradation of phasic muscle contractile proteins with most muscle disorders. In addition, changes in both calcium storage [16] and ATP concentrations [17] have been noted in the PLD during atrophy following removal of neurotrophic influence. However, the problem of protease regulation in muscle still remains unclear, since the precise intracellular location of these proteolytic enzymes as well as their activators and inhibitors (other than ions and ATP) is not known.

References

[1] Bird, J. W. C., and W. N. Schwartz: Fedn Proc. Fedn Am. Socs exp. Biol. **36**, 555 (1977)
[2] Dayton, W. R., D. E. Goll, M. G. Zeece, R. M. Robson, and W. J. Reville: Biochemistry **15**, 2150 (1976)
[3] Mayer, M., R. Amin, R. J. Milholland, and F. Rosen: Exp. molec. Path. **25**, 9 (1976)
[4] Pennington, R. J. in: Muscle Diseases. J. N. Walton, N. Canal, and G. Scarlato (Eds.). Excerpta Medica, Amsterdam 1970, p. 252.
[5] Katunuma, N., E. Kominami, K. Kobayashi, Y. Hamaguchi, Y. Banno, K. Chichibu, T. Katsunuma, and T. Shiotani in: Intracellular Protein Turnover. R. T. Schimke and N. Katunuma (Eds.). Academic Press, New York 1975, p. 187
[6] Stauber, W. T., A. M. Hedge, and B. A. Schottelius: Life Sci. **18**, 1441 (1976)
[7] Hess, A.: J. Physiol., Lond. **157**, 221 (1961)
[8] Goldberg, A. L., and R. Odessey in: Exploratory Concepts in Muscular Dystrophy II. A. L. Milhorat (Ed.). Excerpta Medica, Amsterdam 1974, p. 187
[9] Stauber, W. T., and B. A. Schottelius: Cytobios **14**, 87 (1975)
[10] Anson, M. L.: J. gen. Physiol. **20**, 565 (1937)
[11] Blackwood, C., and I. Mandl: Anal. Biochem. **2**, 370 (1961)
[12] Lowry, O. H., N. J. Rosebrough, A. L. Farr, and R. J. Randall: J. biol. Chem. **193**, 265 (1951)
[13] Wrogemann K., and S. D. J. Pena: Lancet **1976**/I, 672
[14] Mayer, M., R. Amin, and E. Shafrir: Archs Biochem. Biophys. **161**, 20 (1974)
[15] Jakubiec-Puka, A., W. Drabikowski, and A. Gorecka in: Intracellular Protein Catabolism. H. Hanson and P. Bohley (Eds.). **1**, 409. Martin-Luther-Universität, Halle-Wittenberg 1974/6
[16] Stauber, W. T., and B. A. Schottelius: Exp. Neurol. **48**, 534 (1975)
[17] Malvey, J. E., D. D. Schottelius, and B. A. Schottelius: Exp. Neurol. **33**, 171 (1971)

Acta biol. med. germ., Band 36, Seite 1653—1659 (1977)

Neurology Service, V. A. Lakeside Hospital,
and Department of Neurology, Northwestern University Medical School, Chicago, Illinois 60611, USA

Lysosomal enzyme secretion in rat ventral prostate. Secretagogue action of testosterone and dibutyryl cyclic AMP

H. Koenig, C. Y. Lu, and R. Bakay

Summary

Rat ventral prostate slices, when incubated in vitro, secrete protein, lysosomal enzymes and newly phosphorylated components in a time- and temperature-dependent manner. Testosterone and dibutyryl cyclic AMP immediately stimulate secretion and $^{32}P_i$ incorporation. Acid phosphatase and β-N-acetylhexosaminidase are secreted as acidic isoenzymes presumably contained within primary lysosomes.

Introduction

The prostate is an androgen-dependent accessory sex gland in the male which delivers a complex secretion product containing, inter alia, citric acid, spermine and related polyamines and various enzymes, notably acid phosphatase and proteases, into the seminal plasma [1]. The prostate secretes small amounts of fluid at frequent intervals under basal conditions ("resting" secretion) and much larger volumes upon stimulation of its nerve supply, administration of muscarinic cholinergic drugs, and sexual stimulation ("stimulated" secretion) [2]. It has been variously suggested on cytological grounds that secretion by the prostate involves a pinching off of the luminal cytoplasm (apocrine secretion) [3], exocytosis of secretion granules originating in the Golgi apparatus [4, 5] and containing acid phosphatase [5] (merocrine secretion), or a combination of apocrine and merocrine secretion [3]. Biochemical studies of the prostate have focused largely on the androgenic stimulation of biosynthetic processes [6] and the mechanism of uptake and metabolism of androgens by prostatic cells [7]. However, the biochemical and molecular aspects of prostatic secretion have received little or no attention.

We previously found that testosterone in vivo rapidly produced a decrease in the equilibrium density of lysosomes and an increase in their size in the rat ventral prostate [8], and coincidently stimulated the formation and discharge of apocrine secretion granules containing lysosomes and mitochondria into the acinar lumen [9]. We now report that testosterone and dibutyryl cyclic AMP stimulate the rat ventral prostate to secrete protein, several lysosomal hydrolases, and phosphoryated constituents.

Materials and methods

Incubation procedure

Prostatic secretion was studied in a slice-incubation system. For each incubation experiment the ventral prostates from three male Sprague-Dawley rats (180—250 g) were cut into slices 0.5—1.0 mm thick. The incubation medium was Krebs-Ringer buffer with a full complement of amino acids [10] in a ratio of 1 g of tissues per 100 ml of medium. The slices were preincubated in the medium with $^{32}P_i$ (50 μCi of $Na_3\,^{32}PO_4$ per 100 ml of medium) for 15 min at 37 °C with constant shaking in an atmosphere of 95% O_2 – 5% CO_2, rinsed in cold isotope-free medium and distributed equally between 4 flasks in the same incubation medium without isotope (1 g/100 ml) equilibrated with 95% O_2 – 5% CO_2. Flasks containing dibutyryl cyclic AMP (1 mM) and testosterone (10 μM) and a control flask containing only the solvent (0.2 ml ethanol) were incubated at 37 °C with continuous shaking for 4 hrs. A fourth flask was kept at 0°. Supernatant samples were removed at regular intervals. At the end of the incubation the tissues was removed by centrifugation (1000 × *g* for 10 min).

Analytical procedure

Protein, acid phosphatase (orthophosphoric monoester phosphohydrolase, EC 3.1.3.2), β-N-acetylhexosaminidase (β-2-acetamido-2-deoxy-D-glucoside acetamidodeoxyglucohydrolase, EC 3.2.1.30), and arylsulfatase (aryl sulfate sulfohydrolase, EC 4.1.6.1) were assyed as previously described [11]. For measurement of ^{32}P radioactivity, the proteins were precipitated and washed with 10% trichloracetic acid (TCA), taken up in 0.5 N NaOH and 10 ml of Aquasol (New Englang Nuclear Corp., Boston, Mass.) was added for counting in a Beckman LS-250 liquid scintillation system. Lysosomal enzymes in the incubation medium and the tissue were characterized by isoelectric focusing in a *p*H 10–3 ampholine gradient in an LKB Model 7100 column (Legend to Fig. 2 and ref. [12]). In some experiments the native prostatic "juice" or secretion was collected by centrifuging gland slices cut at 0.35 mm in a Model TC-2 tissue chopper (Sorvall, New Town, Conn.) at 400 × *g* for 10 min and similarly analyzed.

Results

During incubation at 37 °C without added hormones, control prostate slices spontaneously discharged protein, enzymes and TCA-insoluble ^{32}P into the medium (Fig. 1). The spontaneous discharge of protein, hydrolases and TCA-insoluble ^{32}P began at once at a maximum rate and then slowed down after about 1 h. The spontaneous discharge of protein, hydrolases and TCA-insoluble ^{32}P was substantially reduced by incubating slices at 0 °, indicating that secretion is dependent on energy production by oxidative phosphorylation. Testosterone and dibutyryl cyclic AMP produced a 50—60% increase in the discharge of protein, acid hydrolases and TCA-insoluble ^{32}P during the first 0.5 to 1 h of incubation.

Figs. 2 and 3 compare the isoelectric focusing pattern of the acid phosphatase and β-N-acetylhexosaminidase in unincubated ventral prostate slices with that of the enzymes discharged into the medium by prostate slices incubated in the presence of 5α-dihydrotestosterone (10 μM) for 30 min. In this experiment the androgen stimulated the release of protein by 62% and acid hydrolases by 25—30% as compared with the 37 °C control. Both hydrolases occurred in multiple molecular forms with *p*Is ranging between 4.1 and 8.6. The medium contained mostly isoenzymes with low *p*Is, whereas the tissue contained mostly isoenzymes with high aIs. Thus the acidic isoenzymes of acid phosphatase (*p*I 4.7 and *p*I 6.1) and of β-N-acetylhexosaminidase (*p*I 4.9 and *p*I 6.1) comprised 100 and 70% respectively of the total activity in the medium. In the tissue the more basic isoenzymes of acid phosphatase (*p*I 6.8 and *p*I 7.9) and β-N-acetylhexosaminidase (*p*I 6.8 and *p*I 8.6) comprised 54 and 79% of the total activity and the *p*I 4.7—4.9 components were rudimentary. The *p*I 4.7 and 6.1 components of acid phosphatase in the medium and the *p*I 5.8 and 6.8 components in the tissue were not inhibited by 1 mM tartrate, but the *p*I 7.9 form of the enzyme in the tissue was inhibited by 80% by this agent. The isoelectric focusing pattern of the A_{280nm} of

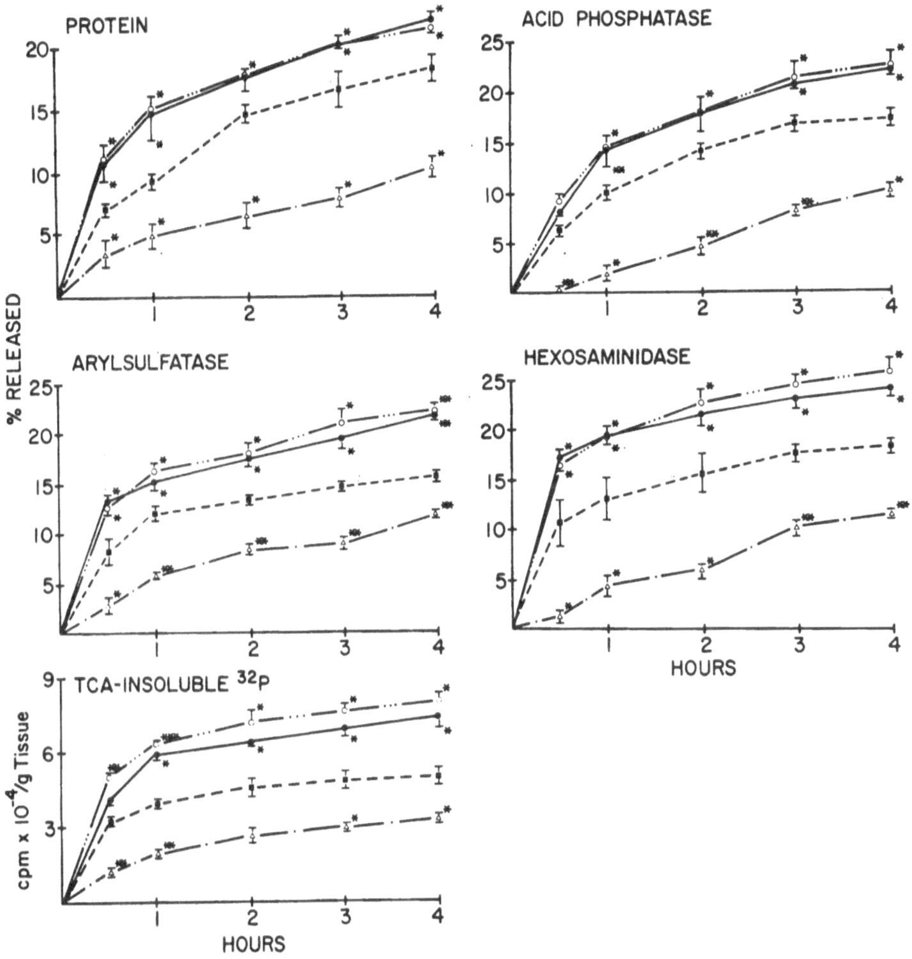

Fig. 1. Effect of temperature, testosterone and dibutyryl cyclic AMP on the release of protein, lysosomal acid hydrolases and TCA-insoluble ^{32}P by rat ventral prostate during incubation in vitro.

Ventral prostate slices from intact rats were preincubated with $^{32}P_i$ for 15 min, rinsed and incubated at 37 °C in an isotope-free chase medium for 4 hrs in the presence of 10 μM testosterone (○——○), 1 mM dibutyryl cyclic AMP (●——●) or without added hormones ■——■). A fourth flask was maintained at 0° (△——△). Supernatant samples were removed at stated intervals for analysis. The results are the means ± S.E.M. of three experiments. $*P < 0.05$; $**P < 0.01$; $***P < 0.001$ compared with the 37 °C control.

the incubation medium and the tissue extract also differed substantially, indicating differences in their overall protein composition. Similar results were obtained with the enzymes and protein that were released spontaneously into the medium by control prostate slices.

In the "resting" secretion collected from the unstimulated rat ventral prostate the acid phosphatase also occurred predominantly as acidic isoenzymes with *p*I values of 5.1 (62%) and 5.7 (37.5%) (Fig. 2A), whereas a substantial portion of the β-N-acetylhexosaminidase, 42% of the total, occurred in a basic form with a *p*I

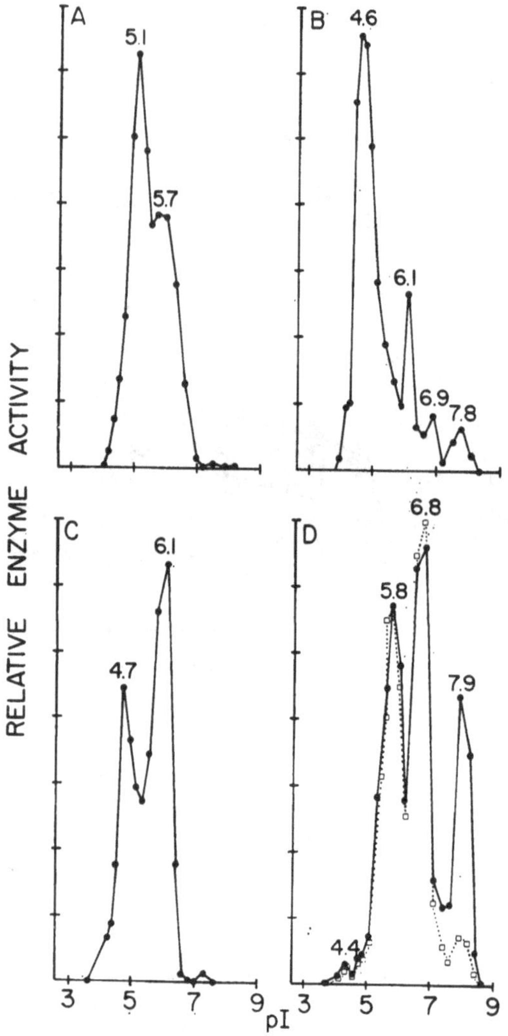

Fig. 2. Isoelectric focusing patterns of prostatic acid phosphatase in the "resting" secretion (A), "stimulated" secretion (B), incubation medium (C), and tissue (D).

A) "Resting" secretion collected from unstimulated ventral prostate slices by low speed centrifugation. B) "Stimulated "secretion collected from ventral prostate slices removed from rats 10 min after pilocarpine administration. C) The incubation medium was collected after ventral prostate slices had been incubated in the presence of 10 µM 5α-dihydrotestosterone for 0.5 h at 37 °C. The enzymes were concentrated by pressure dialysis against 0.05 M glycine-NaOH buffer, *p*H 8.7, with an Aminco UM-10 membrane. D) The tissue enzymes were extracted from unincubated ventral prostate slices [12]. The isoelectric points (*p*I) of the fractions are given in the abscissa. Tissue acid phosphatase assayed in the presence of 1 mM sod. tartrate (□——□)

value of 9.1 (Fig. 3A). However, the "stimulated" secretion collected 10 min after the administration of pilocarpine, a cholinergic agent which provokes prostatic secretion [1, 2], revealed a more striking preponderance of the acidic forms of these enzymes. Thus, 82 and 11% of the acid phosphatase was present in components with *p*I values of 4.6 and 6.1 (Fig. 2B); and 71% of the β-N-acetylhexosaminidase was present in a component with a *p*I value of 4.9, and 28% in a less basic component with a *p*I value of 8.7 (Fig. 3B).

Discussion

The present study has shown that during incubation in vitro rat ventral prostate slices spontaneously secreted protein, three lysosomal hydrolases and TCA-insoluble ^{32}P into the medium in a time- and temperature-dependent manner. Testosterone and the dibutyryl analog of cyclic AMP stimulated the release of all these

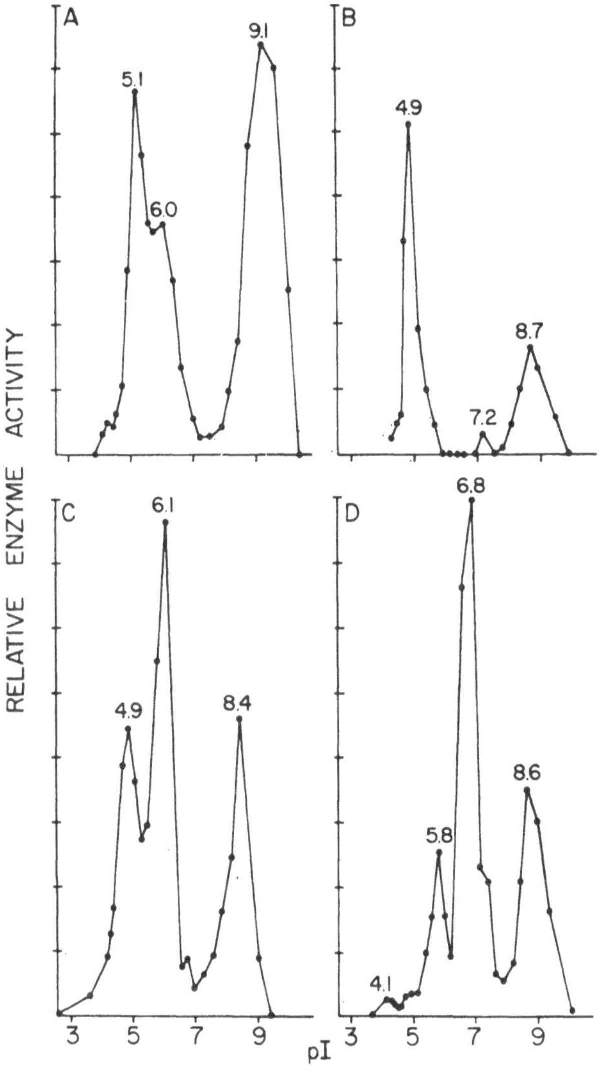

Fig. 3. Isoelectric focusing patterns of prostatic β-N-acetylhexosaminidase in the "resting" secretion (A), "stimulated" secretion (B), incubation medium (C), and tissue (D). See legend to Fig. 2 for additional details

constituents. Nonspecific leakage of cytoplasmic constituents from injured cells can be ruled out as a significant factor in the incubation experiments by the finding that the isoelectric focusing patterns of the proteins and lysosomal enzymes released into the incubation medium were markedly different. Further, the isoelectric focusing patterns of the hydrolases in the medium closely resembled those in the natural prostatic secretion. It can therefore be concluded that the in vitro discharge of protein and lysosomal enzymes in the slice-incubation system is a reliable indication of secretory activity.

Our results appear to be the first demonstration that androgenic steroids serve as a secretagogue, directly stimulating secretion in the ventral prostate. The finding that dibutyryl cyclic AMP also stimulated prostatic secretion in vitro suggests that the secretagogue action of androgens may be mediated by the adenyl cyclase-cyclic AMP system. Cyclic AMP has been implicated as a mediator of several other androgenic effects in the rat ventral prostate [13]. We have also found that androgens and dibutyryl cyclic AMP stimulate secretion in the rat seminal vesicle [14].

Our experiments call attention to the lysosomal hydrolases as important constituents of the prostatic secretion. It is noteworthy that acid phosphatase and β-N-acetylhexosaminidase were secreted into the incubation medium mostly as acidic isoenzymes, whereas they occured in the glandular tissue as less acidic and basic isoenzymes. These hydrolases also are present as acidic isoenzymes in the natural secretion expressed from the rat ventral prostate under basal conditions and they are even more acidic after stimulation of the gland by pilocarpine and testosterone (C. Y. LU and H. KOENIG, unpublished findings). VANHA-PERTTULA et al. [15] have previously shown that the secretory form of acid phosphatase in the rat ventral prostate is an acidic, tartrate-resistant form of the enzyme. It can therefore be concluded that these two lysosomal hydrolases are secreted as acidic isoenzymes. After secretion these enzymes tend to become more basic, probably as a result of autolytic degradation. Similar alterations have been observed during in vitro incubation of prostatic secretion (C. Y. LU and H. KOENIG, unpublished findings) as well as lysosomal extracts [16, 17]. The phosphorylated components in the prostatic secretion have not yet been characterized, but may include protein-associated phospholipids and phosphoproteins.

We have previously reported that the nascent lysosomal hydrolases are sialylated in the Golgi apparatus [18—21] and that the completed hydrolases are packaged in primary lysosomes as acidic sialoglycoproteins [12, 16]. However, secondary lysosomes contain both acidic and basic forms of these enzymes [12, 16, 17]. The secretory protein in the rat ventral prostate is known to be transported through the Golgi apparatus for packaging in secretory granules before discharge [4]. The acidic character of the secreted prostatic hydrolases is therefore consistent with the view that the newly synthesized enzymes are processed in the Golgi apparatus and packaged in primary lysosomes [3—5], and that the latter correspond to the acid phosphatase-reactive particles previously found to be discharged into the acinar lumen within apocrine secretion granules [9]. It seems possible that some constituents of small molecular weight present in the prostatic secretion, e. g., amino acids, prostaglandins, glycerophosphorylcholine, are not secreted as such, but are generated by lysosomal digestion of secreted lipoprotein and glycoprotein constituents in the acinar lumen.

Acknowledgements

Dr. R. BAKAY participated in this research during his free quarter as a Senior Medical Student. We thank Dr. ALFRED GOLDSTONE for helpful discussion. This research was supported in part by the Veterans Administration and NIH grant HD 09729.

References

[1] MANN, T. in: The Biochemistry of Semen and of the Male Reproductive Tract. John Wiley and Sons, New York 1964

[2] HUGGINS, C.: Harvey Lect. **42**, 158 (1947)

[3] BRANDES, D. in: Male Accessory Sex Organs. D. BRANDES (Ed.). Academic Press, New York 1974, p. 17 and p. 183
[4] FLICKINGER, C. J.: Anat. Rec. **180**, 427 (1974)
[5] HELMINEN, H. J., and J. L. E. ERICSSON: J. Ultrastruct. Res. **33**, 528 (1970)
[6] SINGHAL, R. L., and D. J. B. SUTHERLAND in: Molecular Mechanisms of Gonadal Hormone Action. Advances in Sex Hormone Research. **1**, 225. J. A. THOMAS and R. L. SINGHAL (Eds.). University Park Press, Baltimore 1975
[7] TVETER, K. V., V. HANSSON, and O. UNHJEM in: Molecular Mechanisms of Gonadal Hormone Action. Advances in Sex Hormone Research. **1**, 17. J. A. THOMAS and R. L. SINGHAL (Eds.). University Park Press, Baltimore 1975
[8] KOENIG, H., R. KNIGHT, R. NAYYAR, and C. HUGHES,: J. Cell Biol. **67**, 220a (1975)
[9] KOENIG, H., and C. HUGHES, J. Cell Biol. 220a (1975)
[10] EAGLE, H.: Science, N.Y. **130**, 432 (1959)
[11] GOLDSTONE, A., H. KOENIG, R. NAYYAR, and C. HUGHES: Biochem. J. **132**, 259 (1973)
[12] GOLDSTONE, A., and H. KOENIG: FEBS Lett. **39**, 176 (1974)
[13] AHMED, K. in: Molecular Mechanisms of Gonadal Hormone Action. Advances in Sex Hormone Research. **1**, 129. J. A. THOMAS and R. L. SINGHAL (Eds,). University Park Press, Baltimore 1975
[14] KOENIG, H., C. Y. LU, and R. BAKAY: Biochem. J. **158**, 543 (1976)
[15] VANHA-PERTTULA, T., R. NIEMI, and H. J. HELMINEN: Invest. Urol. **9**, 345 (1972)
[16] GOLDSTONE, A., and H. KOENIG: Biochem. J. **141**, 527 (1974)
[17] NEEDLEMAN, S. B., and H. KOENIG: Biochim. biophys. Acta **379**, 43 (1975)
[18] GOLDSTONE, A., and H. KOENIG: Life Sci. **11**, 511 (1972)
[19] NAYYAR, R., A. GOLDSTONE, H. KOENIG, and C. HUGHES: Proceedings of the 4th International Congress of Histochemistry and Cytochemistry, Kyoto 1972, p. 335
[20] GOLDSTONE, A., and H. KOENIG: Biochem. J. **132**, 267 (1973)
[21] NEEDLEMAN, S. B., H. KOENIG, and A. GOLDSTONE: Biochim. biophys. Acta **379**, 57 (1975)

Acta biol. med. germ., Band 36, Seite 1661–1666 (1977)

Instituto de Investigaciones Citológicas, Caja de Ahorros y Monte de Piedad de Valencia, Valencia, Spain
and Department of Biochemistry, University of Kansas Medical Center, Kansas City, Kansas 66103 U.S.A.

Evidence pointing to the main role of lysosomes in mitochondrial proteolysis at neutral *p*H

V. Rubio, J. Rivas, J.-L. Iborra, and S. Grisolia

Summary

Recombination experiments using radioactive mitochondria and mitoplasts, and non-radioactive lysosomes or digitonin-soluble fraction of mitochondria, show equal rates of proteolysis and of inactivation of carbamyl phosphate synthetase; the amount of lysosomal protein was equal in both cases on the basis of N-acetyl-β-glucosaminidase activity. Therefore, lysosomes seem to be responsible for all the proteolytic activity exhibited by the digitonin soluble fraction of mitochondrial preparations. Since this fraction contains ca. 90% of the proteolytic activity present in mitochondrial preparations, most of the proteolysis can be attributed to lysosomal contamination. These findings and stability characteristics "in vitro" and "in vivo" of some matrix enzymes are presented and discussed in relation to protein turnover.

Introduction

Although there have been a number of reports indicating marked proteolysis at neutral *p*H in mitochondrial preparations [1], lysosomal involvement, while considered, has remained unclear, mainly due to technical difficulties in preparing mitochondria free of lysosomes.

In a recent publication [2] we have demonstrated that most of the neutral protease activity of mitochondrial preparations is present in the digitonin-soluble compartment (outer membrane, intermembrane space and contaminating organelles, such as lysosomes). Moreover, the N-acetylglutamate dependent carbamyl phosphate synthetase, which is present in the matrix of rat liver mitochondria, was inactivated by macromolecular components present in the digitonin-soluble compartment. Also, separation of mitochondrial populations yielded higher proteolytic activity and faster CPS inactivation in the "light" mitochondria, which contain a much higher proportion of lysosomes, than in the "heavy" mitochondria. While these results strongly suggest that lysosomes are responsible for the bulk of neutral proteolytic activity shown by mitochondria, the participation of the outer membrane and intermembrane space of mitochondria could not be excluded. In the present paper we present further evidence favoring a prominent role of lysosomes in the proteolysis of rat liver mitochondria at neutral *p*H. Differences in stability "in vitro" and "in vivo" of some matrix enzymes will also be discussed and its possible relation to the clarification of turnover of proteins.

Abbreviations used: NaβGase, N-acetyl-β-glucosaminidase; CPS, carbamyl phosphate synthetase; MDH, malate dehydrogenase; GDH, glutamate dehydrogenase; SDS, sodium dodecyl sulphate; BSA, bovine serum albumin; MSH, mercaptoethanol

Materials and methods

L-[^{14}C] Leucine (324 Ci/mol) was purchased from Schwarz/Mann. All other chemicals were of the best commercial grade available.
Rat liver mitochondria were obtained and fractionated with digitonin [3]. The „soluble" fraction (containing the outer membrane and the intermembrane space plus contaminating organelles, including lysosomes) was concentrated with dry Sephadex G-25 coarse. Digitonin was then removed by gel filtration on Sephadex G-25 superfine, using buffer A or B (see below). Fractions containing the protein were pooled and concentrated with Sephadex to 70–80 mg protein/ml. Radioactive mitochondria and mitoplasts were obtained from rats (ca. 250 g) injected intraperitoneally with 100 µCi of [^{14}C]leucine 10 hrs before sacrifice.
Mitochondria and mitoplasts were washed with buffer A (70 mM sucrose, 220 mM D-mannitol, 5 mM K-phosphate, 5 mM MSH, *p*H 7.4) and after suspension in buffer B (5 mM K-phosphate, 5 mM MSH, *p*H 7.4), to ca. 100 mg protein/ml were disrupted by freezing and thawing 10 times using a dry ice-acetone bath.
Lysosomes prepared according to Ragab et al. [4] were suspended in buffer B to ca. 100 mg/ml and disrupted as described for mitochondria.
Unless otherwise specified incubations were at 37 °C and carried out immediately after preparation of mitochondria or fractions thereof. At the indicated times, a portion was taken and diluted 1:5 in cold 5 mM mercaptoethanol. One half was centrifuged at 46.000 × *g* for 10 min. Enzyme activities were assayed in the supernatant. The other half was precipitated with 10% trichloroacetic acid, and radioactivity was measured in the precipitate and supernatant. Unless specified, the radioactivity in the supernatant is expressed as % of the radioactivity present in the acid insoluble protein at 0 time.
SDS-polyacrylamide gel electrophoresis of mitochondria and mitoplasts was performed according to Clarke [5], in 7.5% gels containing 0.1% bisacrylamide and 0.1% SDS.
CPS was measured spectrophotometrically [6]. Malic dehydrogenase was assayed by a standard procedure [7]. Monoamine oxidase, glutamic dehydrogenase and NAβGase were assayed essentially as described by Schnaitman et al. [3], Godinot and Lardy [8], and Findlay et al. [9], respectively. Protein was assayed by the biuret method in 10% trichloroacetic acid precipitates (dissolved in 0.2 N KOH). The biuret-dexycholate technique [10] was used to ascertain the concentration of mitochondrial protein. BSA (Fraction V, Sigma Chemical Co.) was used as a standard.

Results

As depicted in Fig. 1 equal rates of release of acid soluble radioactivity were found in disrupted (frozen and thawed) mitochondria, and with a mixture of boiled mitochondria and lysosomes (containing the same NAβGase activity as it was present in the unboiled mitochondrial preparation). These results support the idea that the proteolytic activity exhibited by mitochondrial preparations can be accounted for by lysosomal contamination. Since boiled mitochondria may not be attacked by proteases at the same rate than the non-boiled organelles, attempts were made to solve this problem by using mitoplasts.
These particles have much less proteolytic activity "per se" and thus are a good substrate for proteases located in the digitonin-soluble compartment. Radioactive and non-radioactive mitochondria were subfractionated with digitonin, and non-radioactive lysosomes were simultaneously isolated. Then, radioactive mitoplasts were incubated with non-radioactive digitonin soluble fraction or with enough lysosomes to restore the entire NAβ Gase activity of the mitochondrial preparation. Boiled lysosomes or non-radioactive digitonin soluble fraction were added as specified in Fig. 2 (to yield equal concentrations of protein in all tubes). A control with mitoplasts mixed with boiled lysosomes and digitonin soluble fraction was

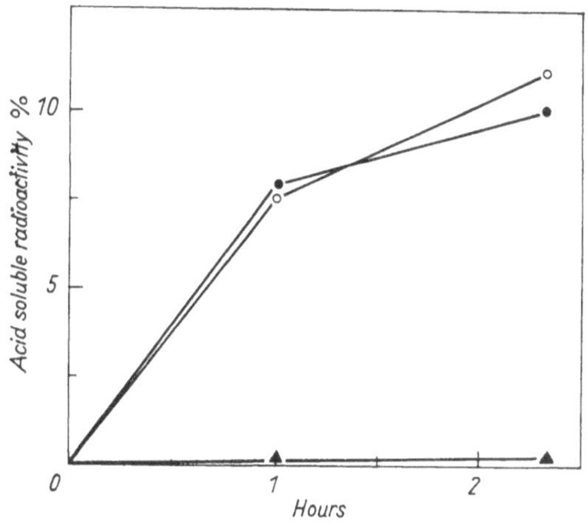

Fig. 1. Release of acid-soluble radioactivity by mixtures of mitochondria and lysosomes.

Radioactive mitochondria (45 mg of protein, about 70000 dpm) and non-radioactive lysosomes (1.8 mg of protein) were incubated in 0.5 ml of buffer B. (●) Mitochondria + boiled lysosomes; (○) boiled mitochondria + lysosomes; (▲) boiled mitochondria + boiled lysosomes. The amounts of mitochondria and lysosomes used were adjusted to give the same NAβGase activity

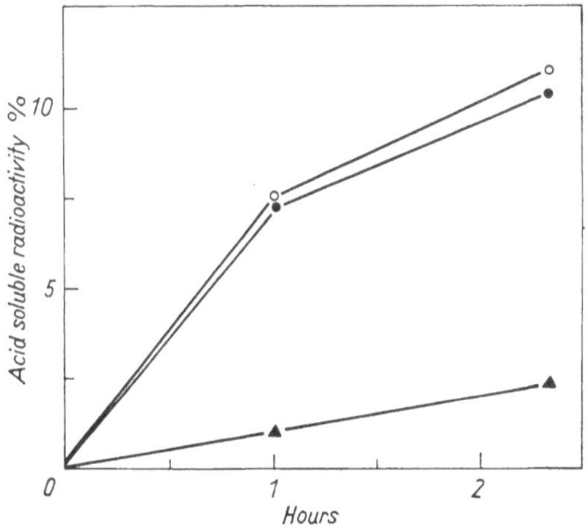

Fig. 2. Release of acid-soluble radioactivity by mixtures of mitoplasts, lysosomes and digitonin-soluble fraction of mitochondria.

Radioactive mitoplasts (35 mg of protein, about 55000 dpm), and non-radioactive digiton-insoluble fraction (10 mg of protein) and lysosomes (1.6 mg of protein) were incubated in 0.5 ml of buffer B. (○) Mitoplasts + digitonin-soluble fraction + boiled lysosomes; (●) mitoplasts + boiled digitonin-soluble fraction + lysosomes; (▲) mitoplasts + boiled digitonin soluble fraction + boiled lysosomes. Equal NAβ-Gase activity was present in the amounts of digitionin-soluble fraction and lysosomes used

also prepared. As it can be seen in Fig. 2, equal rates of proteolysis of mitoplasts were observed with digitonin-soluble compartment or with an equivalent amount of lysosomes (in terms of NAβGase content). Moreover, as presented in Fig. 3, CPS was inactivated at the same rate in mitochondria and in mixtures of mitoplasts with lysosomes (enough to restore the NAβGase activity of the mitochondrial preparation) and heat inactivated digitonin soluble fraction. As shown also in the figure, the addition of boiled lysosomes did not change the rate of CPS inactivation in mitoplasts [2].

It must be pointed out that CPS degradation could be also followed by SDS gel electrophoresis of mitochondria or of mitoplasts. While not presented here, the amount of Coomassie stain in the CPS band [5] was progressively reduced with time, on incubation of mitochondria or of mitoplasts under conditions leading to CPS inactivation. Simultaneously material of lower molecular weight accumulated in the area corresponding to peaks Ia and II (see CLARKE [11]).

These results demonstrate that lysosomal contamination alone can account for the entire proteolysis exhibited by the digitonin-soluble fraction of mitochondria,

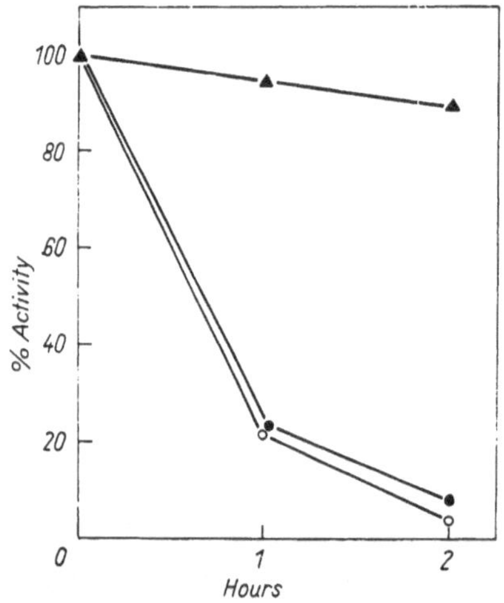

Fig. 3. Decay with time of CPS activity in mixtures of mitochondria, mitoplasts, digitonin-soluble fraction and lysosomes.

Mitochondria (45 mg of protein), mitoplasts (35 mg of protein), digitonin-soluble fraction (10 mg of protein) and lysosomes (1.6 mg of protein), were incubated when indicated in 0.5 ml of buffer B. (●) Mitochondria + boiled lysosomes; (○) mitoplasts + boiled digitonin soluble fraction + lysosomes; (▲) mitoplasts + boiled digitonin-soluble fraction + boiled lysosomes. Equal NAβGase activity was present in mitochondria and in the mixture of mitoplasts, unboiled lysosomes and boiled digitonin-soluble fraction. Mitoplasts contained ca. 10% NAβGase activity of mitochondria

which represents ca. 90% of the proteolytic activity present in mitochondrial preparations. The origin of the residual proteolysis (ca. 10%) associated with mitoplasts is uncertain. Since approximately 10% of all NAβGase activity present in mitochondria remains associated with mitoplasts, it seems reasonable to postulate also a lysosomal origin for this activity.

Rate of inactivation of several matrix enzymes in mitochondria and in mitoplasts

It seemed also of interest to compare the rate of inactivation in mitochondria and in mitoplasts, of several matrix enzymes which have different $t_{1/2}$ "in vivo". As presented in Fig. 4 there was not direct relationship between stability "in vivo" of CPS, malate dehydrogenase and glutamate dehydrogenase ($t_{1/2}$ ca. 7, 2 and 1 day respectively [12]) and rate of inactivation of these enzymes in isolated mitochon-

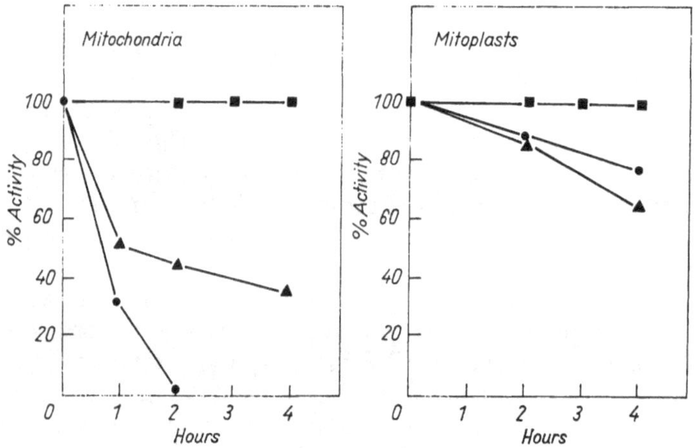

Fig. 4. Effect of time on CPS (●), malate dehydrogenase (▲) and glutamate dehydrogenase (■) activities in disrupted mitochondria or mitoplasts. 80 mg protein/ml of mitochondria or mitoplasts in buffer B were incubated. Activities are expressed as % of those at 0 time.

dria or mitoplasts. Indeed the decay of CPS was much faster in mitochondria. Malate dehydrogenase was also more stable in mitoplasts. On the other hand, as also illustrated in the figure, glutamate dehydrogenase, which is located in the same mitochondrial compartment, is, as expected [13], very stable in both mitochondria and mitoplasts.

Discussion

It is well established that mitochondrial preparations show marked proteolysis at neutral *p*H [1]. While lysosomes are known to be present in these preparations, their possible role in determining this proteolysis, while considered, has not yet been clarified. Indeed, it has been demonstrated that the proteases responsible for the inactivation of pyruvate dehydrogenase in mitochondrial preparations are present in the digitonin-soluble fraction. Also lysosomes can inactivate this enzyme at neutral *p*H [14].

We have recently demonstrated that the bulk of the neutral protease activity of rat liver mitochondria is extracted with digitonin. Since most lysosomes are also solubilized by this treatment [15], it was unclear if these proteases were located in the outer mitochondrial compartment or if they were lysosomal.

The data presented here clearly demonstrate that lysosomes alone can account for the entire proteolytic activity of the digitonin-soluble fraction of mitochondrial preparations. The activity remaining associated with mitoplasts (ca. 10%) can probably be also attributed to lysosomes, since mitoplasts contain still some NAβ-Gase.

In contrast to their stability "in vitro", the "in vivo" half-lives of CPS, malate dehydrogenase and glutamate dehydrogenase are ca. 7, 2 and 1 day, respectively [12]. The stability of glutamate dehydrogenase in isolated mitochondria, (stable for nearly 24 hrs in the presence of antibiotics) is interesting, particularly since it is not stable in homogenates [13]. Possibly GDH turnover is determined by factors other than those operating at the proteolytic level, including translocation or the modification of the enzyme, thereby making it more susceptible to intracellular proteases as it is to trypsin in the presence of NADPH [16]. Of course, cytoplasmic proteases may also be responsible, with or without cofactors, for GDH degradation; and finally GDH may be sensitive to inactivation by lysosomes at low *p*H.

Further experiments are required to clarify these questions; however, their extension should shed light on the important problem of protein turnover.

Acknowledgement

This work was supported by Grant AMO 1855 from the National Institutes of Health.

References

[1] Bartley, W., and L. M. Birt in: Essays in Cell Metabolism. P. 1. W. Barltey, H. L. Kornberg, and J. R. Quayle (Eds.). John Wiley and Son, New York 1970
[2] Rubio, V., and S. Grisolia: FEBS Lett. **75**, 281 (1977)
[3] Schnaitman, C., G. Erwin, and J. W. Greenwalt: J. Cell Biol. **32**, 719 (1967)
[4] Ragab, H., C. Beck, C. Dillard, and A. L. Tappel: Biochim. biophys. Acta **148**, 501 (1967)
[5] Clarke, S.: J. biol. Chem. **251**, 950 (1976)

[6] CHABAS, A., S. GRISOLIA, and R. SILVERSTEIN: Eur. J. Biochem. **29** 333 (1972)
[7] Biochimica Catalogue, C. F. Boehringer and Soehne Gmbh., Mannheim, FRG 1968
[8] GODINOT, C., and H. A. LARDY: Biochemistry **12**, 2051 (1973)
[9] FINDLAY, J., G. A. LEVY, and C. A. MARSH: Biochem. J. **69**, 467 (1958)
[10] JACOBS, E. E., M. JACOBS, D. R. SANADI, and L. B. BRADLEY: J. biol. Chem. **223**, 147 (1956)
[11] CLARKE, S.: J. biol. Chem. **251**, 1354 (1976)
[12] NICOLETTI, M., C. GUERRI, and S. GRISOLIA: Eur. J. Biochem. (in press)
[13] SALINAS, M., R. WALLACE, and S. GRISOLIA: Eur. J. Biochem. **44**, 375 (1974)
[14] WIELAND, O. H.: FEBS Lett. **52**, 44 (1975)
[15] LOEWENSTEIN, J., H. R. SCHOLTE, and E. M. WIT-PEETERS: Biochim. biophys. Acta **223**, 432 (1970)
[16] GRISOLIA, S., M. FERNANDEZ, R. AMELUNXEN, and C. L. QUIJADA: Biochem. J. **85**, 568 (1962)

Acta biol. med. germ., Band 36, Seite 1667—1672 (1977)

Department of Biochemistry, University of Kansas Medical Center, 39th and Rainbow Blvd., Kansas City, Kansas 66103 U.S.A.

Increased susceptibility of carbamylated glutamate dehydrogenase to proteolysis

W. Hood, E. de la Morena, and S. Grisolia

Summary

Glutamate dehydrogenase is very susceptible to carbamylation which results in loss of activity. The effect of a number of proteolytic enzymes (pronase, trypsin and chymotrypsin) on native and carbamylated glutamate dehydrogenase was tested. In all cases, the carbamylated enzyme was at least twice as susceptible to proteolysis as the native enzyme. Antibodies were prepared against glutamate dehydrogenase and carbamylated glutamate dehydrogenase; the carbamylated enzyme was antigenically indistinguishable from the native enzyme. Preliminary experiments indicate that the carbamylated glutamate dehydrogenase is taken up by ascites tumor cells while glutamate dehydrogenase is not. It seems possible that the effects described can be extrapolated to degradation by lysosomes and to other covalently modified enzymes.

Introduction

Based on the fact that enzymes, due to ligand binding and/or covalent modification, may be more or less stable and susceptible to a number of agents including proteolysis, the elastoplasticity theory was proposed to explain some "in vivo" phenomena. Recognition of proteins via elastoplastic effect will result in selective degradation and thus be of importance in protein turnover [1, 2]. In as much as glutamate dehydrogenase (GDH) is very susceptible to carbamylation [2, 3], we tested the effect of a number of proteolytic enzymes on native and carbamylated GDH with pronase, trypsin and pepsin. In all cases, the carbamylated enzyme was much more susceptible to proteolysis than the native enzyme. Antibodies were prepared against GDH and carbamylated GDH; the carbamylated enzyme was antigenically indistinguishable from the native enzyme.

Materials and methods

Bovine liver GDH Type 1, trypsin, pronase, chymotrypsin and carbamyl phosphate were Sigma products. [^{14}C]-KCNO was obtained from Amersham Searle Co. Freund's (complete) adjuvant was from Calbiochem. All other chemicals were of analytical grade. Mice inoculated with ascites cells were obtained from the National Institutes of Health, Bethesda, Md. The method of Lowry et al. [4] was used for determining protein and protein hydrolysis. Bovine serum albumin was used as a standard. Radioactivity was measured in a Nuclear Chicago Isocap/300 liquid scintillation system.

Carbamylation of GDH

Since crystalline GDH is supplied in a suspension in ammonium sulfate, 4.0 ml (80 mg) were centrifuged at 10,000 × *g* for 10 min. The precipitate was taken in 2.0 ml of 250 mM carbamyl phosphate. After 1 h at 38 °C the mixture was loaded onto a 3 × 35 cm Sephadex G-25 fine column (kept at 4 °C) and eluted with 0.02 M NaCl at a flow rate of 12.0 ml per h. The appearance of the carbamylated GDH was monitored by the method of Hunninghake and Grisolia [5]; the bulk appeared at the void volume. To obtain ^{14}C-labelled carbamylated

GDH, the above procedure was followed throughout except that the pelleted GDH was taken into 2.0 ml of 30 mM KCNO containing 5 μCi of [^{14}C]-cyanate and that the incubation was for 0.5 h at 25 °C. Under the conditions described above, the carbamylated GDH retained approximately 3.0% activity.

Proteolysis of native and carbamylated GDH

Incubation mixtures contained 100 μmoles potassium phosphate, *p*H 7.0, 700 μg carbamylated or native GDH and chymotrypsin, trypsin or pronase in 1.0 ml. After incubation for 0.5 h at 37 °C, the mixtures were deproteinized with 5% perchloric acid and centrifuged. An aliquot of the supernatant was taken and acid-soluble material measured by the procedure of Lowry et al. [4]. When using ^{14}C-carbamylated GDH, 4.5 mg of ^{14}C-carbamylated GDH (200 cpm/mg) were incubated (with shaking) with 250 μmoles potassium phosphate buffer, *p*H 7.0, and 300 μg of either trypsin or pronase in 4.6 ml at 37 °C. At 0 time and 20, 40 and 60 min, 1.0 ml aliquots were withdrawn and deproteinized with 0.1 ml 30% perchloric acid. Aliquots, 0.4 ml, of the supernatants were then used to measure radioactivity; other 0.4 ml aliquots from the supernatants were used to estimate acid-soluble materials by the method of Lowry et al. [4].

Preparation of mouse ascites tumor cells

0.3 ml of Ehrlich ascites tumor cells were injected i.p. into 30 g mice. Approximately 5 ml of cell suspension were removed immediately prior to the experiment from a mouse in which the ascites cells had been growing from 10–14 days. The ascites cells were centrifuged at 500 × *g* for 2 min and then washed twice in 5 ml of Krebs Ringer phosphate. They were then suspended in 5 ml of Krebs Ringer phosphate (~20 mg protein/ml) and used as such.

Production of antibodies against GDH

5 rabbits were used. They were each injected in the toe pad with 4 mg GDH in complete Freund's adjuvant. After 2 weeks, the animals were each given a further injection of 1 mg GDH. 4 days later approximately 35 ml of blood were removed from the ear vein of each animal. After 3 more weeks, blood was again collected from each animal.

Production of antibodies against carbamylated GDH

5 rabbits were used. They were each injected in the toe pad with 3 mg carbamylated GDH in complete Freund's Adjuvant. After 2 weeks, each animal was given a further injection of 1 mg enzyme. Since little antibody production occurred, the animals were injected i.p. with 10 mg carbamyl GDH in complete Freund's adjuvant. 1 week later approximately 40 ml of blood were collected from the ear vein of each animal. After 3 more weeks, blood was again collected from each animal.

Preparation of blood sera

Freshly collected blood was kept at room temperature for 2 hrs, the clot was removed and then centrifuged at 3000 × *g* for 15 min. The sera was stored at −20 °C until used.

Gel diffusion

The gel diffusion technique of Ouchterlony [6] was used to visualize antigen-antibody reactions. Petri dishes containing 1% agar in 0.05 M sodium phosphate buffer, *p*H 7.4, were used. All diffusions were carried out at 4 °C.

Quantitative precipitin curves

A series of tubes were prepared containing 100 μl of sera and 0 to 300 μg of native or carbamylated GDH in 0.4 ml of 0.15 M NaCl, buffered with 0.02 M potassium phosphate buffer, *p*H 7.0. After 1 h incubation at 37 °C, the tubes were stored at 4 °C for 2 days. They were then centrifuged at 5000 × *g* for 15 min, and the precipitate was washed three times with buffered saline. It was dissolved in 0.5 ml of 0.05 M NaOH and a portion assayed by the procedure of Lowry et al. [4].

Results

Cross reactivity of antibodies

Precipitin lines were observed between anti-GDH sera and both GDH and carbamylated GDH. Reactivity appeared to be approximately equal. Anti-carbamylated GDH sera also reacted with both native GDH and carbamylated GDH.

Quantitative precipitation

It was difficult to obtain precipitin curves with carbamylated GDH because of its insolubility. However, good precipitin curves were obtained when anti-native GDH and anti-carbamylated GDH sera were titrated against native GDH. Because of the precipitation of the carbamylated GDH, it was difficult to obtain quantitative results regarding the cross reactivity of the two sera. There was complete precipitation of 25 μg of GDH by 100 μl of anti-GDH serum and there was also complete precipitation of 25 μg of carbamylated GDH with 100 μl of anti-carbamylated GDH serum.

Proteolysis of native and carbamylated GDH

As illustrated in Figs. 1—3, there was increased proteolysis of both native and carbamylated GDH with increasing concentrations of chymotrypsin, trypsin and pronase. Moreover, as shown, the carbamylated enzyme was, in the range tested, at least 4 times more susceptible to degradation than the native GDH with chymotrypsin and with pronase. It was also at least twice as susceptible to trypsin. It should be pointed out that likely the sensitivity is higher at lower levels of hydrolysis; in the experiments presented in Figs. 1—3 the hydrolysis was very extensive. It should be noted as illustrated in Figs. 4 and 5 with chymotrypsin and pronase, respectively, that the degradation of carbamylated GDH increases with time of incubation almost linearly up to $\sim 25\%$ hydrolysis. Interestingly, and as shown, the proteolytic activity assessed by acid-soluble protein or hydrolysis products by colorimetric methods coincides fairly well with that estimated by radioactive measurements.

The above findings clearly indicate the greater susceptibility of carbamylated GDH to proteolysis. This is of much interest since after administration of carbamyl

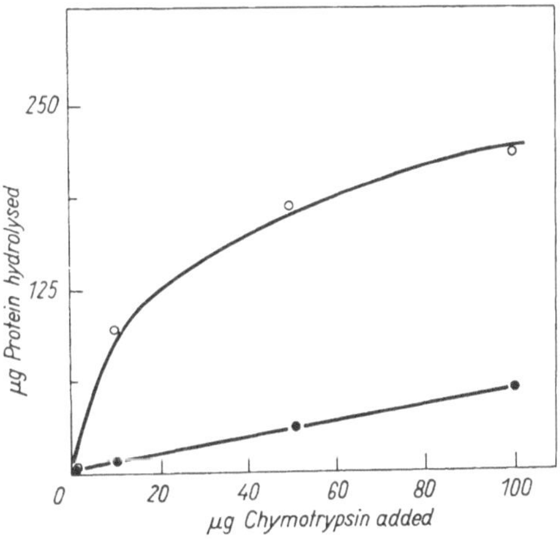

Fig. 1. Effect of chymotrypsin on native (●) and on carbamylated (○) GDH

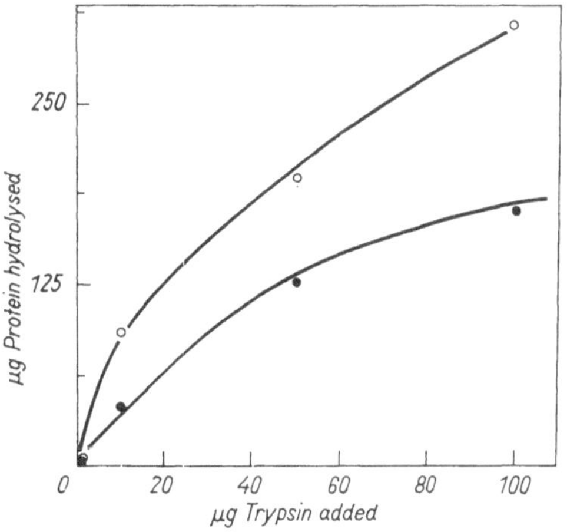

Fig. 2. Effect of trypsin on native (●) and on carbamylated (○) GDH

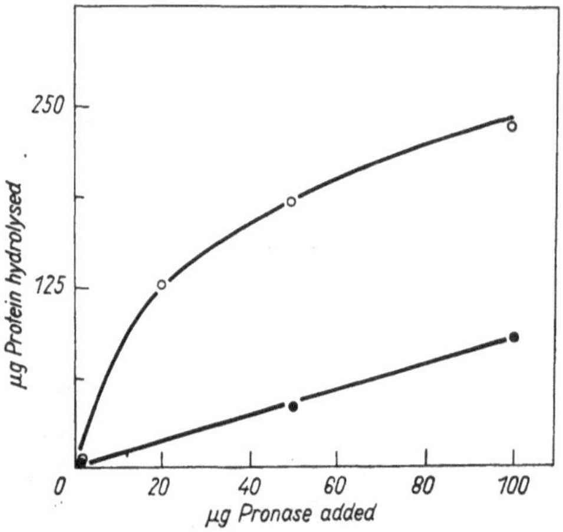

Fig. 3. Effect of pronase on native (●) and on carbamylated (○) GDH

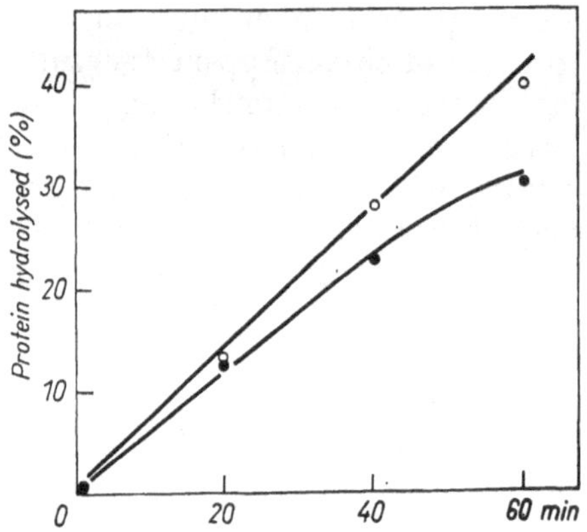

Fig. 4

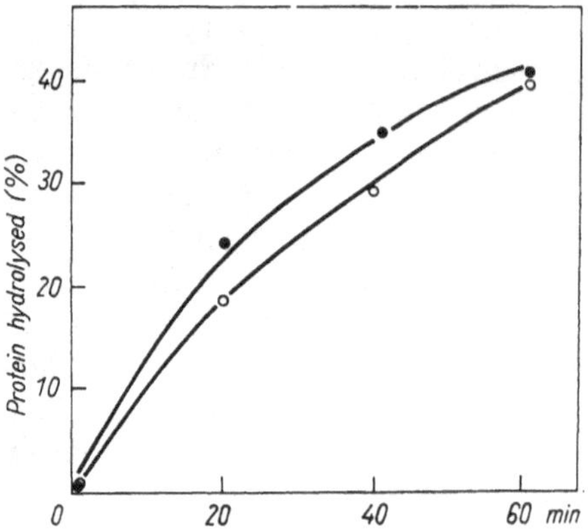

Fig. 5

Fig. 4. Effect of time of incubation on the proteolysis of carbamylated glutamate dehydrogenase by chymotrypsin and trypsin. The extent of proteolysis was measured by radioactive measurements (●) or colorimetrically (○) [4]

Fig. 5. Effect of time of incubation on the proteolysis of carbamylated glutamate dehydrogenase by chymotrypsin and pronase. The extent of proteolysis was measured by radioactive measurements (●) or colorimetrically (○) [4]

phosphate or cyanate to animals, some brain proteins seem to turn over very slowly [7], while on the other hand, carbamylated proteins injected are eliminated from the circulatory system of rats at a much lower rate than non-carbamylated native proteins [8]. It was therefore of interest to compare the behaviour of native and carbamylated GDH in another system of somewhat less complex organization than the whole animal. To that end, we attempted to measure possible differences in the uptake of GDH and carbamylated GDH by ascites tumor cells.

Uptake of native and carbamylated GDH by ascites tumor cells

Washed ascites tumor cells were incubated with several concentrations of GDH and then centrifuged. As shown in Fig. 6, the enzymic activity in the supernatant

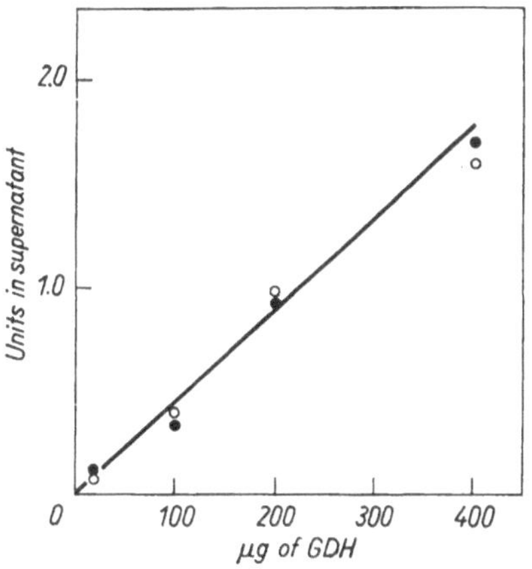

Fig. 6. Incorporation of glutamate dehydrogenase by ascites tumor cells.

A number of flasks containing washed ascites tumor cells (approximately 20 mg protein) were incubated with 0.02–0.04 mg of GDH in Krebs Ringer phosphate in 2 ml at 37 °C with shaking. At 0 time and after 1 h, aliquots from each flask were centrifuged (5,000 × *g* for 5 min) and the enzymic activity determined in the supernatant. (○) zero time values; (●) after 1 h at 37 °C

was identical both at 0 time and after 1 h incubation, clearly illustrating that little or no GDH is taken up by ascites cells.

Ascites tumor cells were then incubated with carbamylated GDH. However, due to the poor solubility of carbamylated GDH, it would be difficult to assess uptake if this was small. Therefore, controls containing carbamylated GDH or ascites cells alone were also incubated, and then samples were withdrawn at intervals and treated with chymotrypsin and pronase as described above. In all cases, the protein content of the supernatants of the incubation mixtures containing ascites cells and carbamylated GDH was lower than the sum of supernatants of carbamylated GDH and ascites cells controls. These results are shown in Figs. 7 and 8.

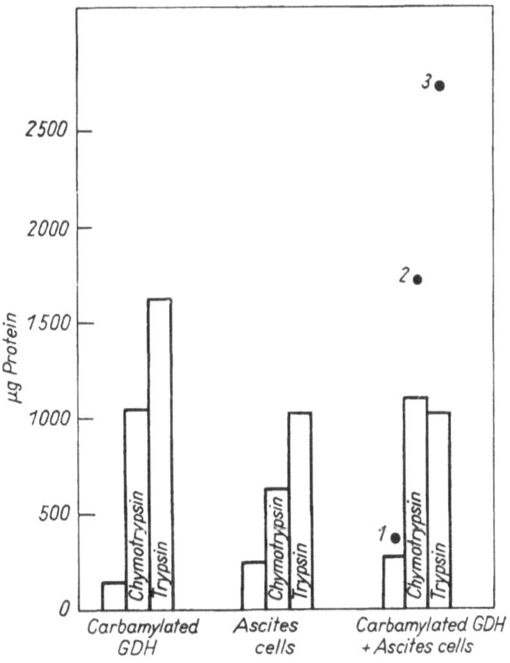

Fig. 7. Incorporation of carbamylated glutamate dehydrogenase by mouse ascites tumor cells. Ascites cells containing approximately 50 mg of protein were incubated (with shaking) with 3 mg of carbamylated GDH in 7 ml of Krebs Ringer phosphate for 0.5 h at 37 °C. Two controls were also set up containing ascites cells only and carbamylated GDH only. At the end of the incubation, three 1 ml aliquots were removed from each tube. To one aliquot was added 0.1 ml of chymotrypsin (3 mg/ml), to another 0.1 ml of trypsin (3 mg/ml), and nothing was added to the third aliquot. After 0.5 h incubation with shaking at 37 °C the mixtures were deproteinized by addition of 0.1 ml of 30% perchloric acid and the acid soluble protein material was measured in the supernatant by the method of Lowry et al. [4]. The numbered points represent the theoretical values for the sum of the values of the tubes containing carbamylated GDH and ascites cells

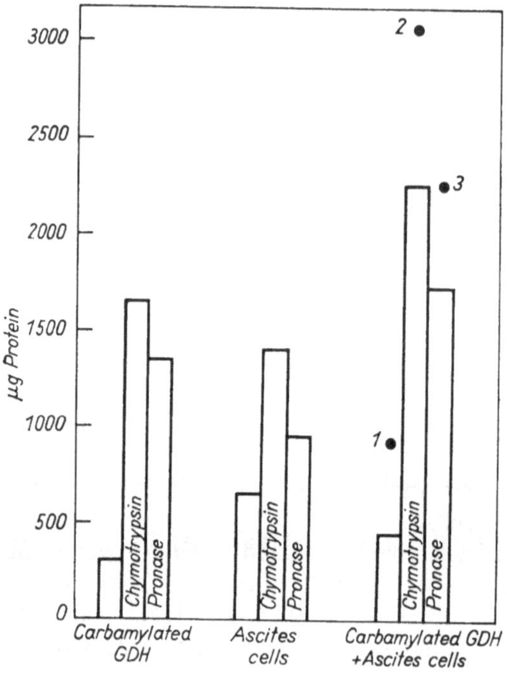

Fig. 8. Incorporation of carbamylated glutamate dehydrogenase by mouse ascites tumor cells. The conditions were as those for Fig. 7, except that chymotrypsin and pronase at the same concentration were used. The numbered points represent the theoretical values for the sum of the values of the tubes containing carbamylated GDH and ascites cells

Discussion

The findings presented here clearly illustrate the difference in stability of carbamylated GDH and GDH to a number of proteolytic enzymes and to the uptake by ascites cells. It would be most interesting to find out the susceptibility of carbamylated GDH and of other enzymes to lysosomal enzymes, as well as to the uptake by lysosomes. Such experiments are in progress. The experiments presented here, together with experiments from us and others, illustrate the importance of modification of proteins, including covalent modification [2], which was predicted by Grisolia [1] over ten years ago.

Acknowledgement

These studies were supported by grant AMO1855 from the United States Public Health Service.

References

[1] Grisolia, S.: Physiol. Rev. **44**, 657 (1964)

[2] Hood, W., and S. Grisolia in: Biochemical Regulatory Mechanisms in Eukaryotic Cells. E. Kun and S. Grisolia (Eds.). John Wiley and Son, New York 1972, p. 137

[3] Gonzalez, P., E. Ventura, and T. Caldes in: The Urea Cycle. S. Grisolia, R. Baguena and F. Mayor (Eds.). John Wiley and Sons, New York 1976, p. 73

[4] Lowry, O. H., N. J. Rosebrough, A. L. Farr, and R. J. Randall: J. biol. Chem. **193**, 265 (1951)

[5] Hunninghake, D., and S. Grisolia: Anal Biochem. **16**, 200 (1966)

[6] Ouchterlony, O.: Acta path. microbiol. scand. **25**, 186 (1948)

[7] Fando, J., and S. Grisolia: Eur. J. Biochem. **47**, 389 (1974)

[8] Grisolia, S., M. Salinas, R. Wallace, and G. K. Singh: Phys. Chem. Phys. **8**, 37 (1976)

Acta biol. med. germ., Band 36, Seite 1673—1680 (1977)

Department of Biochemistry, University of Kansas Medical Center, 39th and Rainbow Blvd., Kansas City, Kansas 66103 U.S.A.

Acetyl glutamate — a model of signals for intracellular proteolysis

J. Rivas, A. Reglero, and S. Grisolia

Summary

The proteolysis at neutral *p*H of mitochondria from liver and brain is more marked in isolated preparations than "in vivo", indicating activation of proteases or inactivation of repressors during isolation. Acetyl glutamate (AG), found in liver mitochondria of ureotelic animals, plays a crucial role as activator of carbamylphosphate synthetase. Since AG levels change under a number of conditions, we checked for an AG deacylase in mitochondria, for otherwise AG must be exported and destroyed by cytosol deacylases. We noted on incubation of mitochondrial extracts with AG an increase in trichloroacetic acid-soluble ninhydrin-reacting material but not in acetate liberation, indicating activation of proteases. This was checked with ^{14}C-labelled mitochondria. Uncer certain conditions AG and other acyl aminoacids stimulate ~5 to 20% the proteolysis with rat liver and with brain mitochondria.

Introduction

Acetyl glutamate is present in liver mitochondria of ureotelic animals, where it plays an important role as an activator of carbamyl phosphate synthetase, key enzyme of the urea cycle [1]. The acetyl glutamate synthetase is located in mitochondria where, in turn, it is subject to metabolic regulation by arginine [2]. Since the "in vivo" levels of acetyl glutamate are reported to change under a number of conditions [2] and since it does not seem to penetrate mitochondria [3], it was of interest to check whether there was acetyl glutamate deacylase in liver mitochondria. We found apparent activity but there were discrepancies depending on whether amino acid or acetate liberation was measured. These discrepancies led to the discovery of a new unsuspected effect. N-acetyl-glutamate and other acyl derivatives of aminoacids can, under certain conditions, stimulate moderately the proteolysis at neutral *p*H of rat liver mitochondrial preparations [4]. This effect possibly reflects the existence of metabolites that serve as signals to initiate the proteolysis of mitochondrial proteins. This communication documents briefly a preliminary account of these findings.

Materials and methods

[^{14}C]-Leucine (50 µCi/ml, 312 mCi/mmol) was purchased from Schwarz-Mann, Orangeburg, New York. Aquasol (scintillation solution) was obtained from New England Nuclear, Boston, Mass. Pyruvate kinase [E.C. 2.7.1.40] (rabbit muscle, type III, lyophilized, salt-free powder), bovine serum albumin (Fraction V, powder) and N-acetyl-L-glutamic acid were purchased from Sigma Chemical Company, St. Louis, Mo. All other chemicals were of analytical grade.
Male Holtzman rats, weighing 300—350 g, were fasted overnight and then sacrificed either by cervical dislocation or by decapitation. The livers were quickly removed and placed in

Abbreviations used: AG, N-acetyl-L-glutamate; CPS, carbamylphosphate synthetase.

ice-cold 0.25 M sucrose. Unless specified otherwise, liver and brain mitochondria were prepared by the method of SCHNEIDER [5], except that a third wash in 0.15 M KCl was done. The mitochondria were suspended in cold distilled water (50–100 mg protein/ml) and broken either by homogenization for 20 s with an Ultra-turrax or by freezing and thawing 10 times using a dry ice-acetone bath. Broken mitochondria could be kept frozen at −20 °C for several days.

Mitochondria were fractionated with 12 mg digitonin/100 mg protein, as described by GREENAWALT [6]. Mitoplasts were washed once with 70 mM sucrose, 220 mM mannitol, 5 mM potassium phosphate buffer, *p*H 7.4, and then resuspended in 5 mM potassium phosphate buffer, *p*H 7.4, to give 75 mg protein/ml. They were broken by freezing and thawing 10 times using a dry ice-acetone bath. The soluble fraction (containing the outer membrane and intermembrane space plus contaminating components from other organelles, e.g. lysosomes) was fractionated with cold acetone as follows: A portion was mixed rapidly into −20 °C acetone to give a 20% concentration (v/v). After centrifugation (all centrifugations were carried out at −10 °C for 10 min at 10,000 × *g*), the supernatant was brought to 40% acetone. After centrifugation and separation of the precipitate, the supernatant was brought to 60% and then to 80%, with separation of precipitates. The precipitates were brought to onehalf the starting vol with 5 mM potassium phosphate buffer, *p*H 7.4, to yield Fractions A, B, C, and D, respectively. For Experiment 2, the fractionation was carried out in the same manner, except that the first fraction corresponded to a final concentration of acetone of 45% (Fraction A'), the second to 65% (Fraction B'), and the third to 85% (Fraction C').

^{14}C-labelled mitochondria were prepared as follows: Rats were given intraperitoneal injections of 1 to 2 ml of [^{14}C]-leucine and were killed 4 to 8 hrs later.

Protein was determined by a biuret method [7]; bovine serum albumin was used as a standard. Amino acids were determined with ninhydrin by the method of SPIES [8] using leucine as a standard. Ornithine was measured as described by RATNER [9]. Acetate was determined by the method of KUO and YOUNATHAN [10], except that the procedure was scaled down 10fold.

Unless specified otherwise, proteolysis measurements were carried out with mitochondria or fractions thereof at *p*H 7.4 and at 37 °C. The reactions were stopped by the addition of cold trichloroacetic acid (TCA) solutions (final concentration 10%). After centrifugation, ninhydrin-positive material was measured in a portion of the supernatant, previously filtered through glass wool. When using radioactive mitochondria, the precipitates were washed once with 10% TCA, resuspended in 0.2 M KOH and then kept overnight at 37 °C. The dissolved proteins were neutralized with 0.3 M HCl and then counted. Filtered (glass wool) aliquots of TCA-soluble fractions were taken. 10 ml of Aquasol were added to the samples in counting vials and radioactivity measured in a Nuclear of Chicago Isocap 300 scintillation counter. All samples were counted long enough to give results within 5% statistical error or less. Protein hydrolysis is expressed either as % of radioactivity initially in protein that is converted to a trichloroacetic acid-soluble form or as ninhydrin-positive material. It should kept in mind that the apparent hydrolysis calculated, on the basis of radioactivity soluble in TCA was consistently 3.6 to 3.7 higher than by ninhydrin measurements (calculated on the basis of complete hydrolysis yielding 10 μmoles amino acid per mg protein) reflecting the fact that the neutral proteolysis was ~30% complete. When measuring acetate liberation, reactions were carried out under the same conditions as when measuring ninhydrin-positive material liberation, but they were stopped by heating at 100 °C for 5 min. After removing insoluble protein by centrifugation, acetate was determined in aliquots of the supernatant. All zero time values have been subtracted from the values given in the Tables and Figures.

Results and discussion

As illustrated in Table 1, evidence for apparent deacylase activity as judged by an increase in ninhydrin-positive material for acetyl glutamate was noted with rat liver mitochondria. As shown, mitochondrial preparations, under our conditions, had no activity with N-acetyl-ornithine, which is a good substrate for the deacylase of rat liver cytosol [11]. Therefore, the activity could not be due to cytosol contamination of the mitochondrial preparation. We then estimated the deacylase

Table 1
Apparent deacylase activity of rat liver mitochondria

N-acetyl amino acid added	Increase in Amino acid as Leucine	Increase in Amino acid as Ornithine	Acetate
	(nmoles/mg protein)		
None	30.3	4.8	0
Glutamate	52.7	—	1.9
Ornithine	—	4.5	—

Reaction mixtures contained in 1.0 ml 50 μmoles potassium phosphate buffer, *p*H 7.4, and when indicated 10 μmoles N-acetyl-glutamate. With N-acetyl-ornithine, 50 μmoles Tris-Cl^-, *p*H 9.6, were used. The following amounts of protein (liver mitochondria) were used: 7 mg with acetyl glutamate, 30 with acetyl ornithine and 32 when measuring acetate liberation. 1 h incubation.

Table 2
Effect of several acyl amino acids on proteolysis of rat liver mitochondria.

Addition	Radioactivity liberated (% of total)	Amino acid liberated (μmoles/mg prot.)
None	3.2 ± 0.6 (7)	0.049 ± 0.016 (12)
N-acetyl-glutamate	4.1 ± 0.6 (7)	0.069 ± 0.023 (8)
N-formyl-methionine	4.3 ± 0.4 (2)	—

Reaction mixtures contained in 0.5 ml of 0.05 M potassium phosphate buffer, *p*H 7.4, radioactive mitochondria (1.4—3.2 mg protein, 150—900 counts/min/mg protein) or non-radioactive mitochondria (1.5—3.5 mg protein) and 20 mM of the indicated acyl amino acids (at *p*H 7.4) were incubated for 1 h. Data are given as mean ± standard deviation; number of experiments are given in parentheses.

activity by measuring acetate production [10]. The values obtained, as illustrated in Table 1, were much lower than those obtained by the ninhydrin method. This suggested that the discrepancy was due to a stimulatory effect of N-acetylglutamate on the neutral proteolysis of mitochondrial preparations [12].

In order to further elucidate this effect, we prepared mitochondria from rat liver labelled with ^{14}C; these were incubated both in the absence and in the presence of several amino acid derivatives. Again, an increase in radioactivity and in the ninhydrin-positive material in the soluble TCA supernatant of mitochondrial preparations undergoing proteolysis was noted when N-acetyl-glutamate or N-formyl-methionine were added (Table 2). The following compounds (up to 20 mM) were without effect: glutamine, folic acid, N-acetyl-aspartate, N-acetyl-glucosamine, carbamyl β-alanine and α-ketoglutarate.

The neutral proteolysis exhibited by mitochondrial preparations is, in all likelihood, largely due to lysosomal contamination [12]. As illustrated in Fig. 1, increasing protein concentration yields increasing proteolysis per mg of protein, i. e. specific activity, to a maximum value; mercaptoethanol increases the activity

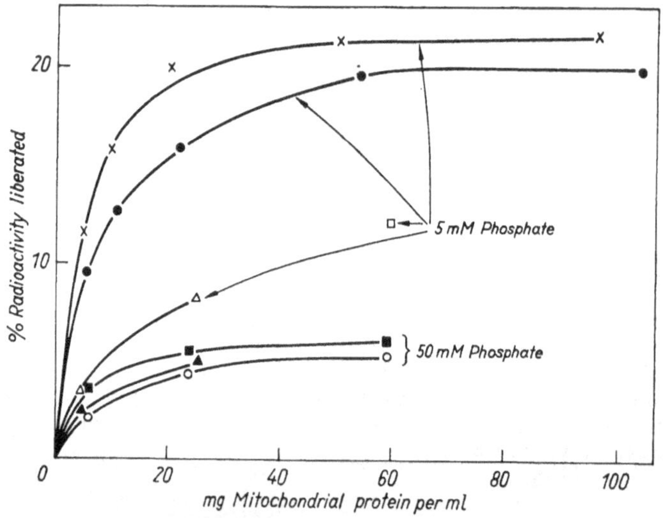

Fig. 1. Effect of protein concentration and method of preparation on the neutral proteolytic activity of mitochondrial preparations.

Reaction mixtures contained potassium phosphate buffer, *p*H 7.4, and radioactive mitochondria, as indicated. ×, 5 mM mercaptoethanol. At 0 time and after 1 h incubation, aliquots were taken, diluted to 5 mg protein/ml with cold buffer and then precipitated with trichloroacetic acid. For the experiments marked (× and ●), mitochondria were prepared by the method of Greenawalt [6], then washed with a solution containing 220 mM mannitol, 70 mM sucrose and 5 mM potassium phosphate buffer, *p*H 7.4, and resuspended in 5 mM potassium phosphate buffer, *p*H 7.4, without (●) or with (×) 5 mM mercaptoethanol, and then broken by freezing and thawing. For the other experiments (○, ■, □, ▲ and △) mitochondria were prepared and broken with an Ultra-turrax (○, ▲ and △) or by freezing and thawing (■ and □)

slightly. Again, as illustrated in Fig. 1, the extent of proteolysis varies with the two types of preparations used, probably reflecting their lysosomal contamination; while the method of preparation influences it, the method of breaking the mitochondria influences little the extent of proteolysis. The increase in the "specific activity" of proteolysis which, as shown, increases with protein concentration, may reflect the increase of the protein substrate and/or the increase of small metabolites, including endogenous acetyl glutamate. Unfortunately, it was not possible to clarify this by dilution, because it is technically difficult to work at very low levels of protein (in addition to being less physiological); below 3 mg protein/ml the relative value of the zero time is large, while the total counts become too low for accurated estimation. As is illustrated more extensively below, Figure 1 typifies also the inhibition of proteolysis by salt.

As illustrated in Figs. 2 and 3, working at fairly low protein concentrations there is an appreciable increase in proteolysis with time, as judged by both radioactive and colorimetric measurements, and in both cases the proteolysis increases on the addition of N-acetyl-glutamate.

The effect of acetyl glutamate is, within certain limits, concentration dependent, indeed, it is inhibitory at high levels. Therefore, most work was carried out at 10 to 20 mM. The inhibitory effect on proteolysis of increasing the ionic strength is

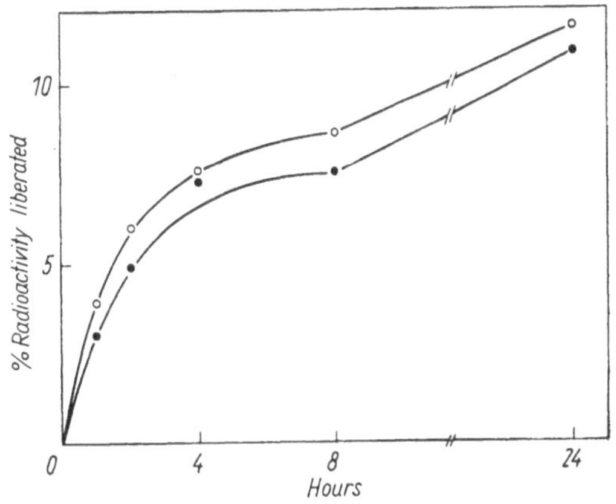

Fig. 2. Proteolysis of ^{14}C-labelled rat liver mitochondrial preparations with and without N-acetyl-glutamate.

Reaction mixtures contained, in 4.0 ml, 0.05 M potassium phosphate buffer, *p*H 7.4, ^{14}C-labelled mitochondrial preparation (25.5 mg protein, 9850 counts/min) and, when used, 20 mM N-acetyl-glutamate. Mitochondria were broken in an Ultra-turrax. ●——●, controls; ○——○ acetyl glutamate present

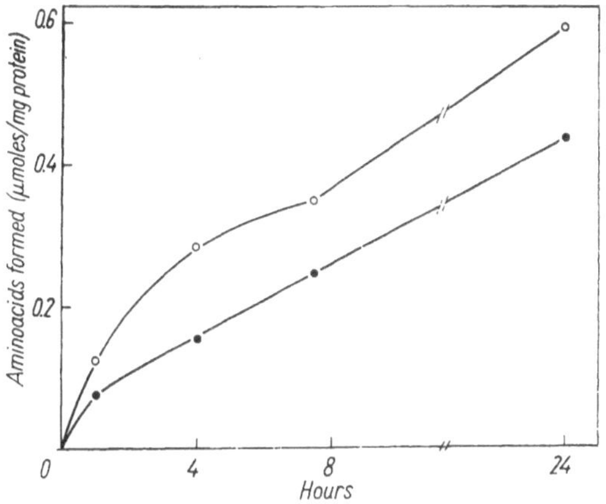

Fig. 3. Kinetics of proteolysis of rat liver mitochondrial preparations either in the absence or in the presence of N-acetyl-glutamate.

Conditions were as for the experiment of Fig. 2, except that 14 mg protein of the mitochondrial preparations were used and that the extent of proteolysis was judged by measuring ninhydrin-positive material. ●——●, control; ○——○, acetyl glutamate present

Table 3
Effect of phosphate on neutral proteolysis of rat liver mitochondria with and without N-acetyl-glutamate.

Expt.	Mitochondria broken by	Mitochondrial protein (mg/ml)	Acetyl-glutamate	Phosphate (mM) 5	50	900
				(% Protein hydrolyzed)		
1	Ultra-turrax	5	0	3.5 ± 0.1	2.4 ± 0.1	—
			20 mM	2.5 ± 0.2	3.1 ± 0.1	—
2	Ultra-turrax	25	0	8.1 ± 0.7	4.95 ± 0.55	—
			100 mM	5.15 ± 0.15	3.7 ± 0.7	—
3	Freezing-thawing	5	0	—	2.35 ± 0.05	1.85 ± 0.05
			20 mM	—	2.6 ± 0.2	1.85 ± 0.05
4	Ultra-turrax	5	0	—	2.2 ± 0.1	1.65 ± 0.15
			20 mM	—	2.4 ± 0.2	1.45 ± 0.25

The conditions were as those of Fig. 1, except as indicated. For experiments 3 and 4, due to the high phosphate concentration, the final concentration of trichloroacetic acid was 20%. The mitochondria used had 500 counts/min/mg protein. 1 h incubation. Data are given as mean ± standard deviation. All experiments were carried out in duplicate.

Table 4
Proteolysis in rat liver mitochondrial fractions and activation by acetyl-glutamate

Fraction	N-Acetyl-glutamate None	N-Acetyl-glutamate 20 mM
	Radioactivity liberated (% of total)	
Mitochondria	3.2	4.9
Soluble portion	1.3	1.4
Particulate portion	2.8	3.2
Soluble + particulate portions	2.0	2.8

0.8 ml of ^{14}C-labelled mitochondria (22.5 mg protein, 20,500 counts/min) were centrifuged at 20,000 × *g* for 10 min. The pellet obtained was taken in 0.8 ml H_2O and, after centrifugation, resuspended in water to 1.6 ml. Both supernatants were combined and brought to 1.6 ml. Proteolysis was determined under the conditions described in Table 2, using 50 µl of mitochondrial preparation or 100 µl of soluble and/or particulate portions, thereof. 1 h incubation.

Table 5
The effect of acetyl glutamate on the proteolytic activity of submitochondrial fractions.

Experiment	Acetone fraction added	N-Acetyl-glutamate added −	N-Acetyl-glutamate added +
		(µmoles aminoacid formed)	
1	None	0.09	—
	A	0.11	—
	B	0.11	—
	C	0.20	0.22
	D	0.25	0.28
	A to D	0.33	—
	A to D*	0.07	0.07
2	None	0.07	0.08
	B′	0.19	0.21
	C′	0.25	0.27
	A′ to C′	0.30	0.35

Reaction mixtures contained in 1.25 ml 62.5 µmoles potassium phosphate buffer, 3.75 mg mitoplast protein and, when indicated, acetone fractions of the digitonin-soluble fraction (see Methods) in equal proportion to the mitoplasts as in the original mitochondria. 10 mM acetyl glutamate was used. At 0 time and after 2 h incubation, 0.5 ml portions were taken and assayed. * without mitoplasts.

illustrated in Table 3, which also shows that the effect of acetyl glutamate at low or very high levels of phosphate was inhibitory.

Attempts were carried out in several ways to minimize the endogenous proteolysis (likely due to lysosomal contamination) and thus to clarify the activation by N-acetyl-glutamate, e. g. by heat. Also, separation by gross solubility was tested. It was found that the proteolytic activity as well as the stimulation by N-acetyl-glutamate were fairly stable to heat (up to 60 °C for 5 min), but there was no increase of effect. As illustrated in Table 4, proteolysis is lower in each fraction than in the starting mitochondria; the fractions are practically devoid of activation by N-acetyl-glutamate, but it is restored when the fractions are recombined. Since the proteolysis could not be reduced sufficiently by these methods so that the effect of acetyl glutamate would possibly become more marked, we attempted separatation of the mitoplasts and the outer membrane and intermembrane fraction (containing lysosomal components). As illustrated in Table 5, some success has been obtained. Perhaps by combination of this technique, the use of heavy mitochondria (i. e. with lower contamination of lysosomes) and the use of higher specific activities, an assay system may be developed for the physiological signals (by fractionations of large amounts of mitochondria) and may clarify the problem of neutral protease and mitochondrial degradation.

We tested proteolysis in rat brain mitochondria and the effect of several amino acid derivatives on it. An increase in radioactivity and in ninhydrin-positive material in the soluble TCA supernatant was noted when N-acetyl-glutamate was added (Table 6). Acyl-amino acids were without effect on proteolysis in rat intestinal mucosa (checked in the 600 $\times$ *g* to 8500 $\times$ *g* fraction) and doubtful in rat kidney mitochondria and rat skeletal muscle (checked in the 600 $\times$ *g* to 8500 $\times$ g fraction).

Table 6
Effect of several acyl amino acids on proteolysis of rat brain mitochondria.

Addition	Radioactivity liberated (% of total)	Amino acid liberated (µmoles/mg protein)
None	1.3 ± 0.7 (3)	0.028 ± 0.011 (3)
N-acetyl-glutamate	1.7 ± 0.4 (3)	0.045 ± 0.011 (3)
N-acetyl-aspartate	2.0 ± 0.2 (3)	–
N-carbamyl-glutamate	1.7 ± 0.3 (2)	–

Experimental conditions were the same as for Table 2, using radioactive brain mitochondria (5 to 10 mg protein/ml). 1 h incubation.

It is known that acetyl glutamate induces conformational and stability effects on carbamyl phosphate synthetase [13] and due to the fact that this enzyme makes up nearly 20% of the protein of the mitoplast, it could explain some of the findings presented here. On the other hand, it is self-evident that neutral proteolysis and intracellular protein degradation are very complex [14].

The findings presented here, although possibly obscured by the extensive proteolysis manifested "in vitro", indicate that small molecular weight metabolites may serve as physiological initiators, inhibitors or controllers for intracellular protein degradation.

Acknowledgement

This work was supported in part by grants AMO 1855 and 1-FO5-TWO-2154-01 from the National Institutes of Health.

References

[1] Grisolia, S., and P. P. Cohen: J. biol. Chem. **204**, 753—757 (1953)
[2] Tatibana, M., K. Shigesada, and M. Mori in: The Urea Cycle. S. Grisolia, R. Baguena and F. Mayor (Eds.). John Wiley and Sons, New York, 1976, p. 95—105
[3] Charles, R., J. M. Tager, and E. C. Slater: Biochim. biophys. Acta **131**, 29—41 (1967)
[4] Rivas, J., A. Reglero, and S. Grisolia in: The Urea Cycle. S. Grisolia, R. Baguena and F. Mayor (Eds.). John Wiley and Sons, New York, 1976, p. 155
[5] Schneider, W. C.: J. biol. Chem. **176**, 259—266 (1948)
[6] Greenawalt, J. W.: Meth. Enzym. **31**, 310—323 (1974)
[7] Jacobs, E. E., M. Jacob, D. R. Sanadi, and L. B. Bradley: J. biol. Chem. **223**, 147 to 156 (1956)
[8] Spies, J. R.: Meth. Enzym. **3**, 468—471 (1957)
[9] Ratner, S.: Meth. Enzym. **5**, 843—848 (1962)
[10] Kuo, S. C., and E. S. Younathan: Anal. Biochem. **55**, 1—8 (1973)
[11] Rivas, J., A. Reglero, and S. Grisolia: Unpublished.
[12] Rubio, V., and S. Grisolia: FEBS Lett. **75**, 281—284 (1977)
[13] Grisolia, S.: Physiol. Rev. **44**, 657—712 (1964)
[14] Nicoletti, M., C. Guerri, and S. Grisolia: Eur. J. Biochem. **75**, 583 (1977)

Acta biol. med. germ., Band 36, Seite 1681–1690 (1977)

Université Catholique de Louvain, Laboratoire de Chimie Physiologique
and International Institute of Cellular and Molecular Pathology, Avenue Hippocrate, 75
B-1200 Bruxelles, Belgium

Flow and shuttle of plasma membrane during endocytosis

P. Tulkens*, Y. J. Schneider, and A. Trouet

Summary

A striking feature of endocytosis is the large amount of surface membrane that is brought into the cells through the formation of endocytic vesicles. Little is known about the fate of this membrane material. It is implausible that it would be destroyed in lysosomes, as the rate of turnover of the constituents of plasma membrane is much too low with respect to the rate of endocytosis in all cells studied so far. Conversely, plasma membrane fragments, internalized by endocytosis cannot merely be incorporated in lysosomes, as these organelles have been shown to maintain their size, despite continuous and active endocytosis. We present evidence that plasma membrane antigens, detected by means of specific antibodies, are internalized during endocytosis and reach lysosomes. They are thereafter returned back to cell surface. These results indicate the existence of a *shuttle* of membrane elements between the cell surface and lysosomes.

Introduction

Cytoplasmic membranes are involved in high flux transport of material from or to cells, during the processes of secretion or endocytosis. This transport is made through a network of vesicles, which continuously fuse and exchange entrapped material, until this is either discharged outside cells or ends up in lysosomes. The importance of this cellular activity should not be underlooked, as it seems to be the only way that allows important passage of macromolecules between the intra-cellular and extracellular media. In this paper, we will study the mechanism of endocytosis and focus our attention on the fate of the membranes that are involved in it.

Endocytosis consists in the formation of a vesicle, called an endocytic vesicle, at the expenses of the pericellular membrane, around a droplet of the external medium.

Endocytosis is usually distinguished into *phagocytosis*, in which particulate material (of a size generally larger than 1 μm) is taken up, and *pinocytosis*, in which only fluid, or very small particles of less than 1 μm are engulfed. These two processes share many features, although definite differences in metabolic requirements have been reported [1]; furthermore, phagocytosis is accomplished only by certain specialized cells, such as macrophages, whereas pinocytosis is observed in almost all cells [2]. In this paper, we will restrict our study to pinocytosis, and the term endocytosis that we will use throughout, will refer only to this cellular activity.

Endocytic vesicles arising from the cell surface fuse with one or several lysosomes; this results in the formation of digestive vacuoles (secondary lysosomes), where hydrolytic enzymes may exert their actions.

* Chargé de Recherches of the Belgian Fonds National de la Recherche Scientifique.

Extracellular constituents taken up by endocytosis, are usually digested, soon after they reached lysosomes, and this aspect of cell physiology is very well documented [2]. Little is known, however, about the fate of the membrane material that accompanies the endocytozed constituents. It is unlikely that this material would be merely incorporated in lysosomes, as the plasma membrane and the lysosome membrane are of distinct composition [2]; mechanisms should therefore exist to deal with it and we will try to unravel them. We will first review the available data regarding the rate of apparent membrane consumption involved in endocytosins and the rate of turnover of the constituents of the plasma membrane. We will thereafter present experimental data which support the idea that endocytosis involves a shuttle of membrane elements between the plasma membrane and lysosomes. The consequences of such a mechanism will be discussed.

Review

Rate of plasma membrane internalization during endocytosis

Material entering cells by endocytosis may either be taken simply in solution, by bulk phase ((*fluid endocytosis*) or may adsorb on the pericellular membrane, and be thereafter internalized during the formation of the endocytic vacuole (*adsorptive endocytosis*) [1]. Fluid endocytosis can maintain high rate of substrate capture for long periods [6, 7]: considering the amount of material taken up [8] and the dimension of the endocytic vesicles (100—200 nm diameter [9, 10]), internalization of large amounts of plasma membrane should be observed. For instance, it has been calculated that endocytosis of sucrose by Chang's cells requires the use of 30% of the cell membrane every hour [11]; similarly, the endocytosis of Triton WR 1339 by liver should "consume" 37% of the plasma membrane per hour [12, 13]. Using the direct approach offered by stereological studies of peroxidase endocytosis, STEINMAN et al. [8] have reported influx rates of 50 to 200% of the cell surface per hour.

The membrane influx associated with adsorptive endocytosis is more difficult to calculate, because of uncertainties regarding the density of binding sites and the association constant towards their ligands. The data of the adsorptive uptake of low density lipoprotein [14], lysosomal enzymes [15] or asialo-glycoproteins [16, 17] indicate that the internalization rate of the binding sites is quite fast, between 50 to 300% of all available sites per hour. Unless those sites are internalized without any appreciable part of the pericellular membrane, an implausible hypothesis, the rate of plasma membrane influx should be important.

In all these studies, it is noted that cells maintain the integrity of their surface membrane and that the size of lysosomes does not increase in relation with the calculated or observed membrane influx. During endocytosis, cells must therefore not only restore their surface membrane or surface binding sites but must also eliminate the excess of membrane material brought to lysosomes. This last point is all the more evident, as the membrane area surrounding lysosomal bodies is only a fraction of the area of the plasma membrane [13].

Two basic mechanisms may be envisaged to account for these requirements: (i) degradation of internalized membrane and binding sites in lysosomes, associated with a corresponding synthesis of new plasma membrane constituents.

(ii) recycling of membrane constituents, involving the restitution to the cell surface of the membrane fragments or subunits that have been internalized during endocytosis.

The first mechanism differs completely from the second in that it implies a very high rate of turnover of all the plasma membrane constituents. It is therfore of interest to examine available data of this turnover.

Turnover rate of plasma membrane

The rate of turnover of the plasma membrane proteins is not much different from that of the proteins of the other subcellular membranes [18, 19]. In cultured mammalian cells, their mean half life is comprised between 25 and 100 hours [20—24]; longer half life have been reported for highly dividing cells [20, 23]. It is controversial whether the various proteins are degraded individually, or if the membrane is renewed in large structural units; in liver [18], pancreas [19] or monkey epithelial cells [25], markedly heterogeneous turnover rates have been reported for proteins, with regard to their molecular size, the largest ones being degraded and resynthetized faster than smaller ones. On the contrary, in hepatoma tumor cells [22], human fibroblasts or Chinese hamster ovary cells [24], all plasma membrane proteins display similar rates of turnover. Little is known about the turnover of other membrane constituents; available reports indicate that glycoproteins are renewed at a rate similar to that of proteins [20, 21], whereas marked heterogeneity has been observed in the rate of turnover of phospholipids and cerebrosides [26, 27].

Materials and methods

Our experiments were conducted on rat embryo fibroblasts. Cells are incubated with endocytozable substances or antibodies (labelled with $^{14}C/^{3}H$ acetic anhydride or fluorescein isothiocyanate), harvested and fractionated by isopycnic centrifugation in sucrose gradients. The distributions of several marker enzymes of lysosomes (N-acetyl-β-glucosaminidase, cathepsin D) or plasma membrane (5'-nucleotidase, nucleoside diphosphatase) are established and compared with those of the antibodies or endocytozed molecules.

Antibodies were raised in rabbits against purified plasma membrane from rat liver or fibroblasts and purified by immunoadsorption on homologous membrane, followed by specific elution and subsequent adsorption on heterologous membranes. These antibodies (anti-PM-IgG) react specifically with isolated plasma membranes and inhibit strongly 5'-nucleotidase. Details on these procedures have been given in previous publications [3—5].

Results

In order to obtain direct information on the fate of the plasma membrane during endocytosis, we have compared the behaviour of different ligands of this membrane, namely (i) substances entering cells by adsorptive endocytosis and (ii) antibodies directed against constituents of the plasma membranes. Rat fibroblasts constitute a priviledged material for this study, as isopycnic centrifugation allows a clear analytical resolution between plasma membrane, detected by 5'-nucleotidase, and lysosomes (N-acetyl-β-glucosaminidase, cathepsin D), the former equilibrating at a buoyant density of about 1.15 g/cm^3 and the latters at about 1.20 g/cm^3 [3].

Endocytosis in fibroblasts

In a first step, we incubated rat fibroblasts in presence of rabbit IgG, labelled with fluorescein, obtained from control animals (F-IgG). As shown previously [4], fibroblasts take up F-IgG by a process of adsorptive endocytosis. This was demonstrated as follows. Cells were incubated for increasing periods of time with F-IgG, collected and fractionated by isopycnic centrifugation. At short times, intracellular IgG displayed a density distribution pattern similar to that of 5′-nucleotidase, marker enzyme of plasma membrane. When incubation was prolonged, label was observed in increasing amounts in fractions rich in cathepsin D, a lysosomal enzyme, evidencing the transfer of F-IgG from plasma membrane to lysosomes. Table 1 shows the absolute quantities of F-IgG found associated to 5′-nucleotidase or cathepsin D in those experiments. Assuming that the whole surface of the cell is involved in the endocytosis of F-IgG, it can be calculated that fibroblasts internalize the equivalent of their plasma membrane every hour. Studies of adsorptive endocytosis of DNA or dextran [28] indicate a similar rate of membrane

Table 1
Subcellular distribution of control fluorescein-labelled IgG (F-IgG) accumulated by cultured fibroblasts

Incubation time (hrs)	Amount of intracellular F-IgG (in µg/mg of total cell protein) assignable to	
	5′-nucleotidase	Cathepsin D
1	0.16	0.08
3	0.14	0.41
36	0.14	1.20

Cells were cultured in presence of F-IgG (100 µg/ml), harvested and fractionated by isopycnic centrifugation [3, 4]. Assignment of F-IgG was made by resolving the distribution patterns of F-IgG into two subpatterns, following those of 5′-nucleotidase and cathepsin D respectively, by means of double regression analysis. The amount of IgG that could not be assigned did not exceed 10% of the intracellular IgG.

influx. It is striking that this rate is of the same order of magnitude as that found for *fluid endocytosis* in L cells [8], in HTC cells [29] or Chang's cells [11]. This supports the idea that *adsorptive endocytosis* and *fluid endocytosis* are not two separate phenomena, and that binding of F-IgG or other compounds to the surface membrane does not act as a signal for endocytosis; the surface membrane would be continuously internalized, but would convey external substances to lysosomes at different rates, depending of their concentration and their possible affinity for binding sites.

The fate of plasma membrane during endocytosis

The fate of the constituents of the cell surface was thereafter studied by means of anti-plasma membrane IgG (anti-PM-IgG). Anti-PM-IgG is accumulated by cells to concentrations 5—30fold higher than that of unspecific IgG. In fractionation experiments, all anti-PM-IgG is found exclusively associated with 5′-nucleotidase. Providing low concentration of antibody is used, no untoward effect of anti-PM-

Table 2
Subcellular distribution of anti-PM-IgG (labelled with [^{3}H] acetic anhydride) and control IgG (labelled with fluorescein isothiocyanate) accumulated by fibroblasts after 24 hrs incubation

	Amount of IgG (in % of the total intracellular IgG) assignable to	
	5'Nucleotidase	Cathepsin D
Anti-PM-IgG	78.9	20.6
Control IgG	7.2	89.4

Cells were cultured in presence of anti-PM-IgG (10 μg/ml) and control fluorescein-labelled IgG (100 μg/ml), harvested and fractionated by isopycnic centrifugation. Same method of calculation of the assignment as in Table 1.

IgG on endocytosis of F-IgG, dextran or peroxidase was noticed. This allowed the following observations to be made: (i) cells incubated 24 hrs in presence of both anti-PM-IgG and unspecific F-IgG display anti-PM-IgG consistently at their surface, whereas F-IgG is found almost exclusively in lysosomes, as expected from data of Table 1. This is illustrated in Table 2, where are indicated the amounts of each type of IgG assignable to 5'-nucleotidase or cathepsin D, during these experiments. Localization of anti-PM-IgG on plasma membrane and of unspecific F-IgG in lysosomes was confirmed by fluorescence microscopy. All along these experiments, it was checked that label represented intact IgG, and that only minimal degradation of accumulated IgG occured.

Results of Table 1 and Table 2 may be explained in two different ways:
(i) anti-PM-IgG and F-IgG react with distinct constituents of the plasma membrane; only the last ones are involved in endocytosis [30, 31],
(ii) the whole plasma membrane is actually involved in the formation of endocytic vesicles, but most of the membrane material, carrying anti-PM-IgG is restituted to the surface of the cell, after coming into contact with lysosomes [4].

To test between these two possibilities, an experiment was designed to evidence possible direct interaction between anti-PM-IgG and lysosomal constituents. Cells were incubated with fluorescein labelled goat (anti-rabbit) IgG (FG-IgG). Like F-IgG, FG-IgG is taken up by endocytosis and after 24 hrs, are found almost exclusively in lysosomes. Cells were then washed, incubated in presence of rabbit anti-PM-IgG for 4 or 24 hrs and fractionated. In comparison with a control experiment, in which cells were incubated with unspecific fluorescein labelled goat IgG, we observed [23]:(i) abnormal distribution patterns of both 5'-nucleotidase and anti-PM-IgG, which partially equilibrated at a buoyant density close to that of lysosomal N-acetyl-β-glucosaminidase; (ii) a reciprocal alteration of the distribution pattern of FG-IgG, which was partially recovered at the buoyant density of normal plasma membrane; (iii) the appearance of substantial amounts of FG-IgG in the culture fluid, with an apparent molecular weight larger than 160,000, suggesting the release of antigen-antibody complexes between FG-IgG and rabbit anti-PM-IgG in the external medium. The distribution of lysosomal enzymes was

Table 3
Distribution of fluorescein labelled goat IgG (FG-IgG), rabbit anti-PM-IgG and 5′-nucleotidase in fibroblasts and in the extracellular medium

	Amount (in % of the total intracellular amount) assignable to (1)		Amount found in the extracellular medium (in % of the total intracellular amount) (2)
	Plasma membrane	Lysosomes	
Control (3)			
FG-IgG	7	91	0.0
Anti-PM-IgG	89	11	—
5′-nucleotidase	100	0	—
Exp. 1 (4)			
FG-IgG	11	87	8.6
Anti-PM-IgG	53	47	—
5′nucleotidase	78	10	—
Exp. 2 (5)			
FG-IgG	18	79	27.2
Anti-PM-IgG	76	24	—
5′-nucleotidase	81	12	—

(1) Assignment is made by comparison with the distribution patterns of 5′-nucleotidase (plasma membrane) and N-acetyl-β-glucosaminidase (lysosomes) of the control experiment; same method of calculation as in Table 1.
(2) Material of a molecular weight equal or higher than 160,000 daltons.
(3) Cells incubated 24 hrs in presence of control FG-IgG, and subsequently in presence of anti-PM-IgG (mol. ratio of intracell. goat IgG/rabbit IgG = 1.82).
(4) Cells incubated 24 hrs in presence of anti-rabbit FG-IgG, and subsequently 4 hrs in presence of anti-PM-IgG (mol. ratio of intracell. goat IgG/rabbit IgG = 4.88).
(5) Cells incubated 24 hrs in presence of anti-rabbit FG-IgG, and subsequently in presence of anti-PM-IgG for 24 hrs (mol. ratio of intracell. goat IgG/rabbit IgG = 1.70).

unaffected. These results are summarized in Table 3, where are indicated the amounts of 5′-nucleotidase, anti-PM-IgG and FG-IgG, assignable to plasma membrane and lysosomes, by comparison with distribution patterns of 5′-nucleotidase and N-acetyl-β-glucosaminidase of control cells. The intracellular concentration of rabbit anti-PM-IgG, relatively to that of FG-IgG, influences markedly the results. If cells contain less anti-PM-IgG than FG-IgG (exp. n°1), the amounts of anti-PM-IgG assignable to lysosomes are important; conversely when cells contain more anti-PM-IgG than FG-IgG (exp. n°2), the distribution of anti-PM-IgG is not so markedly affected, whereas the amounts of FG-IgG assignable to the plasma membrane, or found in the extracellular fluid become very large.

Discussion

Endocytosis involves a rapid influx of membrane material from the surface of the cell to lysosomes. Available data on the turnover rate of the plasma membrane proteins make very unlikely the possibility that this material is physiologically broken down in lysosomes and resynthesized. Our own data, obtained with anti-plasma membrane antibodies indicate that antigens of the plasma membrane are apparently stable for at least 24 hrs at the cell surface, despite active endocytosis. It could be proposed that endocytic vesicles could be made up of only a very limited number of constituents that would turn over very rapidly. Available evidence is however that endocytic vesicles and plasma membrane share several constituents [33, 34]; furthermore, turnover studies do not reveal any very fast turning protein in plasma membranes.

The "shuttling" membrane, as a model for endocytosis

The experiments summarized in Table 3 indicate that direct interaction between a ligand of the surface membrane, such as a rabbit anti-PM-IgG and a compound stored in lysosomes, like goat (anti-rabbit) IgG, can be observed. We suggest that our results are compatible with the following hypothesis: during endocytosis, anti-PM-IgG, located at the surface of the cell, is internalized and reaches lysosomes, where reaction with FG-IgG occurs. If goat (anti-rabbit) IgG is in excess, it will bind most of the incoming rabbit anti-PM-IgG and this will result in the accumulation of this last IgG in lysosomes; it is noteworthy that some 5′-nucleotidase is trapped as well, which is a clear indication that constituents of the plasma membrane have come into contact with lysosomes, and we propose that they are trapped therein through anti-PM-IgG. Conversely, if anti-PM-IgG is in excess, it draws goat (anti-rabbit) IgG along on its way back to the surface membrane, where exchange may occur with anti-PM-IgG present in large amounts in the culture fluid.

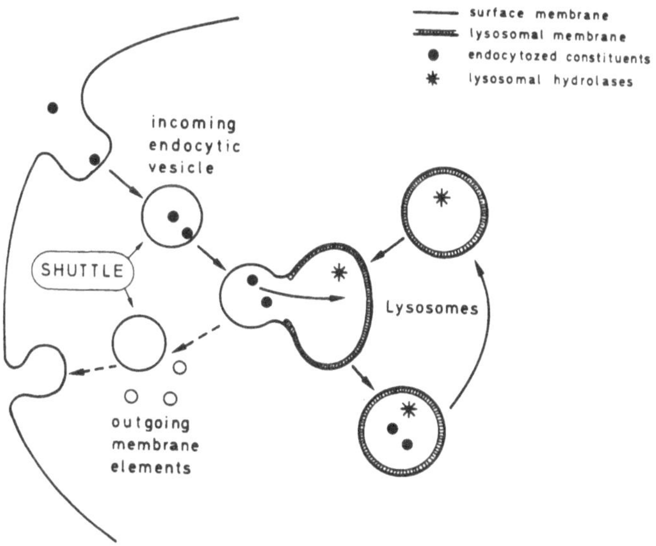

Fig. 1. A proposed mechanism for endocytosis. It involves a permanent shuttle of membrane elements between the cell surface and the lysosomes. Incoming arc is constituted by endocytic vesicles. Efferent arc is of unknown nature, but should accomodate the transport and the correct re-location at the cell surface of antigens of the plasma membrane that have been internalized by endocytosis

Accordingly we propose that endocytosis involves a permanent *shuttle* of membrane elements, between the cell surface and lysosomes. This model is schematically depicted in Fig. 1. The incoming arc is constituted by endocytic vesicles, conveying to lysosomes endocytozed substances, free or adsorbed. Efferent arc is of an unknown nature. Conceivably, phospholipids could return to surface membrane individually, as recently suggested [35]. But the transport "en bloc" of proteins, like surface antigens, carrying anti-PM-IgG, and through those last goat (anti-rabbit) IgG, suggests that the efferent arc of the shuttle is an organized membranous structure, perhaps small vesicles.

Some implications of the endocytosis "shuttle"

If the model of endocytosis presented here is confirmed for other cell types, we believe that it offers a satisfactory explanation for the contradictory features of endocytosis that have been underlined here, mainly the large influx of membrane involved and the apparent stability of the constituents of the cell surface. Several implications can be deduced and we will discuss some of them.

First of all, the shuttle allows to differentiate the fate of the content and the container of endocytic vesicles, and to spare the last for cellular economics. This concept is not new and has been proposed in many processes involving large flux of membrane, such as hormonal secretion [36] or neurotransmitter release [37].

Second, the accumulation of a substance in lysosomes would not only depend on its ability to bind to the surface of cells, or on the cell endocytic rate. In our model, molecules present in endocytic vesicles distribute between lysosomes and the returning vesicles according to their relative affinity for either structure and to the law of action of masses. This would explain why different constituents accumulate in various concentrations in lysosomes, even though they are internalized at similar rates. Susceptibility of these constituents to lysosomal hydrolases should however also be taken into account. The strength of the finding to lysosomes need not to be very great for substances entering cells by fluid endocytosis; for those adsorbed on plasma membrane, affinity towards lysosomes should be much larger; the drop of pH, which occurs when endocytic vesicles fuse with lysosomes [38], or the action of acid hydrolases may contribute to the release of some ligands of plasma membrane and their subsequent reassociation to lysosomes. As transfer to lysosomes is a necessary step to hydrolytic degradation, this mechanism of exchange of material between endocytic vesicles and lysosomes may prove of great importance in the regulation of the catabolism of exogenous substances, and amongst them the various ligands of the plasma membrane such as hormones, lipoproteins or asialo-glycoproteins. Conceivably, similar mechanisms could operate for autophagy and play a key role in the regulation of catabolism of intracellular constituents.

Another important implication is that lysosomal enzymes must somehow be retained in lysosomes, failing which cells would lose their hydrolases very rapidly. We have no direct information regarding the mechanism which retains acid hydrolases; it has however been demonstrated that lysosomal membrane binds "in vitro" several lysosomal enzymes, as would do an acidic ion exchanger [39]. This may physiologically prevent enzymes to leak out and it may be speculated that exocytosis, as observed in many pathological situations, could be provoked by a failure of this ionic retention mechanism. Here again, the shuttle of membrane would have important regulatory properties on the catabolic activities of lysosomes.

Concluding remarks

Flow and recycling of membranes have often been called in as hypothesises in many processes in which vesicular transport is involved [8, 19, 36, 37]. The experimental data presented here, and in our previous publications [4, 28, 32] support this concept in the case of endocytosis and show that the surface of the cell is in continuous contact with the content of lysosomes, through a shuttle of membrane elements, most probably vesicles, that arise from the plasma membrane, fuse temporarily with lysosomes and return to the pericellular membrane. This shuttle constitutes a direct link, in both directions, between extracellular and intralysosomal media. Exchange of material between these two compartments must be subjected to stringent regulation, the study of which may shed new lights on various aspects of cellular physiology and pathology.

Acknowledgements

This work was supported by the Belgian Fonds de la Recherche Scientifique Médicale and Service de la Programmation et de la Politique Scientifique.

References

[1] JACQUES, P. in: Lysosomes in Biology and Pathology. J. T. DINGLE and H. B. FELL (Eds.) **2**, 395. North-Holland Publ. Co., Amsterdam 1969
[2] HOLTZMAN, E. in: Lysosomes: a Survey. Springer, Wien, New York 1976, p. 244
[3] TULKENS, P., H. BEAUFAY, and A. TROUET: J. Cell Biol. **63**, 383 (1974)
[4] TULKENS, P., Y. J. SCHNEIDER, and A. TROUET in: Intracellular Protein Catabolism. V. TURK and N. MARKS (Eds.). **II**, 73. Plenum Press, New York 1977
[5] SCHNEIDER, Y. J.: Ph. D. Thesis, University of Louvain, Belgium 1977
[6] WILLIAMS, K. E., E. M. KIDSTON, F. BECK, and J. B. LLOYD: J. Cell Biol. **64**, 113 (1975)
[7] EHRENREICH, B. A., and Z. A. COHN: J. Cell Biol. **38**, 244 (1968)
[8] STEINMAN, R. M., S. E. BRODIE, and Z. A. COHN: J. Cell Biol. **68**, 665 (1976)
[9] ALLISON, A. C., and P. DAVIES: Symp. Soc. expl Biol. **27**, 419 (1974)
[10] STEINMAN, R. M., J. M., SILVER, and Z. A. COHN: J. Cell Biol. **63**, 949 (1974)
[11] WAGNER, R., M. ROSENBERG, and R. ESTENSEN: J. Cell Biol. **50**, 804 (1971)
[12] WATTIAUX, R.: Ph. D. Thesis, University of Louvain, Belgium 1966
[13] DE DUVE, C., Th. DE BARSY, B. POOLE, A. TROUET, P. TULKENS, and F. VAN HOOF: Biochem. Pharmac. **23**, 2495 (1974)
[14] GOLDSTEIN, J. L., S. K. BASU, G. Y. BRUNSCHEDE, and M. S. BROWN: Cell **7**, 85 (1976)
[15] STAHL, P., P. SCHLESINGER, J. S. RODMAN, and T. DOEBBER: Nature, Lond. **264**, 86 (1977)
[16] MORELL, A. G., R. A. IRVINE, I. STERNLIEB, I. H. SCHEINBERG, and G. ASHWELL: J. biol. Chem. **243**, 155 (1968)
[17] BERG, T., and H. TOLLESHAUG: Abstracts of this symposium 9 (1977)
[18] DEHLINGER, P. J., and R. T. SCHIMKE: J. biol. Chem. **246**, 2574 (1971)
[19] MELDOLESI, J.: J. Cell Biol. **61**, 1 (1974)
[20] WARREN, L., and M. C. GLICK: J. Cell Biol. **37**, 729 (1968)
[21] KAPLAN, J., and M. MOSKOWITZ: Biochim. biophys. Acta **389**, 290 (1975)
[22] TWETO, J., and D. DOYLE: J. biol. Chem. **251**, 872 (1976)
[23] ROBERTS, R. M., and B. O. CHING-YUAN: Biochemistry **13**, 4846 (1974)
[24] ROBERTS, R. M., and B. O. CHING-YUAN: Archs Biochem. Biophys. **171**, 234 (1975)
[25] KAPLAN, J., and M. MOSKOWITZ: Biochim. biophys. Acta **389**, 306 (1975)
[26] PASTERNAK, C. A., and J. S. BERGERON: Biochem. J. **119**, 473 (1970)

[27] HAKOMORI, S.: Proc. natn. Acad. Sci. U.S.A. **67**, 1741 (1970)
[28] TULKENS, P., Y. J. SCHNEIDER, and A. TROUET: Biochem. Soc. Trans. **5**, 1809 (1977)
[29] QUINTART, J.: Ph. D. Thesis, University of Louvain, Belgium 1977
[30] SCHNEIDER, Y. J., A. TROUET, and P. TULKENS: Hoppe-Seyler's Z. physiol. Chem. **335**, 84 (1975)
[31] SCHNEIDER, Y. J., A. TROUET, and P. TULKENS: Archs int. Physiol. Biochim **83**, 997 (1975)
[32] SCHNEIDER, Y. J., P. TULKENS, and A. TROUET: Biochem. Soc. Trans. **5**, 336 (1977)
[33] HUBBARD, A. L., and Z. A. COHN: J. Cell Biol. **64**, 438 (1975)
[34] HUBBARD, A. L., and Z. A. COHN: J. Cell Biol. **64**, 461 (1975)
[35] HARRIS, A. K.: Nature, Lond. **263**, 781 (1976)
[36] DOUGLAS, W. W., and J. NAGASAWA: J. Physiol., Lond. **218**, 94 (1971)
[37] HEUSER, J. E., and T. S. REESE: J. Cell Biol. **57**, 315 (1973)
[38] JENSEN, M. S., and D. F. BAINTON: J. Cell Biol. **56**, 379 (1973)
[39] HENNING, R., H. PLATTNER, and W. STOFFEL: Biochim. biophys. Acta **330**, 61 (1973)

Acta biol. med. germ., Band 36, Seite 1691—1694 (1977)

Institute of Pathology, University of Würzburg, Luitpoldkrankenhaus, 8700 Würzburg, GFR

Inhibition by insulin of the physiological autophagic breakdown of cell organelles

U. Pfeifer

Summary

By using electron microscopic morphometry it was found that the fractional volume of autophagic vacuoles in the cytoplasm of liver cells decreases rapidly after administering 5 units insulin per kg body weight to otherwise untreated rats. From the decay which appears to follow first order kinetics a half-life of 9 min was found for the compartment of autophagic vacuoles. The rates of autophagic breakdown calculated were different for the different cytoplasmic components, indicating that selecting mechanisms are involved in the process of segregation which is the first step in autophagy.

Among the possible mechanisms of the intracellular degradation of the cell's own proteins cellular autophagy [1—3] is the only one for which there exists a clear-cut morphological correlation: the autophagic vacuole (AV). It consists of a bit of cytoplasm segregated from the remaining cytoplasm by a membraneous border. The term AV comprises two stages: the pre-lysosomal autophagosome and, after fusion with a pre-existing lysosome, the autolysosome which represents the place where the enclosed material is degraded into low molecular compounds. Since these two stages cannot always be clearly distinguished by routine electron microscopy, the AV is defined in this paper as the dynamic entity which is formed by segregation, and whose existence is terminated by destruction (Fig. 1), that means degeneration of the enclosed cytoplasmic structures to a stage where they can no longer be identified with the electron microscope.

Because of the well known fact that AV occur in differentiated cells already under physiological circumstances [2, 3] the question has been often discussed, to which extent cellular autophagy contributes to the intracellular turnover, as it can be measured biochemically. The morphometric approach presented in this paper is based on the model shown in Fig. 1.

Assuming steady state conditions it can be deduced from this model that two parameters are required if the rate, $1/t_{cyto}$, at which cytoplasmic components are broken down by cellular autophagy has to be calculated: 1) the volume fraction of the compartment AV in relation to the remaining cytoplasm (V_{AV}/V_{cyto}), 2) the average life time of an AV (t_{AV}). Since there does not exist any method to label specifically the contents of an AV, the only appropriate way seemed to inhibit the formation of new AV as completely and as abruptly as possible, and to calculate then t_{AV} from the decay of the volume fraction of AV.

This work was supported by Deutsche Forschungsgemeinschaft, Sonderforschungsbereich 105. The technical assistance of Hannelore Bergeest and Evelyn Werder is greatfully acknowledged.

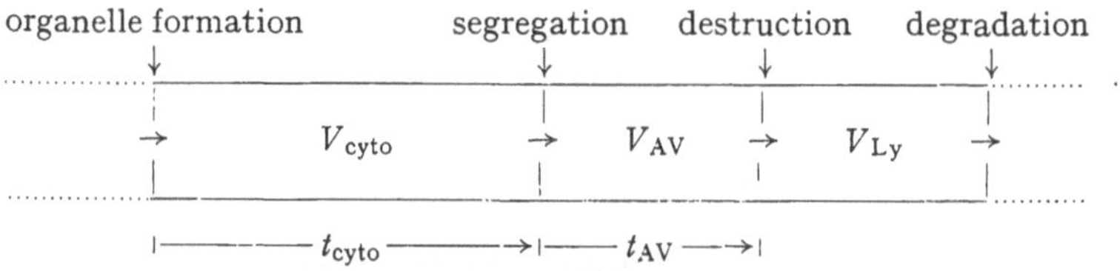

V_{cyto}: Volume of the total cytoplasm except that enclosed in AV.
V_{AV}: Volume of the whole compartment AV
t_{cyto}: mean time interval between the formation of a cytoplasmic structure and its segregation = life time of this structure
t_{AV}: mean time interval between the segregation of a cytoplasmic structure and its destruction = life time of an AV

Under stready state conditions the following equations are valid:

$$V_{AV}/V_{cyto} = t_{AV}/t_{cyto} \quad \text{(I)}$$

$$1/t_{cyto} = (V_{AV}/V_{cyto}) \cdot (1/t_{AV}) \quad \text{(II)}$$

Fig. 1. Model explaining the relationship between static and kinetic parameters which are required for a calculation of $1/t_{cyto}$ which is the rate to which cytoplasmic constituents are broken down by autophagy

Since glucagon is known to stimulate the formation of AV [4, 5] in liver cells, insulin which acts as an antagonist to glucagon with respect to protein degradation [6] was tested as a possible inhibitor of cellular autophagy.

In repeated experiments a total of 46 male adult Sprague Dawley rats were injected i. p. with 5 units insulin per kg body weight between 10.30 and 11.00, the time interval during which in the liver the amount of AV is still increasing in the course of the physiological diurnal cycle [7, 8]. The animals were killed either immediately or at different time intervals, up to 33 min, after the injection. The liver tissue was fixed by immersion with 1.5% OsO_4, dehydrated, and embedded in epon.

By point counting electron micrographs taken at random [9] the volume fractions of the following components in relation to the whole cytoplasm were determined: Mitochondria (Mito), microbodies (Mb) = peroxisomes, endoplasmic reticulum together with ground substance (ERGS), and glycogen (Glyco). The mean values obtained at time zero (16 animals) are shown in column 2 of Table 1. After insulin administration the only significant alteration observed was a decrease of the volume fraction of glycogen to about 65% of the initial value at the end of the experimental time interval.

Using a modified morphometric technique [10] the AV were counted and measured directly at the screen of the electron microscope. According to their main contents different types of AV, containing Mito, ERGS, Mb, or Glyco, could be distinguished. At time zero the volume fraction of all AV amounted to a value of $2.1 \cdot 10^{-4}$. The values for the volume fractions of the different types of AV in relation to the whole cytoplasm are shown in column 3 of Table 1, whereas in column 4 the volume fractions of the different types of AV are given in relation to the respective cytoplasmic component.

After insulin the number of AV profiles per test area of cytoplasm as well as the volume fraction of the compartment AV in relation to the whole cytoplasm showed

Table 1
Morphometric and kinetic parameters of cellular autophagy in rat liver parenchymal cells

1 Cytoplasmic component	2 V_{comp}/V_{cyto}	3 V_{AV}/V_{cyto} $(\cdot 10^{-4})$	4 V_{AV}/V_{comp} $(\cdot 10^{-4})$	5 $t\,1/2_{AV}$ (min)	6 $1/t_{comp}$ (day^{-1})
Total	1.000	2.11	2.11	9.0	0.023
Mito	0.200	0.79	3.95	10.1	0.039
Mb	0.014	0.09	6.42	7.2	0.089
ERGS	0.554	0.81	1.47	11.5	0.013
Glyco	0.214	0.42	1.95	18.0	0.011

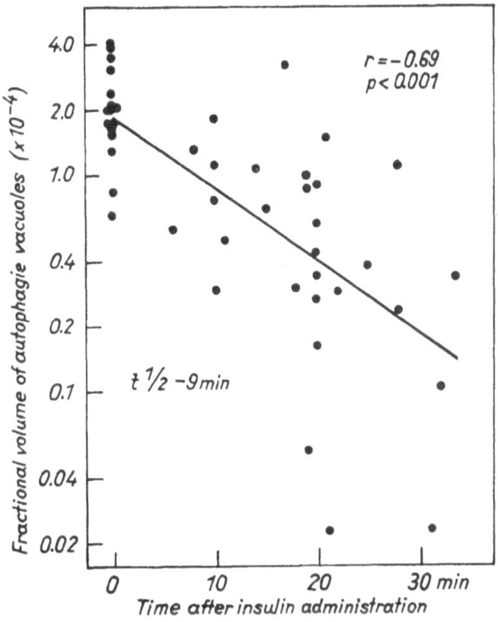

Fig. 2. Decay after insulin administration (5 units per kg bd.wt.) of the fractional volume of autophagic vacuoles in relation to the whole cytoplasm. The negative correlation between the fractional volume of the autophagic vacuoles and the time interval after insulin administration is statistically highly significant as shown by Student *t*-test. A half-life of 9 min was found from the regression line

a rather rapid decrease (Fig. 2) which by regression analysis turned out to be highly significant ($p < 0.001$) for all AV, and also for the different types of AV, except the AV containing glycogen, whose decrease in volume fraction was significant only at the 5% level ($p < 0.05$). The best fitted regression lines were obtained when the values were plotted in a semilogarithmic coordinate system. This suggests that the decay of the AV volume fraction follows first order kinetics which could be explained by the assumption that the process of destruction which, as defined, terminates the "life" of an AV takes place independently of the "age" of an AV. This would be true if destruction depended largely on the presence of lysosomal enzymes, and if fusion between autophagosomes and lysosomes took place at random [11].

The apparent half-life calculated from the decay of the volume fraction of all AV amounted to a value of only 9 min. The values of the half-life of the different types of AV are shown in column 5 of Table 1. Assuming that the average life time equals the half-life divided by ln 2, the values for the rates of breakdown by autophagy for the different cytoplasmic components were calculated according to Fig. 1. They are shown in column 6 of the Table.

It can be seen that the rates of autophagic breakdown are not the same for the different cytoplasmic components. Mitochondria, for instance, are removed from the cytoplasm by autophagy to a rate of about 4% per day, whereas the rate of autophagic breakdown of the microbodies amounts to a value of 9% per day. Similar differences have been reported for the intracellular degradation of mitochondrial and peroxisomal proteins [12, 13]. It can be concluded that selecting mechanisms are involved in the process of segregation by which the autophagic vacuoles are formed.

The absolute rates found for the autophagic breakdown are lower than the biochemical rates of degradation. A possible explanation would be that the formation of AV is not completely inhibited by insulin; consequently the rates of autophagic breakdown could be underestimated. On the other hand may exist mechanisms of protein degradation other than cellular autophagy. It seems to be evident, however, that cellular autophagy plays an important role for the intracellular turnover.

As for the inhibition of protein breakdown the results of the present experiment suggest that insulin acts at the pre-lysosomal level by inhibiting the formation of autophagic vacuoles. This mode of inhibition has to be distinguished from those concerning the process of intralysosomal digestion which is inhibited, for instance, by chloroquine [14] or by ammonia [15].

References

[1] De Duve, C., and R. Wattiaux: A. Rev. Physiol. **28**, 435–492 (1966)
[2] Ericsson, J. L. E. in: Lysosomes in biology and pathology, J. T. Dingle and H. B. Fell (Eds.). Vol. **2**, 345–394. North-Holland, Amsterdam 1969
[3] Pfeifer, U.: Verh. dt. Ges. Path. **60**, 28–64 (1976)
[4] Ashford, T. P., and K. R. Porter: J. Cell Biol. **12**, 198–202 (1962)
[5] Deter, R., and Ch. de Duve: J. Cell Biol. **33**, 437–449 (1967)
[6] Mortimore, G. E., and C. E. Mondon: J. biol. Chem. **245**, 2375–2383 (1970)
[7] Pfeifer, U.: Virchows Arch. B Cell Path. **12**, 195–211 (1973)
[8] Pfeifer, U., and J. Bertling: Virchows Arch. B Cell Path. **24**, 109–120 (1977)
[9] Weibel, E.: Int. Rev. Cytol. **26**, 235–302 (1969)
[10] Pfeifer, U.: Quantification of rarely acurring structures in electron microscopy. NBS Special Publ. 432 Proceedings of the 4th International Congress of Stereology 1976, p. 411–414
[11] Deter, R. L.: Expl Cell Res. **94**, 122–126 (1975)
[12] Poole, B., F. Leighton, and C. de Duve: J. Cell Biol. **41**, 536–546 (1969)
[13] Doyle, D., and J. Tweto: Meth. Cell Biol. **10**, 235–260 (1975)
[14] Wibo, M., and B. Poole: J. Cell Biol. **63**, 430–440 (1974)
[15] Seglen, P. O., and A. Reith: Expl Cell Res. **100**, 276–280 (1976)

Acta biol. med. germ., Band 36, Seite. 1695—1703 (1977)

Central Institute for Diabetes „Gerhardt Katsch", Department of Experimental Research, 2201 Karlsburg, GDR;
University of Halle, Institute of Physiological Chemistry, Halle, GDR[1]
and the University of Chicago, Department of Biochemistry, Chicago, Ill., USA[2].

Proteolytic and transhydrogenolytic activities in isolated pancreatic islets of rats

H. ZÜHLKE, K.-D. KOHNERT, H. JAHR, S. SCHMIDT, H. KIRSCHKE[1], and D. F. STEINER[2]

Summary

In homogenates and subcellular fractions of pancreatic islets of Wistar rats we could demonstrate three groups of protein degrading enzymes. The proteinases of group 1 are characterized by both trypsin-like and carboxypeptidase B-like specificities with slightly acid *p*H optima (*p*H 5.5—6.5) and seem to play important roles in the conversion of proinsulin into insulin. The properties suggest that these enzymes localized in the secretion granule/mitochondria fraction are related to the tissue cathepsins. Group 2 enzymes are thiol-depending proteinases with a *p*H optimum at 7.0 occuring mainly in the cytosol and to a lesser extent in the fraction of nuclei and cell debris. Group 3 represents the thiol protein oxidoreductase with a *p*H optimum of 7.0. This enzyme degrading disulfide bonds could also be important in the formation of the disulfide bonds during protein folding after synthesis.

Introduction

About 20% of diabetics need exogenous insulin. The reason should be at least: 1. deficiency of the insulin biosynthesis and/or secretion, 2. high rate of cleavage of insulin, 3. disturbance of the action of insulin in the periphery (muscle, fat cells etc.).

Much effort has been devoted to understand the specific processes of protein biosynthesis. However, we know very little about the reverse mechanism of intracellular degradation of proteins. The two processes go on simultaneously in tissues with opposite net results, and one is not less important than the other. This might be true also with respect to the biosynthesis and degradation of insulin.

The biosynthesis of insulin takes place in the pancreatic islets of Langerhans. About 1—2% of the whole pancreas consist of islets containing 60—80% of β-cells, the place of the synthesis of insulin (review see [1]). With the discovery of proinsulin by STEINER and OYER [2] it was recognized that limited proteolysis plays an important role in the biosynthesis of insulin [1]. Proinsulin can be converted into insulin in vitro by appropriate mixtures of trypsin and carboxypeptidase B as concluded from the proinsulin sequence [3]. In order to detect these proteolytic enzyme activities in pancreatic islets of rats (homogenates or subcellular fractions) we have developed highly sensitive assays for both trypsin-like and carboxypeptidase B-like enzymes [4, 5].

Morphological results on pancreatic islets of various mammals [6] under special conditions (e. g. inhibition of insulin secretion) demonstrate an enhanced activity of granulolysis despite a high synthesis rate. The intracellular insulin catabolism seems to play an important part in regulating the insulin content of islets. The insulin destruction in homogenates of islets takes place in a stepwise manner first by the action of thiol-protein disulfide oxidoreductase (TPO) and second by proteinases [7]. In this paper, proteinases possibly involved in the conversion of proinsulin into insulin at *p*H 5.5—6.5, insulin and glucagon degrading proteinases at *p*H 7.0 and the TPO of islets are characterized in more detail.

Material and methods

Sources of substrates and reagents: Hippuryl-L-arginine was purchased from Becton, Dickinson and Co., Orangeburg, New York, Cbz-Gly-Gly-Arg-4-methoxy-β-naphthylamide from Bachem Inc., Marina Del Rey, Calif., 90291, (2-Prolyl-3,4-[^{3}H](N)-bradykinin from NEN, Boston, Mass., fluorescamine (Fluram) from Hoffmann-La-Roche Inc., Nutley, New York, collagenase (Type IV) from Worthington Biochemical, Freehold, New Jersey, bovine insulin (crystallized twice) from VEB Berlin-Chemie, GDR, crystallized glucagon from Eli Lilly GmbH, FRG, BANA (N-α-benzoyl-D,L-arginine-2-naphthylamide hydrochloride) and dimethylcasein from Serva, FRG, were used. Carboxypeptidase B was from Boehringer, Mannheim, FRG, Ficoll from Pharmacia Fine Chemicals, Uppsala, Sweden, ninhydrin, bovine serum albumin, 2-mercaptoethanol, iodoacetamide, N-ethyl maleimide diisopropyl fluorophosphate (DFP), and trypsin from Sigma Chemical Corp. St. Louis, Mo., soy-bean trypsin inhibitor from Nutritional Biochemicals Corp., Cleveland, Ohio, a partial sequence of porcine proinsulin Pro-Lys-Ala-[^{14}C]Arg-Arg-Glu-Ala was synthesized by and a generous gift from Dr. H. D. JAKUBKE, Halle/Saale (GDR) [8]. Thin layer plates without fluorescence (No. 6064) were from Kodak Comp. Rochester, N. Y. 14650. Antiserum against TPO isolated from rat liver was the generous gift of Dr. ANSORGE, Institute of Physiological Chemistry, University of Halle (GDR). Antisera against highly purified rat liver thiol-protein disulfide oxidoreductase were obtained by immunization of rabbits with 1 mg of enzyme protein in 0.9% sodium chloride and complete Freund's adjuvant [10].

Islets of Langerhans were isolated from pancreas of Sprague-Dawley rats (280—320 g), injected with pilocarpine (0.25 ml, 4%) 2 hrs before decapitation, by collagenase digestion according to LACY and KOSTIANOVSKY]11], by using density centrifugation in ficoll (15—25%) and isolated by means of the stereo microscope. Batches of 50—200 islets were gently homogenized in 20 µl Hanks solution in a micro tube (400 µl content) with a teflon pestle. The homogenates were diluted with deionized and twice distilled water up to 200 µl. 1—3 µg of whole protein were used for the enzymic assays. [^{125}I]-labelled insulin and glucagon were prepared using the ICI method [9]. The homogenate of about 500 pancreatic islets was centrifuged as described elsewhere [12]. The marker enzyme of the subcellular fractions (glutamate dehydrogenase, 6-phosphogluconate dehydrogenase, malate dehydrogenase, acid galactosidase, acid phosphatase) were determined according to [13].

The proteolytic degradation products of unlabelled insulin and glucagon were measured after addition of Fluram and fluorimetric detection (see [14]).

Carboxypeptidase B-activity was determined with hippuryl-L-arginine as substrate. Incubations were carried out in dimethylarsinate buffer for 6—9 hrs. Fluorescamine was then added to detect free amino groups fluorometrically (for details see [15]). Homogenates of islets of Langerhans were incubated for 90 min at 37 °C in 10 mM dimethylarsinate buffer with [^{3}H] prolyl-bradykinin as a substrate. Products were resolved by thin layer chromatography. Des-Arg-bradykinin migrates faster than bradykinin in propanol/ammonia (3:2) as solvent (for details see [15]).

Islet homogenate (10—15 µg protein) was incubated in 40 µl 0.03 M citrate or phosphate buffer, *p*H 6.5, containing 5 mg/ml heptapeptide for 7—9 hrs at 37 °C. In this assay cathepsins H, L und B_1, respectively, isolated from rat liver [16] were used in an amount of 5 µg whole protein. The split products were separated by thin layer chromatography in propanol/ammonia (2:3) as solvent.

Results

Highly sensitive assays (pg-range) for both trypsin-like and carboxypeptidase B-like enzymes in homogenates and subcellular fractions of pancreatic islets were developed (for details see Material and methods). For the detection of trypsin-like activity the substrate Cbz-Gly-Gly-Arg-(4-methyl-2-naphthyl)amide was used (Fig. 1). There are 2 *p*H-optima at 5.5 and 6.5, respectively. Both activities are stimulated by 2-mercaptoethanol. Soy-bean trypsin inhibitor and DFP have no influence.

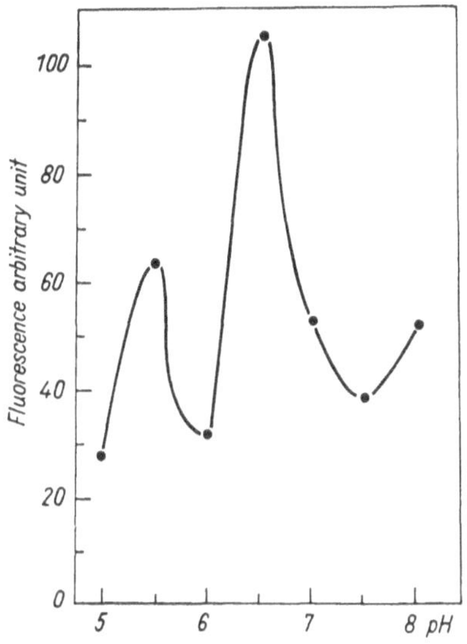

Fig. 1

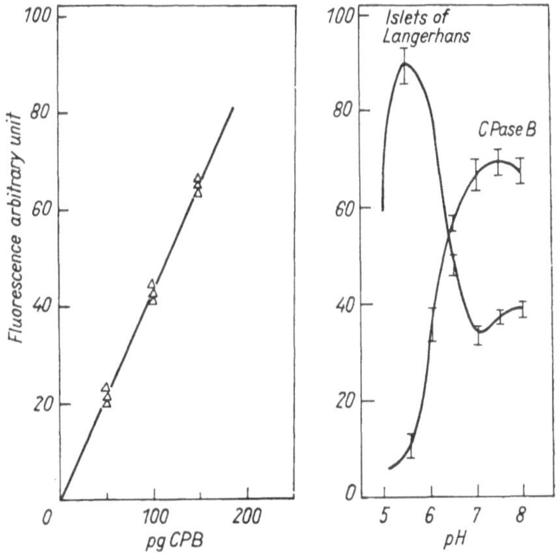

Fig. 2

Fig. 1. Determination of trypsin-like activities in homogenates of pancreatic islets with Cbz-Gly-Gly-Arg-(4-methyl)β-naphthylamide. *p*H-dependence curve

Fig. 2. Determination of carboxypeptidase B activity with hippuryl-L-arginine as substrate and the free arginine released is detected by means of fluorescamine (left pannel). *p*H-dependence curve (right pannel) for homogenates of pancreatic islets and pancreatic carboxypeptidase B (CPase B)

Hippuryl arginine is split by carboxypeptidase B-like activity. With this method to compare the *p*H dependence of pancreatic carboxypeptidase B (CPB) and the corresponding activity in homogenated islets, it can be seen that their optima differ: pancreatic CPB has a *p*H optimum of 7.0—7.5 but the activity in islets homogenate has an optimum *p*H between 5.5 and 6.0 (Fig. 2). The activity in the homogenates is inhibited by EDTA and o-phenanthroline, whereas 2-mercaptoethanol, DFP and iodo acetamide have no influence.

A second assay for carboxypeptidase B-like activity is based on the splitting of 2-prolyl-3,4-[^{3}H](N)-bradykinin into des-Arg^9-bradykinin and Arg separated by thin layer chromatography.

After incubation of islet homogenates with [^{3}H]-bradykinin in the *p*H-range between 5 and 6 a radioactive component with the R_F value of des-Arg-bradykinin

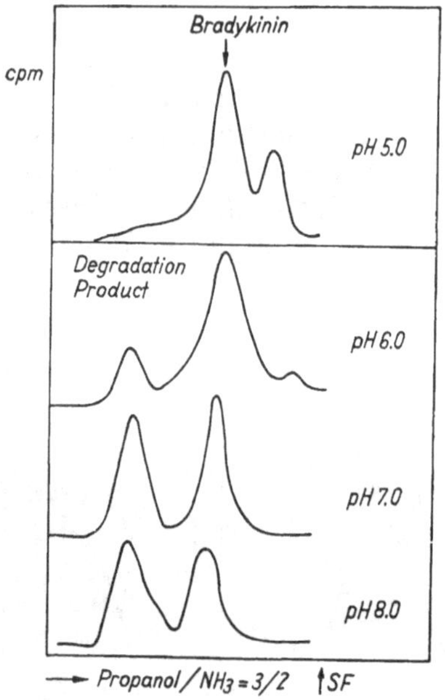

Fig. 3. Assay for carboxypeptidase B-like activity in homogenates of pancreatic islets with [^{3}H]prolyl-bradykinin as a substrate. Products were resolved by thin layer chromatography. The faster migration component is des-Arg-bradykinin. SF = solvent front

is observed (Fig. 3), whereas in the range of *p*H 6 to 8 another radioactive spot appears. EDTA as well as EDTA + 2-mercaptoethanol stimulate the formation of the des Arg-bradykinin at *p*H 6.0, N-ethyl maleimide inhibits, STI and DFP have no influence.

The release of free [^{14}C]Arg from the synthetic heptapeptide (partial sequence of pork insulin) after incubation with homogenates of islets is given in Fig. 4. The split products of the heptapeptide depend on the *p*H: at lower *p*H the highest radioactivity contains Ala-Arg and at *p*H 6.5 Arg only. EDTA inhibits the formation of Arg, EDTA and 2-mercaptoethanol give an increase of Ala-Arg.

Using the proinsulin heptapeptide as a substrate for cathepsins H, L and B_1, respectively, from rat liver we can see from Fig. 5 that cathepsin L in the presence of 2-mercaptoethanol and EDTA behaves as the converting enzyme: [^{14}C]Arg is released in contrast to cathepsins H and B_1.

We incubated homogenates of pancreatic islets and subcellular fractions respectively at *p*H 6.5 with bovine proinsulin. Proinsulin and its split products were separated in a micro polyacrylamide disc electrophoresis in capillaries. The gel was stained with Coomassie Blue R 250 [12]. The main degradation product in the secretion granule/mitochondria fraction is a protein with the R_F value comparable with insulin (Fig. 6). EDTA inhibits the conversion, pancreatic trypsin inhibitor and soy-bean inhibitor have no influence.

In Fig. 7 is shown the titration curve of a constant amount of antiserum to thiol-protein disulfide oxidoreductase with pancreatic islet homogenate.

TPO antibodies, iodo acetamide and p-chloromercuribenzoate respectively inhibit the degradation of insulin.

Table 1 shows the proteolytic degradation of insulin and glucagon by islet homogenates. At *p*H 7.0 the breakdown of glucagon is about five times higher than

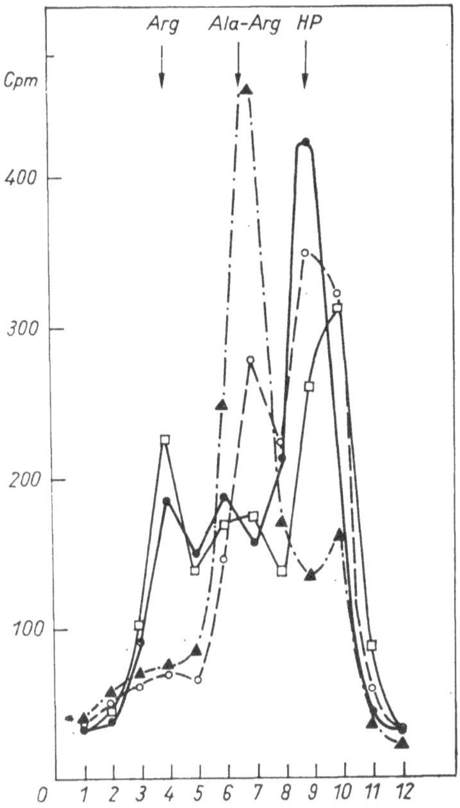

Fig. 4

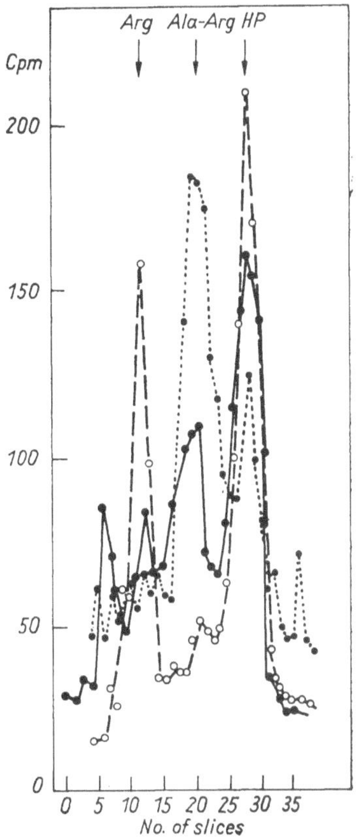

Fig. 5

Fig. 4. Determination of proteinase activity in homogenates of pancreatic islets (*p*H 6.5) with a synthetic heptapeptide (HP) (partial sequence from porcine proinsulin) Pro-Lys-Ala-[^{14}C]Arg-Arg-Glu-Ala (abscissa: relative ^{14}C radioactivity). The split products are separated by thin layer chromatography. 2-ME = 2-mercaptoethanol. ●, islets; □, islets + 2-ME; ○, islets + EDTA; ▲, islets + 2-ME + EDTA

Fig. 5. Incubation of cathepsins H, L and B_1 respectively from rat liver with a synthetic heptapeptide (HP, cf. Fig. 4) in presence of 2-mercaptoethanol and EDTA (see legend to Fig. 3). ●—●, cathepsin H; ○--○, cathepsin L; •···•, cathepsin B_1

Table 1

Degradation of insulin an glucagon by homogenates of pancreatic islets of rats.

$$\text{Specific activity} = \frac{\text{pmol TCA-soluble NH}_2}{\mu\text{g homogenate protein} \cdot \text{min}}$$

	Insulin		Glucagon	
	*p*H 7.0	*p*H 5.5	*p*H 7.0	*p*H 5.5
Islets	27.5	19.0	140.1	47.0
Islets + EDTA	24.8	—	64.8	—
Islets + 2 ME	85.3	19.5	142.5	38.8

2 ME = 2-Mercaptoethanol

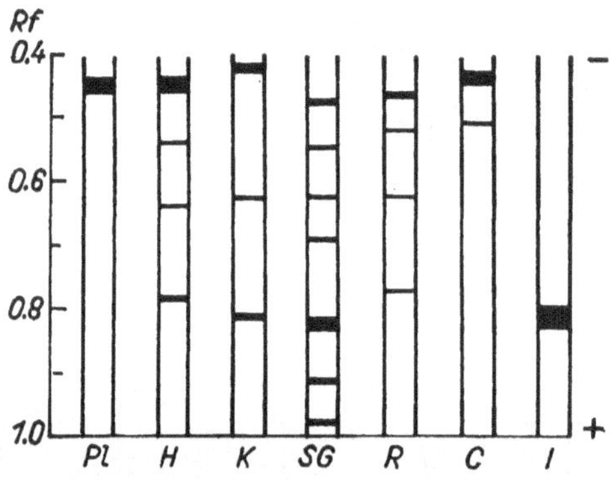

Fig. 6

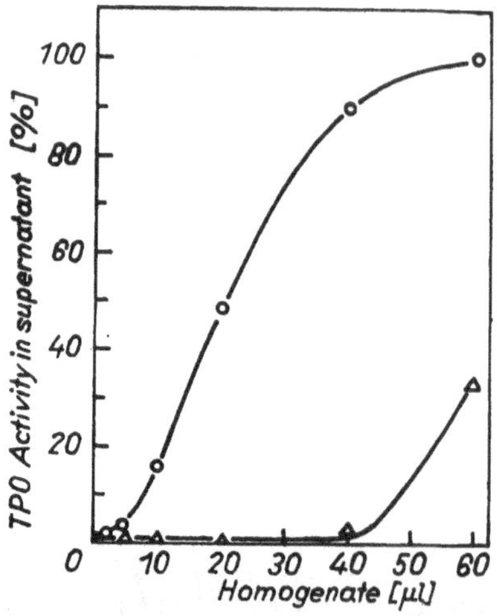

Fig. 7

Fig. 6. Degradation of bovine proinsulin by homogenates of pancreatic islets and its subcellular fractions at *p*H 6.5. Separation of the split products in the micro polyacrylamide disc electrophoresis (details for the method see [12]). PI = proinsulin, H = homogenate, K = nuclei-, SG = secretion granules/mitochondria-, R = microsomal fractions, C = cytosol, I = insulin

Fig. 7. Titration curve of a constant amount of antiserum to rat liver TPO with pancreatic islet homogenate. △, with TPO antiserum; ○, no antiserum

Table 2

Effect of thiols, thiol reagents, and chelating agents on proteolytic activities of pancreatic islets homogenates

Substrate	*p*H	Thiols	Thiol reagents	Chelating agents
α-N-benzoyl-D,L-arginine	5.5	↑	not tested	=
2-naphthylamide	7.0	↑		↓
Cbz-Gly-Gly-Arg-4-methyl-β-naphthylamide	5.5	↑	↓	=
Hippuryl-L-arginine	5.5–6.0	=	=	↓
Bradykinin	6.0	=	↓	↓
Pro-Lys-Ala-Arg-Arg-	6.0–6.5 [^{14}C] Arg	↑	not tesred	↓
Glu-Ala	6.0–6.5 Ala-[^{14}C] Arg	↑ [1]	not tested	↑ [1]
Proinsulin	6.0–6.5	=	not tested	↓
[^{125}I]-glucagon	7.0	↑	↓	↓
[^{125}I]-insulin[2]	7.0	↑	↓	↑

↑ Activation; ↓ Inhibition; = no difference

[1] 2-mercaptoethanol + EDTA; [2] 75 µg insulin per incubation

that of insulin. EDTA has no influence on insulin degradation whereas glucagon is split to a lesser extent. 2-mercaptoethanol stimulates the insulin degradation at *p*H 7.0 only.

In Table 2 the results are summarized. The islets contain at least three groups of enzymes:

1. Thiol-depending proteinases with a *p*H optimum between 5.5 and 6.5.
2. Thiol-depending proteinases with a *p*H optimum at 7.0.
3. Thiol-protein disulfide oxidoreductase with a *p*H optimum at 7.0.

Discussion

Although it has been possible to detect activities which produce insulin-like material from proinsulin in extracts of whole pancreas [17], in homogenates of islets of Langerhans [12, 18—22] or in its subcellular fractions [12, 23—26], the intracellular origin and mechanism of action of these enzymes remain uncertain. Many polypeptide hormone precursors, as well as other protein precursors have two or more residues of lysin or arginine at the cleavage site(s), a fact which leads to the supposition that the cellular processing enzymes have properties similar to pancreatic trypsin and carboxypeptidase B [27]. An important unanswered question is whether all the various pro-proteins which have paired basic residues at their cleavage sites are converted by similar or identical proteinases within their cells or alternatively whether specific enzymes exist in each specialized tissue. In order to detect and characterize appropriate proteolytic enzyme activities in islets of Langerhans we have developed highly sensitive assays for trypsin-like and carboxypeptidase B-like enzymes ([4]; see also [15]).

All these results summarized in Table 2 demonstrate the occurrence in islets of both carboxypeptidase B-like activity requiring a metal ion such as zinc and trypsin-like activity having a lower *p*H optimum than pancreatic carboxypeptidase B and trypsin. Several carboxypeptidases active in the acid *p*H region have been reported including catheptic carboxypeptidase B [28] possibly associated with cathepsin B_2 [29] and bradykinase [28]. Moreover, the similarity of the tryptic activity observed in the islet homogenates to cathepsin B_2, which is known to have trypsin-like specificity and a *p*H optimum near 6.5 [30], leads to the suspicion that this activity may arise from lysosomes disrupted during homogenization. However, the possibility must be borne in mind that the converting enzymes could be similar to some lysosomal cathepsins.

On the other hand, EDTA and other chelating agents such as o-phenanthrolin inhibits the cleavage of hippuryl-L-arginine as well as the formation of [^{14}C]Arg from synthetic heptapeptide (Fig.2, Fig. 4). These results cannot be explained by the presence of catheptic enzymes. Moreover, using the heptapeptide as a substrate for cathepsins H, L, and B_1 respectively from rat liver we can see from Fig. 5 that cathepsin L in the presence of 2-mercaptoethanol and EDTA behaves as a converting enzyme: [^{14}C]Arg is released, in contrast to cathepsins H and B_1 being in aggreement with results of Friedrich et al. [31]. But we have to emphasize that cathepsin L needs 2-mercaptoethanol and EDTA releasing labelled Arg whereas in the presence of EDTA homogenates of pancreatic islets do not form [^{14}C]Arg. Therefore, cathepsin L seems not to be identical with the enzyme system in the islets responsible for the proinsulin conversion. Further work will be necessary to implicate these enzymes directly in the conversion process occuring probably in the granules. An important limitation to further progress has been the lack of suitable methods for preparing highly purified secretion granules free of lysosomes.

At the second symposium on Intracellular Protein Catabolism 1975 we could demonstrate that homogenates of islets and their subcellular fractions degrade [^{125}I]-insulin by cleavage of the interchain disulfide bonds, followed by proteolysis of the resulting A and B chains [7, 14]. This sequential degradation in particular VARANDANI [32] measured in a variety of other mammalian tissues. The TPO-activity is completely inhibited by antiserum to rat liver TPO (Fig. 7). By means of the two dimensional immune electrophoresis we were able to calculate the amount of TPO present in pancreatic islets to about 1.5% of the whole islet protein (manuscript in preparation). TPO activity mainly located in the microsomal fraction might play an important part in the last step of the proinsulin biosynthesis, the correct formation of the disulfide bonds. We cannot yet describe the total phenomenon of protein folding after synthesis [33], but we should take into consideration that TPO might possess this important function.

We are not yet able to answer the question which of these enzymes are involved in the biological regulation of the biosynthesis and/or the degradation of insulin in vivo. Nevertheless, further characterization of these enzymes in vitro is necessary.

References

[1] STEINER, D. F., W. KEMMLER, J. L. CLARK, P. E. OYER, and A. H. RUBENSTEIN in: HANDBOOK of Physiology – Endocrinology I. D. F. STEINER and N. FREINKEL (Eds). Williams and Wilkins, Baltimore 1972, pp. 175–198

[2] STEINER, D. F., and P. E. OYER: Proc. natn. Acad. Sci. U.S.A. **57**, 473 (1967)

[3] KEMMLER, W., J. D. PETERSON, and D. F. STEINER: J. biol. Chem. **246**, 6786 (1971)

[4] ZÜHLKE, H., and D. F. STEINER: Fedn Proc. Fedn Am. Socs exp. Biol. **34**, 657 (1975)

[5] ZÜHLKE, H., D. F. STEINER, A. LERNMARK, and C. LIPSEY in: Polypeptide Hormones: Molecular and Cellular Aspects. Ciba Foundation Symposium 41. Elsevier, Excerpta Medica, North-Holland, Amsterdam 1976, p. 183

[6] RENOLD, A. E.: Diabetes **21**, Suppl. 2619 (1972)

[7] KOHNERT, K. D., H. JAHR, S. SCHMIDT, H. J. HAHN, and H. ZÜHLKE: Biochim. biophys. Acta **422**, 254 (1976)

[8] NEUBERT, K., and H. D. JAKUBKE in: Peptides 1972. H. HANSON and H. D. JAKUBKE (Eds). North-Holland Publ. Comp., Amsterdam 1973, p. 235

[9] ANSORGE, S., and B. KAISER: Wiss. Z. Karl-Marx-Univ. Lpz., Math.-naturwiss. R. **18**, 559 (1969)

[10] ANSORGE, S., P. BOHLEY, H. KIRSCHKE, J. LANGNER, B. WIEDERANDERS, and H. HANSON in: Intracellular Protein Catabolism. H. HANSON and P. BOHLEY (Eds). Wiss. Beitr. Martin-Luther-Univ. Halle, Vol. **1**, p. 319 (1974)

[11] LACY, P. E., and M. KOSTIANOVSKY: Diabetes **16**, 35 (1967)

[12] ZÜHLKE, H., H. JAHR, S. SCHMIDT, D. GOTTSCHLING, and B. WILKE: Acta biol. med. germ. **33**, 407 (1974)

[13] JAHR, H., and H. ZÜHLKE: Acta biol. med. germ. **35**, 1477 (1976)

[14] SCHMIDT, S., K. D. KOHNERT, H. JAHR, H. ZÜHLKE, B. WILKE, H. KIRSCHKE, and H. FIEDLER in: Intracellular Protein Catabolism II. V. TURK and N. MARKS (Eds). Plenum Press, New York-London 1977, p. 131

[15] ZÜHLKE, H., and D. F. STEINER: in preparation

[16] KIRSCHKE, H., J. LANGNER, B. WIEDERANDERS, S. ANSORGE, and P. BOHLEY: Eur. J. Biochem. **74**, 293 (1977)
[17] YIP, C. C.: Proc. natn. Acad. Sci. U.S.A. **68**, 1312 (1971)
[18] SMITH, R. E.: Diabetes **21**, 581 (1972)
[19] SORENSEN, R. L., R. D. SHANK, and A. W. LINDALL: Proc. Soc. exp. Biol. Med. **139**, 652 (1972)
[20] ZÜHLKE, H., K. D. KOHNERT, H. J. HAHN, and M. ZIEGLER: Mod. Probl. Endokrin. **4**, 132 (1972) (Russian)
[21] ZÜHLKE, H., H. JAHR, K. D. KOHNERT, H. J. HAHN, B. WILKE, and S. SCHMIDT in: Peptides 1972. H. HANSON and H. D. JAKUBKE (Eds). North-Holland Publ. Comp. Amsterdam 1973, p. 398
[22] SMITH, R. E., and R. M. VAN FRANK: Endocrinology **94**, A190 (1974)
[23] KEMMLER, W., and D. F. STEINER: Biochem. biophys. Res. Commun. **41**, 1223 (1970)
[24] KEMMLER, W., D. F. STEINER, and J. BORG: J. biol. Chem. **248**, 4544 (1973)
[25] SUN, A. M., B. J. LIN, and R. E. HAIST: Can. J. Physiol. Pharmac. **51**, 175 (1973)
[26] ZÜHLKE, H., H. JAHR, S. SCHMIDT, and H. KIRSCHKE in: Early Diabetes, 8th Karlsburg Symposium 1974 H. BIBERGEIL, H. FIEDLER and U. POSER (Eds). 1974, p. 421
[27] STEINER, D. F., W. KEMMLER, H. S. TAGER, A. H. RUBENSTEIN, A. LERNMARK, and H. ZÜHLKE in: Proteases and Biological Control. **2**, 531 E. REICH, D. B. RIFKIN and E. SHAW (Eds). Cold Spring Harbor Laboratory, Cold Spring Harbor, New York 1975
[28] GREENBAUM, L M., and K. YAMAFUJI: Life Sci. **4**, 657 (1965)
[29] NINJOOR, V., S. L. TAYLOR, and A. L. TAPPEL: Biochim. biophys. Acta **370**, 308 (1974)
[30] OTTO, K. in: Tissue Proteinases. A. J. BARRETT and J. T. DINGLE (Eds). North-Holland, Amsterdam and London, American Elsevier, New York 1971, p. 1
[31] FRIEDRICH, K., H. KIRSCHKE, and S. ANSORGE: Acta biol. med. germ. **36**, 1723 (1977)
[32] VARANDANI, P. T.: Biochim. biophys. Acta **371**, 577 (1974)
[33] FREEDMANN, R. B., and H. C. HAWKINS: Biochem. Soc. Trans. **5**, 348 (1977)

Acta biol. med. germ., Band 36, Seite 1705–1712 (1977)

Departments of Biochemistry and Medicine, St. Thomas's Hospital Medical School, London, Sel 7eh, U.K.
and Deutsches Wollforschungsinstitut, Aachen, Federal Republic of Germany

Studies on the relationship between the molecular structure and the catabolism of insulin

D. Papachristodoulou, D. Brandenburg*, D. I. Dron, R. H. Jones, P. H. Sönksen, and J. H. Thomas

Summary

The catabolism of insulins modified at the A_1, B_1 or B_{29} positions or containing a synthetic crosslink between the A_1 and B_{29} positions has been studied in vivo and in vitro. The metabolic clearance rates (MCR) of insulin, proinsulin and chemically modified insulins have been measured by a priming-dose constant infusion technique in greyhounds. Insulins modified at A_1 and B_{29}, particularly the crosslinked materials, had markedly lowered MCR's whilst B_1 analogues did not differ from insulin. Proinsulin and the A_1-B_{29} crosslinked materials showed a markedly lowered degradability by glutathione-insulin transhydrogenase.

Introduction

The availability of insulins chemically modified at specific sites on the molecule is making possible the study of the relationships between the structure and function of the hormone [1]. The study of the behaviour of these analogues both in vivo and in vitro will help to define not only the characteristics of the insulin molecule essential for biological activity but also to identify a site or sites involved in its degradation.

Materials and methods

The analogues used in these studies have been prepared and characterized by Dr. D. Brandenburg in Aachen [2–4] and Dr. D. Lindsay in Sussex [5–7].
The modifications are at the N-terminal glycine of the A chain, the ε-NH_2 group of B_{29} lysine or at the N-terminal phenylalanine of the B chain. (Fig. 1.) Some analogues had a synthetic crosslink between A_1 and B_{29} and these were originally chosen in view of their similarity to proinsulin which was also investigated. There is a considerable body of information on the chemical and biological properties of A_1B_{29} modified insulins. These residues lie on the surface of the molecule in close spatial proximity [8] and it has been suggested that they may be intimately concerned with binding to the receptor site [9].

Method of assay

In all the studies both in vivo and in vitro the concentrations of insulin, proinsulin and the analogues were measured by radioimmunoassay [10]. By screening 23 antisera raised against insulin we were able to select one or more for the assay of each analogue. These varied in their susceptibility to modifications at different sites of the insulin molecule and were used in the estimation of analogue concentrations both in biological fluids and the in vitro assays. A tracer technique was not employed as iodination of the analogues might affect their metabolism [11].

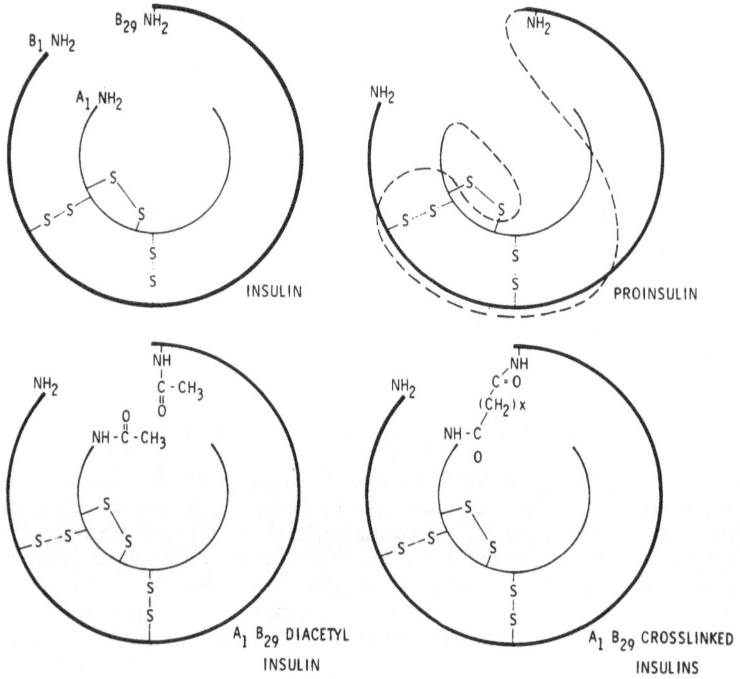

Fig. 1. Diagrammatic representation of insulin, proinsulin and the chemically modified materials studied. The crosslinked analogues have an aliphatic link between the free amino groups of A_1 glycine and B_{29} lysine. A_1, B_{29} diacetyl insulin has no synthetic crosslink, but the free amino groups are chemically modified in a comparable fashion

In vivo experiments

In vivo studies were conducted in anaesthetised greyhounds fasted overnight. The experimental protocol is shown in Fig. 2. The external jugular vein was canulated for blood sampling. Urine was collected through a urethral catheter. After 30 min of baseline sampling (period I) the material under study, insulin or analogue, was infused into a hind limb vein. The rate of infusion was doubled every 30 min (periods II—V) until at the end of the fifth period the pump was stopped to allow estimation of the decay time ($T\frac{1}{2}$). Each infusion was preceded by a priming dose to achieve rapid equilibration. Blood glucose concentrations were also measured. The metabolic clearance rate (MCR) was calculated:

$$\mathrm{MCR}(\mathrm{ml\ kg^{-1}\ min^{-1}}) = \frac{\text{Infusion rate (pmol kg}^{-1}\text{ min}^{-1})}{\text{Steady-state plasma concentration (pmol ml}^{-1})}$$

In vitro experiments

Glutathione-insulin transhydrogenase (EC 1.8.4.2) was prepared from rat liver "microsomes" by the method of ANSORGE et al [12] and incubated at 37 °C with insulin, proinsulin or analogue (final concn. 1 µM) in the presence of GSH (1 mM) and EDTA (12.5 mM) for periods up to 1 h. Samples were removed at various time intervals and the reaction stopped by dilution in the presence of N-ethyl maleimide (2 mM). The degradation was measured by loss of immunoreactivity, corrected for non-enzymatic degradation and expressed as a percentage of the amount of insulin degraded under identical conditions after 30 min.

Results and discussion

The metabolic clearance rates (MCR) for insulin are shown in Fig. 3. At no time does the MCR fall below 10 ml kg^{-1} min^{-1}. There is a fall in MCR with increasing steady state concentration indicating the presence of a saturable as well as a linear component. The results for proinsulin and examples of five different ana-

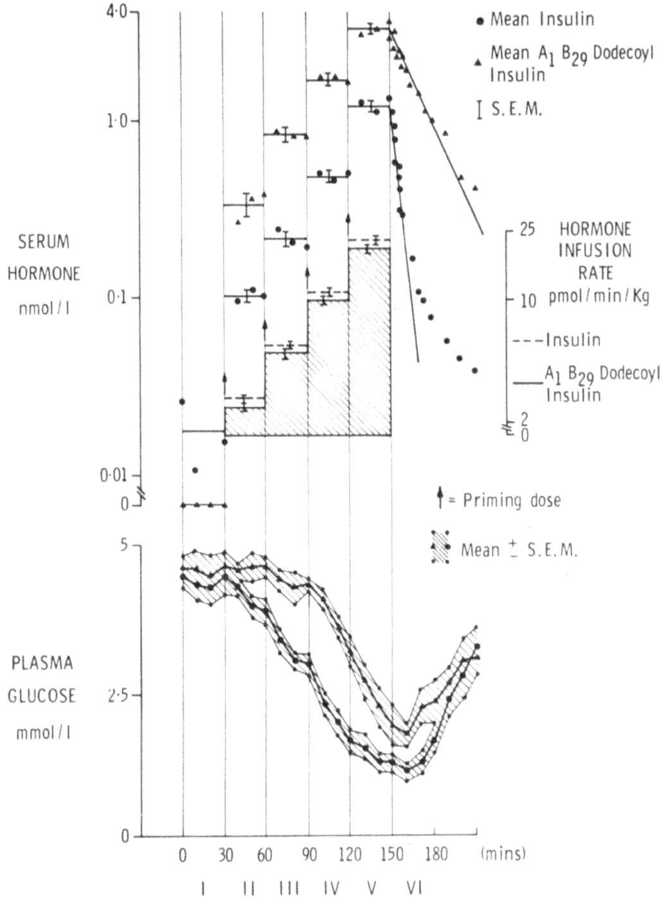

Fig. 2. Experimental design. (1) Each experiment was divided into six periods I – V of 30 min each, and VI of 90 min. (2) Insulin or analogue was administered by continuous infusion during periods II – V. The infusion rate was doubled at the end of each period. (3) Serum samples were estimated for insulin or analogue by radioimmunoassay. The diagram demonstrates the steady-state concentrations achieved during the infusion periods II – V and the decay after the infusion was stopped. (4) Plasma glucose was measured throughout the experiments

logues are shown in Figs 4—8. Fig. 4 shows the results of six experiments with proinsulin. The values never reach 10 ml kg^{-1} min^{-1} but there seems to be an element of saturation. The results of one of the crosslinked analogues, A_1—B_{29} oxalyl insulin, are shown in Fig. 5. Values are again less than 2 standard deviations from the mean for insulin but no saturable component is evident. A_1—B_{29} dodecoyl insulin (Fig. 6) shows slightly higher values than oxalyl insulin especially at low steady state levels but they are still significantly lower than the results obtained with insulin. A small component of saturation is present. Fig. 7 shows the results obtained with diacetyl insulin which is modified at A_1 and B_{29} but without a crosslink. The MCR is lowered compared to insulin but not to the same extent as when A_1 and B_{29} are crosslinked. There is no evidence of saturable clearance. In marked contrast are the results of B_1 modified insulins such as B_1 carbamyl (Fig. 8). The

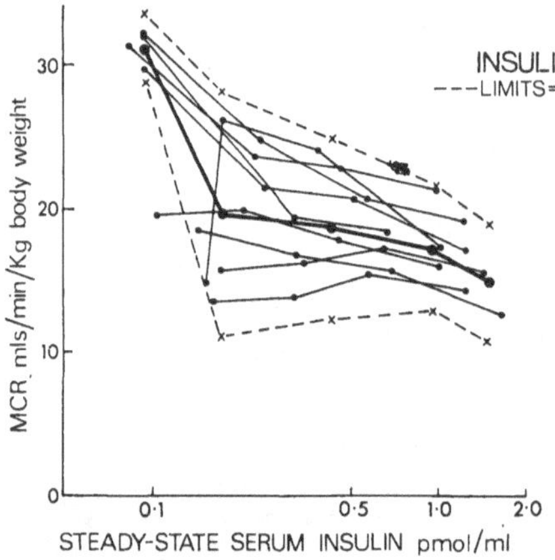

Fig. 3. Metabolic clearance rate (MCR) of insulin at various steady-state serum concentrations.

The thin lines represent the individual experiments, the heavy line the mean and the dotted lines the 95% confidence limits

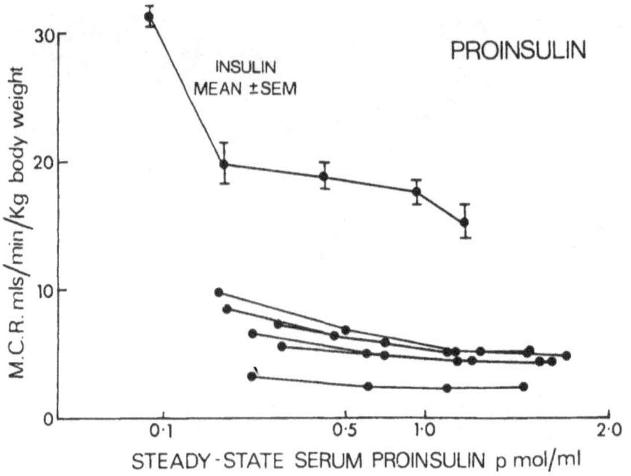

Fig. 4. Metabolic clearance rate (MCR) of proinsulin at various steady-state serum concentrations

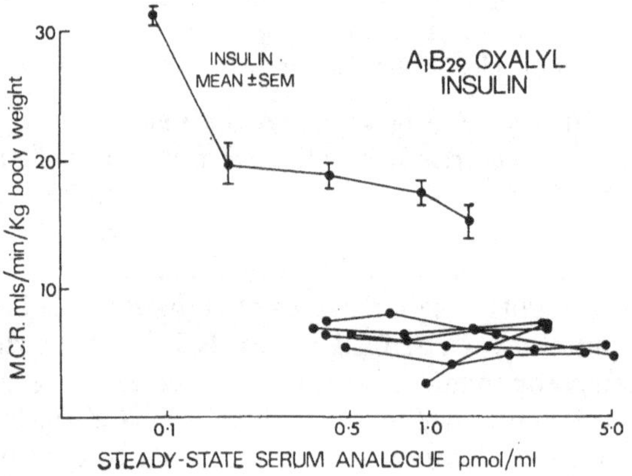

Fig. 5. Metabolic clearance rate (MCR) of A_1-B_{29} oxalyl insulin at various steady-state serum concentrations

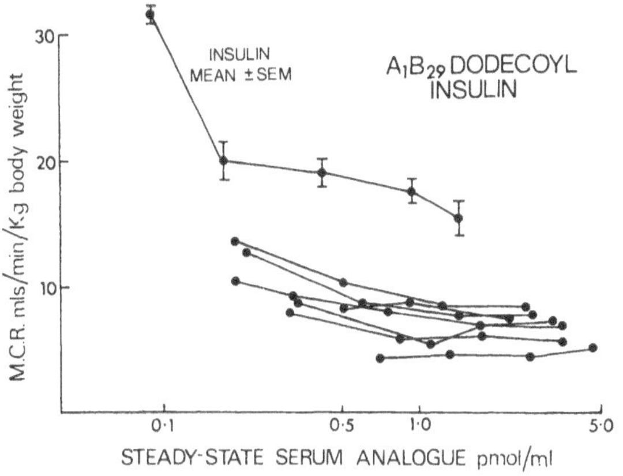

Fig. 6. Metabolic clearance rate (MCR) of A_1-B_{29} dodecoyl insulin at various steady-state serum concentrations

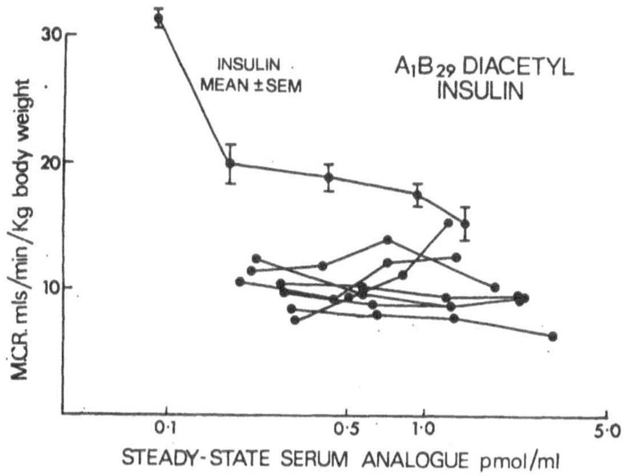

Fig. 7. Metabolic clearance rate (MCR) of A_1, B_{29} diacetyl insulin at various steady-state concentrations

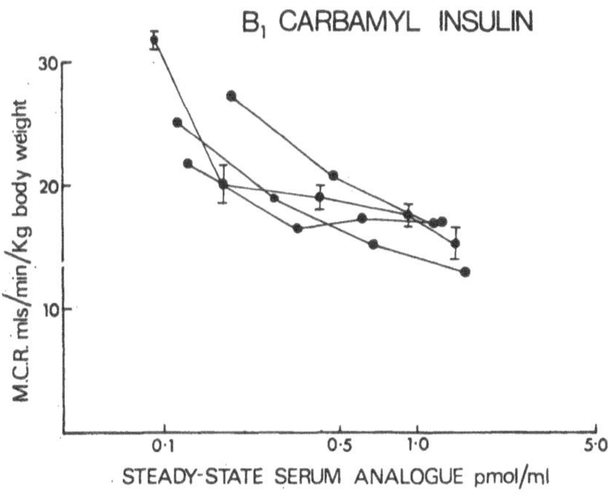

Fig. 8. Metabolic clearance rate (MCR) of B_1 carbamyl insulin at various steady-state serum concentrations

Table 1
Reduction in metabolic clearance rate (MCR) of proinsulin and analogues related to insulin. The analogues are listed in order of ascending biological activity

	Potency % (Fat cells)	Modification A_1	B_{29}	B_1	Reduction in MCR	Saturable clearance
Pork Proinsulin	8.8	*——	(*)		+++	+++
A_1-B_{29} Oxalyl	5.1	*——	*		+++	0
A_1-B_{29} Suberoyl	5.4	*——	*		++	0
A_1-B_{29} Dodecoyl	6.0	*——	*		+++	+++
A_1 Succinyl	17	*			+++	++
A_1-B_{29} Diacetyl	32	*	*		+	0
A_1 Carbamyl	35	*			++	+
A_1 Acetyl	41	*			+	+
B_{29} Succinyl	82		*		++	+++
B_{29} Acetyl	87		*		+	+
B_1 Acetoacetyl	87			*	0	++++
Insulin	100					++++
B_1 Diiodotyrosine	106			*	0	++++
B_1 Carbamyl	115			*	0	++++

plots completely overlap with those for insulin. Table 1 gives a summary of the results of the analogues examined to date. They are listed in order of ascending biological activity as assayed by a standard laboratory method which measures lipogenesis in isolated fat cells [13].

To quantitate the MCR's requires mathematical analysis and resolution of the data into a saturable and a linear component as mentioned above and this is being currently undertaken. Table 1 presents a qualitative estimate of MCR's relative to insulin obtained from graphical data as those shown in Figs. 3—8. It is evident that the MCR of the crosslinked analogues was decreased whereas modifications at the A_1 and B_{29} residues without a crosslink decreased the MCR to a lesser degree. Single A_1 or B_{29} modifications had a small effect whereas alterations at B_1 had no effect whatsoever in this respect. It is also clear from the table that crosslinked analogues which had the lowest biological activity had the lowest MCR and those with the highest biological activity such as the B_1 modified ones had MCR's like insulin. The A_1 or B_{29} analogues which had intermediate biological activity also exhibited a moderate decrease in MCR compared to insulin. The interpretation of the degree of saturable clearance is less clear but it is evident that those analogues whose biological activity and MCR resembles insulin, that is the B_1 analogues, exhibited a saturable clearance component similar to insulin.

The MCR of insulin may depend on excretion, the presence and activity of degrading enzymes and the access the hormone has to its degradation sites. It was decided to examine one of these factors viz. the enzymatic degradation of insulin. If highly specific structural requirements have to be met for binding and activation, should we expect a similar specificity at the molecular level for degradation? There is evidence [14] that the enzymatic degradation of insulin by rat liver occurs in a stepwise manner: firstly a splitting of the insulin at the disulphide bonds by glutathione-insulin transhydrogenase followed by hydrolysis of the resulting A and B chains. Thus it would appear that glutathione-insulin transhydrogenase is the rate controlling enzyme in the degradation by the liver. The rates of degrada-

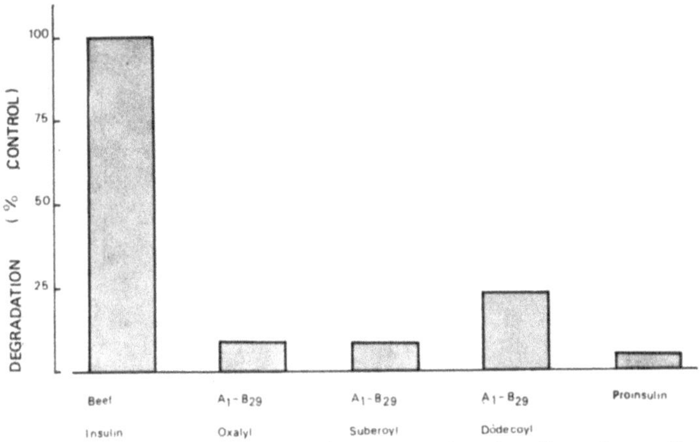

Fig. 9. Degradation by GSH-insulin transhydrogenase of proinsulin and crosslinked analogues relative to insulin

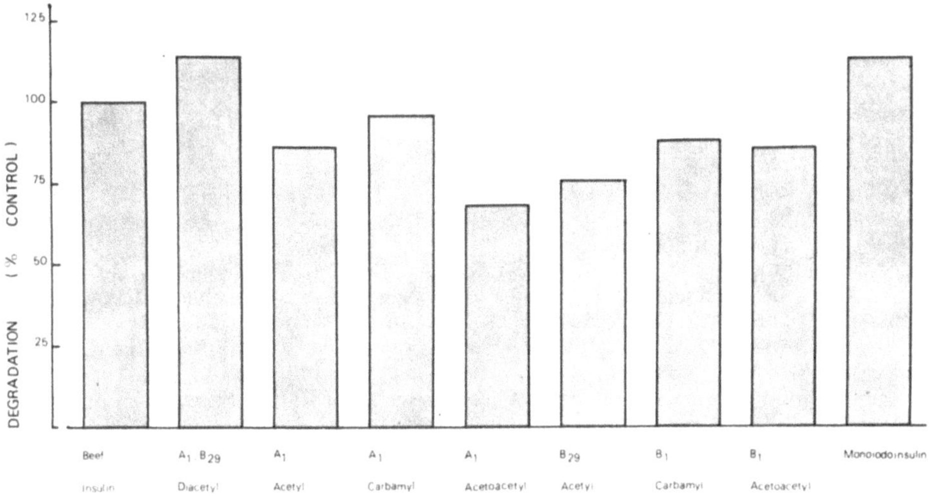

Fig. 10. Degradation by GSH-insulin transhydrogenase of insulin modified at A_1, B_{29}, B_1 and monoiodo-insulin relative to insulin

tion of insulin, proinsulin and the analogues by glutathione-insulin transhydrogenase have been measured.

The findings of these preliminary experiments are shown in Figs. 9 and 10. The degradation of proinsulin and the analogues with a synthetic crosslink between A_1 and B_{29} was markedly impaired compared to insulin (Fig. 9). On the other hand analogues which had no crosslink were degraded at rates similar to insulin even if these analogues were modified at A_1 and B_{29}. It would appear that modification at A_1 and B_{29} without a crosslink lowered the MCR but did not impair the enzymatic breakdown. A good example of this is diacetyl insulin. A_1, B_{29}, and B_1 modified insulins differed in their MCR's but behaved in a similar manner as regards degradation.

It seems that the presence of a crosslink between the A and B chains other than the disulphide bridges whether natural, as in proinsulin, or semisynthetic, lowers the material's susceptibility to degradation by glutathione-insulin transhydrogenase. Single substitution at a number of sites does not seem to impair the ability of the hormone to act as substrate for the enzyme. The pattern of diminished clearance in vivo has some similarities with this but also some important differences. The integrity of the A_1 group has been shown to be essential for binding and biological activity. [9, 15] and as shown here for the retention of normal MCR. A_1 modification did not result in a less rapid degradation by GSH-insulin transhydrogenase unless a synthetic crosslink is present. It would be interesting to study analogues with semisynthetic crosslinks between the A and B chains but not involving the A_1 site on the molecular surface. It would seem from our experiments that the determinants of the clearance rate of an insulin analogue in vivo are not identical to those which define its susceptibility to glutathione-insulin transhydrogenase, suggesting perhaps hat the access to the enzyme is not entirely free and may, as suggested by TERRIS and STEINER [16, 17], be determined by the rate of binding to receptors on the cell surface.

Acknowledgements

The authors are indebted to the Wellcome Research Laboratories, Beckenham, Kent for the gift of insulin antisera. This research was supported by grants from the British Diabetic Association and the Research (Endowments) Committee of St. Thomas' Hospital.

References

[1] PULLEN, R. A., D. G. LINDSAY, S. P. WOOD, I. J. TICKLE, T. L. BLUNDELL, A. WOLLMER, G. KRAIL, D. BRANDENBURG, H. ZAHN, J. GLIEMANN, and S. GAMMELTOFT: Nature, Lond. **259**, 369 (1976)

[2] BRANDENBURG, D., W. BUSSE, H. GATTNER, H. ZAHN, A. WOLLMER, J. GLIEMANN, and W. PULS: Proceedings of the 12th European Peptide Symposium, Reinhardsbrunn Castle, G.D.R. 1972. North-Holland, Amsterdam 1973

[3] BRANDENBURG, D., and I. HOPPE-Seyler: Hoppe-Seyler's Z. physiol. Chem. **353**, 869 (1972)

[4] BRANDENBURG, D., D. G. GATTNER, A. WOLLMER, and I. HOPPE-SEYLER: Hoppe-Seyler's Z. physiol. Chem. **353**, 599 (1972)

[5] LINDSAY, D. G., and S. SHALL: Biochem. J. **115**, 589 (1969)

[6] LINDSAY, D. G., and S. SHALL: Biochem. J. **121**, 737 (1971)

[7] LINDSAY, D. G., O. LOGE, W. LOSERT, and S. SHALL: Biochim. biophys. Acta **263**, 658 (1972)

[8] BLUNDELL, T. L., G. G. DODSON, D. C. HODGKIN, and M. VIJAYAN: Recent Prog. Horm. Res. **27**, 1 (1971)

[9] BLUNDELL, T., G. DODSON, D. HODGKIN, and D. MERCOLA: Adv. Protein Chem. **26**, 279 (1972)

[10] THOMAS, J. H., D. I. DRON, and R. H. JONES: Diabetologia **11**, 379 (1975)

[11] OOMS, H. A.: Emploi des Insulines Radioiodes comme traceurs en biologie. Collection "Medico-Monographies d'Agreges". Editions Arscia S. A., Bruxelles, Librairie Maloine S. A., Paris

[12] ANSORGE, S., P. BOHLEY, H. KIRSCHKE, J. LANGNER, B. WIEDERANDERS, and H. HANSON: Eur. J. Biochem. **32**, 27 (1973)

[13] MOODY, A. J., M. A. STAN, M. STAN, and J. GLIEMANN: Horm. Metab. Res. **6**, 12 (1964)

[14] VARANDANI, P. T., L. A. SHROYER, and M. A. NAFZ: Proc. natn. Acad. Sci. U.S.A. **69**, 1681 (1972)

[15] WOOD, S. P., T. C. BBUNDELL, A. WOLLMER, R. LAZARUS, and R. W. J. NEVILLE: Eur. J. Biochem. **55**, 531 (1975)

[16] TERRIS, S., and D. F. STEINER: J. biol. Chem. **250**, 8389 (1975)

[17] TERRIS, S., and D. F. STEINER: J. clin. Invest. **57**, 885 (1976)

Acta biol. med. germ., Band 36, Seite 1713—1721 (1977)

Institute of Physiological Chemistry, University of Halle, 402 Halle (Saale), Hollystraße 1, and [1]Central Institute for Diabetes, 2201 Karlsburg, GDR

Insulin and glucagon degradation in livers of sand rats (Psammomys obesus)

S. Ansorge, H. Kirschke, [1]E. Köhler, J. Langner, I. Römer, and B. Wiederanders

Summary

Intracellular distribution of insulin degrading enzymes in livers of sand rats (Psammomys obesus) shows a very similar pattern as in livers of Wistar rats. The microsomal insulin degrading activity is due predominantly to the thiol-proteindisulfide oxidoreductase (TPO). Two forms of the microsomal TPO in livers of sand rats and Wistar rats could be separated by the two-dimensional immune electrophoresis in TPO-antibody containing agarose gels.

As in livers of Wistar rats, three enzymes have been identified responsible for insulin degradation in cytosol of livers of sand rats: (a) the insulin and glucagon degrading proteinase (Brush), a metal-dependent enzyme, (b) a solubilized form of the microsomal TPO, and (c) the "small" TPO (mol. wt. 6000—10000).

Besides microsomal fraction and the cytosol, lysosomal fraction may also be involved in breakdown of insulin and glucagon. *p*H-dependence of degradation of insulin and glucagon in the acidic range by homogenates of livers of sand rats resembles strongly that of the soluble lysosomal fraction of livers of Wistar rats.

Comparison of the specific activities of the peptide hormone and protein degrading enzymes of livers of sand rats with those of Wistar rats shows that livers of sand rats exhibit significantly lower activities of the TPO system, the insulin and glucagon degrading proteinase as well as of the lysosomal proteinases (measured with [^{125}I]-glucagon and -insulin at *p*H 4.5 and 5.8, and with azocasein at *p*H 6.0), whereas the activity of cathepsin D seems to be about the same in both species.

Introduction

As demonstrated in previous studies, livers of Wistar rats dispose of a group of enzymes capable of degrading insulin and partially glucagon at pharmacological as well as physiological hormone concentration [1—3]. These enzymes are summarized in Table 1. It has not been clear as yet, however, whether these groups of enzymes are present also in animals which develop diabetes mellitus and whether their activity is changed under diabetes-like conditions.

Egyptian sand rats (Psammomys obesus) develop a diabetes-like syndrome after transfer from their natural environment to laboratory conditions, i. e. higher caloric diet and reduced mobility [4]. Therefore, the sand rat seems to be a suitable model to study insulin and glucagon breakdown under diabetes-like conditions.

The aim of the present study was to investigate the intracellular localization and the nature of insulin and glucagon degrading enzymes present in livers of sand rats as well as to compare their activities with those of livers of Wistar rats.

Most of our experiments were done with "normal" non-diabetic sand rats, which showed no rise in their body weight as well as blood glucose level, or with animals which had not been characterized in respect of the stage of diabetes.

Table 1
Insulin degrating enzymes of rat liver

Enzymes	Bonds cleaved	Localization
1. Thiol-proteindisulfide oxidoreductase (TPO) (Glutathione-insulin transhydrogenase)	Disulfide	Microsomal fraction (Plasma membrane ?) Cytosol
2. Insulin and glucagon degrading proteinase (Insulin-specific protease)	Peptide	Cytosol
3. Cathepsin B Cathepsin H Cathepsin L	Peptide	Lysosomes

Insulin and glucagon degrading enzymatic activities were determined by measuring the formation of radioactive products soluble in 5% trichloroactic acid from ^{125}I-labelled hormones [5].

Results and discussion

Intracellular localization determined at neutral pH

As shown on Fig. 1 patterns of intracellular distribution of insulin degrading enzymes depend on conditions used for the enzyme assay: In the presence of chelating agents (EDTA, o-phenanthroline), at physiological as well as pharmacological insulin concentrations highest specific activity of insulin breakdown is localized in the microsomal fraction, whereas at lower insulin concentrations (1—110 nM) in the absence of chelating agents as well as in the presence of both, chelating agent and manganese ions, highest specific activity of insulin degradation is associated with the cytosol fraction. Same results have been found also with livers of Wistar rats (not shown). This clearly demonstrates that livers of sand rats, like livers of Wistar rats, contain at least two different insulin degrading enzymes acting at neutral *p*H.
The following experiments show that the microsomal activity is due predominantly to the action of the thiol-protein disulfide oxidoreductase system (TPO, glutathione-insulin transhydrogenase) and that the activity of the cytosol determined with low insulin concentrations represents mainly the insulin and glucagon degrading proteinase (insulin-specific proteinase).

Microsomal TPO

When deoxycholate-treated microsomes of livers of sand rats were incubated with monovalent antiserum from rabbit against the purified TPO from microsomes of livers of Wistar rats [6], enzymatic activity measured in supernatants after sedimentation of the TPO-antibody complex was inhibited more than 50% (Table 2). This demonstrates that the TPO is indeed present in the microsomal fraction of livers of sand rats. It is not clear, however, whether the residual activity determined with physiological insulin concentrations is due to an additional non-TPO activity or to non-optimum reaction conditions between the antigen and the antibodies in the assay system.

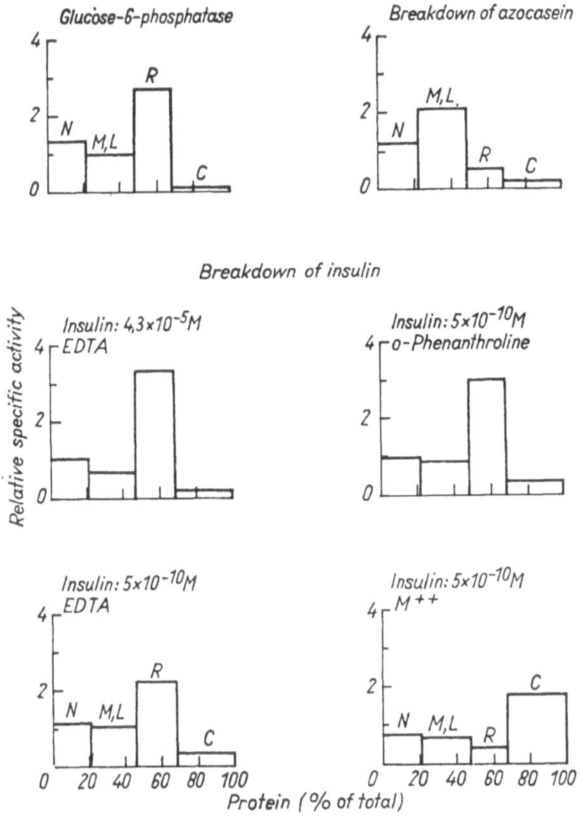

Fig. 1. Intracellular localization of insulin degrading enzymes in livers of sand rats. Enzymatic activities were determined according [5]. The assay of insulin degrading activities with low insulin concentration (0.5–110 nM) was carried out in the presence of 0.1% bovine serum albumin. Final concentrations of EDTA, o-phenanthroline and Mn^{++} in the incubation mixture were 3.3 mM, 2 mM and 1 mM, resp. N, nuclear fraction; M, mitochondria; L, lysosomes; R, microsomal fraction; C, cytosol

Table 2

Inhibition of insulin degradation of the microsomal fraction by rabbit antiserum against the purified TPO from livers of Wistar rats.

TPO activity (% of total) determined at 0.5 nM insulin

Additions	Sands rats Microsomes (30 µg protein)	Wistar rats Microsomes (25 µg protein)	Wistar rats Purified TPO (0,4 µg protein)
Rabbit serum	100	100	100
Rabbit TPO-antiserum	46	32	10

50 µl of the deoxycholate-treated microsomal fraction (diluted to 0.02% deoxycholate) were mixed with either 50 µl of normal rabbit serum or with 50 µl of rabbit antiserum against the purified TPO from Wistar rats. After incubation for 1 h at 20 °C and for 48 hrs at 4 °C the incubation mixture was centrifuged and the activity was determined with 50 µl supernatant using an insulin concentration of about 0.5 nM in the presence of 3 mM EDTA and 1 mM GSH at *p*H 7.5.

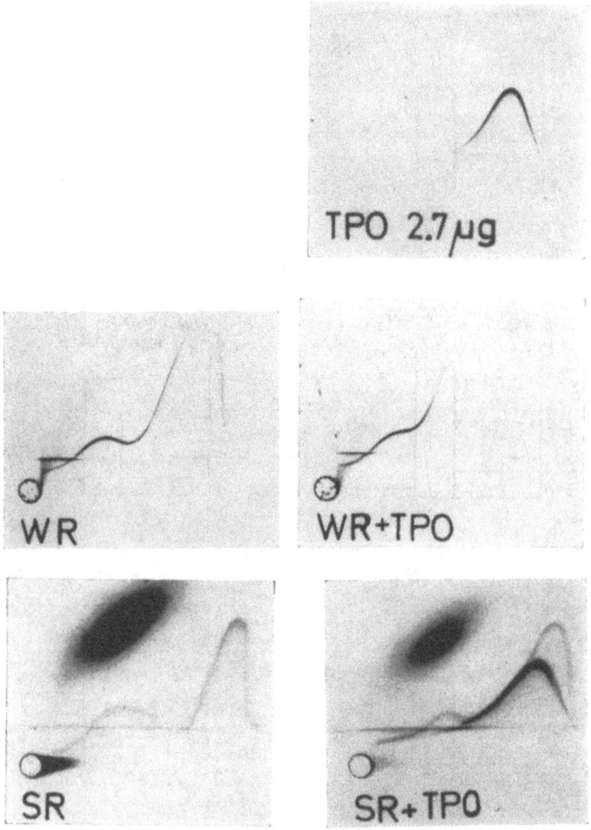

Fig. 2. Laurell-electrophoresis of deoxycholate-soluble supernatants of liver homogenates of Wistar rats and sand rats in TPO-antibody containing agarose gels.

In the first dimension samples of 15 μl of supernatants of 30% homogenates treated with 0.5% deoxycholate were subjected to electrophoresis in agarose gels (5 × 5 cm) at 10 V/cm for 4 hrs (to the right). After this first electrophoresis the agarose from the upper part was substituted by 2.3 ml of agarose containing 150 μl TPO antiserum from rabbits and the second electrophoresis was performed at a right angle to the first direction at 6 V/cm for 18 hrs (upward). Precipitin arcs were stained with Amidoblack 10 B

Additional evidence for the presence of the TPO in livers of sand rats has been produced by the technique of electrophoresis in antibody-containing agarose gel according to LAURELL [7] and RESSLER [8] (Fig. 2). Purified TPO from microsomes of livers of Wistar rats shows a single precipitin line (top curve of Fig. 2) demonstrating that the antiserum used is monovalent. Analyzing the deoxycholate-soluble proteins of livers of sand rats and Wistar rats two different forms of the TPO system are detectable in both (left side of Fig. 2). The faster moving component (main peak) corresponds to the purified TPO from the microsomal TPO used as antigen, whereas the slower moving peak represents a new unknown form of the TPO system present in both species. Both forms of the TPO have also been found in the deoxycholate-soluble part of the microsomal fraction from livers of Wistar rats in same proportions as in the soluble part of the total homogenates. Conclusively, like the faster moving TPO the slower moving form seems to be localized predominantly in the microsomal fraction, too. Co-electrophoreses of liver proteins soluble in deoxycholate together with the purified microsomal TPO from Wistar rats convincingly demonstrate that the TPO forms of sand rats are similar but not identical with the TPOs of Wistar rats (right side of Fig. 2).

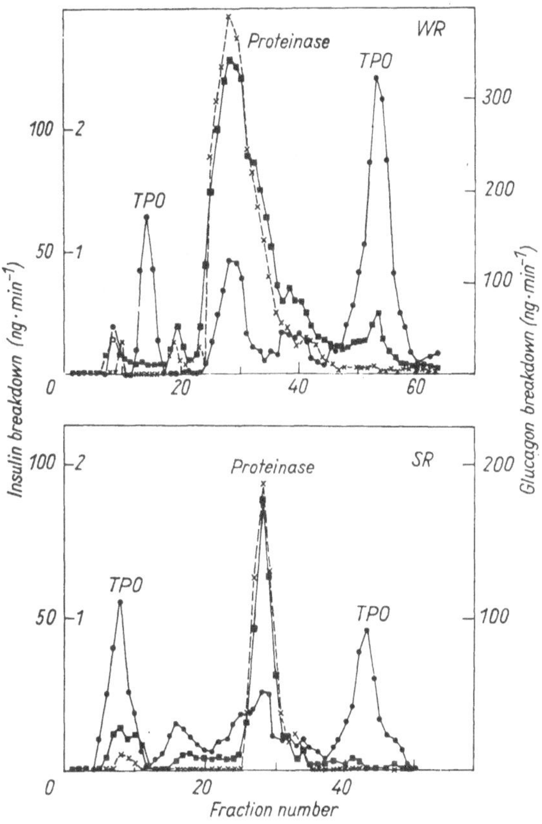

Fig. 3. Chromatography of cytosol of livers of Wistar rats (top) and sand rats (bottom) on DEAE-Sephadex A – 50 at *p*H 7.85.

Top: 20 ml of cytosol from 50% homogenate of livers of Wistar rats were applied to a 450-ml column equilibrated with 0.1 M Tris, 0.1 M KCl, *p*H 7.85. The elution was started with the equilibration buffer and continued with a linear gradient of KCl (0.1 – 0.45 M) in 0.1 M Tris buffer, *p*H 7.85, delivered from two chambers, each containing 800 ml. 25 ml fractions were collected.

Bottom: 17 ml of cytosol from 50% homogenate of livers of sand rats were placed on a 200-ml column equilibrated with 0.1 M Tris, 0.1 M KCl, *p*H 7.85. The elution was started with the equilibration buffer and continued with a linear gradient of KCl (0.1 – 0.36 M) in 0.1 M Tris buffer, *p*H 7.85, delivered from two chambers, each containing 600 ml. 25 ml fractions were collected.

Insulin degradation with 43 μM insulin was determined at *p*H 7.5 in presence of 2 mM GSH and 5 mM EDTA (●). Insulin degradation with 0.11 μM insulin (■) and glucagon breakdown with 12 μM glucagon (×) were measured at *p*H 8.0

Enzymes of the cytosol

Cytosol of rat liver contains a proteinase distinguisghed by a comparable low K_M value for insulin and an apparently high specificity for insulin and glucagon [3]. This so-called insulin and glucagon degrading proteinase (insulin-specific proteinase) can be separated from the small quantities of the two forms of the TPO, which occur in the cytosol, by chromatography on DEAE-Sephadex at *p*H 7.85 (Fig. 3). The TPO eluted in front has a mol. wt. of about 6000—10000, whereas the TPO eluted after the proteinase seems to be a solubilized portion of the microsomal fraction. Both have been demonstrated also after chromatography on Sephadex G-75. They represent about 10—15% of the total TPO activity of the liver [1]. The "small" TPO having a mol. wt. 6000—10000 does not react with antibodies against the microsomal TPO.
In contrast to the TPOs the proteinase is a metal-dependent enzyme which can be inhibited by chelating agents [2]. Comparison of the pattern of chromatography on DEAE-Sephadex of the cytosol of livers of Wistar rats (Fig. 3, top) with that of sand rats (Fig. 3, bottom) clearly demonstrates that both the proteinase and the two forms of the TPO of the cytosol are present in livers of sand rats. The identity of the proteinase is supported by the fact that the relative activities of insulin (solid line) and glucagon breakdown (dotted line) are approximately the same in both species. Moreover, like the proteinase of Wistar rats [2] the enzyme of sand rats can be inhibited by o-phenanthroline (Fig. 4), and the inhibition can be prevented by divalent cations as manganese, zinc and cobalt (not shown).

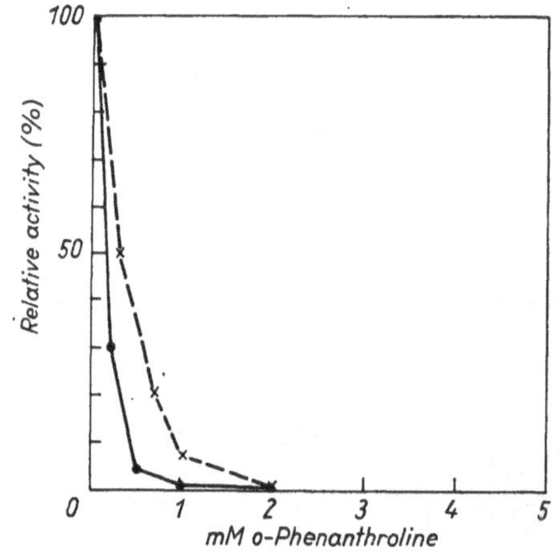

Fig. 4. Effect of o-phenanthroline on the activity of the insulin and glucagon degrading proteinase from livers of sand rats (×) and Wistar rats (•) obtained after chromatography of cytosols on DEAE-Sephadex (compare Fig. 3).
Enzymatic activity was determined with glucagon (12 μM) at *p*H 8.0

Lysosomal proteinases

The last group of enzymes which should be considered here is the group of lysosomal proteinases. At the 2nd Symposium in Ljubljana we have reported that beside the insulin and glucagon degrading enzymes discussed above lysosomal proteinases of livers of Wistar rats exhibit insulin and glucagon degrading activity also at physiogical hormone concentrations [2]. The most active cathepsin has been found to be cathepsin L. We have not studied purified lysosomal proteinases from livers of sand rats. However, *p*H-dependence at the acidic range of degrada-

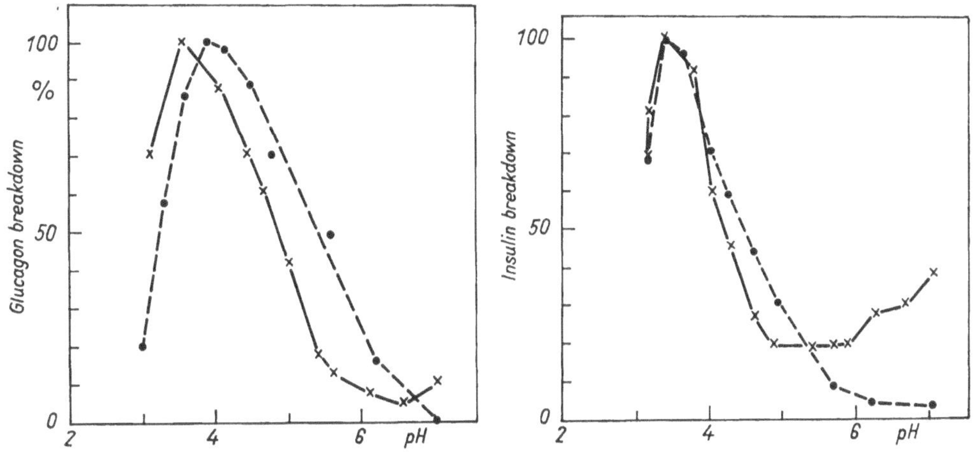

Fig. 5. Effect of *p*H on insulin and glucagon breakdown by lysosomal proteinases from livers of sand rats and Wistar rats. The water soluble part of the lysosomal fraction of livers of Wistar rats (53-fold purified) was prepared according to [9]. The final *p*H of the incubation mixture was adjusted by using 0.1 M citrate-phosphate buffer.

●— — —●, lysosomal fraction from livers of WR; ×———×, liver homogenate from SR

tion of insulin and glucagon by homogenates of livers of sand rats resembles strongly that of the water-soluble part of the lysosomal fraction of livers of Wistar rats (Fig. 5). From this it is highly probable that similar lysosomal cathepsins may also be involved in the breakdown of pancreatic hormones by livers of sand rats as of Wistar rats.

Taking together these results one can state that livers of sand rats contain about the same or very similar groups of insulin and glucagon degrading enzymes as livers of Wistar rats.

The question arises whether the activities of these groups of enzymes are the same or markedly different in both species.

Comparison of hormone degrading activities of livers of Wistar rats and sand rats

Using different assay conditions with respect to hormone concentrations, *p*H, and chelating agents it is possible to determine the TPO, the insulin and glucagon degrading proteinase and the group of lysosomal proteinases side by side in crude liver homogenates. In Table 3 the specific activities of the three different enzyme systems of the livers of both species are summarized. The values clearly demonstrate that the activity of all three enzyme systems are markedly lower in livers of sand rats than in livers of Wistar rats. This finding is valid not only for the degradation of insulin and glucagon under various conditions but also for the degradation of azocasein by lysosomal proteinases at *p*H 6. The only exception found is cathepsin D (determined with azohemoglobin in the absence and in the presence of 2.5 μM pepstatin at *p*H 3.0) which exhibits about the same specific activity in both species (not shown).

Interpretation of these results is difficult, because we cannot decide if these lower activities of sand rats are due to species differences or to a prediabetic stage of sand rats.

Table 3
Insulin and glucagon degradation in liver homogenates of Wistar rats (WR) and sand rats (SR) (ng · min⁻¹ · μg protein⁻¹)

Enzymes	Assay conditions	WR	SR	$\frac{SR}{WR} \cdot 100$
TPO	Insulin *p*H 7.0, 43 μM	2.76 ± 0.11	1.65 ± 0.23	60
Insulin-glucagon degrading proteinase	Insulin *p*H 8.0, 0.11 μM	0.056 ± 0.05	0.039 ± 0.004	71
	Glucagon *p*H 8.0, 12 μM	2.40 ± 0.29	1.35 ± 0.13	56
Lysosomal proteinases	Insulin *p*H 4.5, 43 μM	0.42	0.31	74
	Insulin *p*H 4.5, 0.11 μM	0.010	0.006	60
	Glucagon *p*H 4.5, 12 μM	3.03 ± 0.33	1.55 ± 0.51	51
	Glucagon *p*H 5.8, 12 μM	1.15 ± 0.19	0.25 ± 0.10	22
	Azocasein *p*H 6.0, 1%	3.89 ± 0.21	2.49 ± 0.80	64

Moreover, it must be taken into consideration that probably only a part of the total hormone degrading activities determined in vitro is responsible for insulin degradation, and that the nature and concentration of the effectors and co-substrates of the enzymes determined are different in vivo as compared with the in vitro system used here. In this connection it should be mentioned that the concentration of non-protein-as well as protein-bound sulfhydryl groups were found to be significantly higher in livers of sand rats than in those of Wistar rats [10].

Sand rats develop a diabetes syndrome which is characterized among other phenomena by a hyperinsulinism. As shown by the group of Dr. KÖHLER in Karlsburg the basal level of insulin in blood is in "normal" and protodiabetic sand rats about twice that in Wistar rats [4]. Possibly this hyperinsulinism is due, at least in part, to the markedly lowered insulin degradation in livers of sand rats in the basal state together with an elevated insulin secretion of the pancreas [4].

It should be mentioned, however, that under special conditions insulin inactivation seems to be markedly higher in livers of sand rats than of Wistar rats. As shown by KÖHLER et al. (unpublished) hepatic extraction of insulin in sand rats (measured as portal-peripheral difference of immune-reactive insulin) increases particularly 30—60 min after stimulation of insulin secretion up to values 2—3 times higher than in Wistar rats. During this time the insulin concentration in portal blood of sand rats increases from 90 to about 200 μU/ml plasma, whereas the peripheral concentration remains unchanged. Provided that hepatic extraction of insulin reflects insulin degradation in liver, one could speculate that this phenomenon might be an expression of a safety feed back mechanism of livers of sand rats induced by critical insulin concentrations in portal blood.

References

[1] ANSORGE, S., P. BOHLEY, H. KIRSCHKE, J. LANGNER, B. WIEDERANDERS, and H. HANSON in: Intracellular protein catabolism (I). H. HANSON and P. BOHLEY (Eds). Barth Leipzig 1975, p. 319—336

[2] ANSORGE, S., H. KIRSCHKE, J. LANGNER, B. WIEDERMANDERS, P. BOHLEY, and H. HANSON in: Intracellular protein catabolism (II). V. TURK and N. MARKS (Eds). Plenum Press, New York and London 1977, p. 163–166
[3] BRUSH, J. S.: Diabetes **20**, 140–145 (1971)
[4] KÖHLER, E., S. KNOSPE, H. SCHÄFER, B. ZIEGLER, W. BLECH, B. BIERWOLF, H. HAHN VON DORSCHE, H. D. GOTTSCHLING, H. FIEDLER, and H. BIBERGEIL: Endokrinologie **68**, 198–210 (1976)
[5] ANSORGE, S., P. BOHLEY, H. KIRSCHKE, J. LANGNER, and H. HANSON: Eur. J. Biochem. **19**, 283–288 (1971)
[6] ANSORGE, S., P. BOHLEY, H. KIRSCHKE, J. LANGNER, B. WIEDERANDERS, and H. HANSON: Eur. J. Biochem. **32**, 27–35 (1973)
[7] LAURELL, C. B.: Anal. Biochem. **15**, 45–52 (1966)
[8] RESSLER, N.: Clinica chim. Acta **5**, 795–800 (1960)
[9] BOHLEY, P., H. KIRSCHKE, J. LANGNER, and S. ANSORGE: FEBS Lett. **5**, 233–235 (1969)
[10] SCHWERTNER, R.: Diplomarbeit, Martin-Luther-Universität Halle-Wittenberg, Bereich Medizin 1974

Acta biol. med. germ., Band 36, Seite 1723–1727 (1977)

Institute of Physiological Chemistry University of Halle, 402 Halle (Saale), Hollystraße 1, GDR

Conversion of proinsulin into insulin by cathepsins B and L from rat liver lysosomes

S. Ansorge, H. Kirschke, and K. Friedrich

Summary

Conversion of proinsulin and intermediate forms of proinsulin into insulin were studied with rat liver cell fractions and purified lysosomal proteinases by using the technique of polyacrylamide disc-electrophoresis. Both substrates were degraded very rapidly by homogenates and crude lysosomal fractions to split products not detectable on disc-electropherograms. Neither breakdown nor conversion were detected with the cytosol and the microsomal fraction. With partially purified lysosomal fractions (mol. wt. approx. 25000) or with highly purified cathepsin L or cathepsin B (B_1) proinsulin was converted into products migrating like the intermediate forms and insulin, and the intermediates were converted into products migrating like insulin and deoctapeptide-insulin in disc-electropherograms. The mechanism of conversion seems to be different for both enzymes. The results force us to conculde that lysosomal cathepsins, especially cathepsins L and B might be involved in the process of conversion of proinsulin into insulin and perhaps also of other precursors into biologically active proteins in vivo.

Introduction

As reported by Dr. Zühlke in the preceding paper (see also [1]), enzymes with trypsin-like and carboxypeptidase B-like specificity are believed to play an important role in the intracellular conversion of proinsulin into insulin as well as in the processing of other precursor forms of proteins and peptides. Several authors [2, 3] have considered the possibility that these converting enzymes are related to some of the lysosomal proteinases. This hypothesis has been supported by the findings of Zühlke et al. [1] that indeed islets homogenates contain proteinases exhibiting properties similar to those of thiol-proteinases of lysosomes.

However, purified lysosomal proteinases have not been used as yet to imitate the conversion of proinsulin into insulin in vitro.

The aim of the present communication was to examine the action of lysosomal fractions and of purified lysosomal proteinases of rat liver in the conversion of proinsulin and intermediate forms of proinsulin into insulin (for details see [4]).

Insulin precursors, proinsulin and intermediates from beef were provided by Dr. Zühlke and coworkers (Central Institute for Diabetes, Karlsburg). These substrates were incubated with enzyme fractions and, immediately after the incubation, the samples were analyzed by polyacrylamide disc-electrophoresis at *p*H 9.5.

Results

Using liver homogenates or crude lysosomal fractions both precursors of insulin were degraded very rapidly, mainly to split products not visible on disc-electropherograms. Maximum breakdown occurred at *p*H 6.0 in the presence of GSH and/or EDTA. Neither breakdown nor conversion were detected with the cytosol and the microsomal fraction of rat liver.

First indications of conversion into insulin-like components (migrating like insulin in the disc-electrophoresis) were found with the water soluble fraction of lysosomes, especially with the fraction having molecular weights of 20000—30000, obtained after chromatography on Sephadex G-75. Therefore, in further experiments purified cathepsins from this fraction, cathepsin B, L, H, L20C11 and L20C12, were tested in detail. Preparation of these cathepsins were performed according to the method of Kirschke et al. [5—7].

Among these 5 proteinases cathepsins L and B were found to be capable of catalyzing the conversion of proinsulin and its intermediates into insulin-like components. This is demonstrated in Fig. 1—3.

The rate limiting step of cathepsin L-catalyzed conversion seems to be the conversion of proinsulin into insulin (Fig. 1). Within an incubation time of 60 min

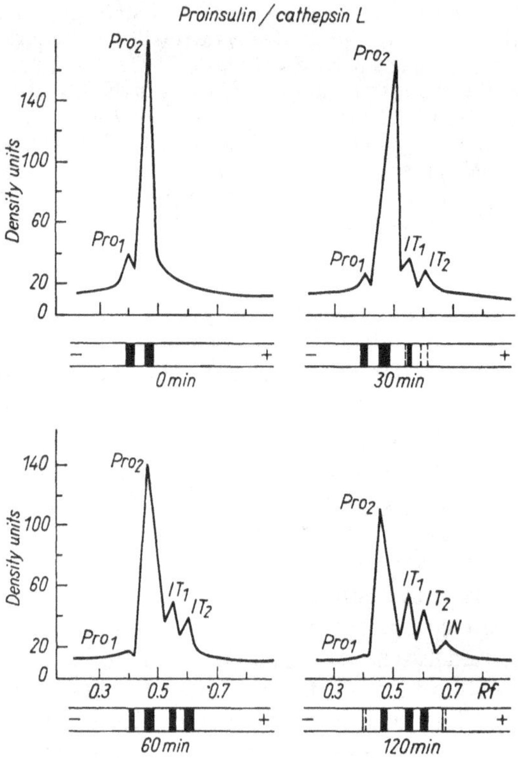

Fig. 1. Conversion of proinsulin into the intermediate forms of proinsulin by cathepsin L. 50 µl of mixtures containing 0.22 mM proinsulin, 0.49 µg cathepsin L and 0.16 M phosphate buffer, *p*H 6.0, were incubated for the given times. Immediately after the incubation at 38 °C 20 µl of the mixtures were analyzed by disc-electrophoresis in 15% polyacrylamide (0.4 × 8 cm) with separation-*p*H of 9.5. Protein bands were fixed with trichloroacetic acid and stained with Coomassie brillant blue G-250 in 12.5% trichloroacetic acid. Densitometry of the stained gels was performed with the "Vitatron" (Dieren, Holland).

Abbreviations: Pro = proinsulin, IT = intermediate forms of proinsulin, IN = insulin, DOPI = deoctapetide-insulin

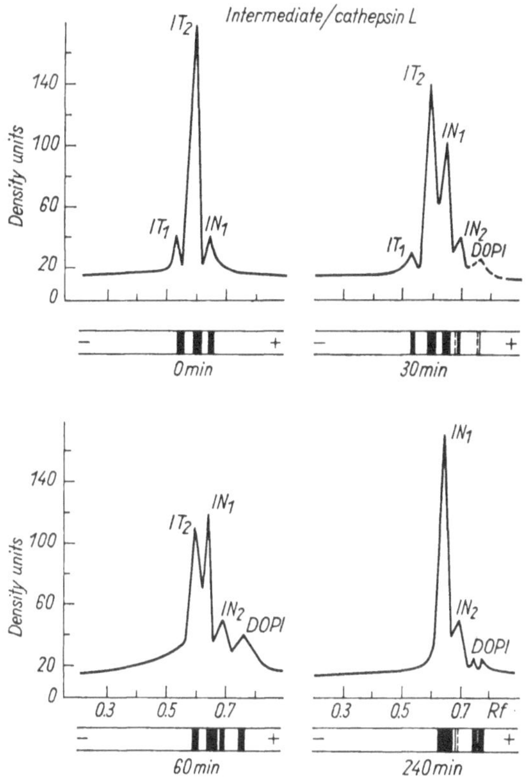

Fig. 2. Conversion of the intermediate forms of proinsulin into insulin by cathepsin L. The experimental conditions were the same as described in the legend of Fig. 1 (0.22 mM intermediates). For abbreviations see also Fig. 1

only a small portion of proinsulin was transformed to the intermediates and insulin, resp., whereas the intermediates of proinsulin were converted to about 50% into insulin (and in part to deoctapeptide insulin) within the same time (Fig. 2). Complete conversion occured after 4 hrs of incubation.

The mechanism of the cathepsin L-catalyzed conversion of proinsulin into insulin seems to be different from that of the cathepsin B-catalyzed reaction. This can be concluded from the time course of the conversion as well as from the pattern of the reaction products generated from proinsulin as well as from the intermediate forms by cathepsin B and cathepsin L. Moreover, the intermediates were transformed more slowlier by cathepsin B than by cathepsin L, and higher concentrations of cathepsin B are necessary, as compared with cathepsin L, to demonstrate the conversion (Fig. 3).

To identify the component that migrates like insulin in the electrophoresis the insulin-like component obtained after treatment of the intermediates with cathepsin L was eluted from the electrophoresis gels and incubated with DCC-trypsin (Fig. 4). The only product obtained after tryptic treatment has been found to be deoctapeptide-insulin. Therefore we conclude that really either insulin or dealaninated insulin are the products of conversion of proinsulin and intermediates by cathepsin L and B.

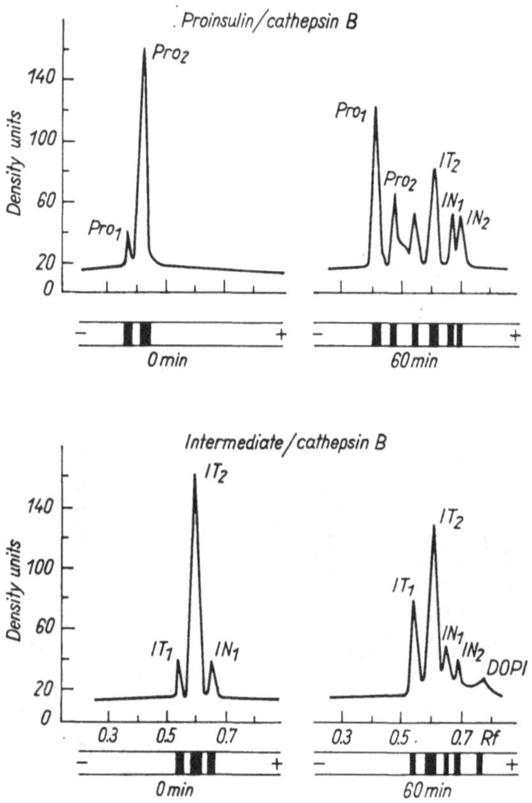

Fig. 3. Conversion of proinsulin into the intermediates (top) and of the intermediates into insulin (bottom) by cathepsin B.

The incubation mixtures contained proinsulin or intermediates (0.16 mM), 18.1 µg cathepsin B and 0.16 M phosphate buffer, *p*H 6.0. Incubations and analyses of the samples were performed as described in Fig. 1

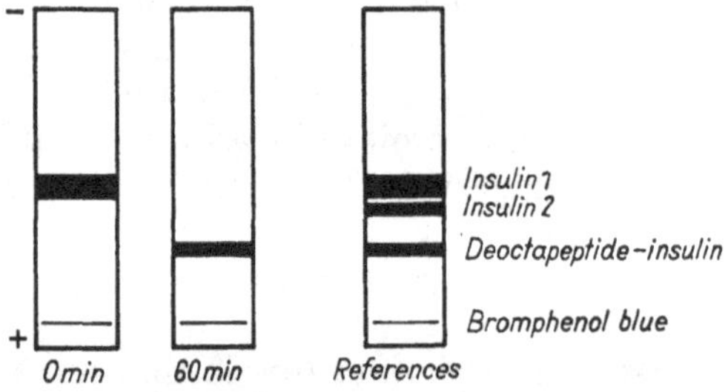

Fig. 4. Tryptic conversion of the insulin-like component into deoctapeptide-insulin.

The insulin-like component generated by the action of cathepsin L on the intermediate forms of proinsulin were collected from 12 electrophoreses by elution of the insulin band, visualized by short treatment with trichloroacetic acid, in 0.01 M hydrochloric acid. After separation of the gel and drying, the eluted material was incubated with 0.3 µg DCC-trypsin at *p*H 7.5. The reaction product was analyzed by disc-electrophoresis

These results force us to conclude that lysosomal cathepsins, especially cathepsins L and B, are true candidates for the conversion of proinsulin into insulin via the intermediate forms of proinsulin, and perhaps also of other precursors to biologically active proteins in vivo.
Our experiments cannot decide, however, if the conversion of proinsulin into insulin could be accomplished alone by these cathepsins. Possibly cathepsins B and/or L act like trypsin [8] in a way that an additional carboxypeptidase B-like activity is necessary in a second step to eliminate a carboxyl-terminal basic amino acid residue remained at the B-chain of insulin after catheptic action.

References

[1] Zühlke, H., D. F. Steiner, A. Lernmark, and C. Lipsay in: Ciba Foundation Symposium 41 (New Ser.), Elsevier, Exerpta Medica, North-Holland, Amsterdam, Oxford, New York 1976, p. 183–195
[2] Steiner, D. F., W. Kemmler, J. L. Clark, P. E. Oyer, and A. H. Rubenstein in: Handbook of Physiology. Endocrinology. D. F. Steiner and N. Freinkel (Eds). Williams and Wilkins, Baltimore 1972, p. 175–198
[3] Smith, R. E.: Diabetes **21**, 581–583 (1972)
[4] Friedrich, K.: Diplomarbeit, Martin-Luther-Universität Halle-Wittenberg, Sektion Chemie, 1973
[5] Kirschke, H., J. Langner, B. Wiederanders, S. Ansorge, and P. Bohley: Acta biol. med. germ. **28**, 305–322 (1972)
[6] Kirschke, H., J. Langner, B. Wiederanders, S. Ansorge. P. Bohley, and U. Broghammer: Acta biol. med. germ. **35**, 285–299 (1976)
[7] Kirschke, H., J. Langner, B. Wiederanders, S. Ansorge, and P. Bohley: Eur. J. Biochem. **74**, 293–307 (1977)
[8] Kemmler, W., J. D. Peterson, and D. F. Steiner: J. biol. Chem. **246**, 6786–6791 (1971)

Acta biol. med. germ., Band 36, Seite 1729—1733 (1977)

[1] Physiologisch-chemisches Institut der Martin-Luther-Universität, DDR 402 Halle (Saale)
[2] Zentralinstitut für Molekularbiologie der AdW der DDR, Abteilung Zellphysiologie, DDR 1115 Berlin-Buch

Presence of an endopeptidase activity in rat liver ribosomes

J. LANGNER[1], S. ANSORGE[1], P. BOHLEY[1], H. WELFLE[2], and H. BIELKA[2]

Summary

Preparation of ribosomes using different procedures (treatment of postmitochondrial-postlysosomal supernatant or microsomes with 1% triton in 0.15 or 0.5 M KCl and subsequent sucrose gradient centrifugation; treatment of microsomes with 1.5% deoxycholate/2% triton) results in purified ribosomes which contain an endopeptidase activity detectable by breakdown of ribosomal proteins to trichloroacetic acid soluble split products. The proteolytic activity can be recovered also in the extracted proteins of whole ribosomes. With ribosomes the *p*H optimum of proteolytic breakdown is at about 7. The inhibition of the activity by leupeptin, DIFP and soya bean trypsin inhibitor suggests a serine type of the proteolytic activity.

Introduction

In 1974 we reported for the first time on the presence of an endopeptidase in rat liver ribosomes [1]. In the meantime, LEVJANT et al. [2] reported similar findings from rat liver, and KORANT [3] on an endopeptidase in HeLa cell ribosomes. The results of these studies taken together provide evidence that ribosomes contain an endopeptidase activity in addition to the exopeptidase activities reported on previously by other authors [4—7].

Material and methods

Preparation of ribosomes

Ribosomes were prepared by the following procedures:

1. Addition of triton to microsomes, 0.15 M KCl: Homogenates (typically from 35—40 Wistar rats, starved for 20 hrs) were prepared in TKM-buffer (50 mM Tris, 25 mM KCl, 5 mM $MgCl_2$, 5 mM β-mercaptoethanol, 0.25 M sucrose, *p*H 7.8) and centrifuged twice at 15 to 20,000 $\times$ *g*, for 10 min each. The postmitochondrial-postlysosomal supernatant was then centrifuged for 150 min at 105,000 $\times$ *g* (max) and the resulting microsomal pellet was washed 2—3 times with TKM buffer (MS 3 in Fig. 1). Ribosomes were detached from the membranes by 1% triton X-100 in 0.15 M KCl solution (including 10 mM Tris, *p*H 7.7, 5 mM $MgCl_2$ and 10 mM β-mercaptoethanol), and sedimented at 105,000 $\times$ *g* for 120 min. The ribosomal pellet was then washed at least once with the same buffer and once with buffer without triton. In Fig. 1, ribosomes prepared according to this procedure are referred to as MS 3 + 1% triton/0.15 M KCl.

2. Addition of triton to microsomes, 0.5 M KCl: This procedure is the same as the first one, except that the treatment with triton was effected in the presence of the higher KCl-concentration, i.e. 0.5 M. In Fig. 1, ribosomes prepared according to procedure 2 are referred to as MS 3 + 1% triton/0.5 M KCl.

3. Addition of triton to microsomes, 0.5 M KCl + additional gradient: Ribosomes prepared according to procedure 2 still showing low activities of the lysosomal marker enzymes acid phosphatase and RNase (tested at *p*H 5.25, 7.5 and 9.1). These activities could be removed below measurable amounts by performing a sucrose gradient as additional purification step:

Ribosomes prepared according to procedure 1 or 2 were layered on top of a discontinous sucrose gradient (0.5 and 1.7 or 2.0 M sucrose, 16–20 hrs at 300,000 × *g*), with or without addition of 1% triton. In Fig. 1, ribosomes prepared according to procedure 3 are referred to as MS 3 + 1% triton/0.5 M KCl + gradient.

4. Addition of triton to postmitochondrial-postlysosomal supernatant: The postmitochondrial-postlysosomal supernatant was made 1% of triton and 0.15 M with respect to KCl and then ultracentrifuged for 150 min at 105,000 × *g* (max). The resulting ribosomal pellet was washed as in procedure 1 (in Fig. 1 these ribosomes are designated as RC + 1% triton/0.15 M KCl) or subjected to treatment with 0.5 M KCl in the presence of 1% triton as in procedure 2.

5. Preparation of free ribosomes was performed by ultracentrifugation of the postmitochondrial-postlysosomal supernatant, made as described in procedure 1, directly and without addition of detergent through a gradient as described in procedure 3 for 16–20 hrs at 300,000 × *g*. The pellet of free ribosomes was washed at least once with 5 mM Tris, 50 mM KCl, 1.5 mM $MgCl_2$, 5 mM β-mercaptoethanol, *p*H 7.8.

6. Alternatively to the microsome preparation in procedures 1–3 the time-saving microsome preparation procedure of KAMATH et al. [9] was used, in which microsomes were precipitated by means of 8 mM $CaCl_2$.

7. Alternatively to the detachment of ribosomes from endoplasmic membranes by means of 1% triton we used also a treatment of microsomes, prepared as in procedure 1, with 1.5% sodium deoxycholate + 2% triton X-100 in TKM-buffer (see proc. 1), followed by ultracentrifugation for 150 min at 105,000 × *g*, resuspension of the ribosomal pellet in TKM + 1.5 deoxycholate/2% triton and recentrifugation for 60 min at 320,000 × *g* (max.) Ribosomes were thereafter washed at least once with 5 mM Tris, 50 mM KCl, 1.5 mM $MgCl_2$, 5 mM β-mercaptoethanol, *p*H 7.8.
Ribosomes purified according to the methods described have A 260/280 ratios of 1.78–1.90 and A 260/235 ratios of 1.65–1.75.

Preparation of ribosomal proteins

Ribosomal proteins were prepared by extraction of the ribosomal pellet with 0.25 N HCl or 2 M LiCl. After sedimentation of the RNA, the proteins were precipitated from the clear supernatant by acetone at −20 °C, washed with cold acetone and ether, dissolved in a small amount of water and lyophilized directly or after dialysis against 200 vol of cold distilled water. The protein preparation thus obtained contained less than 1% of RNA.

Determinations of proteolytic activity

in ribosomal preparations are complicated by two facts: (1) the activities are rather low; (2) azocasein, the substrate mainly used by us, was not split by ribosomes. Since on the other hand ribosomal proteins are very good substrates for proteolytic enzymes [1], we used as a test system the incubation of ribosomes alone, without addition of other substrates. The degradation of endogenous substrate – the ribosomal proteins – was measured by determination of rest-N, amino-N, and Lowry-reactive material in the TCA supernatant [8]. Therefore it is impossible to calculate purification factors. The activity in the autolysis assay is given as percent degradation of protein during the incubation time (up to 10 hrs). This procedure allows the measurement of degradation rates as low as 0.3 to 0.5%.

Results and discussion

Evidence for the presence of the endopeptidase on ribosomes

From the results shown in Fig. 1, it can be concluded that the proteolytic activity is strongly bound to ribosomes. None of the tested variations in the preparation of ribosomes resulted in ribosomal particles without any proteolytic activity. Although the proteolytic activity of ribosomes prepared by the different procedures (see Material and methods) is low in comparison to other cellular proteinases, it is well

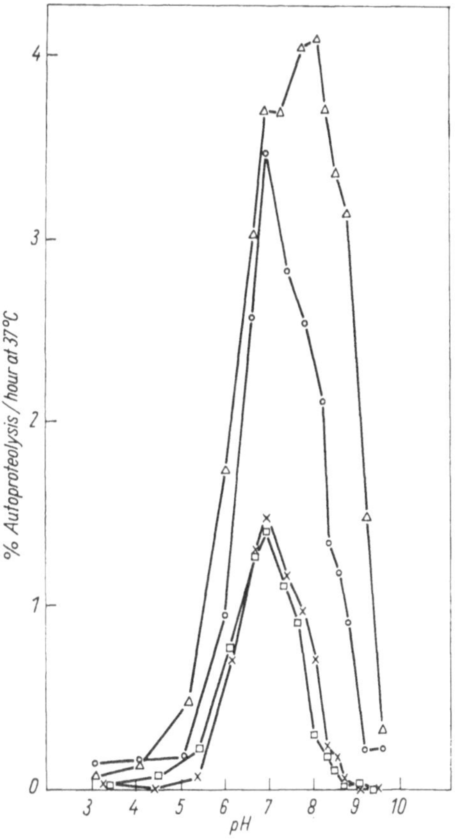

Fig. 1. *p*H activity profiles of the proteolytic activity of ribosomes at different steps of purification using different procedures.

△: Ribosomes obtained from microsomes (washed twice = MS 3) treated with 1% triton X-100, 0.15 M KCl (procedure 1); □: ribosomes obtained from microsomes treated with 1% triton X-100, 0.5 M KCl (procedure 2); ×: ribosomes obtained from microsomes treated with 1% triton X-100, 0.5 M KCl + gradient (0.5–1.7 M sucrose) (procedure 3); ○: ribosomes obtained from the postmitochondrial-postlysosomal supernatant (RC treated with 1% triton X-100, 0.15 M KCl (procedure 4).

All ribosomes were spun down at least $15 \cdot 10^6 \cdot g \cdot$ min and washed at least once with detergent free buffer. Activity determinations: 50 µl ribosomal fraction (containing about 0.1 to 0.4 mg of ribosomal protein) + 100 µl buffer (*p*H 3–7, McIlvaine; *p*H 7.5–9.5, borate) were incubated at 37 °C for 4–8 hrs; Lowry determination in 20 µl TCA supernatante at zero time and after 4–8 hrs at 37 °C. Calculation of % autoproteolysis = % degradation according to [8], cf. this paper Table 1

detectable. The activity is also found on free ribosomes and is recovered also in good yield in the fraction of the ribosomal proteins, where it is stable even after lyophilization.

Nevertheless, convincing evidence demonstrating the real ribosomal nature of the enzyme has yet to be provided. The fact that ist was not possible to obtain ribosomes free of proteolytic activity, however, supports the idea of the ribosomal origin of this proteolytic activity. The results of Korant on HeLa cells presented on this symposium point in the same direction.

The results demonstrated in Fig. 1 indicate that the wash procedures, particularly the increase in KCl concentration up to 0.5 M, remove a substantial part of activity. The nature of the test system did not yet allow to look for this part of activity that is lost in the supernatants during centrifugation procedures. Alternatively, however, these losses in measurable activity might be due to a loss of endogenous substrate. This question awaits further clarification.

pH-activity profiles

One of the most important features of the activity is its *p*H optimum around 7. Fig. 1 shows that at all purification steps a shoulder on the alkaline slope of the profiles exists. Ribosomal proteins (not shown) show the same properties.

Endopeptidase nature of the proteolytic activity

The enzyme is an endopeptidase as revealed by the comparison of amino nitrogen determinations in TCA supernates after and before hydrolysis with hydrochloric acid. The values for the quotient ranged between 8 and 24 (Tab. 1).

Table 1
Amino nitrogen determination before and after hydrolysis with HCl in TCA supernates of autolysis assays as evidence for the endopeptidase nature of the ribosomal proteolytic activity

Amino nitrogen (TNBS method)			LOWRY method	
Increase before hydrolysis	increase after hydrolysis	% degrad. after hydrolysis	Increase	% degrad.
0.016 µg	0.19 µg	3.19	1.61 µg	3.87
$\frac{\text{Amino-N after HCl hydrolysis}}{\text{Amino-N before HCl hydrolysis}} = 11.9$				

Ribosomes were incubated for $5^1/_2$ hrs. at 37 °C, *p*H 7.0 (McIlvaine buffer). 20 µl of TCA supernate was used for TNBS (with or without prior HCl hydrolysis) and Lowry method, resp., resulting in the "increase" figures, given as µg/20 µl TCA supernatant. "% degrad." = increase in % of the amino acid (after HCl hydrolysis) and protein content (Lowry method) in the assay mixture, resp.
The result of the Lowry method from this experiment is given to demonstrate the satisfactory agreement between both methods.

Influence of effectors, KCl and deoxycholate

Using whole ribosomes and the proteins prepared therefrom, respectively, we tested the following effectors without significant influence (10^{-3}M): TLCK, TPCK, pepstatin, pCMB, o-phenanthroline and gluthatione. Using leupeptin, DIFP, and soya bean trypsin inhibitor, however, we got significant inhibitions (ID_{50} $6 \cdot 10^{-6}$M, $5 \cdot 10^{-4}$ M, and $5 \cdot 10^{-2}$ mg/ml, respectively, taken from plots of enzyme inhibition *vs* log effector concentration), pointing to a serine type of the proteinase. The sulfhydryl reagents DTT and DTE caused inhibition by about 50% (5 mM) as did EDTA (10 mM).
Table 2 shows the fair insensitivity of the enzyme against potassium chloride up to 1 M. Deoxycholate in concentrations used for ribosome preparation, however,

Table 2
Influence of KCl and deoxycholate on ribosomal autoproteolysis at *p*H 7.0
(Control without additions = 100%)

KCl		Deoxycholate	
Conc. (M)	Relative activity	Conc. (%)	Relative activity
0.15	100.2		
0.5	99.3	0.5	3.7
1.0	94.0	1.0	0.6
2.0	69.5	2.0	not detectable

A ribosome preparation was made 0.15 M–2.0 M with respect to KCl and 0.5 %–2.0 % with respect to deoxycholate, resp., and the resulting proteolytic activity (McIlvaine buffer, *p*H 7.0, 4 hrs, 37 °C; details see Fig. 1) is compared with that of controls without additions.

Table 3
Recovery of the proteolytic activity of ribosomal preparations after repeated washings to remove deoxycholate

Without deoxycholate	With 1% deoxycholate	After washing centrifugation once	twice	three times
100%	0.6%	31.1%	80.7%	87.9%

One part of a ribosome preparation was tested for proteolytic activity (McIlvaine buffer, *p*H 7.0, 5 hrs, 37 °C; details see Fig. 1) directly (control) or in the presence of 1% deoxycholate. Another part of this ribosome preparation was made 1% with respect to deoxycholate and then by repeated centrifugation (60 min 300,000 × *g*, resuspension of the ribosomal pellets in 5 mM Tris, 50 mM KCl, 1 – 5 mM $MgCl_2$, 5 mM β-ME, *p*H 7.8) deoxycholate was gradually removed and the activity of the 1st, 2nd and 3rd pellet tested as before. The buffer volume used in the three washes resulted in a dilution of about 110fold, the deoxycholate concentration after three washes is therefore expected to be at about 0.01%.

causes complete but reversible inhibition as indicated in Table 3. Table 3 shows that a ribosome preparation in 1% deoxycholate regains activity nearly totally if deoxycholate is removed by several washings with buffer.

Our results extend those of LEVJANT et al. [2] and are in good agreement with their findings, except the insensitivity against TPCK in our experiments. The results from HeLa cells given by KORANT ([3] and this volume, p. 1565) are somewhat more different with respect to the influence of effectors, temperature and *p*H, but KORANT proves the serine type and endopeptidase nature of the activity, too. Part of the reported differences may be due to the different test systems, since KORANT used a procedure without TCA precipitation, and he found that about 70% of the obtained split products were precipitable by TCA.

Acknowledgment

We thank Prof. UMEZAWA for the generous gift of pepstatin and leupeptin. The expert and skilful assistance of Mrs. B. OELKE is greatly appreciated.

References

[1] LANGNER, J., P. BOHLEY, and H. BIELKA: Symposium "Ribosomes and Biosynthesis of Proteins", May 13–16, 1974, Schloß Reinhardsbrunn (GDR)
[2] LEVJANT, M. I., V. S. BILINKINA, M. G. TRUDOLJUBOWA, and V. N. OREKHOVICH: Molek. Biol. **10**, 770 (1976)
[3] KORANT, B. D.: Biochem. biophys. Res. Commun. **74**, 926 (1977)
[4] MATHESON, A. T., and A. J. DICK: FEBS Lett. **6**, 235 (1970)
[5] McCORQUODALE, D. J.: J. biol. Chem. **238**, 3914 (1963)
[6] KERWAR, S. S., H. WEISSBACH, and G. G. GLENNER: Archs Biochem. Biophys. **143**, 356 (1971)
[7] BINKLEY, F.: J. biol. Chem. **236**, 1075 (1961)
[8] LANGNER, J., S. ANSORGE, P. BOHLEY, H. KIRSCHKE, and H. HANSON: Acta biol. med. germ. **26**, 935 (1971)
[9] KAMATH, S. A., and K. A. NARAYAN: Anal. Biochem. **48**, 53 (1972)

Acta biol. med. germ., Band 36, Seite 1735—1745 (1977)

Department of Biochemistry and Biophysics and the Electron Microscopy Laboratory, The University of Connecticut, Storrs, CT. 06268 U.S.A.

Implications of amino acid compartmentation for the determination of rates of protein catabolism in livers in meal fed rats

E. A. Khairallah, J. Airhart, M. K. Bruno, D. Puchalsky, and L. Khairallah

Introduction

In the past several years our laboratory has been using radioisotopes to study meal-related variations in protein metabolism in livers of intact rats. In order to circumvent the uncertainties inherent in isotopic studies in vivo, we devised an assay of protein synthesis which directly measured the specific radioactivity of amino acids on the immediate precursor, amino acyl-tRNA [1—3]. However, as synthesis is only one component of protein metabolism it was also essential to develop an adequate measurement of protein degradation in the whole animal, a technique rapid enough to detect changes from hour to hour and capable of obtaining data without disturbing the process being monitored.

At first glance, a knowledge of net protein accumulation and total synthesis should enable us to measure rates of degradation by difference. Unfortunately, in short term studies one must also consider the liver's active involvement in protein secretion, a component which may be variable following a meal [4—5] and has not yet been adequately assessed in vivo.

Investigators have often evaluated protein degradation by measuring the release of radioactive amino acids from pre-labelled proteins. This technique is valid only if reincorporation into protein can be prevented and the products of protein catabolism are completely recovered. Regretably, [^{14}C]-guanido-arginine, originally thought to be essentially non-reusable, has been shown to generate significant underestimation in vivo [6]. Furthermore, procedures for interpreting decay curves of pulse labelled proteins can require weeks to obtain sufficient data to draw meaningful conclusions [7].

Two techniques that have been used successfully to circumvent the problem of isotope reutilization in perfused livers include the inhibition of protein synthesis by antibiotics like cycloheximide or expansion of the total free pools with an excess of the unlabelled amino acid. Unfortunately, the levels of antibiotics sufficient to suppress protein synthesis can also alter the rates of degradation [2]; while an excess of an amino acid necessary to eliminate reutilization can dramatically alter plasma amino acid levels in vivo and would most likely induce important systemic side effects that would be impossible to control or evaluate. These factors may tend to obliterate the physiological significance of such investigations.

In this paper we suggest yet another approach which developed out of studies in our laboratory on the compartmentation of amino acids [1—3]. In order to determine the source of amino acids for protein synthesis, we had introduced tracer doses of radioactive valine into the circulation and monitored the resulting specific radioactivities of free valine in the hepatic extracellular and intracellular fluids as well as valine esterified to tRNA. The following observations are pertinent to the present discussion: (a) For an amino acid, such as valine, that is neither synthesized nor catabolized in the liver, the net uptake or release of the free amino acid into the circulation is also a direct result of the combined actions of protein synthesis and degradation [8]: (b) When the isotope reached steady stated distribution in the liver, the specific radioactivity of the tRNA-bound valine was always intermediate between the values in the extracellular and intracellular pools [1—3]; (c) The degree of intermediacy of the specific radioactivity of the valyl-tRNA was directly and quantitatively proportional to the amino acid concentrations in the extracellular and intracellular pools [3]; and (d) The tRNA-bound valine acquired label with biphasic kinetics suggesting a brief rapid initial surge to saturate a small intermediate pool followed by a gradual accumulation of isotope exactly paralleling the labelling kinetics of the intracellular valine [2].

Although alternative models have been considered [2] and may accommodate most of the data at hand, the model presented in Fig. 1 appears to have the most predictive value. It is visualized that only the valine in the process of transport within the cell membrane system can serve as a substrate for activation by the tRNA synthetases [1, 3]. The valine molecules within this hypothetical membrane pool are not free per se but are bound to the transport carriers, (*mo* and *mi*) and the tRNA synthetases can then charge valine bound to these carriers without reference to the direction of flow of the amino acid. On the basis of these premises it can be shown that one can calculate physiologically meaningful rates of degra-

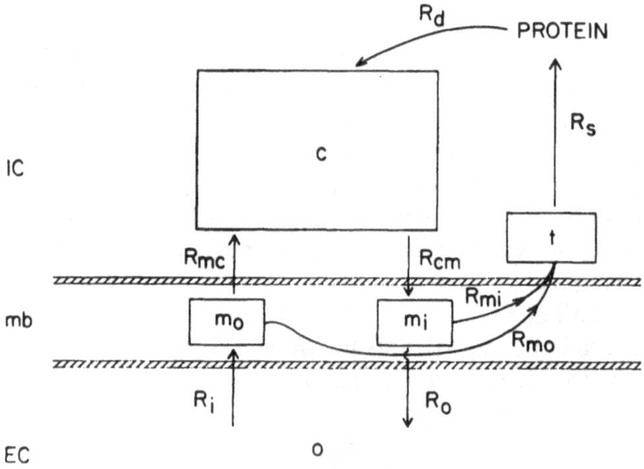

Fig. 1. Model of the relationship between hepatic valine pools.

Pool = the total quantity of valine molecules within designated spatial or metabolic limits. c = the pool of free valine within the liver cells. m_0 = the pool of valine associated with membrane carriers moving from outside to inside the cells. m_i = the pool of valine associated with membrane carriers moving from inside to outside the cells. $m = m_0 + m_i$ = the total pool of valine associated with membrane carriers. t = the pool of valine esterified to tRNA. o = the pool of free valine in the extracellular water of the liver. R = the rate of flow of valine from one pool to another expressed in terms of nmoles of valine/min/liver of a 100 g rat (L_{100})

dation and transport solely from a knowledge of four parameters; (a) The rate of synthesis (Rs); and the steady state specific radioactivities of the (b) Extracellular (Ao) (c) Intracellular (Ac) and (d) t-RNA bound (At) amino acid. A simplified discussion of the efficacy of this model is illustrated below while a more detailed mathematical analysis will be presented elsewhere [9].

Let us assume some typical values for these four easily measurable parameters (eg $Rs = 125$ nmol valine incorporated/min/liver of a 100 g rat (L_{100}); $Ac =$ 900 dpm/nmol; $At = 1620$ dpm/nmol, and $Ao = 2700$ dpm/nmol). Based on the diagram presented in Fig. 1, one can readily assume that for the short duration of the experiments (10—15 min after isotope administration) the intracellular pool (c) and the hypothetical membrane pools (*mo* and *mi*) should maintain a steady state concentration. This would imply that the rates of amino acids flowing into and out of these pools must be equal:

$$Rd = Rcm - Rmc \tag{1}$$

$$Rs = Rmo + Rmi \tag{2}$$

$$Ri = Rmc + Rmo \tag{3}$$

$$Ro = Rcm - Rmi \tag{4}$$

Now the relative specific radioactivity of the intracellular pool (Ac/Ao) specifies the proportion of amino acids coming into the intracellular pool (c) from two sources: the extracellular pool (o) as expressed by the rate, Rmc, and from protein degradation, Rd. Thus an Ac/Ao ratio of 900/2700 in the above example implies that for every molecule coming from outside the cell with a specific radioactivity of 2700 dpm/nmol, two unlabelled molecules are entering the intracellular pool from protein degradation. Hence,

$$Rmc/Rd = 1/2 \text{ or } Rmc = Rd/2 \tag{5}$$

Substituting in equation (1) results in:

$$Rmc = Rd + Rd/2 = 3Rd\ 2 \tag{6}$$

Furthermore, if as recently reported (ref. [3]) the specific radioactivity of the valyl-tRNA can be accurately predicted by combining the extracellular and intracellular values in proportion specified by the trans-membrane concentration gradient, then a specific radioactivity of tRNA-bound valine (At) equal to 1620 dpm/nmol would suggest that for every two molecules charging the tRNA from the extracellular compartment with a specific radioactivity of 2700 dpm/nmol, three valine molecules with a specific radioactivity of 900 dpm/nmol must be arising from the intracellular pool. Hence

$$Rmi/Rmo = 3/2 \tag{7}$$

Given that the rate of protein synthesis (Rs) is equal to 125 nmol valine incorporated/min/L_{100} we can simulataneously solve for Rmi and Rmo by using equations (2) and (7), thus

$$Rmi = 75 \text{ nmol/min/}L_{100} \tag{8}$$

and

$$Rmo = 50 \text{ nmol/min/}L_{100} \tag{9}$$

In addition Rcm/Ri should also equal 3/2 and

$$Ri = 2/3\ Rcm \tag{10}$$

Therefore, substituting in equations (3) and (5) makes

$$2/3\ Rcm = Rd/2 + 50\ \text{nmol/min}/L_{100} \tag{11}$$

and since from (6) $Rcm = 3/2\ Rd$, then

$$(2/3)(3/2)\ Rd - Rd/2 = 50\ \text{nmol/min}/L_{100} \tag{12}$$

Hence

$$Rd = 100\ \text{nmol/min}/L_{100} \tag{13}$$

$$Rcm = 3/2\ Rd = 150\ \text{nmol/min}/L_{100} \tag{14}$$

$$Ri = 2/3\ Rcm = 100\ \text{nmol/min}/L_{100} \tag{15}$$

$$Rcm = Rd/2 = 50\ \text{nmol/min}/L_{100} \tag{16}$$

and

$$Ro = Rcm - Rmi = 75\ \text{nmol/min}/L_{100} \tag{17}$$

Furthermore, the percentage of amino acids arising from protein degradation that can reutilized for synthesis can be calculated as:

$$\text{Reutilization} = 100\left(\frac{R_s}{R_d}\,\frac{A_0 - A_t}{A_0}\right)\left(\frac{A_0 - A_c}{A_0}\right) = 33.3\% \tag{18}$$

Material and methods

In vivo measurements

Male rats from the Lewis strain housed under controlled lighting conditions (dark period from 5:30 pm – 5:30 am) were trained to eat once daily between 6 pm and 9 pm. The rats weighed about 150 g at the time of sacrifice. Detailed procedures for the labelling and isolation of the valine in the intracellular, extracellular as well as esterified to tRNA have been published elsewhere [1 – 3, 10].

Protein synthesis was monitored by measuring the increment in acid insoluble dpms between 10 and 15 min after an intraperitoneal injection of 33 μCi[^{3}H]-valine/100 g body weight, and corrected for the average specific radioactivity of the valyl-tRNA over the same time interval. The rate of degradation was calculated from the rates of synthesis and the specific radioactivities of the three hepatic amino acid pools as illustrated above.

Insulin was assayed by the double antibody procedures of HALES and RANDLE [11], and glucacon was assayed by the radioimmunoassay of FALOONA and UNGER (12].

Electron microscopy of acid phosphatase

Liver slices from rats at 6 and 9 pm were cut from the central lobe regions. The 1 × 3 mm thick sections were fixed in 2% glutaraldehyde buffered at *p*H 7.2 in Na-cacodylate, washed in 0.05 M Na acetate *p*H 5.0 and incubated in Gomori lead medium [13] for 1 h at 25 °C. The substrate used was Na-ß-glycerol phosphate at a final concentration of 0.01 M. Control specimens were run in the same medium lacking the substrate. After washing again in *p*H 5.0 Na-acetate, the specimens were post-fixed in 2% osmium-tetraoxide in 0.05 M Na-cacodylate, *p*H 7.2, and dehydrated in an ascending series of ethanol, cleared in propylene oxide and embedded in DER-334 resin. Thin sections were cut on an LKB-3 Ultratome and studied with a Phillips EM 300 electron microscope.

In vitro measurements

Livers from the 6 and 9 pm time periods from the meal fed rats were homogenized in 3 volumes of 0.33 M sucrose, 0.05 M Na-cacodylate, and 1% NaCl, *p*H 6.0, buffer and as indicated in the legends to the figures were either dounced (5 strokes each with the A and B pestle) or polytroned (15 s at position 4 of the PT-10 Polytron). The rate of release of valine was monitored at both 0 °C and 37 °C, and the valine concentrations were quantitated on a JEOL 6-AH Amino Acid Analyzer. The intracellular pools were corrected for extracellular valine by determining the ^{36}Cl space as described earlier [1, 3]. [^{3}H]-acetyl hemoglobin was used as an exogenous marker to monitor the activity of lysosomal cathepsins released in the presence or absence of 0.2% Triton-x-100 [14].

Results and discussion

The specific radioactivity of valine in the hepatic pools and the rates of protein synthesis and degradation before and after the meal (at 6 and 9 pm) are presented in Table 1. Although the onset of the meal did lead to a four-fold increase in the extracellular valine concentration [3], and a concomitant decrease in the extracellular specific radioactivity, the intracellular specific radioactivity of valine actually increased about 50%. Consequently, the model described in Fig. 1 would predict that in the absorptive rat the elevated extracellular valine must play a proportionately larger role in determining the composition of the membrane pool which charges the tRNA and hence the specific radioactivity of the valyl tRNA actually decreases despite the 50% increase in the specific radioactivity of the intracellular valine.

Furthermore, the ratio of the intracellular to extracellular specific radioactivity of valine increases from a low of about 18% prior to the meal to a high of 77% immediately after the meal. GAN and JEFFAY [15] had earlier viewed the ratio of intracellular to extracellular specific radioactivity as a relative index of internal protein degradation; that is a lowering of the ratio would indicate an increased flow of unlabelled valine arising from protein degradation. However, inspection of Fig. 1 reveals that there could be two other means of altering the specific radioactivity ratio without necessarily affecting intracellular protein degradation. For example, an increased rate of protein synthesis could trap more of the incoming valine before it mixed with the intracellular pool and since the extracellular fluid is the source of the label, the intracellular specific radioactivity would decrease. Alternatively, a decrease in the concentration of extracellular valine or in the rate of transport itself would also diminish the flow of valine into the intracellular compartment. Therefore, conclusions about the rates of protein degradation based solely on the specific radioactivity ratios require reliable measurements of the rates of protein synthesis and amino acid transport in vivo to be definitive. This is what we have attempted to do and the data are presented in Table 1.

Table 1
The specific radioactivity of valine in hepatic pools and the rates of protein synthesis and degradation in vivo in meal-fed rats

	6 pm	9 pm
Extracellular specific radioactivity	6609 ± 186	2416 ± 95
Intracellular specific radioactivity	1182 ± 85	1832 ± 90
tRNA-specific radioactivity	2689 ± 108	2169 ± 67
R_s (nmoles/min/L_{100})	88 ± 2	95 ± 5
R_d (nmoles/min/L_{100})	99 ± 7	25 ± 9
R_i (nmoles/min/L_{100})	45 ± 3	124 ± 11
Reutilization (% of R_s derived from R_d)	59 ± 1	9 ± 3

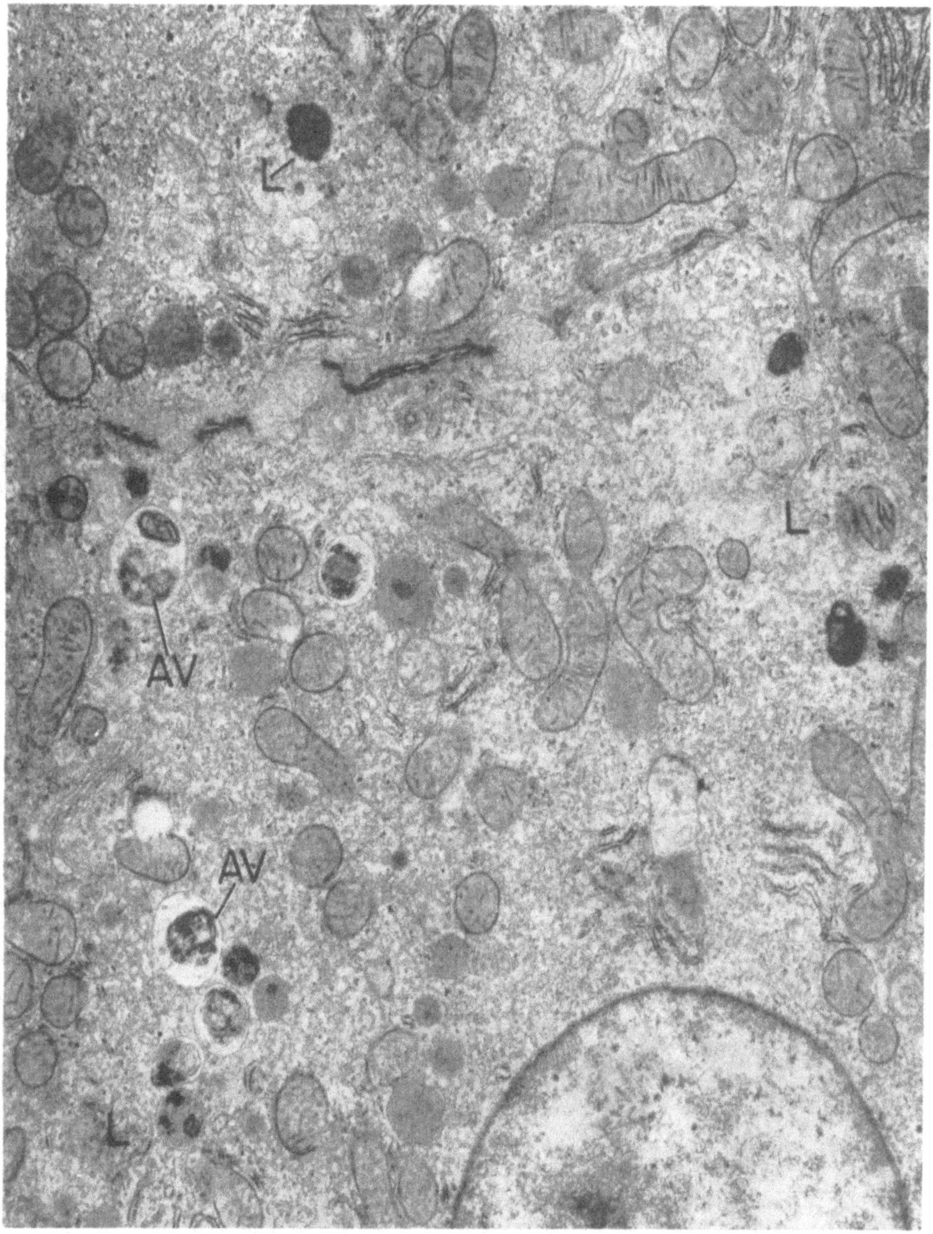

Fig. 2 and 3. Electron micrographs of 1000 square Å sections of hepatocytes from meal-fed rats trained to eat a single meal between 6–9 pm and stained histochemically for acid phosphatase with the lead Gomori technique [13].

Fig. 2 is from a 6 pm rat just prior to feeding; Fig. 3 is from a 9 pm rat immediately following the meal. Note specifically the absence of autophagic vacuoles in Fig. 3 as compared to Fig. 2. Magnification × 14,200

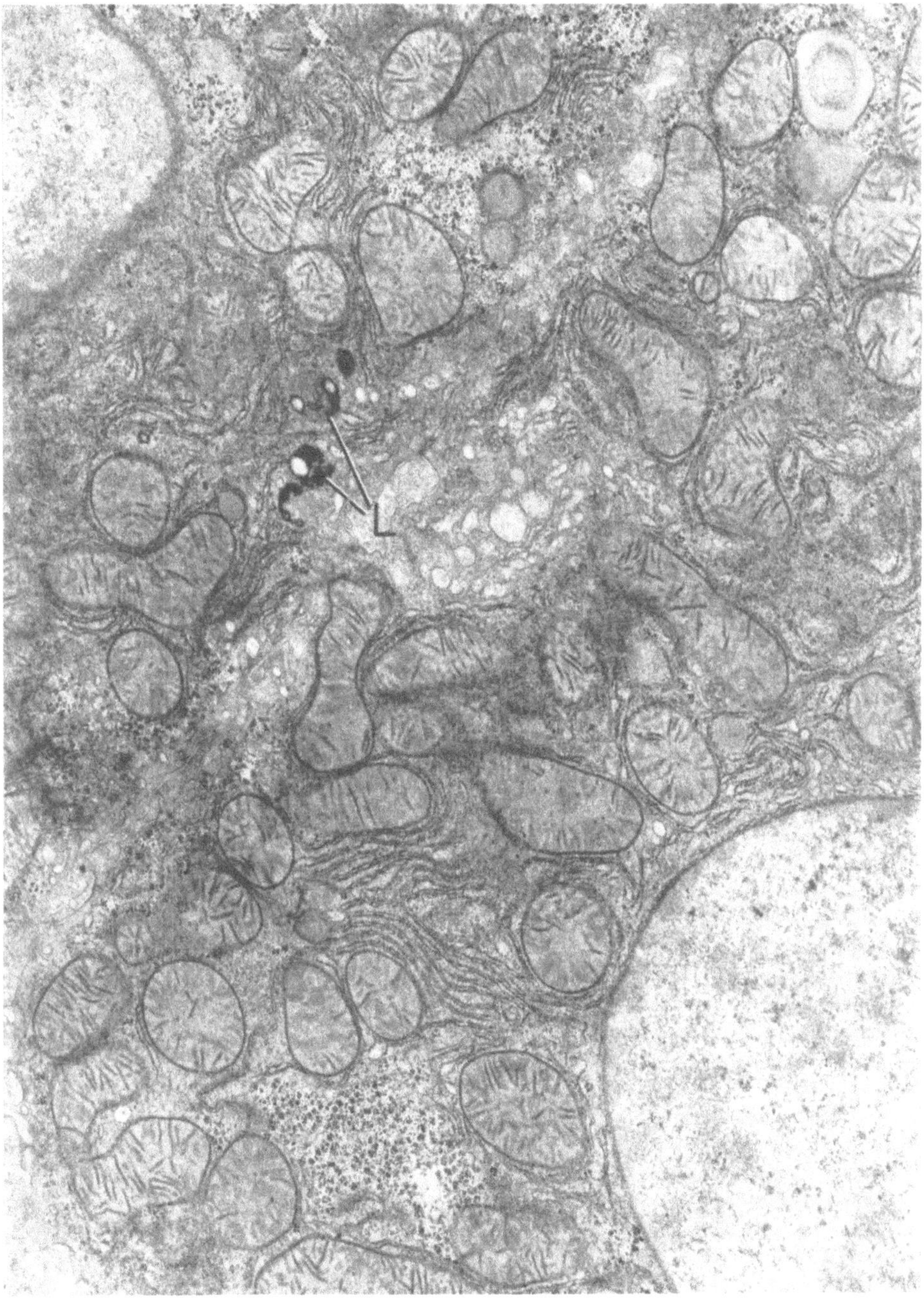

Fig. 3

Table 2
Insulin and glucagon concentrations in the portal blood of meal-fed rats just before (6 pm) and after (9 pm) a meal

	6 pm	9 pm
Insulin (μunits/ml plasma)	31.5 ± 1.5	98.1 ± 6.1
Glucagon (μg/ml plasma)	102 ± 5	104 ± 8
Insulin/Glucagon (molar Ratio)	4.9 ± 9	16.3

The most dramatic observation in vivo was the 4fold decrease in the calculated rate of degradation that can be observed immediately following the meal. Several investigators had alluded to this possibility previously [16, 17], but none had actually noted the magnitude of the altered rate of degradation immediately after feeding, and this despite the fact that protein synthesis is not apparently increased significantly. It should be pointed out that the insulin levels also increase four fold following the ingestion of the meal with an even greater increase in the molar ratio of insulin to glucagon levels in the portal circulation (Table 2). Thus in agreement with observations obtained in perfused livers [18, 19], the increased insulin and amino acid levels immediately after the meal do not alter the rate of hepatic protein synthesis but are closely correlated with a highly significant decrease in the rate of protein degradation in vivo.

In an attempt to demonstrate this altered rate of degradation by other means, we first resorted to study the lysosomal population in the hepatocytes of livers before and after a meal. After histo-chemical staining with the Gomori lead technique specific for acid phosphatase [13], it became very obvious that a shift in the lysosomal population had occurred (Fig. 2 and 3). It is clear in comparing these two micrographs that immediately after the meal the number of autophagic vacuoles virtually disappears, while the number and size of lysosomes are significantly decreased. On sampling over 100 electron micrographs at both time periods, we noted that per unit area the lysosomes had decreased 30% by number and 56% by volume; while the autophagic vacuoles at 9 pm were barely 2% of those detected at 6 pm before the meal (Table 3). These figures perhaps exaggerate the actual differences noted on ingesting a meal since they are expressed per 1000 square Å in area, but it should be noted that the liver weight increases about 12—15%, and the total hepatocyte volume also increases proportionately following the meal. Furthermore, the extracellular hepatic space as judged by the ^{36}Cl distribution is

Table 3
Relative number and size of lysosomes and autophagic vacuoles in hepatocytes of meal-fed rats just before (6 pm) and after (9 pm) eating a meal

	6 pm	9 pm
Lysosomes/1000 square Å		
Number	8.17 ± 0.92	5.81 ± 0.68
Total volume %	0.885 ± 0.081	0.493 ± 0.94
Area/lysosome %	0.104 ± 0.002	0.084 ± 0.004
Autophagic vacuoles/1000 square Å		
Number	2.016 ± 0.25	0.046 ± 0.001
Volume %	0.514 ± 0.042	0.001

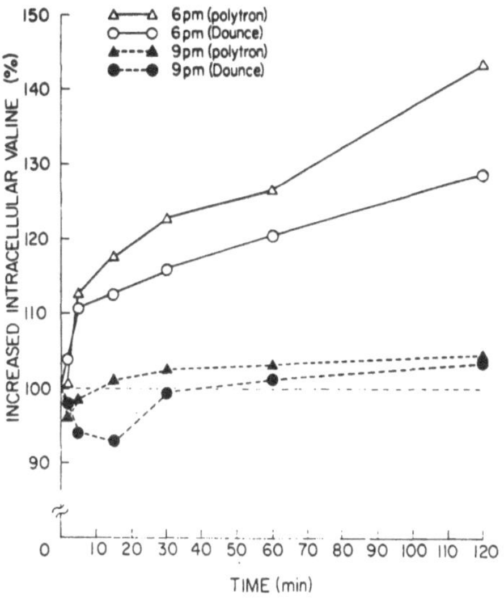

Fig. 4

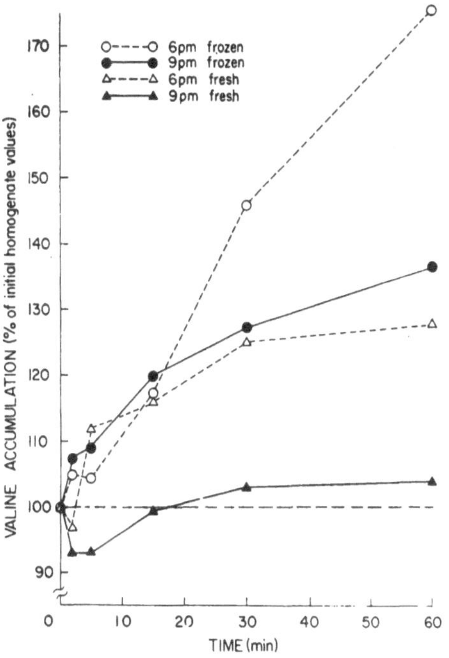

Fig. 5

Fig. 4 and 5. Comparisons of the accumulation of intracellular valine in liver of meal-fed rats just before (6 pm) and after (9 pm) the ingestion of a meal. Fig. 4 compares the effect of homogenization in a Dounce as compared to a Polytron PT-10. Details are provided in the text

decreased by about 25% directly following the meal [3]. Thus even though the decreased number of lysosomes may not actually prove to be significant, it is nevertheless true that their size does decrease significantly and very few autophagic vacuoles are discernable following the meal.

The dramatic decline in the calculated rate of degradation on feeding correlated with the valine concentration in liver homogenates (Figs. 4 and 5) where it could be shown that homogenates obtained from the 9 pm rats indicated only about 5—7% increase in the accumulation of valine, while the pool size from 6 pm rats increased 50% above basal levels. It should be pointed out that a significant 12—15% increase in the intracellular valine pool occurred within 5 min following homogenization of livers from the starved rats, but actually decreased for about 10—15 min in post-absorptive livers. In data not shown here we could also demonstrate that over 90% of the increase after 15 min of incubation of the 6 pm rats arose from an enriched "lysosomal" fraction.

On incubating homogenates in the presence of [^{3}H]acetyl-hemoglobin as an exogenous substrate for catheptic activity, it was noted that even in the presence of 0.2% of Triton X-100 the "lysosomes" from the absorptive rats clearly showed a significantly greater latency as compared to the rats just before feeding (Fig. 6). Thus we can conclude that both the electron microscopic observations and these preliminary in vitro experiments tend to substantiate the rates of degradation calculated on the basis of the compartmental analysis of hepatic amino acids.

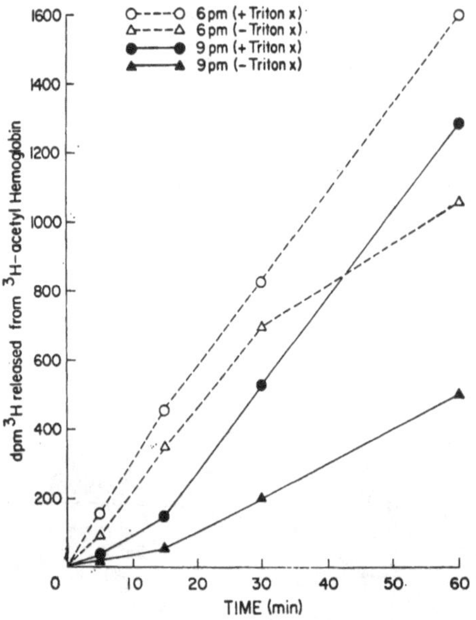

Fig. 6. The release of acid-soluble ^{3}H dpm from [^{3}H]-acetyl hemoglobin incubated with homogenates from livers of meal fed rats just before (6 pm) and after (9 pm) the ingestion of a meal. Triton-X-100 was used at final concentration of 0.2%

Two alternative interpretations of amino acid compartmentation within the cell have recently been proposed. We had reported [2] in agreement with previous observations of MORTIMORE et al. [18—21], the existence of a non-equilibrating lysosomal pool that seemed essential to explain kinetic data obtained in perfused livers. SEGLEN [22] has presented similar data for isolated hepatocytes. In both systems, however, the rates of degradation have been shown to be nearly double those of synthesis [2, 22]. Such a condition clearly cannot exist in vivo where the liver must maintain positive amino acid balance at least to account for the synthesis of secreted serum proteins. Indeed it may be suggested that the rate of protein degradation in vivo may be dependent upon the capacity of lysosomes to release amino acids into the intracellular pool at a rate rapid enough to maintain adequate levels of amino acids for on-going protein synthesis. The loss of this control linking the rate of protein degradation to the rate of protein synthesis may result in the apparent build-up of intralysosomal amino acids seen in perfused livers and hepatocytes. Despite the fact that an intralysosomal amino acid pool has been reported [23], we feel that the evidence that such a pool actually exists in vivo is still an open question.

By contrast several investigators have presented evidence that the tRNA itself may be compartmentalized so that some tRNA species can charge from the general cell pool whereas others charge from some membrane associated compartment [24—26]. Our data to date are compatible with such compartmentation but we feel that both alternative suggestions would have less predictive value than the model proposed above.

We would like to acknowledge with thanks Dr. S. REICHLIN of the New England Medical Center for assistance in the performance of the insulin and glucagon assays and Dr. A. WACHTEL for assistance in interpreting the electron micrographs. This work was supported by grants from the National Institute of Health (AM 15919) and the University of Connecticut Research Foundation.

References

[1] AIRHART, J., A. VIDRICH, and E. A. KHAIRALLAH: Biochem. J. **140**, 539–545 (1974)
[2] KHAIRALLAH, E. A., and G. E. MORTIMORE: J. biol. Chem. **251**, 1375–1384 (1976)
[3] VIDRICH, A., J. AIRHART, M. K. BRUNO, and E. A. KHAIRALLAH: Biochem. J. **162**, 257–266 (1977)
[4] PHILIPPENS, M. H., H. MAYERSBACK, and L. E. SCHEVING: J. Nutr. **107**, 126–139 (1977)
[5] ROSE, P., and E. A. KHAIRALLAH: Unpublished observations
[6] SWICK, R., W., and M. M. IP: J. biol. Chem. **231**, 751–764 (1974)
[7] GARLICK, P. J., J. C. WATERLOO, and R. W. SWICK: Biochem. J. **156**, 657–663 (1976)
[8] MORTIMORE, G. E., K. H. WOODSIDE, and J. E. HENRY: J. biol. Chem. **247**, 5458–5463 (1972)
[9] AIRHART, J., and E. A. KHAIRALLAH: Manuscript in preparation
[10] WALLYN, C. S., A. VIDRKCH, J. AIRHART, and E. A. KHAIRALLAH: Biochem. J. **140**, 545–548 (1974)
[11] HALES, C. N., and J. P. RANDLE: Biochem. J. **88**, 137–146 (1963)
[12] FALOONA, G. R., and R. H. UNGER in: Methods of Hormone Radio-Immunoassay. B. M. JAFFE and H. R. BEHRMAN (Eds.). Academic Press, New York 1974, p. 317–330
[13] HAYAT, M. A.: Electron Microscopy of Enzymes: Principles and Methods. I. Van Nostrand-Reinhold Co., New York 1973
[14] HILLE, M. B., A. J. BARRETT, J. T. DINGLE, and H. B. FELL: Expl Cell Res. **61**, 470 to 473 (1970)
[15] GAN, J. C., and H. JEFFAY: Biochim. biophys. Acta **242**, 125–135 (1971)
[16] GARLICK, P. J., D. J. MILWARD, and P. T. JAMES: Biochem. J. **136**, 935–945 (1973)
[17] OBLED, C., M. ARNAL, and G. FAUCONNEAU: Annls Biol. anim. Biochim. Biophys. **15**, 73–93 (1975)
[18] MORTIMORE, G. E., and C. E. MONDON: J. biol. Chem. **245**, 2375–2382 (1970)
[19] WOODSIDE, K. H., and G. E. MORTIMORE: J. biol. Chem. **247**, 6474–6478 (1972)
[20] NEELY, A., and G. E. MORTIMORE: Biochem. biophys. Res. Commun. **59**, 680–687 (1974)
[21] MORTIMORE, G. E. in: Lysosomes in Biology and Pathology. Vol. **5**, 157–184. J. T. DINGLE and R. T. DEAN (Eds.). North Holland, Amsterdam 1976
[22] SEGLEN, P. O.: Biochem. biophys. Acta **442**, 391–404 (1976)
[23] TAPPEL, A. L., S. SHIBKO, M. STEEN, and J. P. SUSZ: J. Food Sci. **30**, 498–504 (1965)
[24] FERN, E. D., and P. J. GARLICK: Biochem. J. **156**, 189–192 (1976)
[25] ILAN, J., and M. SINGER: J. molec. Biol. **91**, 39–51 (1975)
[26] HOD, Y., and A. HERSHKO: J. biol. Chem. **251**, 4458–4467 (1976)

Acta biol. med. germ., Band 36, Seite 1747—1752 (1977)

Institute for Experimental Gerontology TNO, Rijswijk, The Netherlands

The role of lysosomal enzymes in protein degradation in different types of rat liver cells

D. L. Knook

Summary

Highly purified suspensions of parenchymal, endothelial and Kupffer cells were prepared from the rat liver. The respective roles of these cell classes in the degradation of proteins was investigated by analysing the cellular distribution of two lysomal proteases. The specific arginine naphthylamidase activity was 2 times higher in Kupffer cells compared with the nearly equal activities in endothelial and parenchymal cells. The specific activity of the important endopeptidase cathepsin D in endothelial and Kupffer cells was about 12 and 36 times higher, respectively, than the activity in parenchymal cells. These results are in agreement with an important role of Kupfter and endothelial cells in the degradation of proteins and protein containing material of exogenous origin.

Introduction

The mammalian liver consists primarily of two main cell classes: parenchymal cells or hepatocytes and sinusoidal lining cells. In the liver of the rat of 3 months of age, parenchymal cells constitute about 55—65% of the total number of liver cells and about 85% of the total liver volume. At this age, one third of all liver cells are sinusoidal cells, but they occupy only about 3% of the total liver volume [1]. The most important constituents of the group of sinusoidal lining cells are Kupffer and endothelial cells. Although the sinusoidal cells have often been generally referred to as Kupffer cells, endothelial cells probably outnumber the Kupffer cells by a factor of two or three [2, 3].

Kupffer and endothelial cells play an important role in the clearance of foreign material from the circulation, although the two cell types differ in their mechanisms of endocytosis [4]. Exogenous proteins are generally endocytosed by the sinusoidal cells. However, if high concentrations of proteins are encountered, some of them will escape uptake by the sinusoidal cells and enter the parenchymal cells of the liver or cells in other organs [5]. After endocytosis, the extracellular proteins will be degraded in the lysosomal system. This system may, at least in liver parenchymal cells, also play a role in the turnover of intracellular proteins [6].

The lysosomes in parenchymal and sinusoidal lining cells differ in many respects. Histochemical investigations reveal relative differences in quality and quantity, the lysosomes in Kupffer cells being larger and more densily stained than the lysosomes in parenchymal cells. During the last five years, methods have been developed for the isolation of different types of liver cells based on perfusion and incubation of the liver with various enzymes. As a consequence, data have been presented on the distribution of a number of lysosomal enzymes over parenchymal and sinusoidal cells of the rat liver. The important lysosomal protease cathepsin D appeared to be present in higher concentrations in sinusoidal lining cells than in parenchymal cells [7—9]. In view of the data mentioned above, it is clear that differences may exist in the mechanism of protein breakdown in parenchymal, Kupffer and endothelial liver cells. An investigation of the cellular distribution of cathepsin D and arginine naphthylamidase, two lysosomal enzymes involved in protein degradation, may give an indication of the role of specific liver cell classes in the intracellular degradation of extracellular and intracellular proteins.

Materials and methods

Animals

Inbred female BN/BiRij rats of 3 months of age and weighing 140—170 g were used.

Preparation of liver cell suspensions

Parenchymal cells were isolated by perfusion and incubation of the liver with the enzymes collagenase and hyaluronidase essentially as described previously [11]. The final cell suspension consisted entirely of parenchymal cells, which met several criteria for viability [12, 13].
The isolation of sinusoidal cells, the main constituents in nonparenchymal cell suspensions, was performed as described earlier by perfusion and incubation of the liver with a pronase E containing Gey's balanced salt solution [3, 9, 14].
The Kupffer and endothelial cells in the nonparenchymal cell suspension were further purified by centrifugal elutriation [3, 15].

Cell suspensions were finally obtained which had a purity of at least 90% for Kupffer cells and 95% for endothelial cells as judged from electron microscopic observations and from the peroxidatic activity of the cells [3, 16].

Assays

Lysosomal enzymes were determined in the parenchymal, sinusoidal, Kupffer and endothelial cell suspensions after incubation with 0.05% Triton X-100 for 20 min at 0 °C. The activity of cathepsin D at 37 °C and *p*H of 3.6 with bovine hemoglobin as substrate was determined fluorimetrically on the basis of the liberation of tryptophan [3]. The activity of arginine naphthylamidase (arginine aminopeptidase [17] or aminopeptidase B [18]) at 37 °C was assayed fluorimetrically with L-arginine-β-naphthylamide as substrate [18] in 0.01 M acetic acid with sodium hydroxide adjusted to *p*H 5.8. Protein was determined by the method of Lowry et al. [19] with bovine serum albumin as standard. Cell counts were performed with a hemocytometer.

Results

Cell yield and viability

Parenchymal, sinusoidal, Kupffer and endothelial cell suspensions were prepared from 3-month-old female rats. Yields of about 20—40 $\times$ 10^6 parenchymal cells, $30 \cdot 10^6$ endothelial cells and $8 \cdot 10^6$ Kupffer cells per g liver were obtained (Table 1). The yield of the parenchymal cells corresponds to a recovery of about 20—40% based on the presence of $114 \cdot 10^6$ parenchymal cells per g liver in a 3-month-old rat [20]. According to previous calculations [3], about $42 \cdot 10^6$ endothelial and $12 \cdot 10^6$ Kupffer cells are present per g liver. Thus, the yield of purified endothelial and Kupffer cells corresponds to a recovery of about 70% and 50%, respectively. In this respect, it should be mentioned that a loss up to about 30% of the number of Kupffer cells present in the sinusoidal cell suspensions may occur during the purification procedure. The integrity of the parenchymal, endothelial and Kupffer cells was determined by trypan blue exclusion and electron microscopy. The dye was excluded by at least 90% of the cells in all cell preparations (Table 1). The electron migrographs also showed structurally intact cells [12—15].

Distribution of cathepsin D and arginine naphthylamidase activities

The activities of cathepsin D and arginine naphthylamidase in parenchymal, sinusoidal, endothelial and Kupffer cell suspensions are presented in Tables 1 and 2. (The activities are expressed per mg of protein and per million cells.) A characteristic pattern of distribution can be observed for the cathepsin D activities in parenchymal, endothelial and Kupffer cells. By far, the highest specific activity of cathepsin D was found for Kupffer cells; these were followed by endothelial cells, while parenchymal cells showed a much lower cathepsin D activity per mg of protein. In relative values, the specific cathepsin D activity in Kupffer cells is about 3 times higher than that in endothelial cells and about 35 times higher than the activity in parenchymal cells. Expressed per million cells, the activity of cathepsin D is higher in Kupffer cells and lower in endothelial cells as compared with the activity in parenchymal cells. These results can be explained on the basis of the much higher protein content of about 120 μg per 10^6 cells for purified Kupffer cells compared with about 40 μg per 10^6 cells for endothelial cells [3].
The high specific cathepsin D activity in Kupffer and endothelial cells might be partly a result of the endocytosis of some of the proteolytic enzymes constituting

Table 1
Some characteristics of parenchymal, sinusoidal, endothelial and Kupffer cell suspensions obtained from the livers of 3-month-old female BN/BiRij rats

Cell suspension	Parenchymal cells	Sinusoidal cells	Endothelial cells	Kupffer cells
Yield (cells/g liver)[1]	$20-40 \cdot 10^6$	$38 \cdot 10^6$	$28 \cdot 10^6$	$8 \cdot 10^6$
Purity	99%	—	95%	91%
Viability[3]	90%	97%	95%	90%
Protein content (10^6 cells)	1.3 mg	63 μg	42 μg	119 μg

[1] Average yield; the variation in the yield of parenchymal cells is caused by and depends on the procedures used for the cell isolation [13]
[2] Mixture of mainly endothelial cells ($28 \cdot 10^6$ cells) and Kupffer cells ($9 \cdot 10^6$ cells)
[3] Percentages based on numbers of cells excluding trypan blue

Table 2
Activity of cathepsin D in parenchymal, sinusoidal, endothelial and Kupffer cells isolated from the rat liver

Cell suspension	Cathepsin D act. (nmoles tryptophan) nmoles/min/mg/protein	nmoles/min/10^6 cells
Parenchymal cells	0.52 ± 0.03 (4)	0.66 ± 0.04 (4)
Sinusoidal lining cells	8.44 ± 0.84 (13)	0.51 ± 0.07 (13)
Endothelial cells	6.12 ± 1.22 (3)	0.25 ± 0.05 (3)
Kupffer cells	17.97 ± 2.87 (3)	2.11 ± 0.26 (3)

The values represent the mean ± S.E., with the number of different cell preparations used for the enzyme assay in parentheses.

Table 3
Activity of arginine naphthylamidase in parenchymal, sinusoidal, endothelial and Kupffer cells isolated from the rat liver

Cell suspension	Arginine naphthylamidase act. (nmoles β-naphthylamine)	
	nmoles/min/mg protein	nmoles/min/10^6 cells
Parenchymal cells	7.67 ± 0.95 (4)	9.86 ± 1.32 (4)
Sinusoidal lining cells	10.57 ± 0.96 (3)	0.80 ± 0.04 (3)
Endothelial cells	9.34 ± 1.72 (3)	0.41 ± 0.03 (3)
Kupffer cells	14.60 ± 2.46 (3)	1.67 ± 0.17 (3)

The values represent the mean ± S.E., with the number of different cell preparations used for the enzyme assay in parentheses

the enzyme combination pronase E by these cells. For the following reasons, this possible interference with the determination of the cathepsin D activity could be excluded. The specific cathepsin D activity in Kupffer and endothelial cells was inhibited by 90% and 75%, respectively, when the cathepsin D inhibitor pepstatin was added in a concentration of $1.2 \cdot 10^{-6}$ M [15]. In this concentration, pepstatin did not inhibit hydrolysis of the cathepsin D substrate bovine hemoglobin by the 0.25% pronase E solution used in the preparation of the Kupffer and endothelial cells [21].

Compared with the cathepsin D activity, a less pronounced distribution pattern is observed for the arginine napthylamidase activity (Table 3). Nearly equal specific activities are found in the parenchymal and endothelial cells, whereas the specific activity in Kupffer cells is about two times higher.

Discussion

In studies on protein degradation and turnover, the whole liver has been very often used as a source for tissue extracts and subcellular fractions, including lysosomal preparations or preparations of lysosomal enzymes. These experimental approaches have undoubtedly been based on the assumption that the great majority, if not all, of the liver cells are parenchymal cells. This assumption seems indeed reasonable in view of the fact that the chief nonparenchymal cells, the sinusoidal lining cells, occupy only about 5% of the total cellular volume of the liver [22]. However, the distribution of the lysosomal structures over the predominant types of liver cells shows a completely different picture: only 57—62% of the total lysosomal volume of the liver is found in parenchymal cells; Kupffer cells combined with endothelial cells contribute 37—42% of the volumes of lysosomes in the liver [22]. Since the activities of cathepsin D and arginine naphthylamidase are higher in sinusoidal cells, the importance of proteolytic enzyme activities in sinusoidal cells may be even greater than would be expected from the volumetric contribution of sinusoidal cell lysosomes.

Detailed information concerning the protein breakdown in different types of sinusoidal liver cells has been lacking up to now. Several studies suggest an important participation of sinusoidal cells in the clearance and digestion of particles, such as injected liposomes [23], and protein as modified serum albumin [24].

More information concerning the processes of protein degradation and turnover in Kupffer and endothelial cells can be obtained by using sinusoidal cell suspensions or purified Kupffer and endothelial cells. It has been demonstrated that no changes in the breakdown of high density lipoproteins and low density lipoproteins result from the procedures used for the isolation of parenchymal and sinusoidal cells [25]. An artificially induced increase in the measured proteolytic enzymes in sinusoidal cells as a consequence of the isolation procedure could also be largely excluded [15].
The pattern of proteolytic enzymes in parenchymal, Kupffer and endothelial cells will reflect the types of substrates that are presented to the lysosomes as a consequence of autophagy or heterophagy. The very high specific activity of cathepsin D in Kupffer cells is in agreement with one of the most important functions of these cells, viz. the endocytosis of foreign components including proteins, protein containing microorganisms and particles in large quantities from the blood. Kupffer cells also react to the presence of protein containing material of endogenous origin which has been altered, e. g., senescent erythrocytes. The high cathepsin D activity in Kupffer cells is in agreement with the opinion of some authors [26, 27], who attribute to this enzyme a predominating role in the degradation of foreign proteins.
While the function of arginine naphthylamidase cannot be defined precisely at present, the less pronounced differences in the specific activity of arginine naphthylamidase in the three types of liver cells investigated may suggest no particular role of this enzyme with respect to a specific function of one of these cell types. In this respect, a more general function of this enzyme seems plausible.
No data have been reported on proteolytic enzyme activities in endothelial cells. The results obtained so far demonstrate that these cells contain the same combination of proteolytic enzymes in their lysosomes as do Kupffer cells, although generally in lower quantities. The question may arise as to whether the lower concentration of enzymes in endothelial cells is still higher than is necessary to fulfil the requirements for autophagy in their intracellular environment. A comparison of the specific cathepsin D activity in parenchymal cells which are supposed to contain enzyme activities just sufficient to fulfil the requirements for their intracellular catabolism with the cathepsin D activity in endothelial cells shows that the latter activity is about 12 times higher. This strongly suggests that lysosomes in endothelial cells may carry out an important function in heterophagy by endocytosis of extracellular proteins.

Acknowledgements

The excellent technical contributions of Elisabeth Ch. Sleyster and Florence G. Westerhuis are gratefully acknowledged.

References

[1] Greengard, O., M. Federman, and W. E. Knox: J. Cell Biol. 52, 261 (1972)
[2] Fahimi, H. D.: J. Cell Biol. 47, 247 (1970)
[3] Knook, D. L., and E. Ch. Sleyster: Expl Cell Res. 99, 444 (1976)
[4] Wisse, E.: J. Ultrastr. Res. 38, 528 (1972)
[5] Gordon, A. H. in: Lysosomes in Biology and Pathology. J. T. Dingle (Ed.) 3, 89. North-Holland Publishing Company, Amsterdam and London 1973
[6] Seglen, P. O., and A. Reith: Expl Cell Res. 100, 276 (1976)

[7] ARBORGH, B., H. GLAUMANN, T. BERG, and J. L. E. ERICSSON: Expl Cell Res. **88**, 279 (1974)
[8] KNOOK, D. L.: Hoppe-Seyler's Z. physiol. Chem. **355**, 1217 (1974)
[9] KNOOK, D. L., E. CH. SLEYSTER, and M. J. VAN NOORD in: Cell Impairment in Aging and Development. V. J. CHRISTOFALO and E. HOLECKOVA (Eds.). Plenum Publishing Corporation, New York 1975, p. 155
[10] VAN BERKEL, T. J. C., J. K. KRUYT, and J. F. KOSTER: Eur. J. Biochem. **58**, 145 (1975)
[11] VAN BEZOOIJEN, C. F. A., T. GRELL, and D. L. KNOOK: Biochem. biophys. Res. Commun. **69**, 354 (1976)
[12] VAN BEZOOIJEN, C. F. A., M. J. VAN NOORD, and D. L. KNOOK: Mech. Age Dev. **3**, 107 (1974)
[13] VAN BEZOOIJEN, C. F. A., T. GRELL, and D. L. KNOOK: Mech. Age Dev. **6**, 293 (1977)
[14] KNOOK, D. L., and E. CH. SLEYSTER: Mech. Age Dev. **5**, 389 (1976)
[15] KNOOK, D. L., and E. CH. SLEYSTER: Expl Cell Res. **109**, 317 (1977)
[16] WISSE, E., F. ROELS, D. DE PREST, J. VAN DER MEULEN, J. J. EMEIS, and W. T. DAEMS in: Electron Microscopy and Cytochemistry. E. WISSE, W. T. DAEMS, I. MOLENAAR, and P. VAN DUYN (Eds.). North-Holland Publishing Company, Amsterdam 1974, p. 119
[17] MÄKINEN, K. K. in: 1st International Symposium on Intracellular Protein Catabolism, Reinhardsbrunn 1973. H. HANSON and P. BOHLEY (Eds.). Barth, Leipzig 1974/76, p. 450
[18] HOPSU, V. K., K. K. MÄKINEN, and G. G. GLENNER: Archs Biochem. Biophys. **114**, 557 (1966)
[19] LOWRY, O. H., N. J. ROSEBROUGH, A. L. FARR, and R. J. RANDALL: J. biol. Chem. **233**, 184 (1958)
[20] SEGLEN, P. O.: Expl Cell Res. **82**, 391 (1973)
[21] BUYS, C. H. C. M.: Uptake and Degradation of Circulating Proteins by the Liver. Ph. D. Thesis, Groningen 1976, p. 66
[22] BLOUIN, A., R. P. BOLENDER, and E. R WEIBEL: J. Cell Biol. **72**, 441 (1977)
[23] WISSE, E. J. J. EMEIS, and W. TH. DAEMS in: Enzyme Therapy in Lysosomal Storage Diseases. J. M. TAGER, G. J. M. HOOGHWINKEL and W. TH. DAEMS (Eds.). North-Holland Publishing Company, Amsterdam 1974, p. 95
[24] BUYS, C. H. C. M., A. S. H. DE JONG, J. M. W. BOUMA, and M. GRUBER: Biochim. biophys. Acta **392**, 95 (1975)
[25] VAN BERKEL, T. J. C., J. F. KOSTER, and W. C. HÜLSMANN: Biochim. biophys. Acta **486**, 586 (1977)
[26] HUISMAN, W., L. LANTING, H. J. DODDEMA, J. M. W. BOUMA, and M. GRUBER: Biochim. biophys. Acta **370**, 297 (1974)
[27] WIEDERANDERS, B., S. ANSORGE, P. BOHLEY, U. BROGHAMMER, and L. LANGNER: Acta biol. med. germ. **35**, 269 (1976)

Acta. biol. med. germ., Band 36, Seite 1753—1762 (1977)

Institute for Nutrition Research, School of Medicine, University of Oslo, Blindern, Oslo 3, Norway

Uptake and degradation of asialo-fetuin by isolated rat hepatocytes

H. Tolleshaug and T. Berg

Summary

^{125}I-labelled asialo-fetuin was taken up by isolated rat hepatocytes by a saturable process. Half maximum uptake was seen at about $3 \cdot 10^{-8}$ M asialo-fetuin. Rate of uptake of asialo-fetuin exceeded rate of degradation at all concentrations of asialo-fetuin tested. Degradation of asialo-fetuin, as indicated by release of acid-soluble radioactivity from the cells, was inhibited by NH_4Cl and chloroquine. The intracellular distribution of labelled asialo-fetuin was studied by differential and density gradient centrifuging. The distribution curves for radioactivity indicated that asialo-fetuin was present in lysosomes about 1 h after the uptake had started. Chloroquine and ammonium ions seemed to inhibit the uptake of asialo-fetuin into the lysosomes, possibly by interfering with the fusion between phagosomes and lysosomes.

Introduction

Studies on rat liver have suggested that the lysosomes in this organ are involved in the catabolism of intracellular proteins as well as proteins brought into the cells by endocytosis.

The liver consists of hepatocytes as well as nonparenchymal cells (e. g. macrophages) and this cellular heterogeneity may make it difficult to evaluate the precise role of the lysosomes in hepatic metabolism. Most studies on hepatic protein turnover have been focussed on the hepatocytes, which contain at least 95% of the liver protein [1]. The nonparenchymal liver cells, on the other hand, contain numerous lysosomes. As much as 25% of some of the hepatic lysosomal enzyme activities may be present in these cells [1].

The study of the role of hepatic lysosomes in protein degradation involves — among other things — the use of inhibitors of lysosomal function (chloroquine, protease inhibitors), subcellular fractionation and the introduction into the lysosomes of proteins by way of heterophagy. Studies on whole liver do not differentiate between effects on parenchymal and nonparenchymal cells. The method of collagenase perfusion [2, 3] has, however, opened the possibility of studying the separate roles of the different types of liver cells in protein catabolism under controlled conditions in vitro.

We have tried to study the lysosomal degradation of proteins taken into liver cells by endocytosis. We have previously shown that denatured albumin is taken up mainly by nonparenchymal liver cells in vitro [4]. The present report concerns studies on the uptake, the intracellular distribution and the catabolism of desialylated fetuin (asialo-fetuin). In vivo studies have revealed that fetuin and several other glycoproteins are removed selectively by parenchymal liver cells if galactose units are exposed in the carbohydrate moiety following the removal of terminal sialic acid residues [5, 6]. The high degree of specificity and affinity involved in the binding of asialo-proteins to hepatocytes suggests the use of such proteins for the study of intralysosomal proteolysis in liver parenchymal cells.

Materials and methods

Chemicals

Collagenase (type I), bovine serum albumin, lactoperoxidase, fetuin (type I) and chloroquine were from Sigma. Bovine serum albumin (fraction V) was purified by charcoal treatment [7]. Fetuin was EDTA treated [8] and desialylated by mild acid hydrolysis [8]. ^{125}I-labelled asiolo-fetuin was prepared by the enzymatic technique described by FRANTZ and TURKINGTON [9], using 0.5 mCi Na^{125}I, 1 mg of fetuin and 10 μg of lactoperoxidase in a total volume of 0.5 ml. The reaction mixture was passed through a Sephadex G-50 column, and the fractions containing labelled fetuin collected. The specific activity of the labelled asialo-fetuin was about $26 \cdot 10^6$ cpm/nmole.

Incubation medium

This consisted of 8.00 g NaCl, 0.4 g KCl, 0.06 g $Na_2HPO_4 \cdot 2H_2O$, 0.06 g $KH_2PO_4 \cdot 2H_2O$, 0.2 g $MgSO_4 \cdot 7H_2O$, 0.4 g $CaCl_2 \cdot 2H_2O$, 4.76 g Hepes, 10 g bovine serum albumin and water to 1000 ml. *p*H was adjusted to 7.5 by adding NaOH.

Preparation of purified liver cells

Isolated rat liver cells were prepared from male Wistar rats, 200—250 g, by a modification [10] of the collagenase perfusion method described by BERRY and FRIEND [2]. Purified hepatocytes and nonparenchymal liver cells were prepared by low speed centrifugations from the initial mixed cell suspension [4, 11, 12].

Cell incubations

For the study of asialo-fetuin uptake and degradation by liver cells in vitro, the cells were suspended in incubation medium (5 ml) and incubated in 50 ml Erlenmeyer flasks in a shaking water bath at 37 °C. The cell concentration was $5-10 \cdot 10^6$ cells/ml. To assess cellular uptake and degradation of ^{125}I-asialo-fetuin the cells were separated from the medium by centrifuging through oil [4, 11, 12]. The resulting cell pellets and samples of the medium (above the oil layer) were treated with 2% phosphotungstic acid [8], and acid soluble and acid precipitable radioactivities were determined in a Packard auto gamma spectrometer.

Subcellular fractionation of hepatocytes

Hepatocytes ($25 \cdot 10^6$ cells/ml) were suspended in ice-cold 0.25 M sucrose and homogenized in a Dounce homogenizer with a tight-fitting pestle. Fractionation by differential centrifugation was done according to DE DUVE et al. [13] in a Sorvall centrifuge equipped with a SS-24 rotor. Density gradient centrifugation was performed with linear sucrose gradients with densities ranging from 1.07 to 1.25. 6 ml of postnuclear fractions (about 20 mg protein/ml) were layered on top of the gradients and the tubes (containing 34 ml) were centrifuged with the swinging-bucket SW-27 rotor in a Beckman preparative ultracentrifuge for 4 hrs at 25,000 r.p.m. The gradients were fractionated into 2 ml fractions.

Biochemical determinations

Protein was determined according to LOWRY et al. [14]. *β*-Acetylglucosaminidase was assayed as described by BARRETT [15].

Results

Uptake of asialo-fetuin by isolated liver cells

When purified hepatocytes and nonparenchymal liver cells were incubated with asialo-fetuin in concentrations ranging from 1 nM to 1 μM only hepatocytes were found to take up significant amounts of the labelled protein. The rate of uptake of asialo-fetuin in hepatocytes was close to constant for at least 5 min at these concentrations, and it was therefore possible to obtain information about the effect of increasing concentrations of asialo-fetuin on its initial rate of uptake in hepatocytes. Fig. 1 shows that asialo-fetuin was taken up by a process which reached saturation at an asialo-fetuin concentration of about 100 nM. Half maximum uptake was seen at about $3 \cdot 10^{-8}$ M.

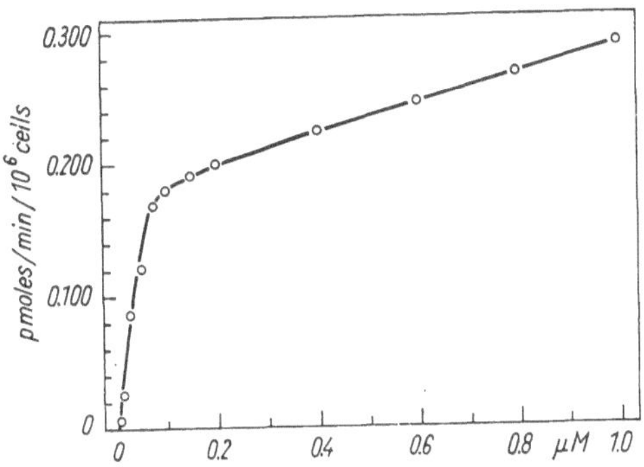

Fig. 1. The effect of increasing concentrations of asialo-fetuin on the initial rate of uptake (pmoles/min/10^6 cells) of asialo-fetuin in rat hepatocytes.

Hepatocytes ($6 \cdot 10^6$ cells/ml) were incubated in presence of varying concentration of ^{125}I-labelled asialo-fetuin. Rate of uptake was determined during the initial phase, when uptake was nearly linear with time (see text)

Information about the specificity involved in asialo-fetuin uptake by rat hepatocytes was sought by adding cold native fetuin (420 nM) to cell suspensions incubated in presence of labelled asialo-fetuin (2 nM), and by measuring the uptake of labelled native fetuin and labelled fetuin which had been desialylated by treatment with neuraminidase. The results of these experiments showed that cold native fetuin had no effects on the uptake of labelled asialo-fetuin, and that insignificant amounts of labelled native fetuin were taken up. Neuraminidase-treated fetuin was, on the other hand, taken up as effectively as fetuin desialylated by mild acid hydrolysis. The rate of uptake of asialo-fetuin was reduced to 10% of control values when hepatocytes were treated for 10 min with neuraminidase (10 mU/ml) prior to the addition of asialo-fetuin.

Our data obtained on isolated rat hepatocytes indicate that asialo-fetuin is taken up by these cells by a process which involves binding sites with high affinity on the hepatocytes and that a prerequisite for this selective uptake is the exposure of galactose units in the carbohydrate moiety of fetuin as well as the presence of terminal sialic acid residues on the cell membrane.

Degradation of asialo-fetuin by rat hepatocytes

One hindrance in the study of degradation of asialo-fetuin in hepatocytes was the occurrence of extracellular proteolytic activity in some of the cell suspensions. We believe that this proteolysis was due to the collagenase-perfusion since extracellular degradation of asialo-fetuin was abolished when the liver was perfused with incubation medium (150 ml) after the collagenase-treatment and when, in addition, the cells were washed 5—7 times to get rid of remaining perfusion-fluid.

Fig. 2 shows typical data for the time-course for uptake and degradation of asialo-fetuin in thoroughly washed hepatocytes. The initial concentration of labelled protein was 35 nM in this particular experiment. Degradation of asialo-fetuin, measured as release of acid soluble radioactivity to the medium, started about

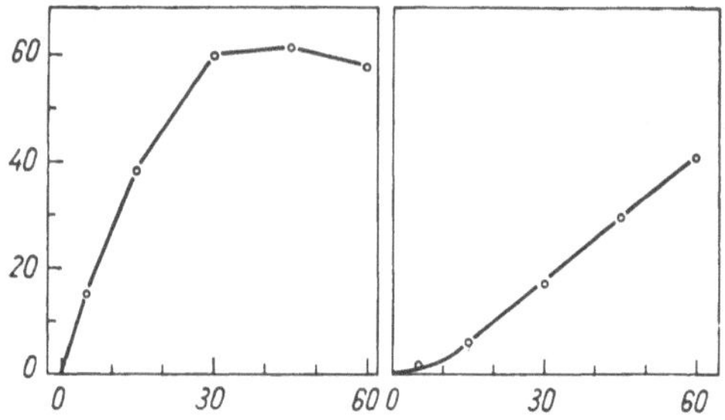

Fig. 2. Time course of uptake and degradation of ^{125}I-labelled asialo-fetuin in isolated rat hepatocytes.

Hepatocytes ($5 \cdot 10^6$ cells/ml) were incubated in presence of 35 nM labelled asialo-fetuin. Uptake was determined as total radioactivity associated with the cells, degradation as acid soluble radioactivity in the medium, and both parameters are presented as percentages of initial acid precipitable radioactivity. The abscissa shows incubation time in min. Uptake: left pannel, degradation: right pannel

15 min after the addition of labelled protein to the cells, and increased thereafter linearly with time for the following hour. Similar data for degradation were obtained at initial concentrations of asialo-fetuin varying between 1 nM and 1 μM. At all concentrations tested, the initial rate of uptake was higher than initial rate of degradation.

Intracellular distribution of asialo-fetuin

In order to follow the intracellular fate of labelled asialo-fetuin in isolated rat hepatocytes the cells were incubated with labelled protein (about 30 nM) for 10 min, then separated from the medium by centrifugations (50 × g for 1 min) and reincubated in fresh medium without asialo-fetuin. Aliquots of cells ($5 \cdot 10^7$) were removed from the incubator after various time intervals, washed free of medium and homogenized in cold 0.25 M sucrose. The homogenates were fractionated either by differential or density gradient centrifuging. Radioactivity and β-acetylglucosaminidase were measured in the subcellular fractions. During the incubation in asialo-fetuin-free medium samples of cell suspensions were also removed for the determination of acid-soluble and acid-precipitable radioactivity in cells and medium. Fig. 3 summarizes the results of these experiments:

During the incubation in asialo-fetuin-free medium about 25% of the initial cell-associated radioactivity was released to the medium in 60 min (Fig. 3A). More than 97% of the released radioactivity was acid-soluble and consisted almost exclusively of free $^{125}I^-$. Acid-soluble radioactivity increased linearly with time from the beginning of the incubation.

Fig. 3B shows the distribution of radioactivity in subcellular fractions prepared by differential centrifugation 0, 15, 30, 60 and 90 min after the start of the incubation in asialo-fetuin-free medium. The distribution of β-acetylglucosaminidase between the different fractions was relatively unaffected by the time of incubation and only data obtained on homogenates prepared after 90 min of incubation are included in Fig. 3B. Radioactivity was initially (10 min after the addition of asialo-fetuin to the cells) found mainly in the soluble and the microsomal fractions.

During incubation there was a relative increase in radioactivity in "heavier" fractions: the nuclear, the mitochondrial and the light mitochondrial fraction. The increase in the latter fraction was particularly evident, and this fraction showed the highest relative specific activity after 30 min of incubation. The distribution pattern was similar, but not identical, to that of β-acetylglucosaminidase after 90 min of incubation. The main difference between the two distribution patterns was that the enzyme activity was relatively more concentrated in the heavier fractions than the radioactivity.

Fig. 3C shows the distribution patterns of radioactivity, and β-acetylglucosaminidase in fractions prepared from sucrose-gradients. The distribution of the lysosomal marker enzyme was independent of the time of incubation of the cells, and only data obtained on homogenates prepared 2 hrs after the start of the incubation are given.

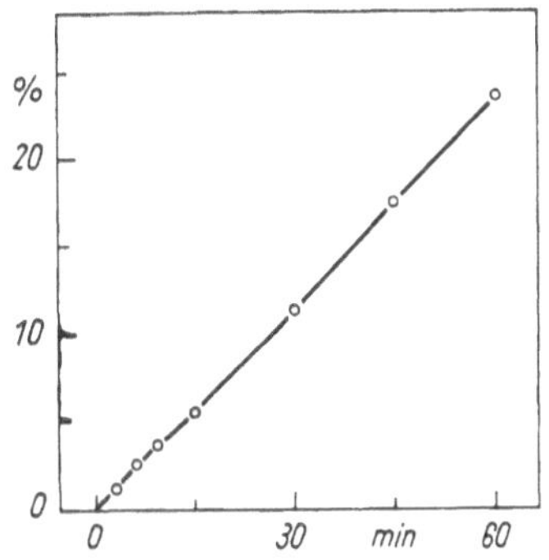

Fig. 3A

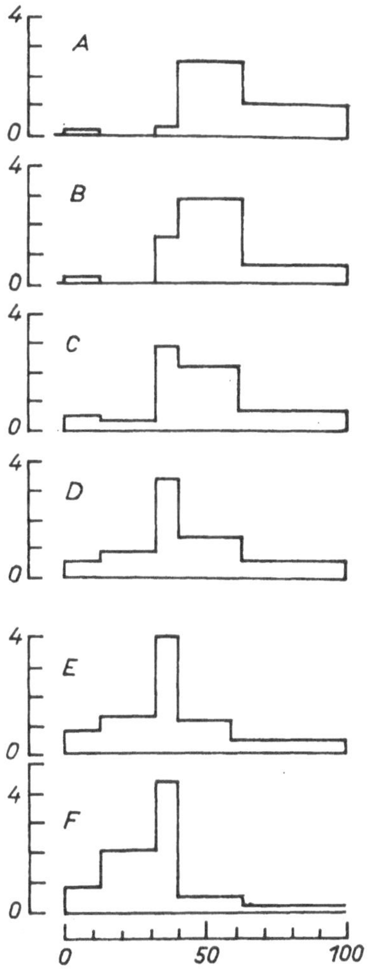

Fig. 3B

Fig. 3. A) Degradation of ^{125}I-labelled asialo-fetuin in hepatocytes which had been preincubated with 30 nM asialo-fetuin for 10 min. Degradation was followed by measuring acid-soluble radioactivity released from the cells during incubation in asialo-fetuin-free medium, and is presented as per cent of the initial cell-associated acid-precipitable radioactivtiy.

B) Intracellular distribution of radioactivity in cells that had been preincubated with 30 nM asialo-fetuin for 10 min. Aliquots of cells ($5 \cdot 10^7$ cells) were taken 0(A), 15(B), 30(C), 60(D) and 90(E, F) min after the start of the incubation in asialo-fetuin-free medium, homogenized and fractionated by differential centrifugation into (from left to right) a nuclear, a mitochondrial, a light mitochondrial, a microsomal and a soluble fraction. The abscissa represents relative protein content (cumulatively from left to right) in fractions as per cent of total recovered protein. The ordinates show relative specific activities (percentage of total recovered activity/percentage of total protein). The lower histogram (F) shows the distribution of the lysosomal marker enzyme β-acetylglucosaminidase after 90 min of incubation.

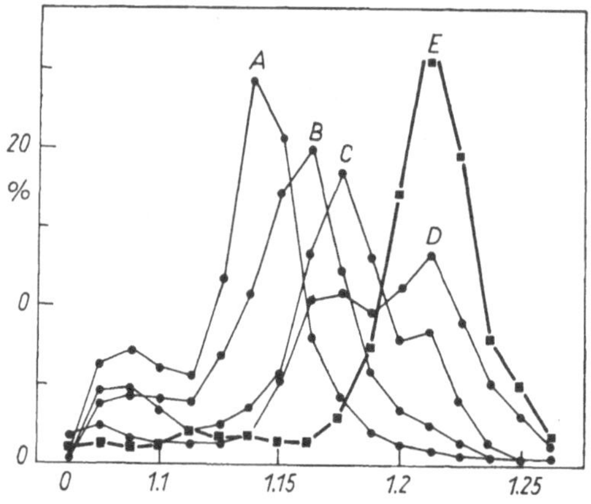

Fig. 3C

C) Distribution of radioactivity and of β-acetylglucosaminidase after centrifuging in sucrose gradients of postnuclear fractions prepared from cells which had been preincubated for 10 min with 30 nM asialo-fetuin and then reincubated in asialo-fetuin-free medium for 0(A), 30(B), 60(C) and 120(D) min. Subfractions are presented in the order of their position in the tube, from meniscus (left) to bottom (right). Measured average densities of the subfractions are given on the abscissa. The ordinate shows radioactivities or β-acetylglucosaminidase (E) in each subfraction as per cent of total recovered activity in the gradient. The curve "E" shows the distribution of β-acetylglucosaminidase after 120 min of incubation

The radioactivity was at the start of the incubation (10 min after the addition of asialo-fetuin to the cells) located mainly in the top fractions of the gradients. The distribution of radioactivity changed progressively to heavier fractions during the first 60 min of incubation in asialo-fetuin-free medium; the peak of the distribution curve after 60 min was at a density of 1.16. About 60 min after the start of the incubation a second peak of radioactivity became apparent in the distribution curve for radioactivity. This peak, which coincided with the distribution pattern of β-acetylglucosaminidase, became relatively larger with continued incubation at the same time as the other peak in the distribution curve for radioactivity decreased. The distribution curves showed, however, two marked peaks even after the cells had been incubated for 3 hrs.

Effects of inhibitors of lysosomal function on the heterophagy of asialo-fetuin

Ammonium ions [16, 17] and chloroquine [18] accumulate in lysosomes and reduce the lysosomal hydrolysis of macromolecules. The effects of these compounds on the uptake, the intracellular distribution and the degradation of asialo-fetuin in hepatocytes were examined in order to get additional information about the role of the lysosomes in the intracellular digestion of asialo-fetuin. Hepatocytes were incubated for 10 min in presence of 30 nM asialo-fetuin, then washed free of medium and reincubated in fresh medium containing chloroquine (0.1 mM) or NH_4Cl (10 mM) or no additions (control). At various time intervals after the start of the second incubation samples of the cell suspension were removed for the determination of acid-soluble and acid-precipitable radioactivity in cells and medium, and for preparing homogenates to be used for differential and density gradient centrifuging. Both ammonium ions and chloroquine reduced the release of acid soluble radioactivity from the cells markedly; after 60 min of incubation control cells had released about twice as much radioactivity as cells incubated with chloroquine or NH_4Cl (Fig. 4A).

Ammonium ions and chloroquine had small, but distinct effects on the distribution of the lysosomal marker enzyme β-acetylglucosaminidase in fractions prepared by differential centrifuging. Both compounds, and ammonium ions in particular, lead to an enrichment of β-acetylglucosaminidase in the microsomal fraction and a concurrent decrease in the enzyme activity in the mitochondrial fractions. The distribution of radioactivity in the subcellular fractions became progessively similar to that of the lysosomal marker with time of incubation in presence of both NH_4Cl and chloroquine. Fig. 4B shows the distribution patterns of radioactivity and β-acetylglucosaminidase in fractions from homogenates prepared after 90 min of incubation. It may be seen that the distribution of radioactivity and of β-acetylglucosaminidase are almost identical in the case of cells incubated in the presence of chloroquine.

Data obtained with sucrose gradient centrifuging showed, in accordance with earlier reports [18], that chloroquine caused a marked decrease in the density of

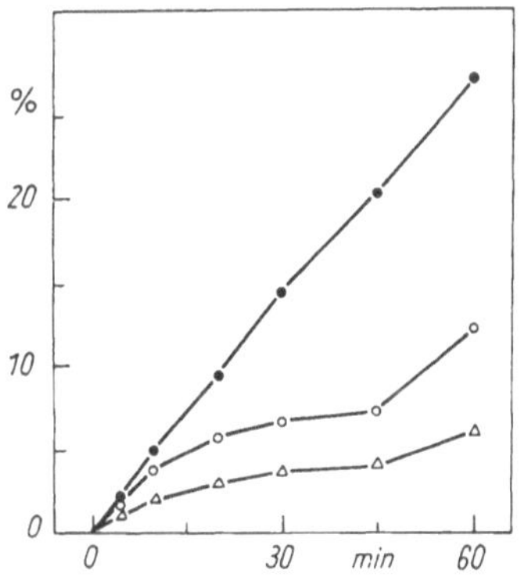

Fig. 4A

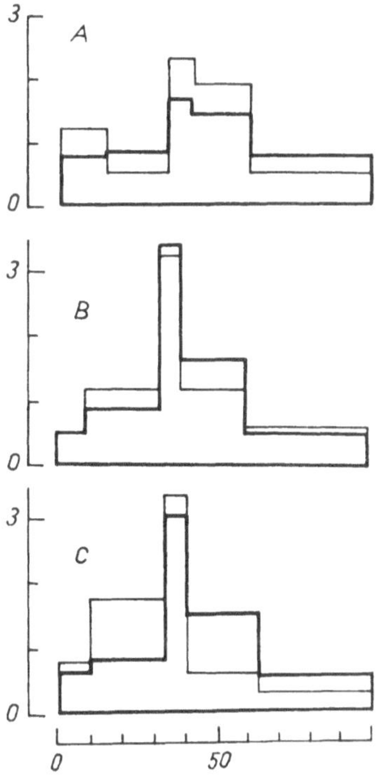

Fig. 4B

Fig. 4. A) The effects of ammonium ions and chloroquine on the degradation of ^{125}I-labelled asialo-fetuin in isolated rat hepatocytes. The cells were preincubated for 10 min with 30 nM asialo-fetuin, then separated from the medium by centrifugation and reincubated in asialo-fetuin-free medium in presence of chloroquine (0.1 mM), NH_4Cl (10 mM) or no addition. Degradation was determined as acid-soluble radioactivity released from the cells to the medium and is presented as per cent of cell-associated radioactivity in the beginning of the reincubation. Control: ●, chloroquine: △, NH_4Cl: ○.

B) Distribution patterns of radioactivity (heavy lines) and β-acetylglucosaminidase (thin lines) in subcellular fractions prepared by differential centrifugation of homogenates obtained from cells which had been incubated in presence of NH_4Cl (10 mM, A) or chloroquine (0.1 mM, B) for 90 min. Distribution patterns in control cells incubated for 90 min are shown in the lower histogram (C).

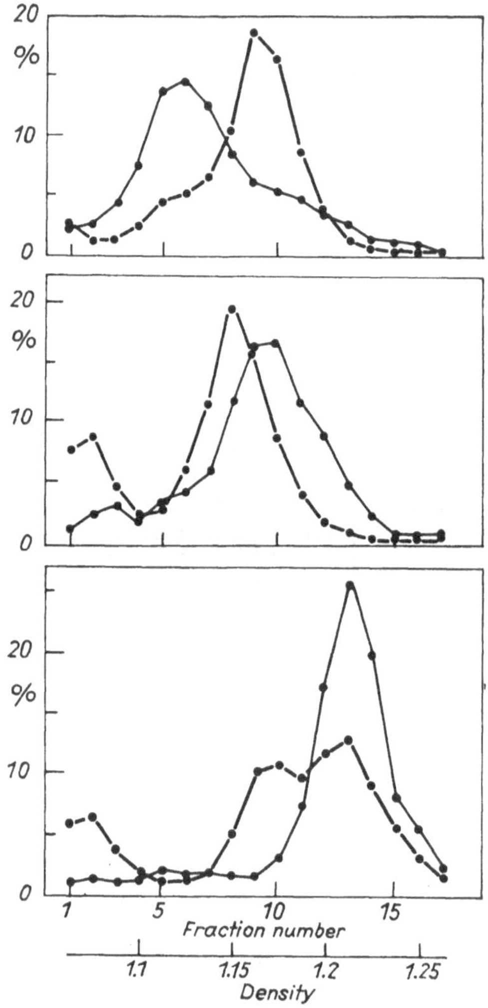

Fig. 4C

C) Density-distribution histograms of β-acetylglucosaminidase and radioactivity after centrifugation in sucrose-gradients of postnuclear fractions prepared from cells incubated for 2 hrs in presence of chloroquine (upper curves) or NH_4Cl (middle curves). Distribution patterns of enzyme and radioactivity in control cells incubated for 2 hrs are shown in the lower histogram. Thin lines: distribution of β-acetylglucosaminidase, heavy lines: distribution of radioactivity. Units on the ordinates are explained in legend to Fig. 3C. Abscissa: Fraction number (from top to bottom of the tubes) or density

lysosomes (as indicated by the distribution curve for β-acetylglucosaminidase). Fig. 4C indicates that the average density of lysosomes 2 hrs after the addition of chloroquine to the cells was about 1.13 as compared to 1.21 for control cells. The density distribution of radioactivity was similar in presence and absence of chloroquine for the first 60 min of incubation. In contrast to data obtained on control cells, however, did no second peak (coinciding with the distribution curve for β-acetylglucosaminidase) appear, even after 3 hrs of incubation. Data obtained with density gradient centrifuging of postnuclear fractions prepared from cells incubated in presence of ammonium ions were in principle similar to those seen with chloroquine treated cells. We may therefore draw the provisional conclusion that chloroquine and ammonium ions prevent the access of asialo-fetuin to the lysosomes.

Discussion

In vivo data have clearly indicated that desialylated glycoproteins are degraded in hepatic lysosomes following the selective endocytic uptake into liver parenchymal cells [6, 8]. That lysosomes are involved in the degradation of asialo-fetuin in isolated rat hepatocytes is likely for the following reasons: (1) There is a time lag between the addition of asialo-fetuin to the cells and the occurrence of extracellular acid-soluble radioactivity. This delay in the release of radioactivity could correspond to the time needed for extracellular asialo-fetuin to be transported by the endocytic route to the lysosomes. (2) Degradation was inhibited by ammonium ions and chloroquine. These compounds are probably selectively concentrated in the lysosomes [17, 18] and may inhibit degradation of asialo-fetuin either by rendering the intralysosomal milieu less favourable for proteolysis or by preventing uptake of asialo-fetuin into the lysosomes. (3) The distribution curve for radioactivity in sucrose gradients revealed a peak that coincided with the distribution curve for β-acetylglucosaminidase.

Although lysosomes are very likely to be involved in the degradation of asialo-fetuin, our present data do not exclude additional factors that may participate in asialo-fetuin-degradation. It is, for example, noticeable that degradation of asialo-fetuin, measured as increase in acid-soluble radioactivity, started at least 30 min before any radioactivity could be demonstrated in the lysosomes. The early degradation of asialo-fetuin may be due to extra-lysosomal proteases, located, for instance in the plasma membrane. Extracellular proteolytic activity is unlikely for reasons explained in the results section. Moreover, the early degradation was also evident in cells that had been preincubated with asialo-fetuin for 10 min and then incubated in asialo-fetuin-free medium. This, and the occurrence of a delay in the release of radioactivity from the cells, clearly indicate that asialo-fetuin degradation is cell-dependent. It could be argued that increased acid-soluble radioactivity may not necessarily be the result of proteolytic activity, but could reflect the action of a dehalogenating system — resulting in the release of free ^{125}iodide. It is difficult, however, to explain how asialo-fetuin could get access to a microsomal [8] dehalogenating system. It is more plausible that the direct source of free iodide is ^{125}I-tyrosine derived through asialo-fetuin-proteolysis. We have recently found that the release of acid-soluble radioactivity from cells incubated with ^{14}C-labelled methylated [19] asialo-fetuin follows a similar time-course as that seen for ^{125}I-labelled asialo-fetuin. This finding, too, indicates that the increase in acid-soluble radioactivity seen in cells incubated with ^{125}I-asialo-fetuin is the (indirect) result of proteolysis.

If asialo-fetuin is degraded solely in the lysosomes then the degradation in these organelles must be so efficient early after the uptake that no labelled protein can be detected (by subcellular fractionation studies) in the lysosome-rich fractions. That asialo-fetuin may reach the lysosomes early after the start of its uptake is indicated by the finding that both ammonium ions and chloroquine inhibited asialo-fetuin degradation very early after their addition to the cell suspensions (Fig. 4A). Due to their selective uptake by lysosomes, it is likely that their inhibitory effects on asialo-fetuin degradation were mediated directly or indirectly through the lysosomes.

Although both chloroquine and ammonium ions probably accumulated in the lysosomes (as indicated by the gradual decrease in the density of these organelles), we do not think that the inhibitory effect of these compounds on asialo-fetuin-degradation was due to reduced rate of hydrolysis of asialo-fetuin intralysosomally. The distribution curves for radioactivity and β-acetylglucosaminidase observed in our density gradient experiments indicated that chloroquine and NH_4Cl rather reduced the uptake of asialo-fetuin into the lysosomes. It is therefore likely that these compounds somehow changed the membranes involved in heterophagy in such a way that fusion between phagosomes and lysosomes was partially or completely prevented. The reduced degradation of asialo-fetuin in presence of chloroquine and ammonium ions could not be due to reduced rate of endocytosis. None of the compounds in the concentrations used affected the initial rate of uptake of asialo-fetuin by the hepatocytes. Moreover, the inhibitory effects on asialo-fetuin degradation could be observed in cells which had taken up asialo-fetuin prior to the treatment with ammonium ions or chloroquine.

Acknowledgements

This investigation was supported by the Norwegian Research Council for Science and the Humanities. The autors wish to express their thanks to Professor KAARE R. NORUM for reading the manuscript and for valuable discussions. The excellent assistance of TURID OSE and KARI HOLTE is gratefully acknowledged.

References

[1] MUNTHE-KAAS, A. C., T. BERG, and R. SELJELID: Expl Cell Res. **99**, 146 (1976)
[2] BERRY, M. N., and D. S. FRIEND: J. Cell Biol **43**, 506 (1969)
[3] SEGLEN, P. O.: Meth. Cell Biol. **13**, 29 (1976)
[4] NILSSON, M., and T. BERG: Biochim. biophys. Acta **497**, 171 (1977)
[5] ASHWELL, G., and A. G. MORELL: Adv. Enzymol. Relat. Areas Mol. Biol. **41**, 99 (1974)
[6] GREGORIADIS, G. in: Lysosomes in Biology and Pathology. J. T. DINDLE and R. T. DEAN (Eds). **4**, 265. North-Holland Publ. Co., Amsterdam 1975
[7] CHEN, R. F.: J. biol. Chem. **242**, 173 (1967)
[8] LA BADIE, J. H., K. P. CHAPMAN, and N. N. ARONSON: Biochem. J. **152**, 271 (1975)
[9] FRANTZ, W. L., and R. W. TURKINGTON: Endocrinology **91**, 1545 (1972)
[10] BERG, T., and J. G. IVERSEN: Acta physiol. scand. **97**, 202 (1976)
[11] DREVON, C. A., T. BERG, and K. R. NORUM: Biochim. biophys. Acta **487**, 122 (1977)
[12] TOLLESHAUG, H., T. BERG, M. NILSSON, and K. R. NORUM: Biochim. biophys. Acta **499**, 73 (1977)
[13] DE DUVE, C., B. C. PRESSMAN, R. GIANETTO, R. WATTIAUX, and F. APPELMANS: Biochem. J. **60**, 604 (1955)
[14] LOWRY, O. H., N. J. ROSEBROUGH, A. L. FARR, and R. J. RANDALL: J. biol. Chem. **193**, 265 (1951)
[15] BARRETT, A. J. in: Lysosomes laboratory handbook. J. T. DINGLE (Ed.). North-Holland Publ. Co., Amsterdam 1972, p. 46
[16] REIJNGOUD, D. J., P. S. OUD, and J. M. TAGER: Biochim. biophys. Acta **448**, 303 (1976)
[17] SEGLEN, P. O., and A. REITH: Expl Cell Res. **100**, 276 (1976)
[18] DE DUVE, C., T. DE BARSY, B. POOLE, A. TROUET, P. TULKENS, and F. VAN HOOF: Biochem. Pharmac. **23**, 2495 (1974)
[19] LA BADIE, W. A. DUNN, and N. N. ARONSON: Biochem. J. **160**, 85 (1976)

Acta biol. med. germ., Band 36, Seite 1763–1776 (1977)

Biochemisch Laboratorium der Rijksuniversiteit, Zernikelaan, Groningen, The Netherlands

Endocytosis and breakdown of proteins by sinusoidal liver cells

T. KOOISTRA, A. DUURSMA, J. M. W. BOUMA, and M. GRUBER

Summary

We studied the uptake of modified forms of bovine pancreatic ribonuclease A (labeled with ^{125}-iodine) by rat liver in vivo. On one hand, these experiments were intended to investigate a possible role of sinusoidal cells in the uptake of plasma proteins; on the other hand, the effect of well-defined modifications of the enzyme on the role of uptake might give us a key to the factors determining life time of plasma proteins. We used nephrectomized rats in most experiments to avoid uptake by the kidneys. Preparations of ribonuclease oligomers prepared by cross-linking with dimethyl-suberimidate enabled us to study a possible relation between uptake and molecular size. This modification does not lead to changes in charge of the protein. Monomer, dimer and polymer fractions were isolated by gel filtration on Sephadex G-75. Of the 11 amino groups in ribonuclease A, 9, 8 and 6 remained unaltered in the monomer, dimer and polymer fraction, respectively. The maintenance of biological activity, the stability of disulfide bonds, and the unchanged susceptibility to endoproteases of the cross-linked products established that gross conformational changes had not occurred. At 1 h after injection, 1% of the monomer, 7% of the dimer and 19% of the polymer were recovered per g of liver protein. Combination of autoradiography, subcellular fractionation, and the determination of labeled ribonuclease derivatives in the spleens showed that the dimer and polymer fractions were mainly present in the lysosomes of sinusoidal cells.

Introduction

In the 1930s, SCHOENHEIMER [1] and his collaborators discovered that in a living animal proteins are subjected to replacement or turnover: they are continually synthesized and degraded. Recent research has convincingly shown that rates of turnover are heterogeneous for different proteins, whether one considers extracellular plasma proteins [2, 3] or intracellular enzymes [4, 5]. Our experiments were undertaken to recognize some of the features of a circulating protein molecule which determine its stability, or relative lability.

Despite a marked growth of interest in the catabolism of circulating proteins in the past few years, little progress has been made in determining the mechanism of turnover of these proteins under normal conditions. Plasma itself can be excluded as a major site of protein breakdown because of its lack of general proteases and the presence of protease inhibitors. Since lysosomal proteases can digest extracellular proteins after their uptake by endocytosis, the lysosomal system may be involved in the turnover of plasma proteins. Other routes, such as excretion in the urine are for the most part quantitatively unimportant.

If lysosomes are the site of breakdown, (selective) adsorption to the cell membrane of the endocytosing cell may well be the rate-limiting and discriminating step in the catabolism of these proteins as has been demonstrated for certain asialo-glycoproteins [6]. These glycoproteins are endocytosed by parenchymal liver cells after attachment to a receptor protein on the plasma membrane.

The quantitative importance of different tissues for turnover is known in detail only for a few materials, but it seems that liver plays an important role in this process. Having a rich vascularization and a large amount of endocytosing cells, it is well equipped for this role. We are especially interested in the "sinusoidal" liver cells (Kupffer and endothelial cells). Kupffer cells (and, to a less extent, endothelial cells too) avidly take up aggregates of denatured proteins or colloidal particles. Buys et al. [7] in our laboratory, however, have shown that aggregation or denaturation is no prerequisite for the uptake of modified serum albumin by these cells. Their results suggest that changes on the surface of the molecule may be sufficient for attachment to receptors on sinusoidal cell membranes.

We now have further studied a possible role of sinusoidal cells of rat liver in the turnover of circulating proteins using (bovine pancreatic) ribonuclease A (m. wt. 13.700) as a probe. Ribonuclease is a very stable enzyme of known amino acid sequence and three-dimensional structure. It can be chemically modified in a number of ways without change in enzymatic activity, and therefore, without gross change of conformation. It is our purpose to relate changes in the rate of uptake by sinusoidal cells to well-defined modifications of the protein.

We used ribonuclease labeled with ^{125}-iodine, which avoids the problem of label reutilization [8]. At different times after injection, radioactivity was determined in plasma, liver and its subcellular fractions, spleen and kidney. Trichloroacetic acid soluble and insoluble radioactivity, as well as total radioactivity were assayed.

Inter-molecular cross-linking of ribonuclease A will result in an increase of the number of membrane-binding groups present per molecule. We expected therefore that a dimer and polymer of ribonuclease would be taken up more readily than the monomer since multiple attachment will enhance binding of molecules to the cell surface. We cross-linked ribonuclease A by a specific reaction of some of the amino groups with the bifunctional reagent dimethylsuberimidate [$CH_3O{-}C({=}\,NH){-}(CH_2)_6{-}C({=}\,NH)OCH_3$] under conditions similar to those described by Hartman and Wold [9] for cross-linking of ribonuclease A by adipimidate. We hoped to obtain ribonuclease derivatives with maintenance of the (enzymic) properties of the native enzyme. To avoid rapid clearance from the blood by the kidney, we did the same experiments with nephrectomized rats.

We investigated cellular and subcellular localization of the ribonuclease derivatives by a combination of autoradiography, subcellular fractionation and the determination of labeled ribonuclease derivatives in the spleens.

Materials and methods

Chemicals

Bovine pancreatic ribonuclease A (salt free; lyophilized; chromatographically homogeneous) was obtained from Miles Laboratories, Slough, England; ^{125}I-Na (carrier-free) from the Radiochemical Centre, Amersham, England; Fluothane (2-bromo-2 chloro- 1:1:1-trifluoroethane with 0.01% w/w thymol added) from I.C.I., Macclesfield, England; Sephadex G-25 and Sephadex G-75 from Pharmacia, Uppsala, Sweden; yeast RNA from Boehringer, Mannheim, FRG.; cytidine 2′:3′-cyclic monophosphate (cCMP) from Miles, St. Louis, Mo., U.S.A. dimethyl suberimidate dihydrochloride from Pierce, Rockford, Ill., U.S.A.; Ready-Solv from Beckman, Fullerton, Ca., U.S.A.; 2, 4, 6-trinitrobenzenesulphonic acid from K & K Laboratories, Irvine, Ca., U.S.A.; dithiothreitol from Calbiochem, San Diego, Ca., U.S.A.; 5,5′-dithio-bis-(2-nitrobenzoic acid) from Fluka, Buchs, Switzerland; bovine serum albumin from Poviet Producten N.V., Amsterdam, the Netherlands; pronase from Calbiochem, San Diego, Ca., U.S.A.; trypsin from Miles-Seravac, Maidenhead, England; α-chymotrypsin from Worthington, Freehold, N.J., U.S.A.; glutaraldehyde from O.C.S., Soesterberg, the Netherlands. All other chemicals used were analytical grade.

Animals and liver fractionations

Male rats of about 200 g of an inbred Wistar strain were used. Rats were injected via the vena femoralis, usually with 0.40 ml of solution per 200 g of rat. The labeled ribonuclease solutions injected, contained 2.0 mg of protein per ml 0.15 M NaCl. At the time of injection, the labeled proteins had a specific activity of about 15 μCi per mg of protein.

Blood samples of 0.15 ml were obtained by means of orbita puncture. After centrifugation, triplicate samples of 20 μl plasma were used for radioactivity measurements and/or enzyme activity determinations.

Rats were nephrectomized by ligating the blood vessels of the kidneys or by removing the kidneys.

After suitable intervals, rats were killed and organs of interest (spleen, kidney and liver) excised, dropped immediately into cold 0.25 M sucrose and homogenized within a short time. All livers had been perfused with ice-cold isotonic 0.15 M NaCl solution until they had become yellowish.

All experiments were done with anaesthetized animals. Anaesthesia was induced and maintained with Fluothane in a mixture of nitrous oxide and oxygen.

Liver fractionations were carried out as described by BOUMA and GRUBER [10].

Protein labeling

^{125}-iodine labeled ribonuclease was prepared by the chloramine-T procedure according to BOCCI [11]: 20–40 mg protein were incubated for 30 min at room temperature in 1.1 ml 0.15 M Tris-citrate buffer, *p*H 8.0, containing about 1 mCi ^{125}-iodide and 0.20 mg chloramine T. The reaction was stopped by adding a fresh solution of 0.12 mg $Na_2S_2O_5$ in 0.1 ml water. Unreacted iodide was removed by dialysis against three changes of about 2 l cold 0.15 M NaCl solution or by Sephadex G-25 gel filtration. A typical product contained 10–20 μCi ^{125}-iodine per mg of protein. Prior to injection, ribonuclease solutions were diluted with 0.15 M NaCl to concentrations suitable for injection.

Determination of protein and enzymes

Protein concentrations were estimated either spectrophotometrically ($E_{280}^{1\%} = 7.3$ [12]), or by the method of LOWRY et al. [13] with ribonuclease as the standard or by the Biuret method.

Enzyme activity towards RNA was determined by the method of CAMPAGNE and GRUBER [14], and towards cytidine 2′:3′-cyclic monophosphate (cCMP) by the method of CROOK et al. [15]. K_m and relative V_{max} values were estimated from Lineweaver-Burk plots of the hydrolysis of cCMP.

Acid phosphatase was measured according to GIANETTO and DEDUVE [16] with β-glycerophosphate as substrate. Glucose-6-phosphatase was assayed by the method of SWANSON [17]

Assay of radioactivity

Radioactivity in plasma was determined after precipitation of protein with trichloroacetic acid at a final concentration of 10% (w/v) in the following way: to 20 μl plasma were added 0.1 ml of a carrier solution containing 10% bovine serum albumin, and subsequently 0.1 ml 22% trichloroacetic acid. Supernatants and precipitates were counted.

Radioactivity in kidney, spleen and liver homogenates, and subcellular fractions was determined either as total counts or after precipitation with trichloroacetic acid (final concentration 10% (w/v)) in the supernatant as well as in the precipitate.

Radioactivity measurements were made with a Nuclear Chicago Mark I liquid scintillation counter. ^{125}-iodine samples were counted as gamma emitters in a heterogeneous system using a metal-loaded liquid scintillator (Ready-Solv VI (Beckman) saturated with lead acetate) [18]. The counting efficiency was about 70%.

To determine total rat plasma radioactivity, a volume of 3.13 ml plasma per 100 g body weight was assumed [19]. Uptake in spleen and kidney was corrected for the amount of radioactivity in residual blood present in the tissues at the time of sampling. Values of 262 μl plasma per g of spleen tissue and 151 μl plasma per g of kidney tissue were taken [19].

Cross-linking of ribonuclease (see Fig. 1)

To a stirred solution of 400 mg bovine pancreatic ribonuclease A in 40 ml 0.1 M sodium phosphate, *p*H 10.0, at 25 °C, 40 mg of dimethylsuberimidate dihydrochloride was added as a solid in five approximately equal portions at 5-min intervals; the *p*H of the solution was maintained at 10 by titration with 0.1 M NaOH. After 1 h, the reaction was stopped by the addition of 2.0 ml of 0.2 M ammonium acetate. Fractions containing monomer, dimer and polymer were separated by gel filtration on Sephadex G-75 in 0.1 M ammonium acetate. The fractions were pooled and lyophilized. They were characterized with respect to the number of lysine residues modified and enzymic activity.

Although the cross-link illustrated in Fig. 1A is an intramolecular one, the formation of intermolecular bridges is similar. The fact that imido-esters hydrolyze under mild conditions [20] could give rise to monofunctionally amidinated ribonuclease species in which one imido-ester group of the dimethyl-suberimidate molecule has reacted with water and the other with the protein (Fig. 1B). The pK_a of the amidines is even higher than that of ε-amino groups, so that an amidinated protein has the same net charge in the acid or neutral *p*H range as the native protein.

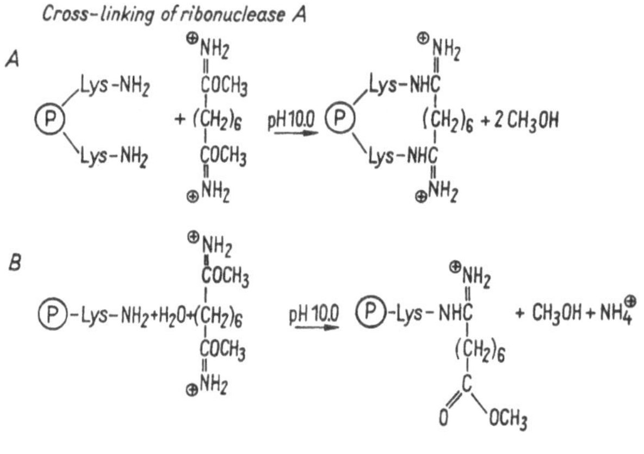

Fig. 1. Reaction scheme of cross-linking by dimethyl-suberimidate

Determination of free amino groups

The number of free amino groups in unmodified and modified ribonuclease was estimated spectrophotometrically with 2,4,6-trinitrobenzene sulphonic acid [21]. Calibration curves were made with native ribonuclease and glycine.

Estimation of conformational changes

Conformational change after chemical modification of ribonuclease was assessed by two criteria: measurements of stability of disulfide bonds to reduction and susceptibility to endoproteases. Reduction of disulfide bonds by dithiothreitol was estimated in the absence or presence of 8 M urea. Free thiol groups were determined spectrophotometrically after reaction with 5,5′-dithio-bis-(2-nitrobenzoic acid), essentially according to ELLMAN [22]. NaCl at a final concentration of 2 M was found to be necessary to make ribonuclease derivatives 10% (w/v) trichloroacetic acid-precipitable after reduction with dithiotreitol in the presence of 8 M urea. For calculation of sulfhydryl content, the net absorbance was employed with a molar absorption value of 13,600 $M^{-1}cm^{-1}$ at 412 nm [22].

Another direct test for conformational change is susceptibility to endoproteases. All incubations were done at 38 °C in stoppered tubes with continuous shaking. Each incubation mixture contained approximately 2 mg of ^{125}-iodine labeled protein (specific activity 0.5 μCi per mg) and 0.11 mg pronase, trypsin or chymotrypsin in 1.1 ml 50 mM sodium phosphate, *p*H 7.2, containing 0.15 M NaCl. At appropriate times, up to 6 hrs, 0.1 ml samples were mixed with 0.1 ml 20% bovine serum albumin used as carrier, and immediately 0.1 ml 30% trichloroacetic acid was added. Samples were kept overnight at 4 °C. After centrifugation, supernatants and precipitates were used for radioactivity measurements. The extent of enzymatic hydrolysis was estimated by the increase in trichloroacetic acid-soluble radioactivity.

Autoradiography

For autoradiography liver was fixed by perfusion with 2% glutaraldehyde in 0.1 M sodium phosphate buffer, *p*H 7.4. The duration of perfusion was about 2 min; the fixative was kept at room temperature. After perfusion, the liver was removed and thin slices were carefully cut into small blocks with a razor blade under the same fixative. These blocks were transferred to fresh fixative and stored for 24 hrs at room temperature under continuous rotation. Tissue sections were dipped into Ilford G 5 liquid emulsion and then dried over silicagel in an desiccator. After exposure at 4 °C for 3–6 weeks and development (Kodak D19 developer) for 10 min at 18 °C, sections were stained through the film with methylene green-pyronine.

Performic acid oxidation of the cross-linked products

Oxidation with performic acid was essentially done according to the procedure described by Hirs [23]. By qualitative analysis of our cross-linked products for amino acid composition, cystine and methionine were absent, but cysteic acid and methionine sulfone could be demonstrated. The oxidation resulted in a notable increase of proteolytic susceptibility, suggesting extensive unfolding.

Amino acid analysis

Amino acid analyses were performed with a Technicon Sequential Multisample amino acid analyser TSM-1, using a special program for the detection of cystine, methionine, cysteic acid and methionine sulfone.

Results and discussion

Labeling of ribonuclease A

Protein labeling with ^{125}-iodine has been extremely useful in biochemical studies. Especially in clearance studies, however, protein denaturation is an ever-present danger because the iodination is carried out in the presence of a powerful oxidizing agent. Denaturation can manifest itself as loss of biological activity and as change in the rate of clearance of the injected protein from the bloodstream. Even an undenatured, iodinated molecule (in the case of ribonuclease about one molecule per 10^4 molecules) might show different behaviour. Therefore, we checked our ^{125}-iodine ribonuclease preparations on enzyme activity and we compared blood-clearance of enzyme activity and radioactivity. The enzyme activity, using RNA as substrate, appeared not to be affected by the iodination procedure. The results of the blood clearance experiments, carried out with untreated and nephrectomized rats, are summarized in Fig. 2. It can be concluded from these curves that enzyme activity and radioactivity are cleared at the same rates. Thus, the iodinated molecules can be used as probes for the unlabeled ones.

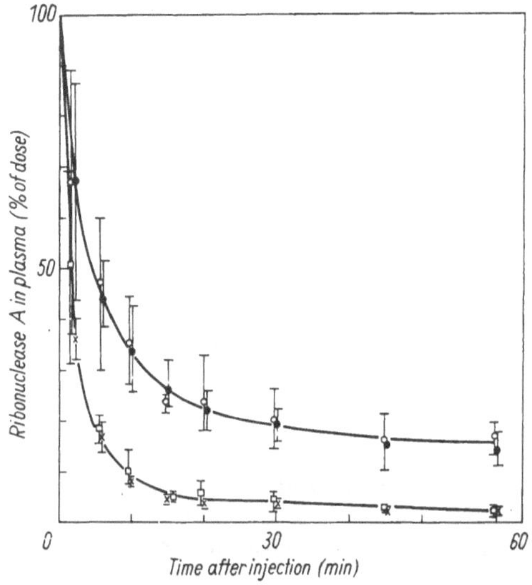

Fig. 2

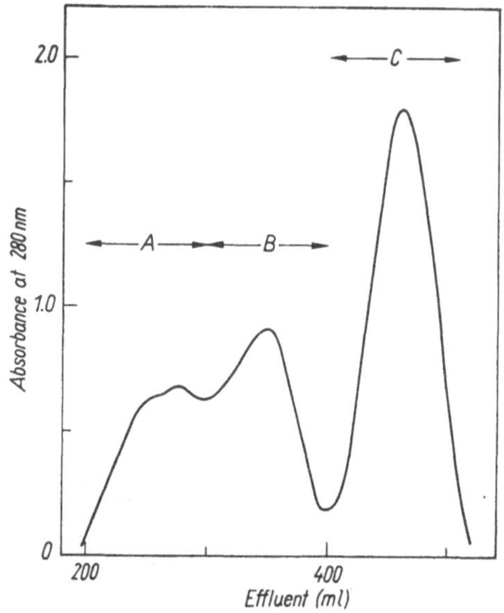

Fig. 3

Fig. 2. Clearance from plasma of trichloroacetic acid-precipitable radioactivity and enzymic activity after intravenous injection of ^{125}-iodine labeled ribonuclease A in normal and nephrectomized rats.

□ enzymic activity, untreated rats; × radioactivity, untreated rats; ○ enzymic activity, nephrectomized rats; ● radioactivity, nephrectomized rats.

Each point represents the mean value for at least three animals. Vertical bars give the range of individual values

Fig. 3. Gel filtration of cross-linking products on Sephadex G-75.

A, B and C refer to the pooled fractions. Experimental details: internal column diameter: 3.2 cm; bed height: 91.5 cm; flow rate: 20 ml/h; eluent: 0.1 M ammonium acetate

Cross-linked derivatives of ribonuclease A

The elution pattern of the cross-linked ribonuclease derivatives after Sephadex G-75 gel filtration is shown in Fig. 3 (A—C refers to the pooled fractions). Enzymatic characteristics of the different fractions are summarized in Table 1.

It is remarkable that amidination of ribonuclease did not result in a change of activity for a small substrate (cytidine 2′:3′-phosphate, cCMP), but in a reduction in the activity towards the other (RNA). HARTMAN and WOLD [9] showed for the monomer of the cross-linking reaction that the most reasonable interpretation for the increased affinity towards cCMP is an alteration or fixation of conformation imposed by the introduced cross-links.

WANG et al. [24] reported that the enzymic properties of the cross-linked dimer are very similar to those observed with the aggregated dimer of ribonuclease A [25, 26] and the naturally occurring dimer from bovine seminal plasma [27].

The maintainance of the biological activity of ribonuclease in the cross-linked products is an indication that gross conformational changes have not occurred. We confirmed this conclusion by direct tests for conformational changes: stability

Table 1
Properties of cross-linked ribonuclease A derivatives

Fraction	% of total	Free NH_2 groups per monomer
A = Polymer	20 ± 2	6.2 ± 0.2
B = Dimer	28 ± 1	8.4 ± 0.3
C = Monomer	52 ± 2	9.4 ± 0.5
Ribonuclease A		11

Fraction	Relative activity		cCMP	
	RNA	cCMP	K_m (mM)	V_{max} (rel.)
A = Polymer	20 ± 6	99 ± 2	0.6 ± 0.2	0.33
B = Dimer	26 ± 7	112 ± 15	0.6 ± 0.2	0.40
C = Monomer	42 ± 4	119 ± 7	0.6 ± 0.1	0.53
Ribonuclease A	100	100	1.7 ± 0.5	1.00

Determinations were carried out as described under Materials and methods. The hydrolysis of cytidine 2′ : 3′ cyclic phosphate was measured with a Zeiss PMQ II spectrophotometer equipped with a recorder (absorbance scale 0 to 0.05) at 284 nm at 25 ± 1 °C. Protein and substrate solutions were prepared in 0.1 M Tris-NaCl, *p*H 7.13. At a given substrate concentration (0.28 mM) preparations of ribonuclease A and its cross-linked derivatives (concentrations up to 35 µg/ml) were assayed by following the progress curve under standard conditions and calculating the initial velocity. Kinetic constants were determined with protein concentrations of 4 µg/ml at substrate concentrations ranging from 0.11 to 0.82 mM. Values are means ± S.E.M. of three separate experiments.

Table 2
Reducible disulfide groups in ribonuclease A and its cross-linked derivatives

Incubation conditions	Free SH-groups per monomer			
	RNAase A	Monomer	Dimer	Polymer
no DTT	0.0	0.0	0.0	0.0
10 mM DTT	0.1	0.1	0.1	0.1
no DTT + 8 M UREA	0.0	0.0	0.0	0.0
10 mM DTT + 8 M UREA	6.9	1.1	1.4	0.6

Free thiol groups were determined after incubation for 2 hrs at room temperature in the presence or absence of 10 mM dithiothreitol and/or 8 M urea. The values are the mean of at least three separate experiments. The cross-linked products had been subjected to the labeling procedure.

of disulfide bonds to reduction by 10 mM dithiothreitol in the absence or presence of 8 M urea (see Table 2) and susceptibility to endoproteases (see Table 3). These results also show that the cross-linking reaction makes the ribonuclease molecule more resistant to unfolding by urea. The results given above were obtained with proteins that had been subjected to the labeling procedure.

Clearance and uptake of ribonuclease A and its cross-linked derivatives in untreated rats

After intravenous injection of radioiodinated ribonuclease A in the rat we found a very rapid clearance of radioactivity from plasma. The enzyme appeared to be

Table 3
Susceptibility of ribonuclease A and its undenatured and denatured cross-linked derivatives to trypsin

Incubation time (min)	Undenatured				Denaturated		
	RNAase A	Monomer	Dimer	Polymer	Monomer	Dimer	Polymer
6	<5	<5	<5	<5	12.5	5.9	8.1
18	<5	<5	<5	<5	32.0	23.0	15.1
60	5.4	<5	<5	<5	36.7	26.4	22.8
360	5.0	<5	7.1	6.6	59.5	46.9	34.2

Determinations were carried out as described under Material and methods. The extent of enzymic hydrolysis was estimated by the increase in trichloroacetic acid-soluble radioactivity and expressed as percentage of trichloroacetic acid-precipitable radioactivity present at the start of the incubation. Values are means of three separate experiments.

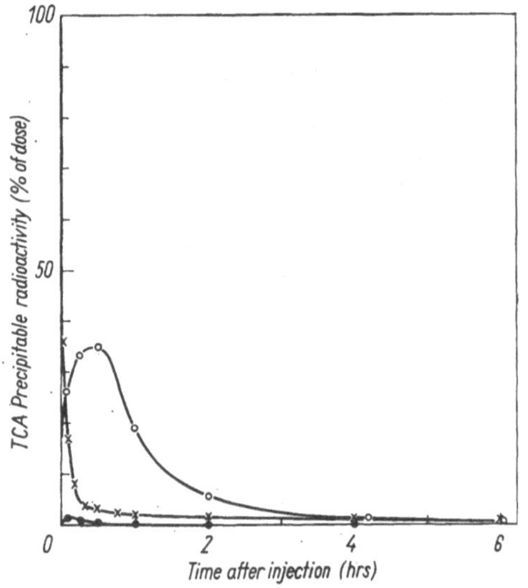

Fig.4. Trichloroacetic acid-precipitable radioactivity in plasma (×), kidney (○) and liver (●) at different times after intravenous injection of ^{125}-iodine ribonuclease A into untreated rats. Each point represents the mean value for at least three animals

rapidly taken up by the kidneys. There was no measurable uptake by the spleen and a negligible uptake by the liver (Fig. 4). These results are in agreement with those of DAVIDSON et al. [28]. In order to study the influence of molecular size on uptake and renal clearance, experiments were done with these larger macromolecules. Results are shown in Fig. 5 and Fig. 6. We conclude from these curves that the larger macromolecules are taken up in the liver more readily than the smaller ones. The data also clearly demonstrate, however, that even the polymer is rapidly cleared from the blood stream and taken up into the kidneys. The sum of label measured in plasma, kidneys, liver and spleen 5 min after injection, was (expressed as percentage of injected dose) 40% for the monomer, 60% for the dimer and 100% for the polymer. Major uptake by some other organ(s) seems unlikely. The discrepancy in the recovery of monomer and dimer probably reflects distribution over extravascular spaces and/or leakage of ribonuclease from capillaries. Leakage is well-known for small proteins and is, for molecules in this size range, probably rapid enough to compete with kidney uptake.

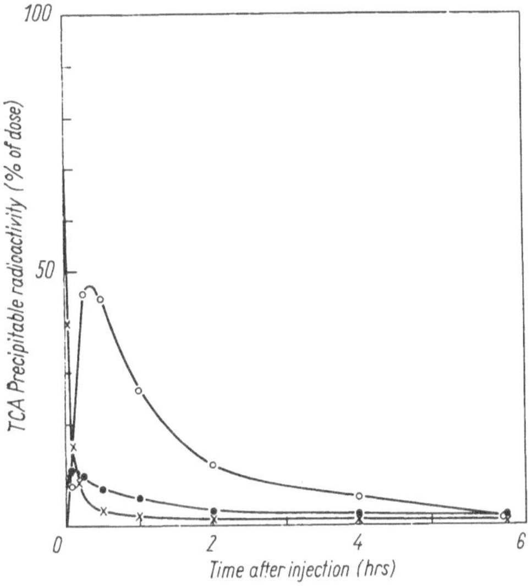

Fig. 5

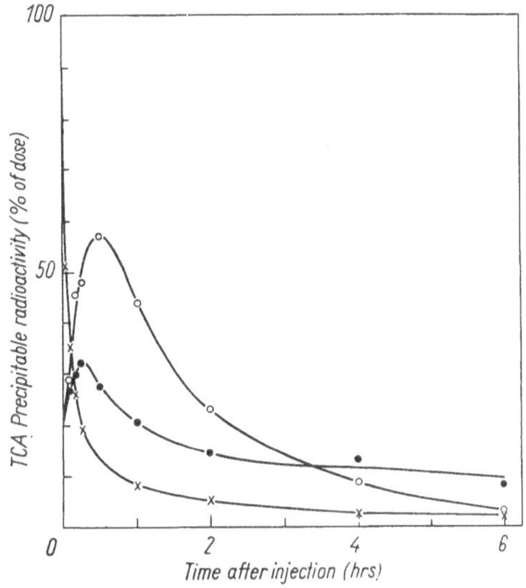

Fig. 6

Fig. 5. Trichloroacetic acid-precipitable radioactivity in plasma (×), kidney (○) and liver (●) at different times after intravenous injection of ^{125}-iodine ribonuclease dimer (fraction B) into untreated rats.

Each point represents the mean value for at least three animals

Fig. 6. Trichloroacetic acid-precipitable radioactivity in plasma (×), kidney (○) and liver (●) at different times after intravenous injection of ^{125}-iodine ribonuclease polymer (fraction A) into untreated rats.

Each point represents the mean value for at least three animals

Fig. 7. Trichloroacetic acid-precipitable radioactivity in liver at different times after intravenous injection of ^{125}-iodine ribonuclease monomer (×), dimer (○) or polymer (●) into nephrectomized rats.

Each point represents the mean value for at least three animals. Vertical bars give the range of individual values

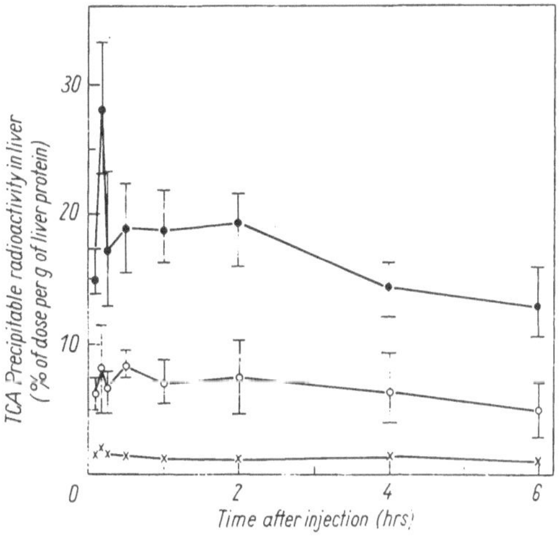

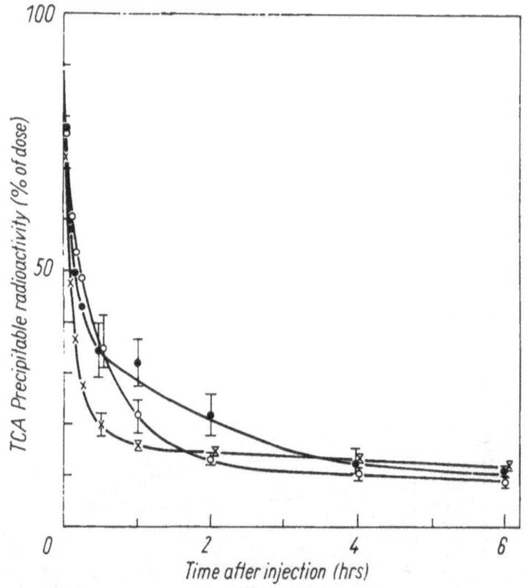

Fig. 8. Clearance from plasma of trichloroacetic acid-precipitable radioactivity after intravenous injection of ^{125}-iodine ribonuclease monomer (×), dimer (○) or polymer (●) into nephrectomized rats.

Each point represents the mean value for at least three animals. Vertical bars give the range of individual values

Clearance and uptake of monomer, dimer and polymer in nephrectomized rats

In order to avoid rapid uptake of our modified proteins from plasma into kidneys, we repeated the above experiments with nephrectomized rats. Essentially, the same results were found but uptake went on for longer time owing to a higher level in plasma. Uptake in liver has been expressed as percentage of dose per g of liver protein to make different experiments comparable (see Fig. 7). The difference in amounts of polymer, dimer and monomer taken up, cannot be attributed to a higher plasma level of the larger molecules since the plasma concentration of monomer, dimer and polymer are very similar at different times after injection (Fig. 8). Different rates of uptake must be due to the molecules proper and not to combination with plasma proteins (results not shown).

Subcellular localization of dimer and polymer

The distribution of labeled dimer and polymer over subcellular fractions was compared with those of the lysosomal marker enzyme acid phosphatase and the microsomal marker glucose-6-phosphatase. Fig. 9 shows the distribution of ^{125}-iodine labeled dimer and polymer after differential centrifugation of liver homogenates 1 h after injection of the proteins in nephrectomized rats. It is evident that the labeled enzyme is in the lysosomes.

Cellular localization of dimer and polymer

An indirect indication for cellular localization can be obtained by comparing the uptake by liver and spleen, expressed per g of tissue protein. Since spleen contains more mononuclear phagocytes per g of tissue than any other organ (including liver), a relatively high uptake by spleen will indicate involvement of sinusoidal cells. We found that uptake by spleen and liver per g of tissue protein was about equal. This points to an important role of the sinusoidal liver cells in the clearance of dimer and polymer.

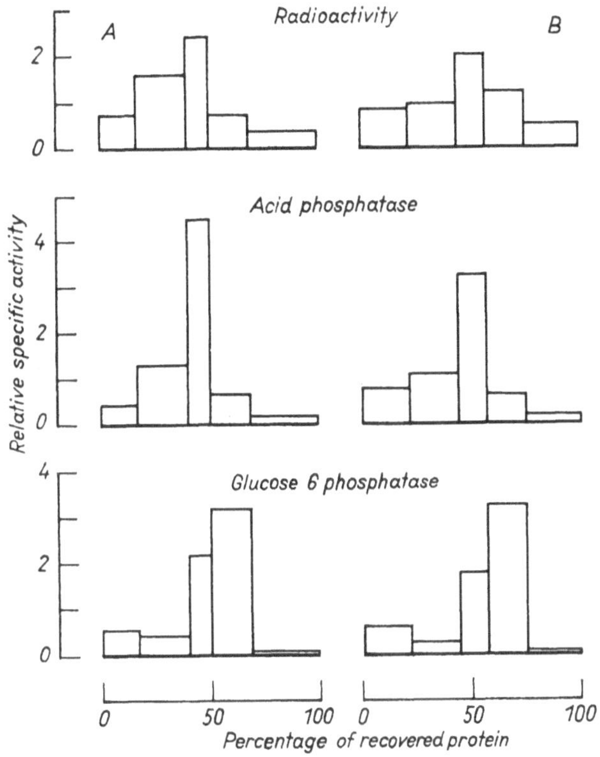

Fig. 9. Distribution of trichloroacetic acid-precipitable radioactivity (A = dimer, B = polymer), acid phosphatase and glucose-6-phosphatase over subcellular fractions.

Livers were homogenized and subdivided into five fractions one hour after injection of radioiodinated dimer and polymer into nephrectomized rats.

Abscissa: Blocks from left to right represent fractions in the order in which they are isolated: nuclear, mitochondrial, lysosomal, microsomal and supernatant fractions. The fractions are presented by their relative protein content, cumulatively from left to right.

Ordinate: Mean relative specific activity = percentage of total activity divided by percentage of total protein. Thus, the area of each block represents the percentage of activity per fraction. Each diagram is the result of two fractionations. Mean recoveries: protein A: 98%; B: 106%, radioactivity A: 97%; B: 97%; acid phosphatase A: 92%; B: 104%; glucose-6-phosphatase A: 102%; B: 89%

Involvement of sinusoidal cells can be shown directly by autoradiography of liver. Liver sections were examined 1 h after injection of ^{125}iodine labeled dimer and polymer in nephrectomized rats. In all cases, grains resulting from radioactive radiation were situated predominantly above the sinusoidal cells. Fig. 10 and Fig. 11 show representative autoradiograms.

Discussion

Our results demonstrate that for an undenatured protein system the rate of uptake by sinusoidal liver cells is correlated to the size of the molecules: polymers of ribonuclease A are taken up more readily than dimer and monomer.

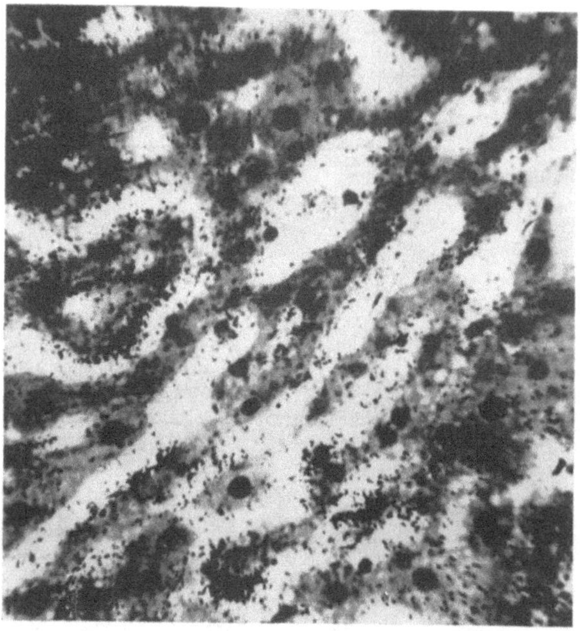

Fig. 10. Autoradiogram of liver section of rat injected with 125-iodine ribonuclease dimer (courtesy of Dr. P. NIEUWENHUIS). Experimentel details are given in the text

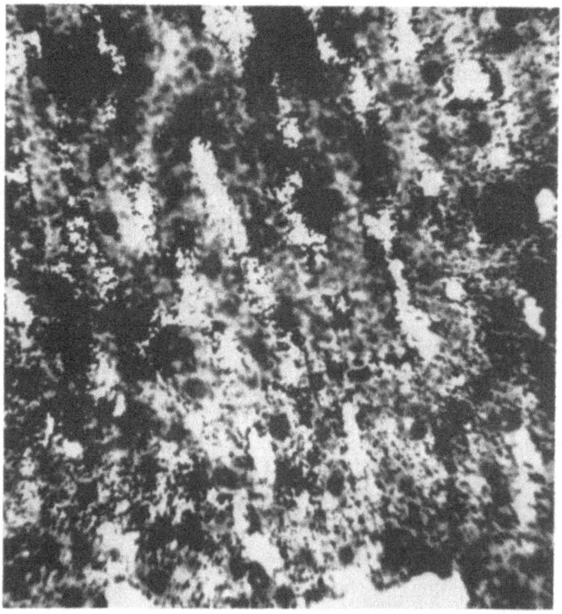

Fig. 11. Autoradiogram of liver section of rat injected with 125-iodine ribonuclease polymer (courtesy of Dr. P. NIEUWENHUIS). Experimental details are given in the text

BARTHOLEYNS and BAUDHUIN [29] have reported similar results for the uptake of ribonuclease dimer and monomer by hepatoma cells in culture.
Probably, ribonuclease A is introduced to the lysosomal system of sinusoidal liver cells by the process of surface endocytosis, i. e. binding to the cell membrane, infolding of a zone of the cell membrane, and sealing-off of this invagination, the endosome [30]. Proteins will then be endocytosed according to the degree of adsorption to the plasma membrane that is being internalized. Since size determines the number of determinant groups per molecule capable of interacting simultaneously with the cell surface, it is clear that inter-molecular cross-linking of ribonuclease will enhance the affinity of the molecule for the cell surface and thus enhance uptake.
The preferential uptake by the sinusoidal cells may have different causes. The rate of entry of a protein into a cell will depend on the rate of pinocytic vesicle (endosome) formation and the affinity of the substrate for the plasma membrane. Pinocytosis is a very prominent activity of sinusoidal cells, but appears to be of less importance in other cells. This fact might explain the cellular localization of dimer and polymer. On the other hand, sinusoidal cells may (also) have more receptive groups at their surface for our proteins. It is also important to remember that rate of endosome formation may itself be altered by the presence of proteins.
What particular group(s) of ribonuclease A have affinity to plasma membranes of sinusoidal cells? Positively charged amino groups of lysine appear to be involved in attachment, since acetylation of amino groups markedly reduced uptake by the liver and succinylation had an even stronger effect (data not shown).
Our results show that uptake of the ribonuclease derivatives is not caused by denaturation. On the contrary, studies with performic acid oxidized monomer, dimer and polymer showed (unpublished results), that these denatured derivatives of ribonuclease did not accumulate in liver at all.
Summarizing, our results suggest that strongly positively charged molecules, even if they are as small as the ribonuclease dimer (m. wt. 27,000) do not survive long in the circulation. In this context it may be significant that most of the (relatively big) plasma proteins are, under physiological conditions, negatively charged.

Acknowledgements

The excellent assistance of J. BOUWER in animal experiments is gratefully acknowledged. Our thanks are also due to Dr. P. NIEUWENHUIS, Histologisch Laboratorium, Groningen for his help in autoradiography experiments. Part of this work was carried out under the auspices of the Netherlands Foundation for Chemical Research (S.O.N.) and with financial aid from the Netherlands Organisation for the Advancement of Pure Research (Z.W.O.).

References

[1] SCHOENHEIMER, R.: The Dynamic State of Body Constituents. Harvard University Press, Cambridge, Mass. 1942
[2] SCHULTZE, H. E., and J. F. HEREMANS: Molecular Biology of Human Proteins with Special Reference to Plasma Proteins. Vol. 1, Elsevier, Amsterdam 1966
[3] DICE, J. F., and A. L. GOLDBERG: Nature, Lond. **262** 514 (1976)
[4] SCHIMKE, R. T. in: Mammalian Protein Metabolism. Vol. **4**, 177. H. N. MUNRO (Ed.) Academic Press, New York 1970

[5] RECHCIGL, M., Jr. in: Enzyme Synthesis and Degradation in Mammalian Systems. M. RECHCIGL, Jr. (Ed.). Karger, Basel 1971, p. 236
[6] MORELL, A. G., G. GREGORIADIS, I. H. SCHEINBERG, J. HICKMAN, and G. ASHWELL: J. biol. Chem. **246**, 1461 (1971)
[7] BUYS, C. H. C. M., A. S. H. DE JONG, J. M. W. BOUMA, and M. GRUBER: Biochim. biophys. Acta **392**, 95 (1975)
[8] COHEN, S., R. C. HOLLOWAY, C. MATTHEWS, and A. S. MCFARLANE: Biochem. J. **62**, 143 (1956)
[9] HARTMAN, F. C., and F. WOLD: Biochemistry **6**, 2439 (1967)
[10] BOUMA, J. M. W., and M. GRUBER: Biochim. biophys. Acta **113**, 350 (1966)
[11] BOCCI, V.: Ital. J. Biochem. **18**, 346 (1969)
[12] RICHARDS, F. M., and H. W. WYCKOFF in: The Enzymes. Vol. 4, 647. P. D. BOYER (Ed.) Academic Press, New York and London 1971
[13] LOWRY, O. H., N. J. ROSEBROUGH, A. L. FARR, and R. J. RANDALL: J. biol. Chem. **193**, 265 (1951)
[14] CAMPAGNE, R. N., and M. GRUBER: Biochim. biophys. Acta **55**, 353 (1962)
[15] CROOK, E. M., A. P. MATHIAS, and B. R. RABIN: Biochem. J. **74**, 234 (1960)
[16] GIANETTO, R., and C. DEDUVE: Biochem. J. **59**, 433 (1955)
[17] SWANSON, M. A.: Meth. Enzymol. **2**, 541 (1955)
[18] ZAK HELMAN, E., and P. TING: Clin. Chem. **19**, 191 (1973)
[19] DITTMER, D. S. (Ed.): Biological Handbooks: Blood and other body fluids. Federation of American Societies for Experimental Biology, Washington, D.C. 1961
[20] ROGER, R., and D. G. NEILSON: Chem. Rev. **61**, 179 (1961)
[21] HABEEB, A. F. S. A.: Anal. Biochem. **14**, 328 (1966)
[22] ELLMAN, G. L.: Archs Biochem. Biophys. **82**, 70 (1959)
[23] HIRS, C. H. W.: J. biol. Chem. **219**, 611 (1956)
[24] WANG, D., G. WILSON, and S. MOORE: Biochemistry **15**, 660 (1976)
[25] LIBONATI, M.: Ital. J. Biochem. **18**, 407 (1969)
[26] LIBONATI, M.: Biochim. biophys. Acta **228**, 440 (1971)
[27] LIBONATI, M., and A. FLORIDI: Eur. J. Biochem. **8**, 81 (1969)
[28] DAVIDSON, S. J., W. L. HUGHES, and A. BARNWELL: Expl Cell Res. **67**, 171 (1971)
[29] BARTHOLEYNS, J., and P. BAUDHUIN: Proc. natn. Acad. Sci. U.S.A. **73**, 573 (1976)
[30] JACQUES, P. J. in: Lysosomes in Biology and Pathology. Vol. **2**, 395. J. T. DINGLE and H. B. FELL (Eds). North-Holland Publishing Co., Amsterdam 1973

Acta biol. med. germ., Band 36, Seite 1777–1788 (1977)

The Rockefeller University, New York, N.Y. 10021

The accumulation of weakly basic substances in lysosomes and the inhibition of intracellular protein degradation

B. Poole, S. Ohkuma, and M. J. Warburton

For the past several years we have been very interested in the mechanism by which cells degrade their own proteins during normal protein turnover and in the mechanism by which certain substances are taken up into cells and concentrated in lysosomes. As we will see these two interests are not completely unrelated. While we do not yet understand all the details of the concentration mechanism in lysosomes, the broad features of the process can be explained by a fairly simple theory [1]. When certain substances have been taken up into lysosomes these substances seem to have fairly profound effects on the process of protein degradation there.

In Fig. 1, a phase contrast micrograph of a rat fibroblast is shown that has been exposed for 2 hrs to medium containing chloroquine at a concentration of 100 μM. The cell is filled with large, easily visible vacuoles. A combination of cell fractionation and microscopy has revealed that these vacuoles are swollen lysosomes [2]. This cell had been exposed to chloroquine, but the morphological picture would be indistinguishable had the cell been treated with a wide variety of weakly basic substances including ammonium chloride, at sufficiently high concentration, and also acidic ionophores like nigericin or X537A. In all cases in which we have been able to make actual measurements of the amount of the substance taken up into

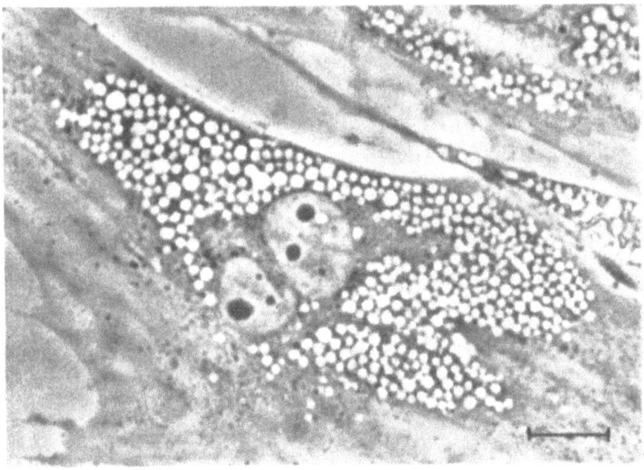

Fig. 1. Phase contrast micrograph of rat fibroblast exposed to 100 μM chloroquine for 2 hrs. The bar represents 10 μm

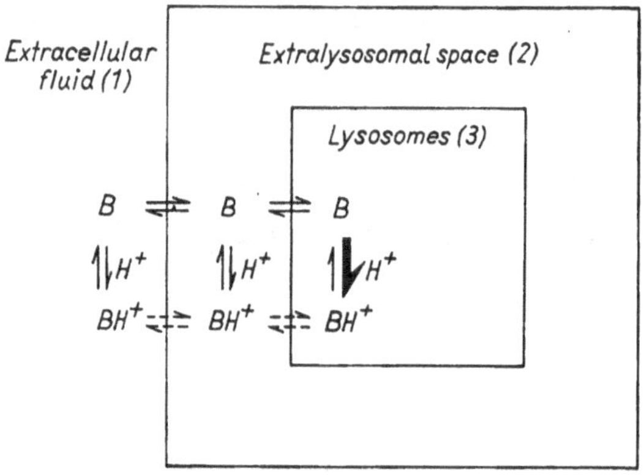

Fig. 2. Model of intralysosomal trapping of weak bases. Taken from [1]

the cells, the measurements were consistent with the hypothesis that these engorged vacuoles contain an isotonic solution of the compound in question.

Fig. 2 shows schematically our theory of the mechanism of intralysosomal accumulation of weakly basic substances. The theory is based on three assumptions. The first is that membranes, both plasma and lysosomal, are freely permeable to the neutral form of these weakly basic substances. It is further assumed that the membranes are impermeable to the protonated form of these same substances. Finally, it is assumed that the *p*H within lysosomes is considerably lower than the *p*H of the medium. It follows from these three assumptions that the concentration of the neutral form of the substance in question will be uniform in all compartments. As a consequence of the high acidity in lysosomes and of simple acid-base equilibrium, there will be an accumulation in the lysosomes of the protonated form of the weak base. As a first approximation, for weak bases with *p*K's above neutrality, the concentration ratio, lysosomes to medium, will be the same for the weak base as it will be for hydrogen ions. When the concentration of the weak base in the medium is sufficiently high that the concentration of the same weak base in the lysosomes approaches isotonicity, then the weak base in the lysosomes will cause the lysosomes to swell osmotically. This we think is the origin of the enormous increase in lysosomal volume observed in cells exposed to weak bases. The concentration in the medium necessary to cause this vacuolation ranges from about 100 μM for substances like chloroquine, quinine and neutral red to about 10 mM for substances like methylamine and ammonia. Thus the concentration ratio, lysosomes to medium, appraoches 1,000 for substances like chloroquine, while it appears to be little more than 10 for substances like ammonia. This suggests that in the presence of high enough concentrations of ammonia, the *p*H within the lysosomes is higher than it was before the cells were treated with this compound. Thus one would expect that treatment with ammonia would interfere with lysosomal function.

We have no experimental evidence concerning the mechanism of vacuolation by the acidic ionophores. However, if the lysosomes contain a system for maintaining their internal acidity, then one would expect that the gradient of hydrogen ion concentration between the lysosomes and the cytoplasm would drive potassium ions to accumulate in the lysosomes in exchange for hydrogen ions. If the hydrogen ions were replaced by some mechanism as they were exchanged out of the lysosomes, then a flow into the lysosomes of potassium ions could be maintained and lead to osmotic swelling.

As shown in Fig. 3, chloroquine, at concentrations such as those occurring in the lysosomes of chloroquine treated cells, is a very effective inhibitor of cathepsin B (formally called cathepsin B1). It is thought that this protease may be one of the more important ones in primary proteolytic attack on native proteins in lysosomes [3, 4]. Thus it would be expected that exposure to chloroquine would have a direct effect on proteolysis in lysosomes.

Indeed, we have allowed mouse peritoneal macrophages to endocytoze a variety of protein substrates and have then studied the effect of chloroquine on the subsequent digestion of these substrates in lysosomes. In all cases, we found that chloroquine had a very strong inhibitory effect on this process. While we cannot exclude the occurrence of some inhibitory effect of chloroquine on the fusion of endocytic vacuoles with lysosomes, kinetic studies have indicated that the chloroquine does exert an inhibitory effect on proteolysis after these endocytic vacuoles have already fused with lysosomes. Significantly perhaps, chloroquine has little effect on the digestion of the endogenous proteins of the macrophages themselves. In order to make as direct a comparison as possible between the intralysosomal digestion of proteins and the digestion of endogenous proteins during normal

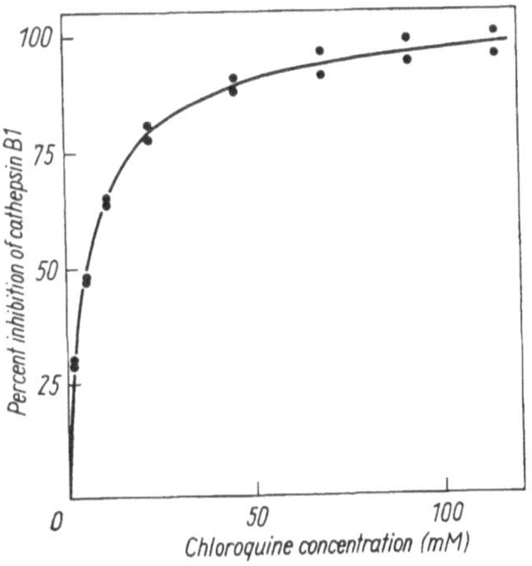

Fig. 3

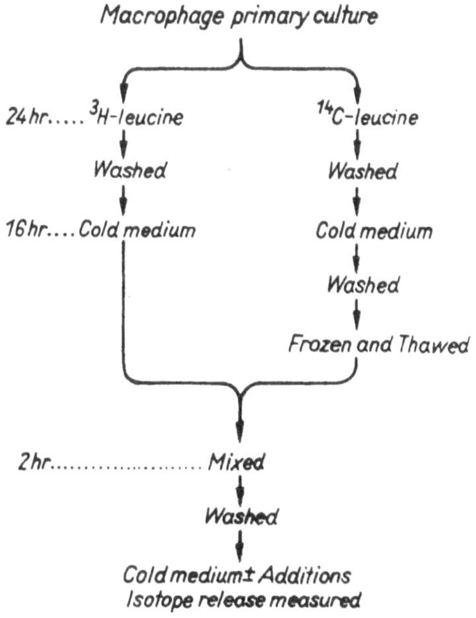

Fig. 4

Fig. 3. Inhibition of cathepsin B by chloroquine.
The enzyme preparation was a postnuclear supernatant from rat liver. Assayed by the method of BARRETT [7] using Z-ala-arg-arg-4-methoxy-2-naphthylamine as substrate [8]

Fig. 4. Experimental procedure for feeding dead to living macrophages

Table 1
Inhibition of the degradation of endogenous and exogenous macrophage proteins in living macrophages fed dead macrophages

	Endogenous %	Exogenous %
Control	0	0
100 μM Chloroquine	4	68
10 mM NH_4Cl	4	60
20 μg/ml X537A	0	32

Parallel cultures were labeled with [^{14}C]leucine or [^{3}H]leucine (2 μCi/ml each) for 24 hrs and then left 14 hrs in unlabeled medium. [^{3}H] labeled cells were harvested and killed by one cycle of freezing and thawing. [^{14}C]Labelled cells were fed for 2 hrs with [^{3}H]labelled dead cell preparation. Washed cells were then incubated in the media shown and the output of trichloroacetic acid-soluble radioactivity was measured after 2 hrs. All values are expressed as a percent of inhibition of digestion within 2 hrs.

protein turnover, we performed the experiment illustrated in Fig. 4. In brief, living macrophages labeled with one isotope of leucine were fed with dead macrophages labeled with another isotope of leucine under exactly the same time schedule. After the labeled living macrophages had been permitted to endocytose the labeled dead macrophages, the digestion of the macrophage proteins from the two sources was measured simultaneously in the same cells under a variety of conditions. Table 1 shows the results of such an experiment. Neither chloroquine, ammonia nor the acid ionophore had significant inhibitory effects on the digestion of the endogenous macrophage proteins. All of these agents, to a greater or lesser extent, inhibited the intralysosomal digestion of the exogenous macrophage proteins. Here again, kinetic experiments demonstrated that at least part of the inhibitory effect of these agents was exerted after the endocytic vacuoles had already fused with lysosomes. This shows us that, whether or not the endogenous macrophage proteins are degraded in lysosomes, these lysosomes cannot be the same lysosomes that are engaged in the digestion of the endocytozed macrophage proteins. We have arranged these experiments in such a way that the cell is degrading approximately the same number of micrograms of protein per minute from the two sources. So, working with the macrophages, we found that we could inhibit severely proteolysis within lysosomes without observing a significant inhibition of the rate of degradation of endogenous macrophage proteins during normal protein turnover.

In the course of our studies on endogenous proteolysis in rat fibroblasts we found something similar. But first, it is pertinent to discuss the background to these experiments which may have interesting implications for the coordination between endogenous protein breakdown and other cellular functions. Some years ago, we discovered that fibroblasts exposed to medium that had been conditioned (depleted?) by exposure to growing fibroblasts, or to medium that was deficient in fetal calf serum, resulted in an increased rate of proteolysis of those cellular proteins that turn over slowly, with no apparent change in the rate of breakdown of those cellular proteins that turn over rapidly. Of course the simplest explanation for these findings was that serum contained some factors that inhibited the breakdown of proteins with slow rates of turnover and that on exposure to cells this factor was somehow inactivated or destroyed. We were very interested in knowing what factor or factors in serum were responsible for this effect. At that time, we entertained the project of fractionating serum to identify the factor or factors. It had been known for many years that serum contained factors necessary for the sustained growth of cells in tissue culture, and that on exposure to cells these factors were depleted. In our opinion it remained possible, but improbable, that the factor or factors responsible for these two phenomena were the same. Consequently, we set out, before doing any serum fractionation, to establish definitively that the two phenomena were unrelated. The results of these studies, which we will now describe, were very surprising to us.

In all of these studies, we have measured, in parallel and in different samples of the same cell population, the rate of protein degradation between the start of the experiment and 2 hrs afterwards and the rate of thymidine incorporation between 8 and 24 hrs afterwards. We first studied the effect, on these two cellular processes, of a deficiency in the medium of a number of different components which are known to be necessary for cell proliferation. In Table 2 we see the results of exposing these cells to media devoid of amino acids, phosphate or glucose in the presence and absence of serum. Whether in the presence or in the absence of serum, none of these deficiencies resulted in a significant inhibition or stimulation of the rate of those proteins that normally turn over rapidly. In the presence of serum each of these deficiencies resulted in a significant stimulation of the rate of breakdown of those proteins that turn over slowly. In the absence of serum, additional deficiencies in the medium caused only very slight, if any additional increases in the rate of breakdown of proteins. We have not shown the thymidine incorporation in the absence of serum because in the absence of serum there was very little thymidine incorporation. However, in the presence of serum these same three medium deficiencies, that caused an increase in the degradation of the proteins that turn over slowly, caused a decrease in the incorporation of thymidine. The results of these preliminary experiments were not in keeping with our hypothesis that in fact there was no real connection between inhibition of thymidine incorporation and stimulation of protein degradation. In order to examine the situation more carefully we studied the dose dependencies of the medium content in serum on these two processes. In this particular experiment we used a subconfluent culture, and we measured not only the rate of protein degradation and the rate of thymidine incorporation but also the increase in the protein content of the culture in terms of micrograms per square centimeter of culture surface. The results of this experiment are shown in Fig. 5. The dose response curves for these three effects of serum are very similar. Even the smallest amount of serum had some effect. All three effects seemed to become maximal at about 3% serum in the medium and the concentration of serum for half-maximal effect was extremely similar. In order to make the relationships between these processes clearer, in Fig. 6 we have plotted the rate of protein degradation against the

Table 2

Effect of omitting various medium components on cellular protein degradation and DNA synthesis

Medium component omitted	Protein degradation				
	Short lived (^{3}H)		Long lived (^{14}C)		[^{3}H-]dT incorporation with serum (%)
	with serum (%)	without serum (%)	with serum (%)	without serum (%)	
None	(22.8 ± 1.3/2hrs) 100	113.6 ± 3.9	(1.92 ± 0.17/2hrs) 100	228.6 ± 7.8	(28900 ± 3000 cpm) 100
Amino acids	98.7 ± 5.7	114.9 ± 6.1	175.0 ± 8.9	281.8 ± 8.9	25.6 ± 10.7
Glucose	103.1 ± 4.8	112.3 ± 7.9	205.2 ± 6.3	210.4 ± 8.3	34.3 ± 3.8
Phosphate	10.39 ± 5.3	113.6 ± 6.1	165.1 ± 4.7	219.8 ± 5.7	22.8 ± 3.5

(a) Protein degradation: Cells were labeled with [^{14}C]leucine (1 μCi/ml) for 50 hrs, left 15 hrs in unlabeled medium, and then labeled for 1 hr with [^{3}H]leucine (10 μCi/ml). Washed cells were incubated in the media shown and the output of trichloroacetic acid-soluble radioactivity was measured after 2 hrs. (b) DNA synthesis: Cells were rendered quiescent by incubating in medium containing 0.25% serum for 48 hrs. Washed cells were incubated for 24 hrs in medium containing 10% dialyzed serum with various medium components omitted. Cells were labeled with [^{3}H]thymidine (1 μCi/ml) for 16 hrs (8–24 hrs after start of treatment). The incorporation of radioactivity into trichloroacetic acid insoluble material was determined. All values are expressed as a percentage of control value. Number in parentheses are the absolute values measured for the controls. Means of 3 ± standard deviations.

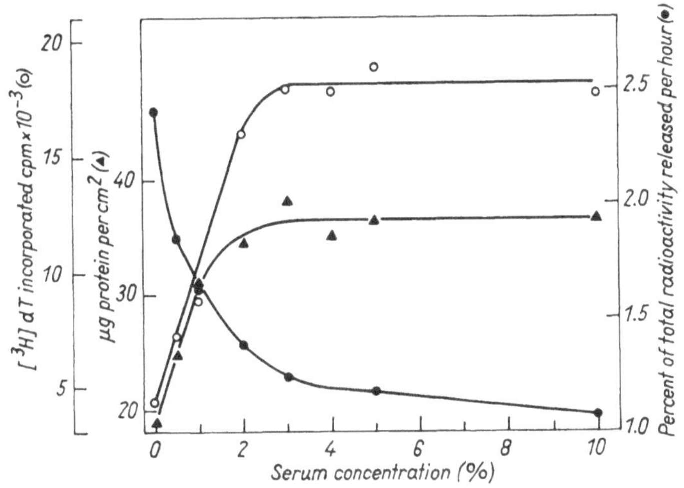

Fig. 5. Effect of serum concentration on DNA synthesis, protein content and protein degradation.
(a) To measure DNA synthesis, cells were rendered quiescent by incubating in medium containing 0.25% serum for 48 hrs. After washing, cells were incubated in fresh medium containing various serum concentrations for 24 hrs. The cells were labelled with 1 μCi/ml [^{3}H]dT for 16 hrs (8–24 hrs after the addition of serum). The incorporation of radioactivity into trichloroacetic acid-insoluble material and the protein content of each culture were determined. (b) To measure protein degradation, cells were labeled with [^{3}H]leucine (1 μCi/ml) for 50 hrs, and then left in unlabeled medium for 15 hrs. Washed cells were incubated in medium containing various serum concentrations and the output of trichloroacetic acid-soluble radioactivity into the medium was measured after 2 hrs. Taken from [9]

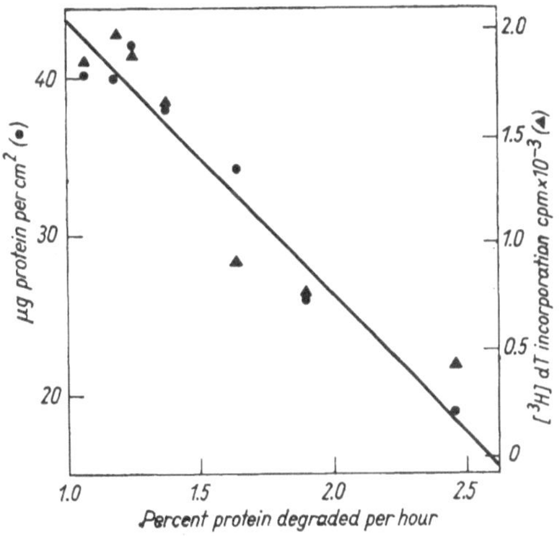

Fig. 6. Correlation diagram between protein degradation and cell growth. Data from Fig. 5. Taken from [9]

extent of thymidine incoporation and the extent of protein accumulation. It is clear from an examination of this figure that there is a very close inverse correlation between the rate of protein degradation on the one hand and on the other hand the extent of thymidine incorporation and the extent of protein accumulation. Here again, we failed to find a dissociation between the effects of medium composition on protein degradation and upon cell proliferation.

In studies that have been made on the factors in serum that support the growth and proliferation of cells it has become obvious that there is not a single serum factor but that a number of serum factors act synergistically to support cell growth [5]. In certain cell types it was shown that a mixture of a bovine pituitary factor, fibroblast growth factor (FGF), insulin and dexamethasone could act synergistically to mimic the effect of serum [6], Consequently, we studied the effect of these three factors, alone and in combination, on thymidine incorporation and on protein degradation. The results of this experiment are shown in Table 3. It is clear that

Table 3
Effect of insulin, dexamethasone and FGF on protein degradation and DNA synthesis

	[^{3}H]dT incorporation into DNA (cpm · 10^{-3})	TCA-soluble radioactivity released per hour (%)
10% serum	28.9 ± 3.1	0.91 ± 0.06
0% serum	4.5 ± 1.1	2.01 ± 0.08
Insulin (50 ng/ml)	6.1 ± 0.6	1.92 ± 0.03
Dexamethasone (0.4 μg/ml)	5.2 ± 0.6	1.99 ± 0.05
Insulin + dexamethasone	8.4 ± 0.9	1.84 ± 0.08
FGF (120 ng/ml)	10.4 ± 0.9	1.69 ± 0.04
Insulin + dexamethasone + FGF	23.2 ± 1.8	1.24 ± 0.06

(a) Protein degradation: Cells were labeled with [^{3}H]leucine (1 μCi/ml) for 50 hrs, left in unlabeled medium for 15 hrs and finally exposed for one hr to serum-free medium. Washed cells were incubated in the media shown and the output of TCA-soluble radioactivity was measured after 2 hrs. All media without serum contained 0.5% BSA. (b) DNA synthesis: Cells were rendered quiescent by incubating in medium containing 0.25% serum for 48 hrs. Washed cells were incubated in the media shown for 24 hrs. Cells were labeled with [^{3}H]thymidine (1 μCi/ml) for 16 hrs (8–24 hrs after the start of treatment). The incorporation of radioactivity into trichloroacetic acid-insoluble material was determined. Means of 3 ± standard deviations.

none of these factors alone or in certain binary combinations had significant effects either on protein degradation or on thymidine incorporation. However, when these three factors were present together they exerted a synergistic effect that was almost, but not quite, the equivalent of the effect of serum itself. At this point in our studies it began to appear obvious that our initial assumption, that the effect of medium composition on protein degradation and on cellular proliferation were independent, was false. We then made one further test. We studied the dose dependency of protein degradation and thymidine incorporation upon the amount of fibroblast growth factor added in the presence of saturating amounts of dexamethasone and insulin. The results of this experiment are shown in Fig. 7. Here again, we found a very close inverse correlation between the amount of protein degraded by the cells and the amount of thymidine incorporated by the cells. And again, as shown in Fig. 8, the inverse correlation between these two effects was very close. Since we measured protein degradation between 0 and 2 hrs after the start of the experiment, while we measured the thymidine incorporation between 8 and 24 hrs after the start of the experiment, it became essential to examine in some detail the kinetics of the two processes. In Fig. 9 we see the results of an

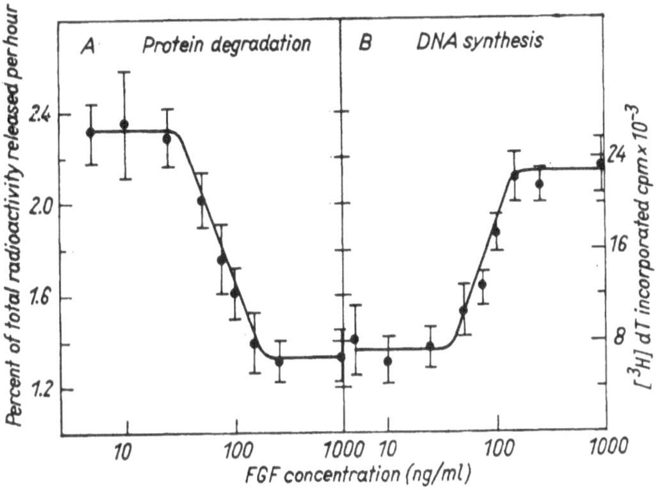

Fig. 7. Effect of FGF concentration on protein degradation and DNA synthesis.
A) Cells were labeled with [^{3}H]leucine for 50 hrs, left in unlabeled medium for 15 hrs and finally exposed for 1 hr to serum-free medium. After washing, the cells were incubated in fresh, serum-free medium containing 0.5% BSA and various concentrations of FGF, insulin (50 ng/ml) and dexamethasone (0.4 μg/ml) for 2 hrs. B) Cells were rendered quiescent by incubating in medium containing 0.25% serum for 48 hrs. After washing, the cells were incubated with varying concentrations of FGF, insulin (50 ng/ml) and dexamethasone (0.4 μg/ml) for 24 hrs. During the last 16 hrs of incubation, [^{3}H]thymidine (2 μCi) and thymidine (2.5 μg) were added to each tube. Taken from [9]

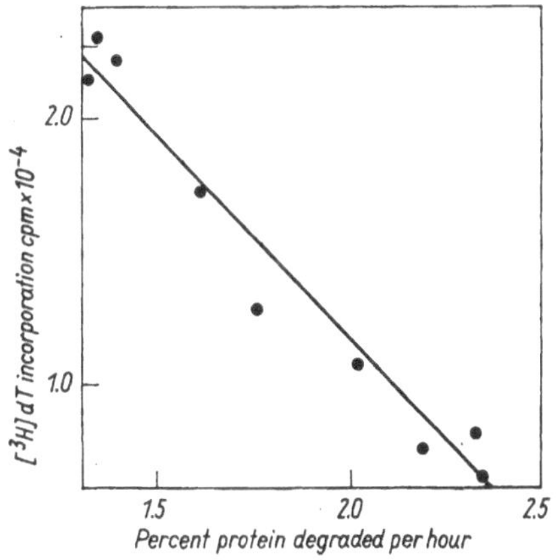

Fig. 8

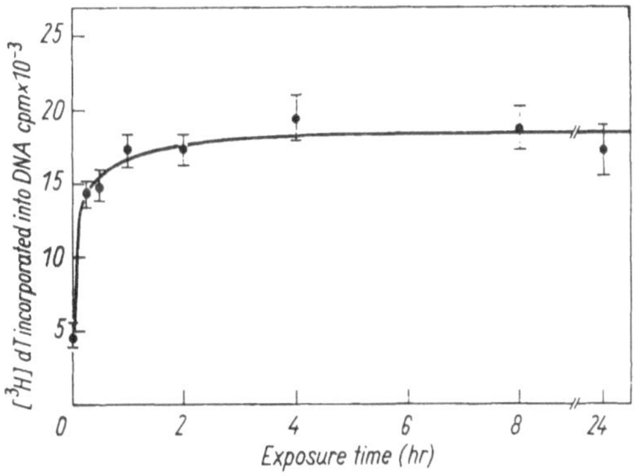

Fig. 9

Fig. 8. Correlation between protein degradation and thymidine incorporation in fibroblasts exposed to various concentrations of FGF. Data from Fig. 7. Taken from [9]

Fig. 9. DNA synthesis in quiescent fibroblasts after a short exposure to serum.
Cells were rendered quiescent by incubating in medium containing 0.25% serum for 48 hrs. After washing, cells were incubated in medium containing 10% serum for the indicated times. After further washing, cells were incubated in serum-free medium. Incubation was continued so that the cells were incubated for 24 hrs after initiation of treatment. All cells were then labeled with 1 μCi/ml [^{3}H]dT for 16 hrs (8–24 hrs after start of treatment). The incorporation of radioactivity into acid-soluble material was determined. Taken from [9]

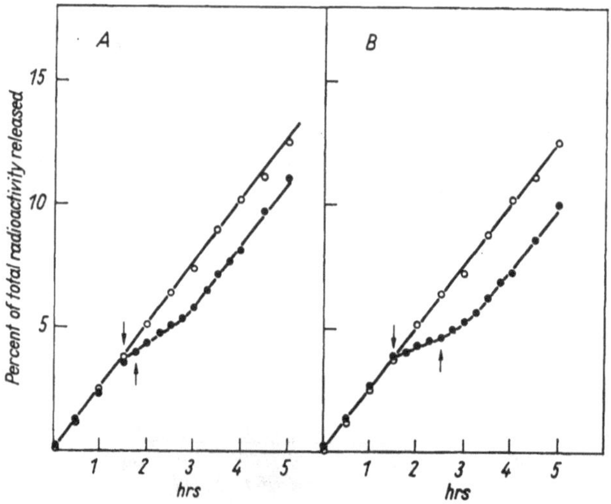

Fig. 10. Effect of a short exposure to serum on the release of trichloroacetic acid-soluble radioactivity into the medium.

Cells were labeled for 50 hrs with [^{3}H]leucine, and then left in unlabeled medium for 15 hrs. A) ○, fresh control medium with serum, changed after 105 min (second arrow); ●, fresh control medium without serum, changed to 10% serum after 90 min (first arrow), changed to fresh medium without serum after 105 min (second arrow). B) ○, fresh control medium without serum, changed after 150 min (second arrow); ●, fresh control medium without serum, changed to 10% serum after 90 min (first arrow), changed to fresh medium without serum after 150 min (second arrow). Taken from [9]

experiment in which cells, exposed to medium deficient in serum for 48 hrs in order to stop DNA synthesis, were exposed to serum for various lengths of time, and then replaced into medium devoid of serum. The thymidine incorporation in these cells was measured between 8 and 24 hrs after their initial exposure to serum. It is clear that very short exposures to serum had very profound effects on the subsequent synthesis of DNA in these cells. An exposure to serum for as short a time as 15 min was almost as effective in stimulating DNA synthesis as was a continuous exposure between 0 and 24 hrs.

In Fig. 10 we see the results of an experiment in which cells in the absence of serum were exposed to serum for 15 min or for 1 hr, and then placed back in serum-free medium. The rate of cellular protein degradation was measured before, during, and after these brief exposures to serum. When the cells were first exposed to serum the rate of protein degradation slowed down by about 50% with no measurable lag period. When the cells were replaced in serum-free medium, protein degradation took some time to regain the rate it had before exposure to serum. However, by 2 hrs after the beginning of serum exposure the cells were again degrading their proteins at the rate characteristic of serum-free medium.

Taken together, the results described above present peculiar features. In a number of very different experimental situations (Tables 2 and 3, Fig. 6 and 8), we have found a very close inverse correlation between the rate of cellular protein degradation and the extent of thymidine incorporation. This correlation can hardly be fortuitous. Consequently, we are forced to conclude that these two cellular processes are tied together by some unknown cellular regulatory mechanism. (We have been unable to demonstrate any involvement of cyclic AMP in these processes.) But, whatever the regulatory mechanism is, it can operate on protein degradation for a very short time and still exert its maximal effect on DNA synthesis many hours later. Another peculiar feature of these observations arises from the presumption that these cells do not synthesize more or less DNA, but rather that they do or do not replicate their genome. Thus, our measurements of thymidine incorporation would be a measure of the fraction of the cells that went on to enter the S phase of the cell cycle. This raises the intriguing possibility that our measurements of the rate of protein degradation could be a measure of the fraction of cells in the population that were or were not converted to a new metabolic state characterized by a different rate of protein degradation. Clearly this problem requires further study.

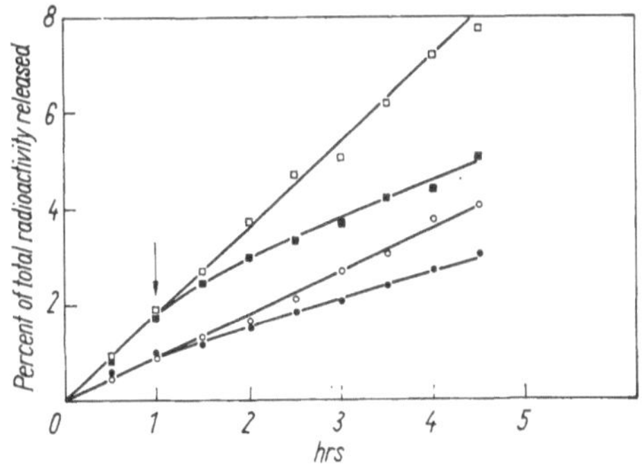

Fig. 11. Effect of chloroquine on protein degradation.

Cells were labeled with [^{3}H]leucine (1 μCi/ml) for 50 hrs and then left in unlabeled medium with serum for 15 hrs and then without serum for 1 hr. After washing, fresh medium, with (○, ●) or without (□, ■) 10% serum, was added to each flask. After 1 hr (arrow), chloroquine (100 μM) was added (○, ■)

However, to return to lysosomotropic substances, we can have cells in two extreme states, most easily achieved by exposing the cells to medium with or without serum. In the absence of serum the rate of protein degradation is higher by a factor of about 2. Fig. 11 shows the results of an experiment in which cells, in the presence or absence of serum, were exposed to 100 μM chloroquine. The chloroquine had a slight inhibitory effect on the protein degradation in the presence of serum. However, in the absence of serum the effect of chloroquine was much more pronounced. After exposure to chloroquine, the rate of degradation was virutually identical in the presence or absence of serum. Here again we have evidence that could be interpreted to mean that a certain part of cellular protein degradation occurs in lysosomes where it is susceptible to inhibition by lysosomotropic agents while the rest of the degradation occurs somewhere else. However, since we have no idea where or what this "other" proteolytic mechanism could be, considerable caution is necessary in the interpretation of such results.

Acknowledgements

The research reported here has been supported by grants AG00367 and AG00609-01 from the U.S. Public Health Service and by grant PCM76-16657 from the National Science Foundation. We are grateful to the U.S. National Academy of Sciences and to the Journal of Cell Biology for permission to reprint copyrighted material.

References

[1] DE DUVE, C., T. DEBARSY, B. POOLE, A. TROUET, P. TULKENS, and F. VAN HOOF: Biochem. Pharmac. **23**, 2495 (1974)
[2] WIBO, M., and B. POOLE: J. Cell Biol. **63**, 430 (1974)
[3] HUISMAN, W., L. LANTING, M. J. DODDENA, J. M. W. BOUMA, and M. GRUBER: Biochim. biophys. Acta **370**, 297 (1974)
[4] BARRETT, A. J.: Biochem. J. **131**, 809 (1973)
[5] HOLLEY, R. W., and J. A. KIERNAN: Proc. natn. Acad. Sci. U.S.A. **71**, 2908 (1974)
[6] GOSPODAROWICZ, D.: J. biol. Chem. **250**, 2515 (1975)
[7] BARRETT, A. J.: Anal. Biochem. **47**, 280 (1972)
[8] DAVIDSON, E., and B. POOLE: Biochim. biophys. Acta **397**, 437 (1975)
[9] WARBURTON, M., and B. POOLE: Proc. natn. Acad. Sci. U.S.A. (in press)

Acta biol. med. germ., Band 36, Seite 1789—1804 (1977)

Department of Tissue Culture, Norsk Hydro's Institute for Cancer Research, The Norwegian Radium Hospital, Montebello, Oslo 3, Norway

Protein degradation in isolated rat hepatocytes

P. O. Seglen and A. E. Solheim

Summary

1. Isolated rat hepatocytes, prepared by the method of collagenase perfusion, are in a highly protein-catabolic state. They degrade their protein at a rate of 3—4% per h, whereas the rate of protein synthesis is only about one-tenth of the degradation rate. The intracellular content of lysosomes and autophagosomes increases rapidly during incubation.
2. Hepatocytes incubated in Dulbecco's cell culture medium under hypoxic conditions have a reduced rate of protein degradation due to the accumulation of ammonia from deaminated glutamine. Ammonia acts as an inhibitor of protein degradation, and up to 90% inhibition can be obtained by the addition of 10 mM NH_4Cl. Ammonia, being a weak base, accumulates in the acidic interior of the lysosomes and elevates the intralysosomal *p*H, thereby rendering the lysosomal proteases inactive. The concomitant osmotic influx of water causes lysosomal swelling, readily observed in the electron microscope.
3. The incorporation of amino acids into protein can be affected by protein degradation in two ways. On the one hand, the proteolytic release of amino acids may cause an isotope dilution which decreases protein labelling; on the other hand, the released amino acids may enhance protein labelling by a stimulatory effect on protein synthesis. In order to obtain constant synthesis and incorporation rates, the cells should be preincubated with amino acids and "swamped" with a radioactive amino acid at sufficiently high concentration to maintain constant specific activity (e. g. 5 mM [^{14}C]-valine).
4. Valine is transported across the liver cell membrane by facilitated diffusion (i. e. carrier-mediated, passive transport); a process which follows Michaelis-Menten kinetics with a K_m of 43 mM, and which is non-concentrative, energy-independent, largely Na^+-independent, temperature-sensitive (E_a = 14 kcal/mol) and subject to counter-transport (accelerative exchange). At 30 °C, the equilibration of valine between the extra- and intracellular medium occurs extremely rapidly (almost complete in 2—3 min).
5. At low temperature (15 °C—20 °C), [^{14}C]-valine transport occurs sufficiently slowly to enable the establishment of different specific activities in the extracellular and the intracellular amino acid pools. Protein labelling follows the intracellular specific activity both during influx and efflux of [^{14}C]-valine, and it can be concluded that the expandable intracellular amino acid pool serves as the precursor pool for protein synthesis.
6. When the hepatocytes are incubated for 1 h with [^{14}C]-valine, acid-soluble radioactivity can be shown to enter a distinct, non-expandable pool in the presence, but not in the absence of, ongoing protein synthesis (i.e. ± cycloheximide). Since this pool can only be labelled by way of protein degradation, it should be regarded as a degradation pool. By sucrose gradient centrifugation, it can be shown that all of the radioactivity in this pool resides in the lysosomal fraction.

Isolated hepatocytes thus appear to have two major valine pools: a general cytoplasmic (expandable) pool, which equilibrates rapidly with the extracellular medium and from which the precursor amino acids for protein synthesis are taken, and a lysosomal (non-expandable) degradation pool which empties into the expandable pool.

Introduction

Rat hepatocytes renew their cellular protein at a rapid rate (1—3% per h) in vivo [1], and are therefore a suitable experimental material for the study of normal protein turnover. By the method of collagenase perfusion [2], intact rat hepatocytes can be isolated in high yield, and such cells have been found to degrade their protein at the same high rate as in vivo [3—5]. It has thus become possible to study protein degradation in a normal cell type under well-controlled in vitro-conditions. In this article various aspects of hepatocytic protein metabolism as investigated in the authors' laboratory will be reviewed.

Material and methods

Isolated hepatocytes were prepared from male Wistar rats (230—300 g), by the two-step method of collagenase perfusion [2, 6] and incubated at 37 °C as a suspension in rapidly shaking centrifuge tubes [7]. After incubation, the cells were either rapidly cooled to 0 °C and separated from the medium by repeated washings in the cold (e.g. for determination of intracellular radioactivity), or the whole sample (cells + medium) was precipitated with perchloric acid directly (for determination of total metabolite levels or protein labelling).
The nitrogen balance was assessed by measuring the net changes in amino acids (ninhydrin-positive material), urea and ammonia during the incubation period. The net loss of nitrogen prevalent in most situations could be taken as a direct measure of protein degradation, the rate of protein synthesis being negligible (in several experiments even completely inhibited by the addition of cycloheximide).
Protein degradation was also measured by pre-labelling the cell protein during a 1 h incubation with [^{14}C]-valine, then removing extra- and intracellular valine by extensive washing of the cells, and finally measuring the net release of acid-soluble radioactivity from the pre-labelled protein.
Protein synthesis was measured by incorporation of [^{14}C]-valine or a [^{14}C]-labelled amino acid mixture (protein hydrolysate) [8, 9]. Amino acid transport was studied by measuring the cellular uptake of [^{14}C]-valine during very short incubation periods (down to 30 s).
For sucrose gradient centrifugations, cell suspensions in 0.25 M sucrose were homogenized with 15 strokes in a Dounce homogenizer. Nuclei were sedimented at 800 × *g* for 10 min, and the post-nuclear supernatant (5 ml) layered directly onto a 35 ml 25—55% sucrose gradient with a 15 ml cushion of 70% sucrose. After centrifugation at 107000 × *g* for 4 hrs, fractions were collected and analysed for radioactivity and β-acetylglucosaminidase activity [10].

Results

Protein-catabolic state of isolated hepatocytes

When suspended in an amino acid-free medium, isolated hepatocytes release large quantities of amino acids (Fig. 1B). This "medium-conditioning" does not represent amino acid leakage, since the intracellular content of amino acids remains constant (Fig. 1 A). In addition to amino acids, the cells release acid-soluble nitrogen in the form of urea (Table 1). In the absence of any exogenous substrate, the released nitrogen can only originate from the degradation of cell protein. The sum of amino acid and urea release represents a total nitrogen loss of about 60 μgatom nitrogen/g cellular wet weight per h, corresponding to the degradation of 3—4% of the cell protein per h. Measurement of the release of [^{14}C]-valine from 1 h prelabelled protein gives a higher value, of 9—10% per h, because protein with rapid turnover is preferentially labelled by a short labelling pulse [11].
The protein-catabolic state of the isolated hepatocytes is probably characteristic of the in vitro situation, in which the cells have become deprived of all the exogenous regulatory factors (hormones, cell contacts and other "differones", cf. refs. [12, 13], which normally maintain the cells in nitrogen equilibrium. In the electron

microscope, the transition into negative nitrogen balance upon incubation of the cells in vitro can be seen to be accompanied by an increased content of autophagosomes and secondary lysosomes intracellularly (Table 2).

The high rate of protein degradation does not reflect cell damage or dysfunction, since the rate actually decreases rapidly with increasing cell damage [14]. Protein degradation requires energy, as indicated by a strong oxygen dependence, and is highly temperature-sensitive (Fig. 10).

The rate of protein synthesis in isolated hepatocytes appears to be low in comparison with protein degradation, since the addition of cycloheximide, an inhibitor of protein synthesis, does not appreciably alter the over-all nitrogen balance (Table 1). An estimation of the protein synthesis rate by incorporation of [^{14}C]-valine (5 mM), assuming that liver protein contains 9% valine [15], gives a variable rate of 0.2—0.5% per h, which can be increased by preincubation of the cells with amino acids (Fig. 6). A considerable fraction of the protein synthesized would presumably be plasma proteins for export, since active protein secretion [16, 17] and nearly normal rates of plasma protein synthesis [18, 19] have been reported in isolated hepatocytes. Synthesis of the cells' own proteins (structural and others) must therefore be almost completely shut off.

The protein-catabolic state apparently does not persist indefinitely in vitro, since hepatocytes in a serum-enriched medium can be maintained in monolayer culture for several days [20, 21].

It would be of great interest to identify the factors (differones) capable of controlling hepatocytic protein metabolism, since this might give important information about growth control in normal cells in general.

Table 1

Lack of effect of amino acids and cycloheximide on nitrogen balance in isolated rat hepatocytes.

The cells were incubated with or without cylohexímide (1 mM) for 60 min at 37 °C with a physiological mixture of amino acids at the concentration indicated, and the net changes in the concentration of amino acids and urea during this period were measured. The nitrogen loss is calculated as the sum of urea and amino acid formation. Each value is the mean ± S.E. of 4 cell samples. From [14].

	Amino acid formation (µmoles/g per h)		Urea formation (µmoles/g per h)		Nitrogen loss (µgatom/g per h)	
	Control	1 mM Cycloheximide	Control	1 mM Cycloheximide	Control	1 mM Cycloheximide
No addition	26.2 ± 0.7	28.8 ± 0.6	17.2 ± 1.0	15.3 ± 0.9	60.6 ± 2.1	59.3 ± 2.0
Amino acids, 2.5 × normal concentration	5.9 ± 2.1	−3.2 ± 1.0	23.0 ± 0.9	26.9 ± 1.0	51.8 ± 2.7	50.7 ± 2.2
Amino acids, 5 × normal concentration	−22.7 ± 0.8	−23.5 ± 0.7	40.6 ± 0.8	41.2 ± 1.2	58.5 ± 1.8	58.8 ± 2.5

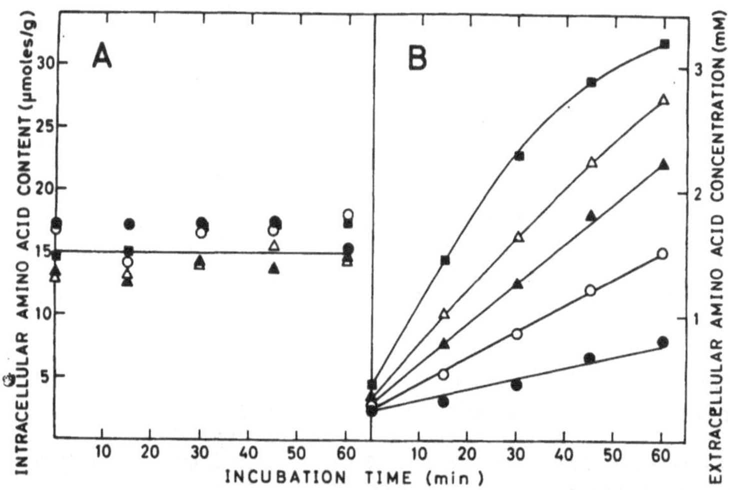

Fig. 1. Effect of cell concentration on the intracellular and extracellular amino acid levels during incubation.

Isolated hepatocytes were incubated at a concentration of 12.5 (●), 25 (○), 50 (▲), 75 (△) or 100 (■) mg cells/ml, and the intracellular (A) and extracellular (B) amino acid contents were measured at various time points after separation of cells from medium. From [8]

Table 2
Morphometric analysis of autophagic/lysosomal vacuole contents (as fractions of cell volume) in isolated rat hepatocytes.
Values represent means ± S.E. of five cell samples. From [5].

Experimental treatment	Autophagic vacuoles (mm^3/cm^3)	Dense bodies (mm^3/cm^3)	Vacuolar lysosomes (mm^3/cm^3)
A) Non-incubated, fixed directly after isolation	2.4 ± 0.9	4.9 ± 1.1	1.7 ± 0.5
B) Control, incubated 1 h without additions	10.9 ± 2.2	12.2. ± 0.8	7.7 ± 2.2
Significance of difference A—B	**P <0.01**	**P <0.001**	**P <0.05**
C) Ammonia-incubated (1 h with 10 mM NH_4Cl)	6.4 ± 1.8	2.6 ± 1.0	133.9 ± 24.4
Significance of difference C—B	**N. S.**	**P <0.001**	**P <0.001**

Regulation of protein degradation: Inhibition by ammonia

In a search for anti-catabolic factors, a physiological mixture of amino acids was first tried, since amino acids have been shown both to stimulate protein synthesis [22—24] and to inhibit protein degradation [25] in the perfused liver. However, although the isolated hepatocytes consumed amino acids rapidly, the amino nitrogen was practically quantitatively converted to urea rather than being incorporated into protein, and the negative nitrogen balance remained essentially unaltered (Table 1). A variety of other factors and conditions (cells from fed or regenerating livers, various sera, hormones and metabolites) were investigated with only limited success, but eventually it was found that incubation in a cell culture

Table 3

Influence of medium composition and cell state on nitrogen balance in isolated rat hepatocytes. The cells were prepared from 16 hrs fasted or ad libitum-fed rats. Incubations with sera were for 2 hrs; other incubations were for 1 h unless otherwise indicated. The values represent the net nitrogen loss (formation of urea + amino acids) from the complete system of cells + medium; each value is the mean ± S. E. of 2–5 cell samples. From [14].

	Nitrogen loss (µg atoms/g per h)
None	67.7 ± 1.8
Glucose, 20 mM	58.4 ± 3.8
Fructose, 20 mM	44.9 ± 1.6
Pyruvate, 20 mM	58.9 ± 3.1
Amino acids (5 × normal concentration)	62.3 ± 1.6
Amino acids (5 × normal) + insulin (10^{-5} M)	65.0 ± 1.8
Pig serum (50%)	61.4 ± 3.3
Horse serum (50%)	55.6 ± 3.2
Calf serum (50%)	55.2 ± 4.4
Foetal calf serum (50%)	37.9 ± 5.7
Fasted rat serum (50%), fasted cells	49.7 ± 5.8
Fed rat serum (50%), fed cells	54.6 ± 3.4
Fasted rat serum (50%), fed cells	42.1 ± 1.9
Fed rat serum (50%), fasted cells	40.6 ± 3.2
20 hrs regenerating cells (70% hepatectomy)	68.7 ± 1.7
Dulbecco's medium, 0–2 hrs	97.1 ± 8.0
Dulbecco's + insulin (10^{-5} M), 0–2 hrs	109.2 ± 10.2
Dulbecco's + foetal calf (2.5%) and horse (15%) serum, 0–2 hrs	64.2 ± 8.3
Dulbecco's medium, 2–4 hrs	17.3 ± 11.0
Dulbecco's + foetal calf (2.5%) and horse (15%) serum, 2–4 hrs	5.8 ± 6.9

medium (Dulbecco's) largely prevented the loss of cellular nitrogen (Table 3). This anti-catabolic effect was strictly dependent upon the incubation conditions: it could only be observed after at least 1 h of incubation in slowly shaking petri dishes (an incubation technique used only for experiments of several hours' duration). Close examination revealed that the crucial process was the rapid de-

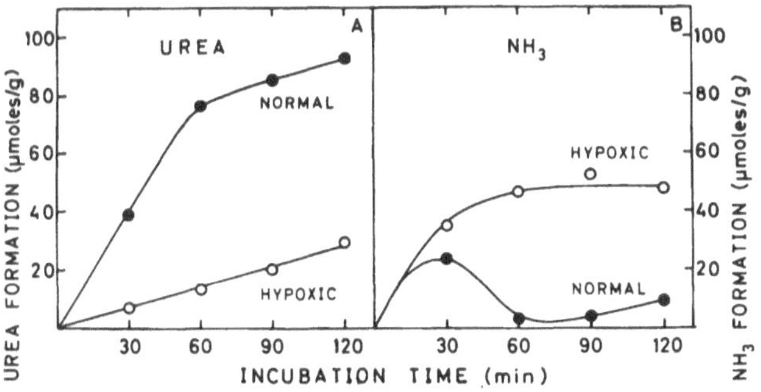

Fig. 2. Formation of urea and ammonia from glutamine under normoxic and hypoxic conditions.

Isolated hepatocytes were incubated at 37 °C with 5 mM glutamine under an atmosphere of air (●) or 5% O_2 (○), and the formation of urea (left panel) and ammonia (right panel) was measured during 2 hrs of incubation. Each point is the mean of two cell samples. From [4] amination by the hepatocytes of medium glutamine to glutamate and ammonia. Under normal conditions ammonia is rapidly converted to urea in isolated hepatocytes, but in the slowly shaking petri dishes the cells became too hypoxic to perform urea synthesis, and ammonia accumulated (Fig. 2). This accumulation of ammonia then resulted in the inhibition of protein degradation [26].

The potency of ammonia as an inhibitor of protein degradation can be readily demonstrated by the direct addition of ammonium chloride to hepatocyte suspensions [3]; a maximal inhibition being seen at 10 mM (Fig. 3). Ammonium chloride is an innocuous substance with a reversible effect, and it is therefore becoming increasingly useful as an inhibitor of protein degradation in a variety of cell types [27—30]. Although ammonia also inhibits protein secretion appreciably, it has little effect on protein synthesis [17].

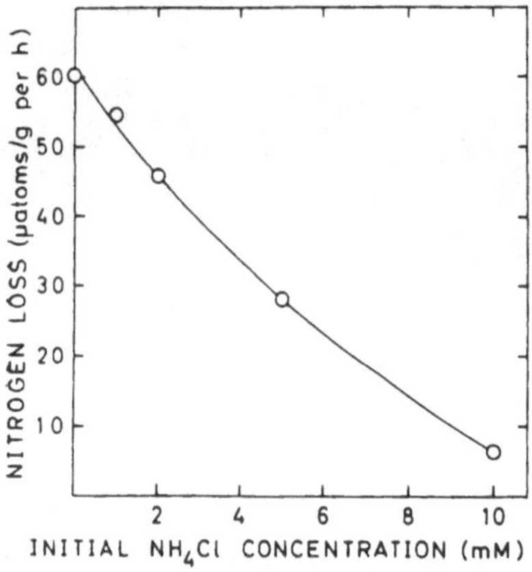

Fig. 3. Dose-dependent inhibition of nitrogen loss from isolated rat hepatocytes by ammonia.

Isolated hepatocytes were incubated at 37 °C for 60 min at the initial concentration of NH_4Cl indicated, and the nitrogen loss (inrease in perchloric acid-soluble nitrogen in the complete system of cells + medium) was calculated on the basis of changes in amino acids, urea and NH_3. From [3]

Since ammonia is one of the natural end-products of amino acid catabolism, its inhibition of protein degradation creates a feed-back cycle which may be physiologically relevant [4]. In tissues other than liver and kidney, there is no conversion of ammonia to urea, and significant amounts of ammonia may accumulate under conditions of rapid proteolysis and transamination. Under tissue culture conditions, there is nearly always a high ammonium concentration in the medium due to spontaneous as well as cell-catalyzed decomposition of glutamine [31], and this could well have some implications for cell growth in vitro.

The inhibition of protein degradation by ammonium chloride in isolated hepatocytes is accompanied by a pronounced swelling of the lysosomes, as seen in the electron microscope (Fig. 4). Being a weak base, ammonia will accumulate in the acidic interior of the lysosomes, causing both an osmotic influx of water (i. e. swelling) and an inhibition of lysosomal proteases due to the elevation of *p*H [5, 32]. The identification of ammonia as a lysosomotropic agent is not a novel discovery; cytoplasmic vacuolization (i. e. lysosomal swelling) of cells incubated in ammonium chloride (or other weak bases) was observed by HEINZ already in 1890 [33]!

Since hepatocytic protein degradation is inhibited up to 90% by ammonia, a lysosomotropic agent, it can be inferred that lysosomes are responsible for the bulk of protein degradation in these cells.

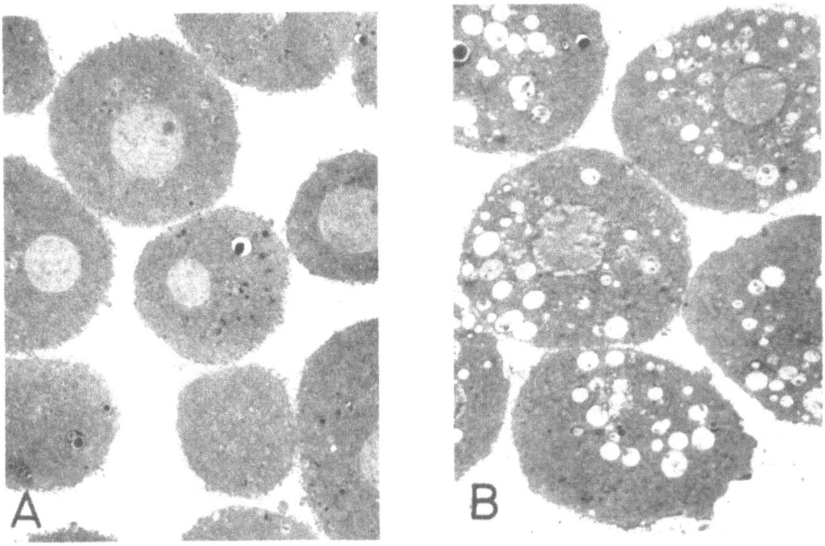

Fig. 4. Induction of lysosomal swelling by ammonia.
Electron micrograph of isolated hepatocytes incubated for 1 h at 37 °C without (A) or with (B) 10 mM NH_4Cl. × 1300. From [5]

Influence of amino acids from protein degradation on amino acid incorporation

Protein synthesis is usually investigated by measuring the incorporation of radioactive amino acids into protein. In Fig. 5, some of the problems of isotope incorporation are illustrated. Although protein labelling follows a near-linear time course, this does not mean that the rate of protein synthesis is constant. The hepatocytes continuously degrade protein and release unlabelled amino acids into the medium, and with only a tracer dose of [^{14}C]-valine present, as is the case here, the specific radioactivity will decline exponentially both extra-and intracellularly (broken line), because valine equilibrates extremely rapidly across the plasma membrane as shown in the figure. Since no corresponding decline in the incorporation rate is observed, the actual rate of protein synthesis must be continuously increasing (dotted line), thus compensating for the decreasing specific activity.

The latter assumption is corroborated by the experiment shown in Fig. 6, where [^{14}C]-valine was given at a sufficiently high concentration (5 mM) to maintain a constant specific activity even in the presence of ongoing proteolysis and amino acid release. It can be seen that the rate of protein labelling (open circles), which in this case should be a direct expression of the rate of protein synthesis, is continuously increasing.

One possible reason for the increase in the rate of protein synthesis might be the accumulation of amino acids from proteolysis, since it has been shown that amino acids stimulate protein synthesis in the perfused liver [22—24]. If so, a preincubation of the cells with amino acids prior to isotope addition would be expected to give a maximal incorporation rate right from the beginning, and this was indeed found to be the case (Fig. 6, closed circles). It can therefore be concluded that

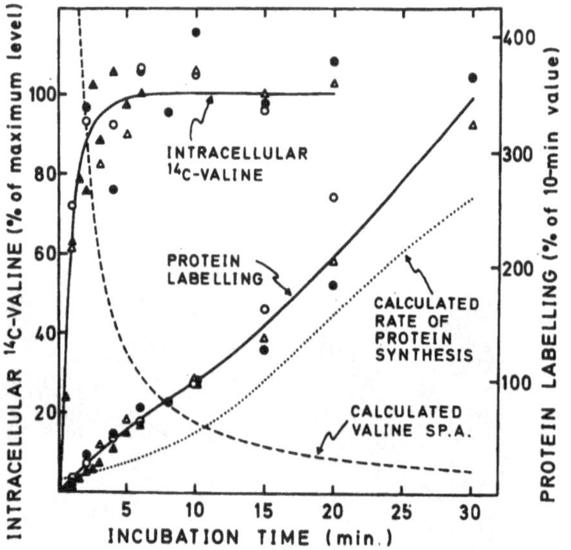

Fig. 5. Time-course of [^{14}C]-valine uptake and protein labelling in isolated rat hepatocytes. The cells were incubated at 37 °C with a tracer dose of [^{14}C]-valine (0.63 μCi/ml, 2.4 μM, 260 Ci/mol), and the net accumulation (0-min value subtracted) of perchloric acid-soluble (i.e. intracellular [^{14}C]-valine) and acid-insoluble (i.e. labelled protein) radioactivity in the cells was measured at various time points (solid lines). The relative specific radioactivity of intracellular valine ([^{14}C]-valine/total valine, broken line), was calculated on the basis of a linear increase in extracellular valine [8, 14] and the uptake curve shown in the figure. The relative rate of protein synthesis (dotted line) was calculated from the assumed valine specific activity and the protein labelling curve shown in the figure (labelling rate = valine sp.a. × synthesis rate).

Data from 4 different experiments (○, ●, △, ▲) are shown; each point is the mean of 2–4 cell samples. Arbitrary scales were chosen for valine sp.a. and rate of protein synthesis, which are relative values. From [9]

amino acids released during protein degradation may exert a stimulatory effect on protein synthesis.

Evidence for the stimulation of hepatocytic protein synthesis by amino acids was previously obtained by incubating the cells with a radioactive amino acid mixture at increasing concentrations [8]. As shown in Fig. 7, both the intracellular amino acid concentration and the intracellular radioactivity increase as a function of the extracellular concentration of radioactive amino acids. However, in addition to this expandable intracellular amino acid pool, there is a basal level of amino acids which can be considered as a non-expandable pool (i. e. a non-exhaustible pool which cannot be depleted by incubation in amino acid-free medium). If this non-expandable pool was mixing completely with the added radioactive amino acids, the intracellular specific activity would increase gradually as a function of the extracellular amino acid concentration, thus accounting for the increase in protein labelling. On the other hand, if there was no such mixing, protein labelling would take place from an amino acid pool of the same, constant specific activity at all amino acid concentrations (the extracellular pool or the expandable intracellular

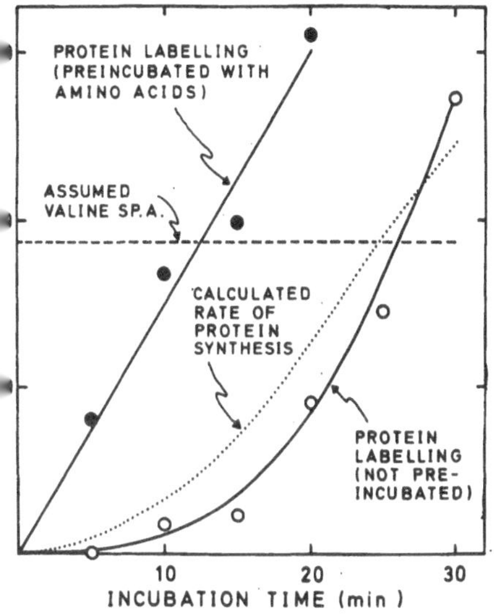

Fig. 6

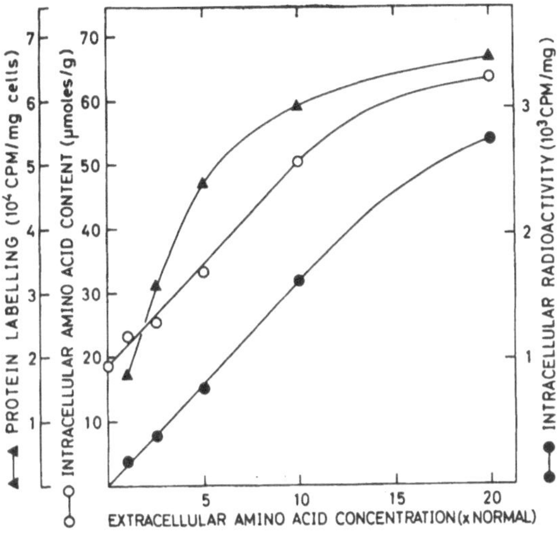

Fig. 7

Fig. 6. Protein labelling at constant [^{14}C]-valine specific activity: effect of amino acids. Isolated hepatocytes were preincubated for 30 min at 37 °C in amino acid-free medium (amino acid-depleted cells, ○) or with a physiological amino acid mixture [8], omitting valine, at 12.5 × normal concentration (amino acid-filled cells, ●). The cells were then re-incubated with 5 mM [^{14}C]-valine (0.63 μCi/ml) in an otherwise amino acid-free medium, and the net incorporation of radioactivity into protein was measured at various time points. The specific radioactivity of valine (broken line) could be assumed to be constant at this high valine concentration, i.e. the rate of protein labelling in the amino acid-depleted cells could be taken as a direct expression of the rate of protein synthesis (dotted line). The rate of protein synthesis in the amino acid-filled cells appears to be constant.

Each point is the mean of two cell samples. Arbitrary scales were chosen for valine sp.a. and rate of protein synthesis. From [9]

Fig. 7. Intracellular radioactivity, intracellular amino acid content and protein labelling as a function of the extracellular amino acid concentration.

Isolated hepatocytes (40 mg cells/ml) were incubated for 30 min with various concentrations of a [^{14}C]-labelled physiological amino acid mixture (100 mCi/mol). Cells were separated from the medium by centrifugation through metrizamide, and the intracellular amino acid content (○), acid-soluble radioactivity (●) and protein labelling (▲) were determined. From [8]

pool), and the stimulation of protein labelling would have to be an effect of amino acids on protein synthesis per se.

Two observations support the latter conclusion: firstly, when the precursor specific activity is held constant by "swamping" the cells with [^{14}C]-valine (5 mM), a mixture of nonradioactive amino acids (minus valine) still stimulate protein labelling. Secondly, the basal (i. e. non-expandable) amino acid pool can be shown by amino acid analysis to have a composition very different from e. g. the amino acid mixture released during proteolysis, suggesting very little mixing. The basal pool is particularly high in glycine, glutamine, taurine and phosphoethanolamine, and very probably represents a composite of different metabolic compartments which do not necessarily have any relationship to protein synthesis or degradation.

In order to learn more about the relationship between protein metabolism and amino acid pools, two questions were posed:

1) Are amino acids for protein synthesis taken from the expandable intracellular pool, or directly (e. g. by tRNA-aminoacylation in the plasma membrane) from the extracellular pool?

2) Is there a distinct "degradation pool" through which amino acids from protein degradation must pass before they equilibrate with the expandable intracellular pool or the extracellular pool?

Evidence for an intracellular location of the amino acid precursor pool for protein synthesis

One way to distinguish between an extracellular and an intracellular precursor pool for protein synthesis (which is a rather controversial question, cf. refs. [8, 9, 34—39]) would be to correlate protein labelling with the gradual influx of a non-

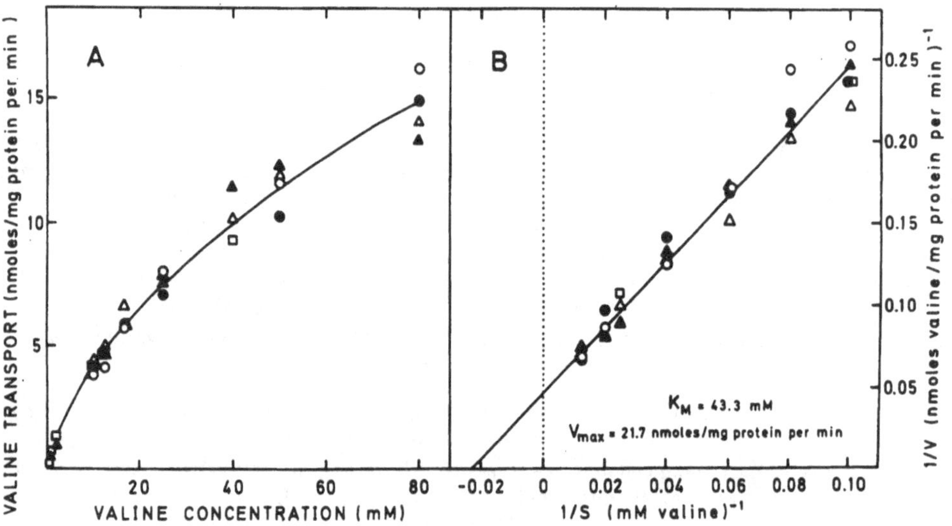

Fig. 8. Michaelis-Menten kinetics of valine transport.

Isolated rat hepatocytes were incubated at 37 °C, and the transport of [^{14}C]-valine at various concentrations (constant specific radioactivity) was measured during influx and efflux. In the influx experiments (●, △, □), the cells were incubated for 1 min with [^{14}C]-valine, and the net accumulation of intracellular radioactivity during this period was determined. In the efflux experiments (○, ▲), the cells were pre-loaded with [^{14}C]-valine during a 30-min preincubation, then washed at 0 °C, and the release of radioactivity into isotope-free medium during a 1 min re-incubation was subsequently measured. Since there were no significant differences between the results from influx and efflux experiments, all data have been combined. Each type of symbol represents a separate experiment; each value is the mean of three cell samples. A) Transport rate as a function of substrate concentration. B) Lineweaver-Burk plot of the 10—80 mM values from A.

The regression line, which was calculated by the method of least squares, gives a K_m of 43 mM and a V_{max} of 22 nmoles · mg protein^{-1} · min^{-1}. From [9]

metabolizable amino acid at tracer concentrations (i. e. constant extracellular specific activity; increasing intracellular specific activity). Unfortunately such studies have given conflicting results(cf. the discussion in ref. [9]), and one of the reasons for this is illustrated in Fig. 5: At 37 °C, the non-metabolizable amino acids (valine, leucine, isoleucine) equilibrate so rapidly across the plasma membrane that no distinction between intra- and extracellular pools can be made. The uptake of valine in isolated hepatocytes was therefore studied in some detail, with the hope of finding conditions which could slow down the uptake rate.
We found that valine transport is carrier-mediated, exhibiting Michaelis-Menten kinetics with a K_M of 43 mM (Fig. 8). The transport is furthermore non-concentrative (Fig. 9), energy-independent and largely Na^+-independent, and is stimulated by counter-transport (accelerative exchange). Valine transport can therefore be characterized as a facilitated diffusion (passive transport) process, similar to the L-system of CHRISTENSEN [40, 41].

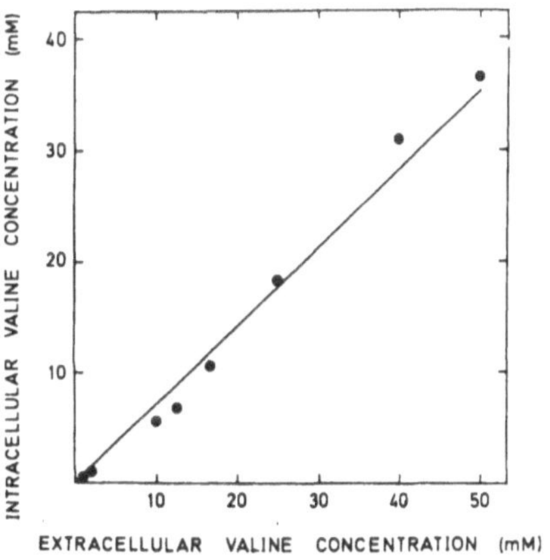

Fig. 9

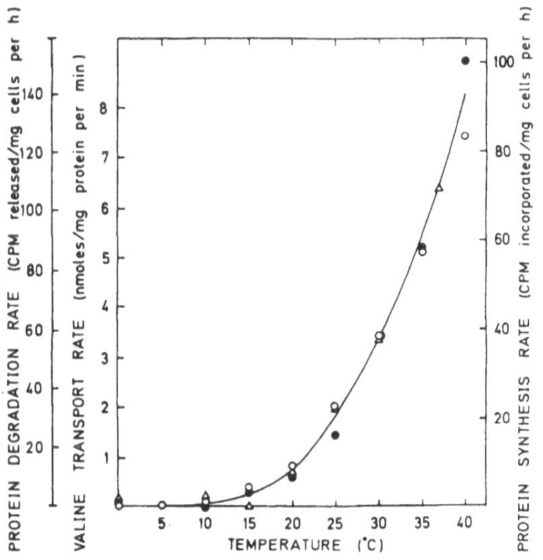

Fig. 10

Fig. 9. Relationship between intracellular and extracellular valine concentration. Isolated hepatocytes were incubated for 30 min at 37 °C with [^{14}C]-valine (16.7 mCi/mol) at the concentration indicated; the cells were then washed at 0 °C and the intracellular [^{14}C]-valine concentration was determined. Each point is the mean of two cell samples

Fig. 10. Effect of temperature on valine transport, protein synthesis and protein degradation. Isolated hepatocytes were incubated at various temperatures, and the rates of valine transport, protein synthesis and protein degradation were determined (in separate experiments) at each temperature. The rate of valine transport (○) was measured as the net uptake of [^{14}C]-valine (20 mM, 62.5 mCi/mol) during a 3 min incubation period. The rate of protein synthesis (●) was measured as the incorporation of [^{14}C]-valine (6 mM, 125 mCi/mol) into protein during a 10 min incubation period (from 15 to 25 min after the start of incubation). The rate of protein degradation (△) was measured as the net release during a 30 min period in the presence of cycloheximide (10^{-3} M) of [^{14}C]-valine from pre-labelled cells (1 h preincubation at 37 °C with 2.4 μM [^{14}C]-valine, 260 Ci/mol). Each point is the mean of 2–4 cell samples. From [9]

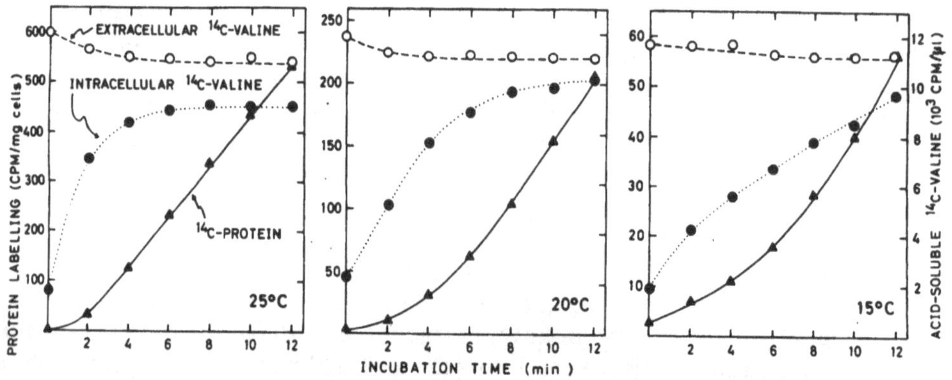

Fig. 11. [^{14}C]-valine uptake and incorporation into protein at different temperatures. Isolated hepatocytes were incubated with a tracer dose of [^{14}C]-valine (24 µM, 260 Ci/mol) at the temperature indicated, and the intracellular content of [^{14}C]-valine (●) and the amount of radioactivity incorporated into protein (▲) was measured at various time points. ○, Extracellular valine concentration. Each value is the mean of two cell samples. From [9]

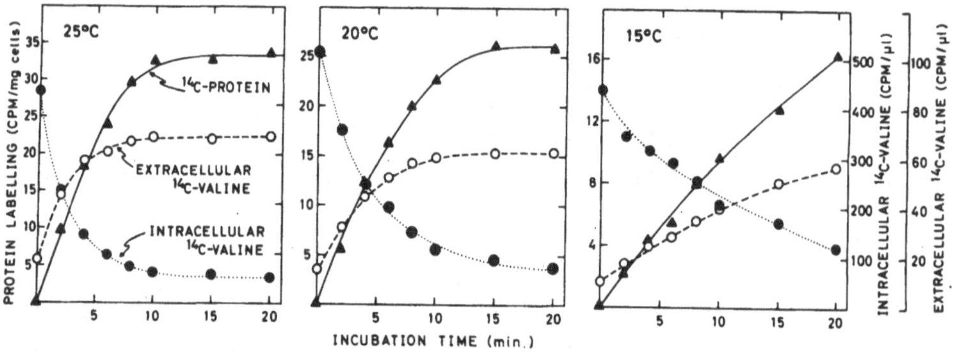

Fig. 12. [^{14}C]-valine efflux and incorporation into protein at different temperatures. Isolated hepatocytes were preincubated for 15 min at 15 °C with [^{14}C]-valine (2.4 µM, 260 Ci/mol), then washed at 0 °C and re-incubated in isotope-free buffer at the temperature indicated. The intracellular (●) and extracellular (○) concentrations of [^{14}C]-valine and the net incorporation of radioactivity into protein (▲, 0-min value substracted) were measured of various time points. Each value is the mean of two cell samples. From [9]

Since valine uptake is carrier-mediated, it is temperature sensitive to the same extent as protein synthesis and protein degradation (Fig. 10), with an activation energy of 14 kcal/mol [9]. By decreasing the incubation temperature, it is therefore possible to slow down valine transport, and at the same time the interference by proteolysis-derived amino acids is diminished due to the reduced degradation rate. The absolute rate of protein synthesis is unimportant, as long as it is measurable.

As shown in Fig. 11, at temperatures from 15 °C to 25 °C a gradual influx of [^{14}C]-valine with time can be observed. Protein labelling exhibits a corresponding lag, i. e. the labelling rate increases in parallel with the intracellular specific activity rather than staying constant like the extracellular specific activity. In a supplementary experiment (Fig. 12), the efflux of [^{14}C]-valine from pre-loaded cells was found to correlate with a parallel decrease in the protein labelling rate, confirming the conclusion [8] that amino acids for protein synthesis are taken from the intracellular (expandable) pool.

Fate of proteolysis-derived amino acids: Evidence for a degradation pool

The liver perfusion experiments of MORTIMORE et al. [42] demonstrated the presence of a non-expandable intracellular valine pool, the labelling characteristics of which suggested that it was derived from protein degradation. Amino acid analysis of isolated hepatocytes has likewise revealed the presence of a basal valine pool, but at such a low concentration ($\simeq$ 0.15 mM) that it could represent the steady state level maintained in the expandable pool (prior to exit into the medium) by continuous protein degradation.

In order to investigate this problem, an attempt was first made to selectively label the putative degradation pool with [^{14}C]-valine. In the experiment shown in Fig. 13, cells were incubated with [^{14}C]-valine for 1 h in the presence and absence of the protein synthesis inhibitor cycloheximide. Then the soluble [^{14}C]-valine in the expandable intracellular pool was extracted by a series of short incubations in isotope-free medium (the cells being allowed to equilibrate with the extracellular pool each time). It can be seen that after extraction of more than 99% of the initial intracellular soluble radioactivity, a distinct pool of [^{14}C]-valine remains in those cells which were allowed to synthesize protein during the incubation with isotope (i. e. in the absence of cycloheximide). Since this pool obviously has derived its [^{14}C]-valine from labelled protein, it could qualify as a true degradation pool.

The possibility that the pool might represent a steady state-level of amino acids in transit through the expandable pool could be discounted by an experiment in which protein degradation was blocked by 10 mM NH_4Cl. This treatment stopped

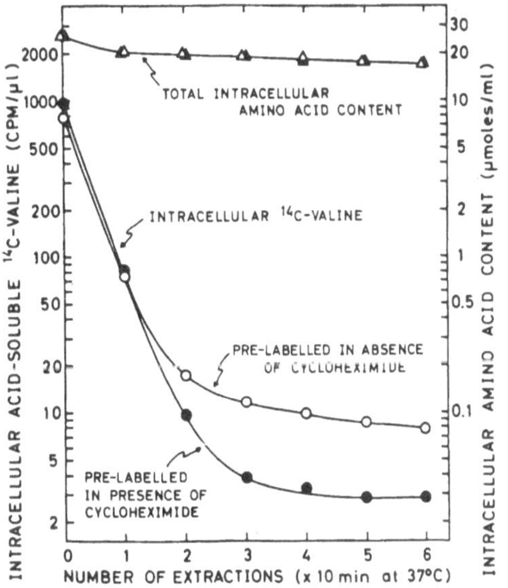

Fig. 13. Selective labelling of a protein degradation pool of valine.

Isolated hepatocytes were incubated for 1 h at 37 °C with [^{14}C]-valine (0.6 µCi/ml) in the presence (●, ▲) or absence (○, △) of cycloheximide (1 mM). After incubation, the cells were washed 6 × in ice-cold buffer; then re-incubated at 37 °C in cycloheximide-containing (1 mM) buffer for 6 consecutive 10 min periods (with change of medium each time) in order to extract as much as possible of the intracellular [^{14}C]-valine. The intracellular contents of [^{14}C]-valine radioactivity (○, ●) and amino acids (total ninhydrin-positive material, △, ▲) was measured in perchloric acid extracts of the cells. Each point is the mean of two cell samples completely the flux of [^{14}C]-valine (and other amino acids) to the extracellular medium during the extractions, but the amount of radioactivity in the putative degradation pool remained essentially unaffected throughout the extraction procedure. This radioactivity therefore does not equilibrate with the extracellular medium, and must consequently be different from the expandable [^{14}C]-valine pool.

Since ammonium chloride blocks protein degradation by a direct effect on the lysosomes [5], one would expect any postlysosomal valine pool to become rapidly depleted during NH_4Cl treatment. The degradation pool is clearly not depleted, and would therefore most probably reside within the lysosomes themselves. Direct evidence for this was obtained by centrifugation of a liver cell homogenate (post-nuclear supernatant) on a sucrose gradient after selective labelling of the degradation pool as described above. As shown in Fig. 14, essentially all of the radioactivity was found in the lysosomal-mitochondrial fraction, coinciding with the sedimentable peak of β-acetylglucosaminidase (a lysosomal marker enzyme) activity. In the presence of cycloheximide, no radioactivity entered the lysosomal fraction.

These results confirm the presence of acid-soluble protein degradation products in liver lysosomes as demonstrated by NEELY and MORTIMORE [43], and furthermore show that this lysosomal pool behaves as a distinct entity within the intact cell. It is perhaps surprising that lysosomes should retain [^{14}C]-valine so well both in vivo and in vitro, and the possibility must be considered that the radioactivity could represent small, acid-soluble [^{14}C]-valine-containing peptides. Alternatively,

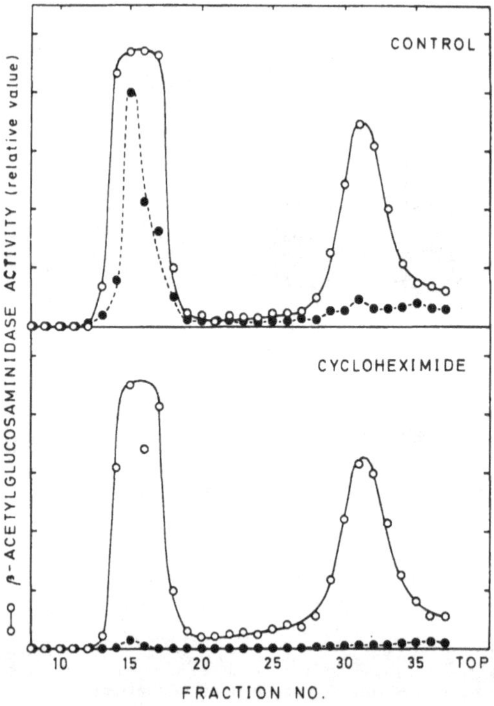

Fig. 14. Lysosomal location of the protein degradation pool of valine.

Isolated hepatocytes were incubated with [^{14}C]-valine in the absence (top panel) and presence (bottom panel) of cycloheximide, then washed and extracted by serial incubations as described in the legend to Fig. 13. The cells were homogenized, and the post-nuclear supernatants centrifuged on sucrose gradients as described in "Materials and methods". [^{14}C]-valine radioactivity (●-----●) and β-acetylglucosaminidase activity (○——○) was measured in the gradient fractions. The left peak indicates the position of intact lysosomes, while the right peak represents material remaining at the top of the gradient the lysosomal membrane may contain transport mechanisms for amino acids, tightly coupled with the proteolytic functioning of the lysosomes. Further experiments, e. g. identification of the radioactive component(s) in the lysosomes will be necessary to resolve this question.

Amino acid pools: General considerations

Our results suggest the presence of two major valine compartments in the liver cell: A lysosomal pool, which contains the immediate protein degradation products, and a general, expandable cytoplasmic pool, which provides the precursor amino acids for protein synthesis, and which equilibrates rapidly with the extracellular medium. The lysosomal pool most probably empties directly into the expandable cytoplasmic pool [42, 44]. Since essentially all of the non-lysosomal [^{14}C]-valine is easily extractable from the intact cells, it would by definition belong to the expandable pool, and any further intracellular sub-compartmentation would have to be within this pool. KHAIRALLAH and MORTIMORE [45] have, on the basis of valyl-tRNA specific activities, postulated the existence of a distinct precursor pool for protein synthesis, and there is even some evidence for different precursor pools for the synthesis of different proteins [46, 47]. Since cells are highly heterogenous with respect to intracellular structure, some micro-heterogeneity in the cytoplasmic (expandable) amino acid pool should perhaps be expected, possibly accounting for some of the anomalies observed in amino acid incorporation experiments. However, the biological significance of such pool micro-heterogeneity remains to be proven.

Acknowledgements

We wish to thank FRANCES DODMAN for her skilful technical assistance, and REIDAR OFTEBRO for his continuous interest. The work was supported by a grant from The Norwegian Cancer Society.

References

[1] GARLICK, P. J., J. C. WATERLOW, and R. W. SWICK: Biochem. J. **156**, 657 (1976)
[2] SEGLEN, P. O. in: Methods in Cell Biology. **13**, 29. D. M. PRESCOTT (Ed.). Academic Press, New York 1976
[3] SEGLEN, P. O.: Biochem. biophys. Res. Commun. **66**, 44 (1975)
[4] SEGLEN, P. O. in: Use of isolated liver cells and kidney tubules in metabolic studies. J. M. TAGER, H. D. SÖLING, and J. R. WILLIAMSON (Eds.). North-Holland, Amsterdam 1976, p. 245
[5] SEGLEN, P. O., and A. REITH: Expl Cell Res. **100**, 276 (1976)
[6] SEGLEN, P. O.: Expl Cell Res. **82**, 391 (1973)
[7] SEGLEN, P. O.: Biochim. biophys. Acta **338**, 317 (1974)
[8] SEGLEN, P. O.: Biochim. biophys. Acta **442**, 391 (1976)
[9] SEGLEN, P. O., and A. E. SOLHEIM: Eur. J. Biochem. (in press)
[10] MUNTHE-KAAS, A. C., T. BERG, and R. SELJELID: Expl Cell Res. **99**, 146 (1976)
[11] POOLE, B., and M. WIBO: J. biol. Chem. **248**, 6221 (1973)
[12] SEGLEN, P. O.: Norwegian J. Zool. **22**, Suppl. 1, 1 (1974)
[13] SEGLEN, P. O. in: Progress in differentiation research. N. MÜLLER-BÉRAT (Ed.). North-Holland, Amsterdam 1976, p. 205
[14] SEGLEN, P. O.: Biochim. biophys. Acta **496**, 182 (1977)
[15] SCHREIBER, G., J. URBAN, J. ZÄHRINGER, W. REUTTER, and U. FROSCH: J. biol. Chem. **246**, 4531 (1971)

[16] WEIGAND, K., and I. OTTO: FEBS Lett. **46**, 127 (1974)
[17] SEGLEN, P. O., and A. REITH: Biochim. biophys. Acta **496**, 29 (1977)
[18] JEEJEEBHOY, K. N., J. HO, G. R. GREENBERG, M. J. PHILLIPS, A. BRUCE-ROBERTSON, and U. SODTKE: Biochem. J. **146**, 141 (1975)
[19] VAN BEZOOIJEN, C. F. A., T. GRELL, and D. L. KNOOK: Biochem. biophys. Res. Commun. **71**, 513 (1976)
[20] BISSELL, D. M., L. E. HAMMAKER, and U. A. MEYER: J. Cell Biol. **59**, 722 (1973)
[21] BONNEY, R. J., J. E. BECKER, P. R. WALKER, and V. R. POTTER: In vitro **9**, 399 (1974)
[22] JEFFERSON, L. S., and A. KORNER: Biochem. J. **111**, 703 (1969)
[23] JOHN, D. W., and L. L. MILLER: J. biol. Chem. **244**, 6134 (1969)
[24] EKREN, T., K. F. JERVELL, and P. O SEGLEN: Nature New Biol. **229**, 244 (1971)
[25] WOODSIDE, K. H., and G. E. MORTIMORE: J. biol. Chem. **247**, 6474 (1972)
[26] SEGLEN, P. O.: Expl Cell Res. **107**, 207 (1977)
[27] KNOWLES, S. E., and F. J. BALLARD: Biochem. J. **156**, 609 (1976)
[28] CARPENTER, G., and S. COHEN: J. Cell Biol. **71**, 159 (1976)
[29] GLIMELIUS, B., B. WESTERMARK, and Å. WASTESON: Expl Cell Res. **108**, 23 (1977)
[30] BERG, T., and H. TOLLESHAUG: Acta biol. med. germ. **36**, 1762 (1977)
[31] GRIFFITHS, J. B., and S. J. PIRT: Proc. R. Soc. B **168**, 421 (1967)
[32] REIJNGOUD, D.-J., P. S. OUD, J. KÁS, and J. M. TAGER: Biochim. biophys. Acta **448**, 290 (1976)
[33] HEINZ, R.: Archs Pathol. anat. Physiol. **122**, 100 (1890)
[34] KIPNIS, D. M., E. REISS, and E. HELMREICH: Biochim. biophys. Acta **51**, 519 (1961)
[35] HIDER, R. C., E. B. FERN, and D. R. LONDON: Biochem. J. **114**, 171 (1969)
[36] VAN VENROOIJ, W. J., H. MOONEN, and L. VAN LOON-KLAASSEN: Eur. J. Biochem. **50**, 297 (1974)
[37] MORGAN, H. E., D. C. N. EARL, A. BROADUS, E. G. WOLPERT, K. E. GIGER, and L. S. JEFFERSON: J. biol. Chem. **246**, 2152 (1971)
[38] LI, J. B., R. M. FULKS, and A. L. GOLDBERG: J. biol. Chem. **248**, 7272 (1973)
[39] WETTENHALL, R. E. H., and D. R. LONDON: Biochim. biophys. Acta **390**, 363 (1975)
[40] CHRISTENSEN, H. N.: Fedn Proc. Fedn Am. Socs exp. Biol. **32**, 19 (1973)
[41] Le CAM, A., and P. FREYCHET: J. biol. Chem. **252**, 148 (1977)
[42] MORTIMORE, G. E., K. H. WOODSIDE, and J. E. HENRY: J. biol. Chem. **247**, 2776 (1972)
[43] NEELY, A. N., and G. E. MORTIMORE: Biochem. biophys. Res. Commun **59**, 680 (1974)
[44] HOD, Y., and A. HERSHKO: J. biol. Chem. **251**, 4458 (1976)
[45] KHAIRALLAH, E. A., and G. E. MORTIMORE: J. biol. Chem. **251**, 1375 (1976)
[46] ILAN, J., and M. SINGER: J. molec Biol. **91**, 39 (1975)
[47] FERN, E. B., and P. J. GARLICK: Biochem. J. **156**, 189 (1976)

Acta biol. med. germ., Band 36, Seite 1805—1813 (1977)

CSIRO Division of Human Nutrition, Kintore Avenue, Adelaide S. A. 5000, Australia

Attempts to relate enzyme inactivation to degradation in vivo

F. J. Ballard, M. F. Hopgood, S. E. Knowles, and G. L. Francis

Summary

Inactivation of liver cytosol proteins has been measured in vitro in the presence of various membranes and disulphides. Inactivation rates correlate with the known degradation rate constants of the enzymes in the intact liver. More extensive studies were carried out with glucose-6-phosphate dehydrogenase (G6PD) and phosphoenolpyruvate carboxykinase (PEPCK) using either cytosol as a source of these enzymes or alternatively highly purified preparations of each enzyme. All membranes purified from liver had a considerable capacity to inactivate the enzymes with higher avtivity found in the hepatocyte plasma membrane. Various lipid preparations or plasma membranes from other tissues were virtually ineffective. Inactivation was dependent on disulphides in the membranes as shown by the inhibition of activity if membranes were pretreated with thiols. Preliminary experiments of the fate of inactivated G6PD or PEPCK show binding to membranes and subsequent proteolysis. A model is proposed for the degradation of labile enymes.

Introduction

Attempts to measure intermediates in the degradation of proteins in vivo, and thus define the sequence of reactions involved, have been limited by two technical restrictions. These are the difficulty of labelling selectively a single protein within intact cells, and the uncertainty as to whether a protein so labelled or inserted into the cells mixes thoroughly with the normal unlabelled protein in the cells. To overcome these problems we have used broken cell preparations where the protein whose degradation is being investigated can be added, in some cases tagged with a radioactive marker. In these experiments as well as with measurements of enzyme activity changes in vitro it is hoped that any controlling factors discovered will be relevant to degradation in vivo. However, any proposed relationship is almost impossible to prove and the most optimistic result is a series of correlations between the two states. Such correlations, if discovered, can perhaps be used as a basis for more direct experiments on degradation in vivo.

Results and discussion

A problem with in vivo analyses of enzyme breakdown is the inability of obtaining the complete degradative pathway in disrupted tissues [1, 2]. Thus overall protein degradation is virtually stopped when tissues are homogenized and incubated at neutral *p*H, or if the energy status of cells is interfered with by the use of metabolic inhibitors. Notwithstanding the problems associated with measuring the total pathway of protein breakdown, it should be possible to perform meaningful experiments with tissue extracts, especially if the assumption is made that the first step in enzyme degradation in vivo is a rate-limiting loss of catalytic activity.

As an indirect test of the hypothesis that enzyme inactivation in vitro may be regulated by the same factors responsible for the control of degradation within intact cells, we selected for study a number of enzymes which were present in the cytosol fraction of rat liver, did not contain prosthetic groups and whose degradation rate constants had been measured in vivo. Enzymes with prosthetic groups were excluded because the rate of cofactor dissociation has been shown to correlate with degradation [3]. We measured the inactivation of two enzymes with long half-lives, lactate dehydrogenase and aldolase; two with short half-lives, phosphoenolpyruvate carboxykinase (PEPCK) and thymidine kinase; and two with intermediate stability, glucose 6-phosphate dehydrogenase (G6PD) and glucokinase. The order of degradation rate constants between the enzymes was approximately reproduced by the relative rates of their inactivation in liver slices and in liver homogenates [4]. Analogous results have found by other workers and correlations have also been reported between degradation rates in vivo and the susceptibility of enzymes to proteolytic inactivation [5, 6].

We have investigated further the inactivation conditions and have sought answers to the following questions:

(1) Where in the cell does inactivation occur?

(2) What is the nature of the reaction or reactions involved in enzyme inactivation and what regulates the rate of the process?

(3) What is the sequence of events following inactivation that leads to the complete breakdown of an enzyme into its constituent amino acids?

Intracellular localization of enzyme inactivation

Initial measurements of inactivation rates in liver homogenates and in other subcellular fractions have shown that the process does not follow simple first order kinetics [4, 7]. Often the enzyme tested, whether it is PEPCK, G6PD or aldolase, remains relatively stable for an initial period and is then inactivated at a continually increasing rate. Such kinetics are difficult to interpret but could possibly represent the gradual activaticn of the degradative pathway. Moreover, rates of inactivation of this type cannot easily be quantified because the initial stabilization may not be constant from one experiment to another.

Inactivation of G6PD by liver plasma membranes is shown in Fig. 1. In this experiment a cytosol fraction was incubated with the membranes and also in the presence of L-cystine. G6PD was stable in the cytosol incubated at neutral *p*H but was inactivated by plasma membranes and at an accelerated rate if 2 mM cystine was also added. Cystine alone did not inactivate the enzyme under the conditions used but was effective at higher concentrations. In most of the following studies on the intracellular distribution of inactivating capacity the process has been followed in a similar manner to that shown in Fig. 1; that is, using cytosol as a source of enzyme and testing the rate of enzyme inactivation in the presence or absence of 2 mM L-cystine. With this approach we discovered initially that G6PD inactivation or PEPCK inactivation in different subcellular fractions of liver homogenates proceeded most rapidly in the presence of a microsomal fraction and did not occur in the cytosol [4, 7]. Nuclear and mitochondrial preparations also had the capacity to inactivate the enzymes.

Further evidence for the microsomal localization of the inactivation capacity came from sucrose gradient analysis of the post-mitochondrial fraction [10]. In these

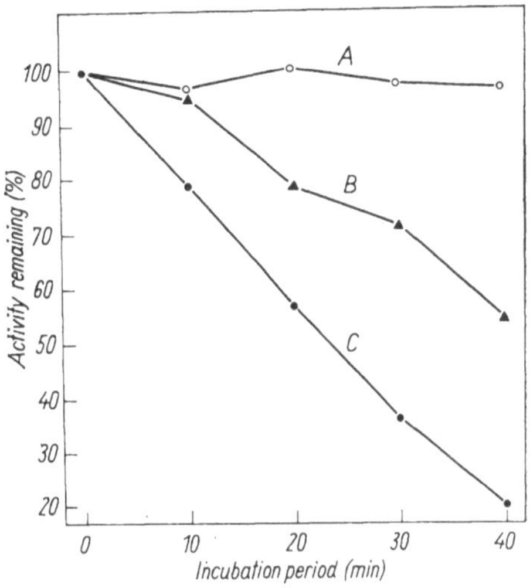

Fig. 1. Inactivation of G6PD by plasma membranes

A cytosol fraction prepared from 0.25 M sucrose homogenates of rat liver by centrifugation at 100,000 $\times g$ for 1 h was incubated at 37 °C in the presence of 20 mM Tris *p*H 8 and (A) 2 mM L-cystine *p*H 8, (B) 0.4 mg/1 ml of purified liver plasma membranes [8], or (C) cystine plus plasma membranes. At different times during the incubation samples were quickly chilled in ice and assayed for residual activity of G6PD [9]

studies the capacity banded with the microsomal marker glucose 6-phosphatase and was well separated from lysosomal or mitochondrial enzymes. Yet centrifugal forces which pelleted glucose-6-phosphatase from liver extracts still left a substantial portion of the inactivation capacity soluble [10], a finding which we interpreted as a localization of the capacity in small membrane fragments distinct from those in the endoplasmic reticulum. This concept was further supported when various membrane fractions were purified and their capacity to inactivate PEPCK and G6PD was tested.

Table 1
Inactivation of G6PD by various membranes

Source of membranes	Relative effect
Liver	
Smooth microsomes	++
Rough microsomes	++
Lysosomes	+
Lysosomal membranes	++
Plasma membranes	+++
Hepatocyte plasma membranes	+++
Reuber Hepatoma plasma membranes	++
Adipocyte ghosts	±
Erythrocyte ghosts	0
Everted erythrocyte ghosts	0
Reticulocyte ghosts	0
Liposomes from microsomal lipids	0
Liposomes from pure lipids	0

Membranes were incubated with a cytosol fraction of rat liver in the presence of 2 mM L-cystine at *p*H 8 and 37 °C. The ability to inactivate G6PD is rated on a scale from no inactivation after 2 hrs (0) to complete inactivation (+++). Different concentrations of membranes and different incubation periods were used in order to determine the relative effect.

In addition to microsomal membranes, inactivation capacity is also present in highly purified lysosomal membranes isolated from livers of Triton WR 1339-treated rats and especially from liver plasma membranes (Table 1). Indeed both these membranes were only slightly contaminated with microsomes as indicated by measurements of marker enzymes [8, 11] and the plasma membrane preparation had a greater capacity to inactivate G6PD than microsomes. Since these results are best interpreted as a generalised membrane localization of the inactivating factor, other membranes were isolated and their ability to inactivate G6PD or PEPCK was measured. Amongst a group of membranes which did not inactivate the enzyme either in the absence or presence of L-cystine were erythrocyte ghosts, everted and resealed erythrocyte ghosts, reticulocyte ghosts, as well as various liposome preparations made from pure lipids or from lipids extracted from microsomes by chloroform-methanol (Table 1). In order to show conclusively that the liver plasma membranes which inactivated G6PD had been isolated from hepatocytes and not from the endothelial cells in liver, hepatocytes were obtained by collagenase digestion of liver [12] and purified by differential centrifugation before being used as a source of the inactivating capacity. Plasma membranes prepared from this source had an ability to inactivate G6PD comparable to that found with plasma membranes from whole liver. Of the non-hepatocyte plasma membranes tested as a source for the inactivating factor, substantial activity was found with membranes obtained from monolayer cultures of Reuber H35 hepatoma cells. These cells retain a number of liver-specific functions, including an inducible PEPCK activity, and are similar morphologically to hepatocytes. Adipocyte plasma membranes had a slight capacity to inactivate G6PD (Table 1) and these cells contain both G6PD and PEPCK. Although very indirect evidence, the finding of inactivating capacity in the membranes of those cell types known to degrade the enzymes at a substantial rate would help validate the membrane factor as being involved in vivo in the degradation of cytosol enzymes.

Nature of the inactivation process

The capacity to inactivate PEPCK is destroyed by heating membranes at 50 °C or higher temperatures, is not extracted from the membranes by high ionic strength buffers and is not altered by incubation of membranes with phospholipase C. This evidence, together with the lack of inactivation capacity of liposomes prepared from liver microsomal lipids or of plasma membranes from erythrocytes, suggests that the inactivation capacity resides in a tissue specific membrane component, probably a protein.

Perhaps the most likely reaction by which enzymes could be inactivated would be by proteolytic cleavage. However, two lines of evidence argue against this:

(1) A wide range of proteolytic inhibitors did not alter the rate of PEPCK inactivation by liver extracts [10]. These inhibitors included those specific for cathepsin B, D, trypsin, and chymotrypsin, as well as broad spectrum inhibitors such as those present in serum.

(2) Inactivation of pure ^{3}H-labelled PEPCK by microsomes occurred by a sequence of events beginning with loss of catalytic activity followed by loss of reactivity towards a specific antibody directed against PEPCK, and finally loss of

solubility of the inactive enzyme [7]. Subsequent experiments showed that this last process was not simply a denaturation-like precipitation of enzyme but reflected the binding of inactive enzyme to the microsomal membranes [10]. Analysis of the radioactive protein on sodium dodecyl sulfate-acrylamide gel electrophoresis at various times during this sequence showed no evidence of either smaller molecular weight portions of PEPCK as would be expected if endoproteolytic cleavage had occurred, or a gradual fall in molecular weight as might be produced by exoproteolytic hydrolysis. Only with very prolonged incubation of ^{3}H-PEPCK with a concentrated microsomal preparation was there any indication of low molecular weight products [7].

If enzyme inactivation does not occur by proteolysis in the system we are studying what other reaction might be involved? As shown in Figure 1, inactivation of G6PD is accelerated by L-cystine. In addition to L-cystine, D-cystine and oxidised glutathione facilitated inactivation of G6PD and PEPCK while the thiol compounds dithiothreitol, reduced glutathione and L-cysteine protected the enzymes from inactivation [10]. Moreover, if liver plasma membranes are treated with dithiothreitol to reduce disulphide bridges and then the dithiothreitol is removed, the modified membranes have completely lost their ability to inactivate G6PD, even in the presence of L-cystine (Table 2). Although the inactivation capacity was partly restored by incubation of membranes in air, reactivation could be prevented by alkylation of the dithiothreitol-treated membranes with iodoacetamide. Unless membranes had been reduced with dithiothreitol, addition of iodoacetamide had no effect on the inactivation capacity.

Our interpretation of these results is shown diagramatically in Fig. 2. We propose that inactivation occurs by reaction of membrane disulphides with enzyme thiols, leading either to the creation of intra-enzyme disulphides or to enzyme-membrane mixed disulphides. The process is prevented by reduction of membrane disulphides with dithiothreitol, and fixed in the inactive state by iodoacetamide. Acceleration

Table 2
Modifications of plasma membranes and the subsequent effect on G6PD inactivation

Membrane treatments	G6PD inactivation (% remaining after 2 hrs)
None	3
Reduced	69
Alkylated	3
Reduced, oxidised	37
Reduced, alkylated, oxidised	100
Alkylated, oxidised	4
No membrane control	100

Purified plasma membranes from rat liver [8] were incubated with a cytosol fraction and 2 mM L-cystine at *p*H 8 and the degree of G6PD inactivation assessed as described in the legend to Fig. 1. Reduction of membrane disulphides with 50 mM dithiothreitol was followed by a washing of membranes by pelleting. Alkylation was accomplished by incubation of membranes in 0.1 M iodoacetamide *p*H 8. Reoxidation was attempted by incubating reduced or reduced and alkylated membranes in air for 2 hrs.

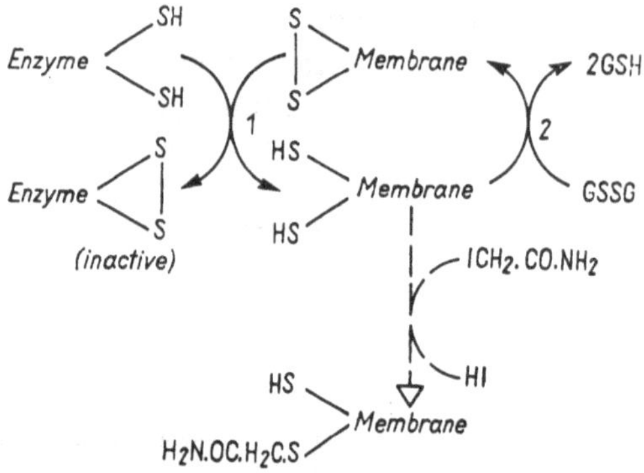

Fig. 2. Possible mechanism for enzyme inactivation by membrane disulphides

Active enzyme is envisaged as being oxidised to an inactive form by membrane disulphides in the presence of an inactivating factor "1". Membrane thiols are reoxcidised by a source of disulphide indicated here as GSSG and catalysed by a second enzyme "2". The site of action of iodoacetamide is indicated

of inactivation by L-cystine or oxidised glutathione could occur by reoxidation of membrane thiols after release of "scrambled" enzymes from the membranes (as illustrated in Fig. 2), or by a direct and perhaps independent oxidation of the enzymes without membranes being involved. Indeed high concentrations of L-cystine do inactivate G6PD in the absence of membranes and also result in the inactivation of liver cytosol enzymes with a selectivity similar to that found for the degradation of the enzymes in the intact liver.

Although many of the experiments described have been carried out with liver cytosol as a source of G6PD or other enzymes, qualitatively similar results are found if pure G6PD is inactivated by plasma membranes. With this more simple system G6PD must be stabilised with low concentrations of NADP in order to keep the enzyme active in the absence of L-cystine or membranes. Since higher concentrations of NADP (1 mM) completely protect G6PD from inactivation by membranes in the presence of L-cystine, it is evident that the ligand is maintaining the enzyme in a conformation not susceptible to disulphide attack. Analogous results are found with PEPCK, which is protected against inactivation by Mn^{2+} or Co^{2+}, the bivalent metal ions which are required for catalytic activity of the enzyme.

A major problem with the proposal for enzyme inactivation described in Fig. 2 is the normally high ratio of thiols to disulphides in cells, as exemplified by a GSH to GSSG molar ratio of at least 10 [13]. This ratio is maintained by the high activity of glutathione reductase (NADPH) and the ready availability of NADPH in mammalian cells. If the oxidation of protein thiols occurs as part of an ongoing system for the degradation of intracellular proteins, then reoxidation of membrane thiols must occur. While this could theoretically occur if there were localised regions of high GSSG to GSH ratio, the problem of regenerating GSSG still remains.

A more reasonable explanation for the reformation of membrane disulphides is a cycle of cystamine reduction to cysteamine with the cysteamine oxidised via the microsomal mixed function oxidase [14]. Cysteamine would not be rapidly reduced since it is not a substrate of glutathione reductase (NADPH). The intracellular concentration of cysteamine is close to the K_m for the mixed function oxidase [14] while the other substrates for the reaction, NADPH and molecular O_2, are readily available. Moreover, the localization of the enzyme on microsomal membranes is consistent with a potential role ancillary to the initial reactions of protein catabolism.

A number of enzymes have been described which catalyse disulphide exchange reactions either in the presence or absence of low molecular weight thiols or disulphides [15]. Such enzymes include the protein disulphide isomerase which catalyses disulphide exchange and the conversion of "scrambled" ribonuclease into the native enzyme, as well as GSH-insulin transhydrogenase which reduces disulphides in insulin and other proteins possibly as a step on the degradation of these extracellular proteins [16]. There is no definitive evidence that the various enzymes involved in disulphide exchange are distinct proteins [15, 17] and certainly we are in no position to equate any activity with the inactivation factor studied in our experiments. However, it does seem reasonable that one or a group of disulphide exchange enzymes could participate both in the correct folding of those membrane or export proteins which normally contain disulphide, and also catalyse the formation of disulphides in intracellular proteins which do not normally contain disulphides in their native configuration. This latter possibility would then reflect a stage in the breakdown of such proteins. Further, low molecular weight or membrane disulphides are envisaged to favour both the stabilization of disulphide-containing proteins and the catabolism of thiol-containing proteins.

Possible reactions following disulphide attack

Radioactive PEPCK that has been inactivated by membranes becomes attached to the membranes [7, 10]. The sequence of events in this process argues for attachment after inactivation, rather as though the membranes are acting as an intracellular fly-paper for "denatured" enzyme. Of course this process of attachment might be a trivial artifact of in vitro studies and may not be related to a degradation sequence in the intact cell. Nevertheless it is useful to consider binding as a potential step in enzyme breakdown because the process can be studied conveniently and the reaction conditions readily assessed. Further, accumulation of "denatured" proteins in vivo has been observed in situations analogous to those relevant to the degradation of enzyme with short half-lives such as PEPCK or G6PD. Thus the creation of abnormal proteins in bacteria or in reticulocytes by incubation of the cells in the presence of amino acid analogs is followed by the appearance of electron-dense inclusions which can be characterised as precipitated protein by disruption of the cells and differential centrifugation [2, 18]. We presume that the inclusions occur because the rate of the initial denaturation-like reaction becomes faster than subsequent proteolytic cleavage. A special example of the accumulation of intermediates in protein breakdown occurs in those erythrocytes with a reduced capacity to generate GSH from GSSG, due to genetic abnormalities in NADPH glutathione reductase, low activities of an NADPH generating system, or the presence of some factor which inhibits these processes [2]. Such data offers further circumstantial evidence for an important role of GSH and a high GSH to GSSG in the maintenance of intracellular protein in stable conformations.

Binding of inactivated enzymes may only be a transient part of the degradation sequence especially if a mixed disulphide between enzyme and membrane occurred

Table 3
Relationships between inactivation, binding to liver plasma membranes and degradation of ^{125}I-G6PD

Membrane treatments	Additions	Activity (% after 3 hrs)	Binding (% after 3 hrs)	Degradation (% after 3 hrs)
None	None	3	9.8	2.33
None	NADP	40	3.0	1.64
None	Cystine	2	11.2	2.03
Reduced, alkylated	None	100	2.7	0.64

Pure G6PD from rat liver was iodinated with ^{125}I-labelled Bolton-Hunter reagent [19] and incubated with liver plasma membranes (0.5 mg/ml) in 50 mM Tris, *p*H 8, at 37 °C. The concentration of other additions were NADP, 1 mM; L-cystine, 2 mM. Reduced, alkylated membranes were prepared as indicated in Table 2. Binding was determined after centrifugation of membranes at 100,00 × *g* for 1 h. Degradation was the percent conversion of radioactivity to trichloracetic acid-soluble material. Zero time values for binding and degradation have been subtracted.

during inactivation. Indeed, experiments with ^{125}I-labelled G6PD or ^{3}H-labelled PEPCK show 15% or 40% binding respectively of the enzymes to membranes even with 100% enzyme inactivation. However, conditions which result in inactivation of G6PD also produce the greatest amount of binding to plasma membranes (Table 3). Further, incubation of G6PD with erythrocyte ghosts, a situation which does not lead to inactivation, gives no binding of the enzyme to the membranes. In addition to the correlation between inactivation rate and binding shown in Table 3, degradation of the enzyme to amino acids is also greatest under conditions when inactivation is most rapid. Although the extent of total degradation is minimal, it is occurring in a highly purified system consisting of G6PD and plasma membranes and offers evidence for the existence of proteolytic enzymes in the membrane fraction. Thus BOHLEY et al. [20] have reported substantial proteolytic activity of intracellular membranes isolated from liver, and both their results and the present findings support the idea that total breakdown of intracellular enzymes can take place on membranes. Although such findings do not prove that total degradation does take place on membranes they do indicate the existence of a degradative pathway outside lysosomes and especially active against intracellular proteins of short half-lives.

Mention has already been made of the rapid breakdown of proteins containing analog amino acids such as canavanine. Recently GOLDBERG and JOHN [2] have reported the complete catabolism of these proteins in cell-free extracts at rates not much slower than found in whole cells. These and comparable results in our laboratory argue for the presence of an extra-lysosomal pathway of protein degradation perhaps analogous to the one proposed here for intracellular enzymes of short half-life. Moreover, the lysosomal system for protein catabolism is regulated by hormones, nutrients and inhibitors of proteolysis or protein synthesis that have little or no effect on the breakdown of abnormal proteins or labile enzymes within intact cells [21]. The two pathways of protein breakdown appear quite distinct, with one, the lysosomal system, responsive to gross stimuli but largely insensitive to the inherent stability of a cellular protein, whereas the second pathway is mostly regulated by the effectiveness of each protein as a substrate for degradation. The present experiments may be relevant to this second pathway.

References

[1] GOLDBERG, A. L., and J. F. DICE: A. Rev. Biochem. **43**, 835 (1974)
[2] GOLDBERG, A. L., and A. C. ST. JOHN: A. Rev. Biochem. **45**, 747 (1976)
[3] LITWACK. G., and A. ROSENFIELD: Biochem. biophys. Res. Commun. **52**, 181 (1973)
[4] HOPGOOD, M. F., and F. J. BALLARD: Biochem. J. **144**, 371 (1974)
[5] BOND, J. S.: Biochem. biophys. Res. Commun. **43**, 333 (1971)
[6] SALINAS, M., R. WALLACE, and S. GRISOLIA: Eur. J. Biochem. **44**, 375 (1974)
[7] BALLARD, F. J., M. F. HOPGOOD, L. RESHEF, and R. W. HANSON: Biochem. J. **140**, 531 (1974)
[8] ARONSON, N. N. Jr., and O. TOUSTER: Meth,. Enzymol. **31A**, 90 (1974)
[9] KORNBERG, A., and B. L. HORECKER: Meth. Enzymol. **1**, 323 (1955)
[10] BALLARD, F. J., and M. F. HOPGOOD: Biochem. J. **154**, 717 (1976)
[11] TROUET, A.: Meth. Enzymol. **31A**, 323 (1974)
[12] BERRY, M. D., and D. S. FRIEND: J. Cell Biol. **43**, 506 (1969)
[13] EGGLESTON, L. V., and H. A. KREBS: Biochem. J. **138**, 425 (1974)
[14] ZIEGLER, D. M., and L. L. POULSON: Trends biochem. Sci. **2**, 79 (1977)
[15] FREEDMAN, R. B., and H. C. HAWKINS: Biochem. Soc. Trans. **5**, 348 (1977)
[16] VARANDANI, P. T., and M. A. NAFZ: Diabetes **25**, 173 (1975)
[17] ANSORGE, S., P. BOHLEY, H. KIRSCHKE, J. LANGNER, J. MARQUART, B. WIEDERANDERS, and H. HANSON: FEBS Lett. **37**, 238 (1973)
[18] PROUTY, W. F., M. J. KARNOVSKY, and A. L. GOLDBERG: J. biol. Chem. **250**, 122 (1975)
[19] BOLTON, A. E., and W. M. HUNTER: Biochem. J. **133**, 529 (1973)
[20] BOHLEY, P., C. MIEHE, M. MIEHE, S. ANSORGE, H. KIRSCHKE, Y. LANGNER, and B. WIEDERANDERS: Acta biol. med. germ. **28**, 323 (1972)
[21] KNOWLES, S. E., and F. J. BALLARD: Biochem. J. **156**, 609 (1976)

Acta biol. med. germ., Band 36, Seite 1815–1820 (1977)

Division of Cell Pathology, Clinical Research Centre, Watford Road, Harrow, Middlesex HA1 3UJ, England

Lysosomes and protein degradation

ROGER T. DEAN

Summary

Evidence from studies on mouse peritoneal macrophages using the inhibitor pepstatin confirms lysosomal involvement in basal protein degradation, and extends its relevance to degradation of long half-life and analogue containing proteins. Studies on the ability of MRC-5 (a limited life-span fibroblast line) cells to selectively degrade analogue-containing proteins are described. These indicate that this capacity is retained even in very old cells; indeed such cells show an increased proportion of rapidly-degradable proteins. Analogue containing proteins bind preferentially to lysosomal membranes, and like liver cytosol proteins of short half-life, are selectively endocytosed and degraded by certain cells in culture. Thus membrane binding allowing selective entry to the lysosomal system may be important in controlling rate of degradation of both intracellular and extracellular protein. A method potentially allowing for determination of the rate of autophagy in cells, is described. This should enable further assessment of the quantitative involvement of lysosomes in protein degradation.

Introduction

This work extends previous work implicating lysosomes in the degradation of intracellular proteins. Further evidence on a hypothesis for selective degradation of lysosomes is also presented, together with studies on the turnover of proteins in cells ageing in vitro.

Materials and methods

Inhibitor experiments: Mouse peritoneal macrophages were collected and cultured as previously [1], with 10% acid-treated fetal calf serum (ATFCS) in Medium 199. Labelling was for 24–72 hrs (according to experiment) with [^{14}C]-leucine-free MEM with 10% ATFCS. After washing with PBS decay was allowed to proceed for 1–4 hrs before the cultures were washed a further three times and placed in MEM-ATFCS with 10 mM-leucine to follow breakdown. Sometimes the cells were labelled during the 1–4 hrs period with [^{3}H]-leucine, in the presence or absence of canavanine. 10 mM-leucine was found to maximise the output of TCA-soluble label, and thus to minimise reincorporation.

MRC-5 human diploid fibroblasts, 3T3 cells, and a rat liver culture line [2], were grown and treated as described [3]. MRC-5s were labelled for two successive 30 min periods with [^{3}H]-valine followed by [^{14}C]-canavanine, or vice versa. After extensive washing between and following the labelling, degradation was measured in the presence of carrier valine and canavanine. The latter was found to have no effect on the turnover of prelabelled material.

In each system, the output of TCA-soluble label was measured, using 5% TCA in the presence of the relevant carrier amino acid(s). TCA-soluble intracellular pools were shown to be satisfactorily depleted by the washings, and to remain approximately constant during the experiments. TCA-precipitable material in cells and medium was also studied. All the cell types release such material continuously; release by 3T3s and MRC-5s was insignificant, but that from macrophages was greater.

To study selectivity of binding and endocytosis, double-labelled dialysed liver cytosol proteins were used [4]; they were obtained from rats labelled as previously so that isotope ratio is an index of average half-life. Other rats were given [^{14}C]valine, or [^{4}H]valine in the presence of 10 mM-canavanine, i.p., and killed 30 min later. Dialysed cytosol and serum protein preparations from one protocol were mixed with equivalent amounts of protein from the other (cytosol with cytosol, and serum with serum). Mixtures were presented to cells in culture after Millipore filtration. Adsorption to the cell surface was measured after 10 min at 4 °C, by washing twice with PBS and counting. Digestion was followed as release of TCA-soluble label. Unilamellar liposomes (microvesicles) were prepared by standard methods [5] using sonication, with sterile solutions throughout; their composition was 10 μmoles phosphatidyl choline, 2.5 μmoles stearylamine, 7.5 μmoles cholesterol (used finally at 20 μmoles lipid per ml.). Labelled sucrose was included within them, and they were purified and freed of non-entrapped by gel filtration. They were supplied at 4 °C to 3T3s for 24 hrs, then removed and the cells washed, and incubated further at 37 °C. Cells were harvested at various times by scraping, and homogenised by sonication for 10 s in an MSE disintegrator at highest energy. Then sedimentability of the sucrose radioactivity at 100,000 × 60 min was assessed.

Results and discussion

Table 1 shows that pepstatin, the inhibitor most diagnostic of lysosomal proteolysis (since it inhibits only carboxyl proteinases, which in most cells are solely lysosomal, and since it does not penetrate cellular membranes, and thus does not distribute itself widely inside cells) inhibits the degradation of proteins of long half-life in macrophages. Inhibition is not detectable at 4 hrs, yet clear by 24 hrs, presumably reflecting the time taken for endocytosis of pepstatin. If pepstatin is only supplied for 30 min and then removed and medium replaced (no washing), no inhibition occurs, confirming that pepstatin does not permeate membranes. Previous work showed inhibition by pepstatin, presented in multilamellar liposomes, of short half-life proteins in perfusion, a situation of accelerated protein degradation. In contrast, the macrophage culture condition seems to be one of basal protein degradation. Macrophage turnover is probably accelerated in the absence of serum, though this dependence is only now under study. Thus lysosomes are probably involved in basal turnover of normal proteins of both short and long half-lives. Table 2 shows that pepstatin also inhibits the breakdown of short half-life proteins labelled in the presence of canavanine, an analogue which is incorporated in place of arginine. Thus lysosomes are involved in the turnover of analogue-containing, and by extension perhaps also of error-containing proteins.

Table 1
Inhibition of macrophage protein degradation by pepstatin

Time (hrs)	Degradation (% release of total label as TCA-soluble fragments)		Degree of Inhibition	Release into medium of TCA-precipitable label (% of total label in system)	
	Control	Pepstatin		Control	Pepstatin
2	4.25 ± 1.2	4.27 ± 0.5	—	4.2 ± 0.5	4.0 ± 0.6
24	39.5 ± 2.0	34.3 ± 1.7	14%	29.2 ± 4.2	25.4 ± 3.6

Pepstatin was used at 20 μg/ml (stock solution, 1 mg/ml in methanol) and controls contained identical amounts of methanol. Cells were labelled with [^{14}C]-leucine for 20 hrs, chased for 2 hrs and then placed in medium with 10 mM-leucine (cold). TCA-precipitable material released comprises both cell death (usually less than 15% as estimated by lactate dehydrogenase release) and secretion, and thus overestimates death.

Table 2
Inhibition of degradation of analogue-containing proteins by pepstatin

	Degradation (release of TCA-soluble label as % of total initial label)		Inhibition		Release of TCA precipitable label (% of total initial label)	
	^{14}C (long-term)	^{3}H (canavanine containing)	^{14}C	^{3}H	^{14}C	^{3}H
Control	56.0 ± 5.0	71.5 ± 4.8	—	—	17.1 ± 3.5	8.6 ± 2.9
Pepstatin	36.7 ± 2.2	45.8 ± 6.5	36%	36%	26.1 ± 2.5	15.6 ± 2.1

Cells labelled with [^{14}C]-leucine for 72 hrs and then with [^{3}H]-leucine in the presence of 1 mM canavanine for 4 hrs. Degradation was measured 24 hrs after the end of labelling. Release of TCA-precipitable material was accelerated by pepstatin, but the selectivity of release (^{14}C rather than ^{3}H) confirms that processes in addition to cell death are involved. The qualitative conclusion is not altered if degradation is expressed as % of (cellular TCA-precipitable label + total TCA-soluble label) at the end of the experiment), rather than as above.

Table 2 also confirms the inhibition of degradation of long half-life proteins by pepstatin. Other lysosomotropic agents (NH_4Cl, chloroquine) also inhibit degradation to varying degrees, as do colchicine and cytochalasin. Inhibition by cytochalasin suggests that microfilaments may be involved in some forms of autophagy, and it is hoped to test this idea using the method outlined below. The effects of these various inhibitors are under scrutiny at present.

It has been suggested that the production of errors in proteins may be important in in vitro senescence [7], and that removal of such proteins may be defective in aged cells. Dr. P. A. Riley and I have therefore assessed the capacity of MRC-5s of various passages to degrade normal and analogue-containing proteins. Both categories of proteins (short labelling) are degraded in two successive exponential phases. An initial brief rapid phase is followed by a more prolonged and slower phase. Canavanine-containing proteins show much shorter half-lives than normals (Table 3), but there are no trends in half-lives of the two phases for either category of proteins during culture senescence. The results are similar whichever labelling sequence is used. However, there is a progressive increase in the proportion of normal protein falling into the first phase (Table 4). The vast majority of cana-

Table 3
Half-lives of proteins in MRC-5 fibroblasts

Passage number	Phase 1 (min)		Phase 2 (hrs)	
	Valine	Canavanine	Valine	Canavanine
22	106	35	33	20
24	123	30	28	—
25	72	56	31	—
25	115	23	31	24
30	127	27	35	—
37	151	32	36	—
38	127	25	27	27
44	132	46	32	—
Mean	119 ± 23	33 ± 11	32 ± 3	24 ± 4

Table 4
Proportion of rapidly degraded protein (phase 1) in MRC-5s

Passage number	Valine (%)	Canavanine (%)
22	12	>91
24	27	>89
25	23	—
25	38	—
30	40	>98
37	46	—
38	52	—
44	57	>98

vanine containing protein always falls into this phase. There seems thus to be no defect in the degradation system for either type of molecule in senescing MRC-5s. Some previous contrary claims may be due to failure to suppress reutilisation [8], while others involve internally conflicting data [9, 10]. If such a deficiency does occur in any case, it seems to be only in the very last passage [9, 10] long after growth retardation has set in.

However, several groups agree that there is an acceleration of breakdown of normal proteins in ageing cells, and we have detected this quite early in the life-span of MRC-5s. There is no direct evidence as to whether this resulted from an increased rate of error production; but there is nothing to suggest that it results from a defect of degradation. Thus it is likely to be at best a secondary effect of ageing.

In assessing lysosomal mechanisms for degradation of analogue containing protein it was first shown that such proteins bind preferentially to lysosomal membranes (using the substrate mixture described in 'Methods' in the protocol of [11]). Then their adsorption to and degradation by cells in culture was studied (Table 5). There seems to be a tendency for preferential adsorption (not shown) and degradation of rapidly-turning over normal proteins and of canavanine-containing

Table 5
Degradation of endocytosed proteins by a rat liver cell line

Time (hrs)	$^{3}H/^{14}C$ ratios			
	Normal cytosol	Normal serum	(Normal + analogue cytosol)	(Normal + analogue cytosol)
Starting Material	3.66	5.53	1.04	0.81
Medium TCA-soluble label				
2	6.1	8.86	1.56	0.82
4	6.4	8.46	1.62	1.24
5	4.27	5.52	1.10	0.63

Each figure is derived from three cultures which gave figures within 10% of the mean. Cultures were in the presence of 10% heat-inactivated FCS. Control experiments show that degradation was not occurring in the medium; the proteinases therein were presumably inhibited by the serum.

proteins, as indicated by the elevated $^3H/^{14}C$ ratios This applies with both extracellular and intracellular proteins, and thus probably represents a general feature of the interaction of proteins with membranes as suggested first by Bohley [12]. This finding may explain the similarities in the characteristics of degradation of intra- and extracellular proteins [13]: the controlling step for both classes of proteins may be membrane bindings. Thus, as proposed earlier, membrane-binding may be the rate limiting step for lysosomal protein degradation [11, 12, 14].

The measurement of autophagy: Table 6 indicates that when 3T3s have been incubated at 4 °C for 24 hrs with microvesicles containing sucrose, the majority of cell associated labelled sucrose is non-sedimentable. There is much current debate on the mechanisms of association of liposomes with cells, but it is clear that fusion predominates when endocytosis is suppressed (as at 4 °C). This allows materials

Table 6
An index of autophagy: the time dependent association of cytoplasmic sucrose with sedimentable structures in 3T3 cells

Time (hrs)	Non-sedimentable radioactivity (% total)	Sedimentable radioactivity (% total)	Increase in sedimentable radioactivity	
			% total	% total non-sedimentable at 0 h
0	80.2 ± 2.7	19.8 ± 0.9	—	—
24	67.7 ± 14.9	32.36 ± 14.8	12.5	15.8
48	60.3 ± 1.9	39.6 ± 1.8	19.8	24.8
72	44.6 ± 3.1	55.5 ± 3.3	35.6	44.4

Figures are based on groups of three cultures.

entrapped in the liposomes to gain access to the cell cytosol, in which the majority should be nonsedimentable, as shown. Since sucrose does not penetrate cellular membranes, changes in its distribution (and thus sedimentability) should reflect primarily sequestration by membranes, i. e. autophagy. Indeed as cultures are incubated further, in the absence of external liposomes and sucrose, the sedimentable fraction of sucrose increases. Thus measurement of the rate of association of sucrose with sedimentable structures may be a valid measure of the rate of autophagy, and unlike morphological assessment, it is a dynamic method, and should include microautophagy. From initial rate measurements by detailed kinetic study, one could estimate the amount of soluble cytoplasmic material undergoing autophagy per hour. The long term data in Table 6 allows a minimum estimate: 16% in 24 hrs; this is a minimum because after joining lysosomal structures and thus becoming sedimentable, sucrose will tend to be transferred to larger more fragile structures, resulting in sedimentability of those molecules. Only 8% or less of the radioactivity initially associated with the cells was released in the medium, over 72 hrs. Extracts of the cells (1 mg/ml protein) were incapable of hydrolysing the sucrose at pHs between three and ten (tested over 2 h hrs and assessed by gel filtration).

An abstract [15] has appeared also reporting the time dependent association of micro-injected proteins with lysosomal structures, consistent with these microvesicle experiments. Different rates of association were observed with different proteins, and thus the earlier proposals of selective autophagy seem to be upheld. Preliminary experiments with the microvesicle system suggest that when double-labelled liver cytosol proteins are placed in the cell cytosol, those of short half-life become sedimentable more rapidly, in agreement with this.

The application of such methods to the study of autophagy should allow more detailed assessment of the quantitative role of lysosomes in protein degradation and of their contribution to specificity.

References

[1] Davies, P., R. C. Page, and A. C. Allison: J. exp. Med. **139**, 1262–1282 (1974)
[2] Paine, A. J.: Biochem. J. **158**, 109–117 (1976)
[3] Canagaratna, M. C. P., and P. A. Riley: J. cell. Physiol. **85**, 271–281 (1975)
[4] Dean, R. T.: Eur. J. Biochem. **58**, 9–14 (1975)
[5] Bangham, A. C., M. W. Hill, and N. G. A. Miller: Meth. Memb. Biol. **1**, 1–68 (1974)
[6] Dean, R. T.: Nature, Lond. **257**, 414–416 (1975)
[7] Orgel, L. E.: Nature, Lond. **243**, 441–445 (1973)
[8] Shakespeare, V., and J. H. Buchanan: Expl Cell Res. **100**, 1–8 (1976)
[9] Schimke, R. T., and M. O. Bradley in: Proteases and Biological Control. Cold Spring Harbor Laboratory, New York 1975, pp. 515–529
[10] Bradley, M. O., L. Hayflick, and R. T. Schimke: J. biol. Chem. **251**, 3521–3529 (1976)
[11] Dean, R. T.: Biochem. biophys. Res. Commun. **67**, 604–609 (1975)
[12] Bohley, P.: Naturwissenschaften **55**, 211–217 (1968)
[13] Dice, J. F., and A. L. Goldberg: Nature, Lond. **262**, 514–516 (1976)
[14] Dean, R. T., and A. J. Barrett: Essays Biochem. **12**, 1–40 (1976)
[15] Stacey, D. A., and V. G. Allfrey: J. Cell Biol. **70**, 3a (1976)

Acta biol. med. germ., Band 36, Seite 1821—1822 (1977)

Institute of Physiological Chemistry,
Martin-Luther-University Halle-Wittenberg,
402 Halle (Saale), GDR

Protein degradation in rat liver cells

P. Bohley, S. Riemann, R. Koelsch, and J. Lasch

Summary

The intracellular protein catabolism in isolated hepatocytes is inhibited by pepstatin and particularly by leupeptin in the presence of liposomes. Leupeptin has an inhibitory action both in the absence and in the presence of liposomes (nearly 40%).

Introduction

The main part of lysosomal and total proteolytic activities in rat liver at *p*H 6.7 in vitro is represented by the thiolproteinases cathepsin B 1, cathepsin L and cathepsin H which can be found in the soluble part of rat liver lysosomes.
In 1971 we demonstrated that these proteinases show in vitro a preference for the degradation of in vivo short-lived proteins [1, 2] and these results were fully confirmed later by Huisman et al. [3] and Segal et al. [4] and recently by Dean [5].
On the other hand, lysosomes contain the acid proteinase cathepsin D, and Dean found in perfused livers a remarkable inhibition of protein catabolism by addition of pepstatin containing liposomes [6].
Using isolated hepatocytes (prelabeled in vivo with [^{14}C]-guanidino arginine) we compared the effect of liposomes containing pepstatin and leupeptin on protein catabolism in the surviving cells.

Materials and methods

Male wistar rats (300—400 g) were narcotized using ether and phenobarbital. Rat liver proteins were labeled in vivo by injection of 250 μCi[^{14}C]-guanidino-arginine via the portal vein. 30 min later the livers were perfused and hepatocytes were prepared according to Seglen [7]. The isolated hepatocytes were incubated for 2 hrs with different kinds of liposomes and inhibitors. Liposomes were prepared according to Dean [6] as described in the following paper by Lasch and Koelsch. Protein degradation was measured as increase in trichloroacetic-acid-soluble radioactivity. About 3—4% of the protein-bound radioactivity became soluble during one hour of incubation.

Results and discussion

As shown in Table 1, the effect of leupeptin (37 ± 4% inhibition of protein degradation) on the intracellular proteolysis is significantly higher than that of pepstatin (only 26 ± 5% inhibition of protein degradation).
Leupeptin inhibits most effectively the thiolproteinases cathepsin B 1 and L and only a small part of lysosomal proteinases can be serine proteinases (compare Z. Salama, this symposium).
Therefore we conclude that cathepsins L and B1 are more important for protein degradation in hepatocytes than cathesin D, but the role for cathepsin D in Kupf-

Table 1
Protein degradation in isolated hepatocytes in % of the control incubation (2 hrs, 37 °C, O_2)

Control (hepatocytes + liposomes)	97 ± 9%
Hepatocytes + liposomes containing pepstatin	74 ± 5%
Hepatocytes + liposomes containing leupeptin	63 ± 4%
Hepatocytes + free leupeptin (10^{-5} M)	62 ± 3%

fer cells (participating in the total protein degradation in DEANS perfusion experiments) may be more important than in hepatocytes (compare D. KNOOK, this symposium).
However, in cell-free systems we found more than 70% inhibition by leupeptin and in the intact hepatocytes only about 40% inhibition. It remains to test other inhibitors in this very suitable system of isolated hepatocytes, but it is possible, too, that the diminished effect of leupeptin in the isolated intact cells is due to transport problems of the inhibitors.
In cell-free systems we found a selective inhibition of the degradation of short-lived cytosol proteins by leupeptin [8]. In particular, cathepsin L [9, 10] degrades preferentially short-lived proteins in vitro [8].
Especially cathepsin L [9, 10] is inhibited by leupeptin and is involved in the degradation of short-lived substrate proteins that are subject to rapid regulation in vivo, too. It seems important to investigate in detail the special functions of cathepsin L in vivo and to compare it with the other cathepsins.

References]

[1] BOHLEY, P., J. LANGNER, S. ANSORGE, M. MIEHE, G. MIEHE, and H. HANSON: Degradation of ^{14}C- and ^{3}H-labeled rat liver cytosol proteins by lysosomal endopeptidases. 7th FEBS Meeting, Varna 1971, 162

[2] BOHLEY, P., C. MIEHE, M. MIEHE, S. ANSORGE, H. KIRSCHKE, J. LANGNER, and B. WIEDERANDERS: Acta biol. med. germ. **28**, 323 (1972)

[3] HUISMAN, W., LINEKE LANTING, H. J. DODDEMA, J. M. W. BOUMA, and M. GRUBER: Biochim. biophys. Acta **370**, 297 (1974)

[4] SEGAL, H. I., J. R. WINKLER, and M. P. MIYAGI: J. biol. Chem. **249**, 6364 (1974)

[5] DEAN, R. T.: Eur. J. Biochem. **58**, 9 (1975)

[6] DEAN, R. T.: Nature, Lond. **257**, 414 (1975)

[7] SEGLEN, P. O.: Expl Cell Res. **82**, 391 (1973)

[8] BOHLEY, P., H. KIRSCHKE, J. LANGNER, B. WIEDERANDERS, and S. ANSORGE: Acta biol. med. germ. **35**, 301 (1976)

[9] KIRSCHKE, H., J. LANGNER, B. WIEDERANDERS, S. ANSORGE, P. BOHLEY, and U. BROGHAMMER: Acta biol. med. germ. **35**, 285 (1976)

[10] KIRSCHKE, H., J. LANGNER, B. WIEDERANDERS, S. ANSORGE, and P. BOHLEY: Eur. J. Biochem. **74**, 293 (1977)

Acta biol. med. germ., Band 36, Seite 1823—1827 (1977)

Institute of Physiological Chemistry,
Martin Luther University Halle-Wittenberg
402 Halle (Saale), GDR

Intracellular protein catabolism

IX. Hydrophobicity of substrate proteins is a molecular basis of selectivity

P. Bohley and S. Riemann

Summary

Double-labeled cytosol proteins from rat liver (^3H in short-lived, ^{14}C in long-lived proteins) were fractionated by using siliconized glass-beads, phenylsepharose and octylsepharose. Always the short-lived proteins are more tightly bound to the hydrophobic matrix. The same distribution was found with monkey liver substrate proteins. Therefore it is concluded that the different degrees of exposure of superficial hydrophobic areas on substrate protein molecules are a molecular basis of selectivity of the intracellular protein catabolism.

Introduction

There are different possibilities to explain the molecular mechanisms of selectivity of intracellular protein catabolism. One of the properties of substrate proteins which determine whether a protein is short-lived or long-lived may be the number of accessible and susceptible peptide bonds. Most of the intracellular proteinases show a similar specificity: they all split preferentially peptide bonds between hydrophobic amino acids (for a review see [1]).

A second property might be the high molecular weight implying more susceptible bonds, more different conformational stages, less stable native conformations and more errors in amino acid sequence [2]. Thirdly a positive correlation between isoelectric points and high turnover rates was found [3, 4], and finally, in 1968 we proposed a hypothetical mechanism of the selectivity of intracellular protein catabolism [5]: Different degrees of exposure of superficial hydrophobic areas of substrate proteins could cause different affinities for lysosomal membranes and/or for proteolytic enzymes. This means that apolar proteins are more susceptible for autophagy and proteinases and therefore short-lived [1, 5].

By using double labeled cytosol proteins [6, 7] we found selective aggregations of short-lived proteins [8, 9] (similar findings in bacteria and reticulocytes are reviewed by Goldberg and St. John [3]) and selective enrichments of short-lived proteins at apolar phases including liver fat [10]. In the last two years our hypothesis has been supported by further evidence from other laboratories. Dean [11] showed the selective binding of short-lived proteins at liposomes, lysosomes and liver membranes. Dice (cit. [3]) found their preferential association with immobilized aliphatic chains and recently similar work was published by Segal [12].

Hydrophobic chromatography without any mixed ion-exchange effects is in our opinion the best suited method to investigate our problem. We used phenylsepharose and octylsepharose and found indeed that the short-lived proteins are more tightly bound to the hydrophobic matrix.

Materials and methods

Double-labeled cytosol proteins from rat liver were prepared as described in [13]. Comparisons of the specific radioactivities (^{3}H-dpm per μg protein-nitrogen) yielded always the same results as the ^{3}H/^{14}C ratios, because the short-lived proteins with high turnover rates are preferentially ^{3}H-labeled. Therefore it was possible to investigate the distribution of short-lived proteins from monkey liver, too. An 8-year-old Rhesus macacus received 1 mCi ^{3}H-valine via the portal vein in phenobarbital narcosis. After 30 min the liver was perfused with 400 ml ice cold 0.9% NaCl-solution and the cytosol proteins were prepared as described in [13] for rat liver. All values for monkey liver are given as ^{3}H-dpm per μg protein-nitrogen. The conditions for hydrophobic chromatography [14] are: Start with 0.15 M KCl and 0.02 M K-phosphate, *p*H 7.1, lowering of KCl to 0.01, finally increasing Triton X 100.

Results and discussion

As shown in the Tables 1—4 short-lived proteins are preferentially bound to the hydrophobic matrix. The proteins with the lowest affinity were eluted by lowering the ionic strength. These proteins are the small part of the long lived ones bound to the sepharoses. Using low detergent concentrations a part of the short-lived proteins can be eluted. There are, however, some minor fractions of long-lived proteins eluted by 2% Triton-X100. The irreversibly bound proteins are mainly the short-lived ones. Better suited than phenylsepharose is octylsepharose (Table 2). We got similar fractionations of double-labeled cytosol proteins by using sili-

Table 1
Hydrophobic chromatography (Phenylsepharose)
of double-labeled proteins from rat liver cytosol
(short-lived proteins ^{3}H-labeled, long-lived proteins ^{14}C-labeled)

	% of total radioactivity		
	^{3}H	^{14}C	^{3}H/^{14}C
Without affinity	16	24	0.66
Eluted with 0.01 M KCl	18	28	0.64
Eluted with 0.2% Triton-X-100	11	8	1.37
Eluted with 5.0% Triton-X-100	3	2	1.50
Absorbed in 5.0% Triton-X-100	52	38	1.37

Table 2
Hydrophobic chromatography (Octylsepharose)
of double-labeled proteins from rat liver cytosol
(short-lived proteins ^{3}H-labeled, long-lived proteins ^{14}C-labeled)

	% of total radioactivity		
	^{3}H	^{14}C	^{3}H/^{14}C
Without affinity	24	35	0.68
Eluted with 0.01 M KCl	13	24	0.54
Eluted with 0.2% Triton-X-100	18	12	1.50
Eluted with 5.0% Triton-X-100	3	2	1.50
Absorbed in 5.0% Triton-X-100	41	27	1.52

Table 3
Fractionation of double-labeled proteins from rat liver cytosol (short-lived proteins ^{3}H-labeled, long-lived proteins ^{14}C-labeled) by use of siliconized glass beads

	% of total radioactivity		
	^{3}H	^{14}C	^{3}H/^{14}C
Without affinity	61	77	0.79
Eluted with 0,03 M KCl	17	17	1.00
Eluted with 0.2% Triton-X-100	6	4	1.50
Absorbed in 0.2% Triton-X-100	16	2	8.00

Table 4
Hydrophobic chromatography of proteins from Rhesus monkey liver cytosol (short-lived proteins ^{3}H-labeled)

	Octylsepharose			Phenylsepharose		
	% ^{3}H	% N	^{3}H/N	% ^{3}H	% N	^{3}H/N
Not bound	30.0	38.0	0.77	29.0	36.0	0.80
Eluted with 0.04 M KCl	30.0	42.0	0.72	27.0	34.0	0.80
Eluted with 0.01 M KCl	4.4	1.6	2.82	5.9	4.1	1.44
Eluted with 2% Triton-X-100	12.7	5.4	2.35	8.2	6.6	1.24
Bound in 2% Triton-X-100	22.9	13.0	1.76	30.0	19.0	1.57

conized glass-beads (Table 3). Finally, Table 4 shows that Rhesus monkey proteins show in principle the same behaviour as rat liver proteins: the short-lived proteins from the cytosol are more tightly bound to the hydrophobic matrix. Incidentally, the monkey liver shows a very low autoproteolysis.

A scheme summarizing our concept of intracellular protein catabolism can be found in [10]. The findings described in this paper support this concept: We propose to distinguish more and less stable conformations with respect to protein breakdown.

As a rule, in newly synthesized proteins the bulk of hydrophobic amino acids is buried (exceptions are membrane proteins and very short-lived proteins) and after dissociation into monomers, dissociation from organelles, dissociation of substrates, dissociation of cosubstrates, splitting of disulfide bonds, splitting of single peptide bonds and other changes, the proportion of superficial apolar amino acids can rise. Therefore, the protein molecule has more susceptible peptide bonds and also more possibilities for random aggregations and precipitation. These aggregates might be autophagized preferentially by lysosomes and after-wards proteolysis can follow. In our opinion, the most important advance of this concept is the possibility to explain regulations of protein catabolism by substrates and cosubstrates on a molecular basis, namely by changes from stable (more polar) to unstable (more apolar) substrate protein molecules.

There remain, however, many unsolved problems. We still do not know whether the regulation of intracellular protein catabolism by substrates and cosubstrates of the proteins depends actually on changes in the amount of superficial hydrophobic areas. Clearly, in the first stage of investigations the use of the whole cytosol containing some hundred different proteins is necessary to get some data of general importance. But, in this case, this terrible mixture cannot be used to test the effects of all substrates and cosubstrates on the affinity of cytosol proteins to apolar groups. To answer this question it seems necessary to test isolated substrate enzymes (compare J. BALLARD, this symposium). Whether these hydrophobic proteins are the big and acidic proteins, too, remains to be investigated. Aggregation and/or membrane binding of apolar short-lived proteins may be preconditions for autophagy. But unfortunately the process of autophagy itself is not very clear. In vivo undoubtedly autophagy occurs, as we know from morphological experiments. But all efforts to simulate autophagy in vitro have not yet been successful. This may depend on the partial energy requirement of intracellular protein catabolism. This energy requirement might allow some first insights into the molecular mechanisms of autophagy, too. Interactions among organelles in autophagy need to be proved, especially the role of resynthesis or rearragement in the Golgi system. There should, however, also be proofs for further causes of this energy requirement (e. g. resynthesis of short-lived activators such as glutathione and in general the maintainance of intralysosomal effector concentrations).

Some general statements

There is a lot of open questions in the field of intracellular protein catabolism that it seemed necessary to make some general statements all people can agree with. In the following list, statement number five was added by R. DEAN. There has not been any objection against this list during the symposium. It should be expressed, however, that the role of lysosomes in general should not be overemphasized. On the contrary, investigations of the primary step of intracellular protein catabolism must include all organelles.

Protein catabolism in rat liver cells:

(1) is necessary for changes in the composition of enzymes;
(2) occurs mainly intracellularly and is very extensive;
(3) has been found in all cell organelles;
(4) is different for different proteins even in the same organelle;
(5) some organelles turn over as an entity;
(6) is selective as to substrate proteins to be degraded;
(7) seems to be random as to the age of each molecule;
(8) may be altered by substrates and cosubstrates of the substrate proteins;
(9) depends on conformational changes of substrate proteins;
(10) is faster fo big, acidic and apolar proteins;
(11) is very rapid for abnormal proteins;
(12) occurs largely in lysosomes by endopeptidases;
(13) is finished in lysosomes and cytosol by exopeptidases.

References

[1] BOHLEY, P., H. KIRSCHKE, J. LANGNER, S. ANSORGE, B. WIEDERANDERS, and H. HANSON in: Tissue proteinases. A. J. BARRETT and I. T. DINGLE (eds.). 187. North-Holland, Amsterdam 1971

[2] SCHIMKE, R. T., and M. O. BRADLEY in: Proteases and biological control. R. REICH, D. B. RIFKIN, and E. SHAW (eds.). 515–531. Cold Spring Harbor Laboratory, USA

[3] GOLDBERG, A. L., and A. C. St. JOHN: A. Rev. Biochem. **45**, 747 (1976)
[4] MOMANY, F. A., J. J. AGUANNO, and A. R. LARRABEE: Proc. natn. Acad. Sci. U.S.A. **73**, 3093 (1976)
[5] BOHLEY, P.: Naturwissenschaften **55**, 211 (1968)
[6] BOHLEY, P., J. LANGNER, S. ANSORGE, M. MIEHE, C. MIEHE, and H. HANSON: Degradation of ^{14}C- and ^{3}H-labeled rat liver cytosol proteins by lysosomal endopeptidases. 7th FEBS Meeting Varna 1971, p. 162
[7] BOHLEY, P., C. MIEHE, M. MIEHE, S. ANSORGE, H. KIRSCHKE, J. LANGNER, and B. WIEDERANDERS: Acta biol. med. germ. **28**, 323 (1972)
[8] BOHLEY, P., H. KIRSCHKE, J. LANGNER, B. WIEDERANDERS, S. ANSORGE, and H. HANSON in: Intracellular protein catabolism. H. HANSON and P. BOHLEY (Eds.). Barth, Leipzig 1974/1976, p. 201
[9] BOHLEY, P., H. KIRSCHKE, J. LANGNER, B. WIEDERANDERS, S. ANSORGE, and H. HANSON: FEBS Meeting Budapest 1974, Abstracts 5256
[10] BOHLEY, P., H. KIRSCHKE, J. LANGNER, S. RIEMANN, B. WIEDERANDERS, S. ANSORGE, and H. HANSON in: Intracellular protein catabolism II. V. TURK and N. MARKS (Eds.). Plenum Press, New York and London 1977, p. 108
[11] DEAN, R.: Biochem. biophys. Res. Commun. **67**, 604 (1975)
[12] SEGAL, H. D. M. ROTHSTEIN and J. R. WINKLER: Biochem. biophys. Res. Commun. **73**, 79 (1976)
[13] BOHLEY, P., H. KIRSCHKE, J. LANGNER, B. WIEDERANDERS, and S. ANSORGE: Acta biol. med. germ. **35**, 301 (1976)
[14] HJERTEN, S., J. ROSENGREN, and S. PALLMANN: J. Chromat. **101**, 281 (1974)

Acta biol med. germ., Band 36, Seite 1829—1831 (1977)

[1] Physiologisch-chemisches Institut der Martin-Luther-Universität Halle, 402 Halle, DDR
[2] Insistut für Physikalische Chemie der Martin-Luther-Universität Halle, 402 Halle, DDR
[3] Pathologisches Institut der Martin-Luther-Universität Halle, 402 Halle, DDR

Pepstatin- and leupeptin-loaded liposomes: A tool in protein breakdown studies

J. Lasch[1], R. Koelsch[1], G. Brezesinski[2], V. Hermann[3], S. Riemann[1], and P. Bohley[1]

Summary

The preparation of proteinase inhibitor loaded "solid" positively charged liposomes is described. Some properties of the vesicle preparations are given and the findings are tentatively summarized in a scheme of liposomophagy.

Introduction

Incorporation of proteinase effectors in liposomes, biodegradable lipid vesicles, offers an intriguing strategy for the intracellular delivery of these compounds to the lysosomal apparatus.

Liposomes are taken up into cells both by endocytosis and by a nonendocytotic mechanism, which involves fusion of vesicles with the plasma membrane [1]. The nonendocytotic pathway predominates in the uptake of vesicles composed of phospholipids that were in the liquid-cristalline phase at experimental temperature. Vesicles prepared from "solid" phospholipids are instead incorporated largely by endocytosis.

Upon addition of sufficiently high amounts of cholesterol to the lipids (above 30 mol%) lecithin-cholesterol clusters are formed trapping nearly all phospholipid molecules which then do not longer take part in the phase transition. Thus cholesterol, by virtue of its solidifying effect, suppresses the ability of liposomes to fuse with plasma membranes [2] and favours endocytotic uptake.

There is ample evidence that the surface charge is also an important factor for the targeting of lipid vesicles to intracellular sites [1, 3] though the singificance of it is not yet fully understood. With positively charged liposomes both mechanisms of uptake (endocytosis and membrane fusion) seem to be operative but the degree to which proteinase inhibitors associated with cationic liposomes are delivered to the garbage system of the cell remains an open question.

This paper describes the preparation and some properties of pepstatin- and leupeptin-loaded positively charged liposomes that were to be used in protein breakdown studies in isolated hepatocytes (cf. the accompanying paper by P. Bohley et al.)

Materials and methods

16.98 mg synthetic lecithin (20 μmole), 8.09 mg cholesterol (20 μmole) and 2.70 mg stearylamine (10 μmole) were dissolved in 4 ml of chloroform/methanol (2:1, v/v). Leupeptin being amphipathic and pepstatin being highly hydrophobic dissolved readily in this solvent. 1 ml of peptide inhibitor solution containing 8 mg leupeptin and 13.1 mg pepstatin, respectively, was mixed with the lipid solution in a homogenator, dried under a N_2 stream und then kept overnight at 13.33 Pa (10^{-1} Torr). Empty liposomes for control experiments had the same composition but peptstatin and leupeptin were omitted. 3 ml of 10 mM potassium phosphate buffer *p*H 7.2, with 137 mM NaCl and 5.2 mM KCl was added to the lipid film and the lipid dispersed by 10 strokes of the homogenator piston. The milky suspension was left for equilibration for about 5 hrs. The lipid dispersions, filled into 3 ml thin-walled spherical glass vessels, were placed into the focus of a sonifier operating at 800 kc [1] and sonicated at varying temperatures (from 55 °C up to 70 °C) for different time intervals (40 to 60 min). Liposomes produced in this way were used for the in situ experiments the same day without further fractionation.

The thermotropic properties of the lipid mixture were determined with a Differential Scanning Calorimeter (Perkin-Elmer DSC-2). Concentrated samples of liposomes were sealed hermetically in aluminium pans and run at a scanning rate of 5 °C/min.

Aliquots of vesicle preparation were mixed with 1% phosphotungstic acid, *p*H 7.0, on 400-mesh Formvar-coated copper grids, blotted, air dried and examined in a SEM 3—2 electron microscope at 60 kV.

Results and discussion

A typical liposome preparation contained lecithin, cholesterol, stearylamine and peptide inhibitor in a molar ratio 6:6:3:5. Thin layer chromatography on silica gel confirmed that no detectable destruction of lipid molecules had taken place. The use of a sonifier operating without disruptor horn avoided contamination by traces of titanium which are usually ejected from the disruptor horn tip and which may have unpredictable effects on the cellular metabolism.

The differential scanning calorimetry revealed the immobilizing effect of cholesterol — phase transitions above 0 °C are completely abolished (cf. fig. 1) — confir-

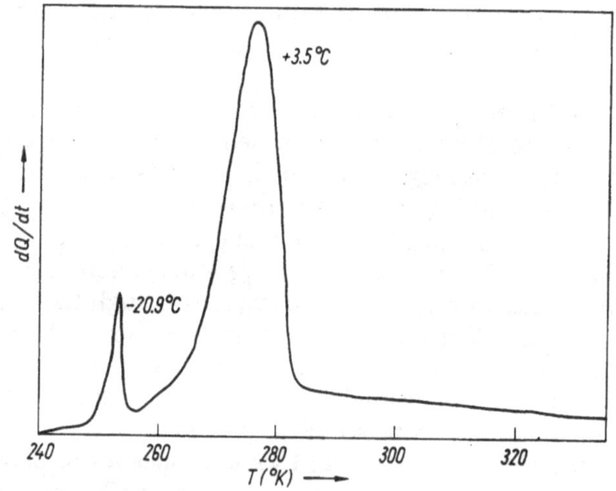

Fig. 1. Thermogram of the lipid mixture of the vesicle preparations.

The lipid suspension prepared in heavy water buffer was concentrated by vacuum dialysis in Sartorius bags 5fold and sealed in the calorimeter pans. The peak at +3.5 °C corresponds to the melting of heavy water. We have no explananation for the peak at −20.9 °C till now. No further endothermic process could be detected up to 120 °C. dQ/dt denotes endothermic heat flow

[1] We wish to thank Doz. Dr. H. FRISCHLEDER and Dr. K. ARNOLD (Physikalisches Institut der KMU Leipzig) for their valuable advice and for placing the sonifier at our disposal.

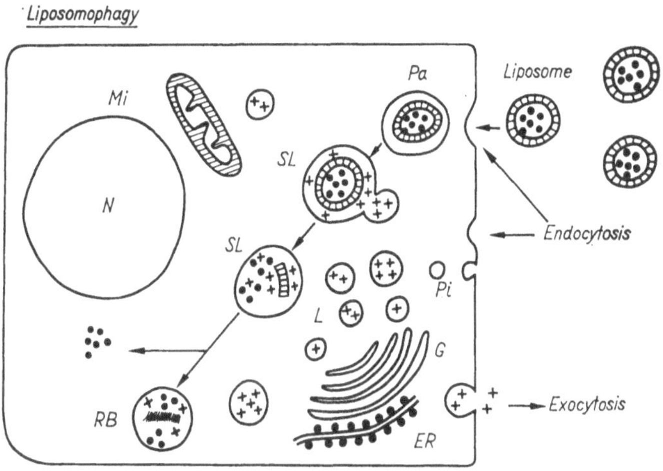

Fig. 2. Diagrammatic representation of endocytotic uptake of liposomes in the lysosomal apparatus

N: nucleus, Mi: mitochondrion, G: Golgi apparatus, ER: ergoplasmic reticulum, L: primary lysosomes, Pi: pinocytotic vesicle, Pa: phagosome, SL: secondary lysosomes and RB: residual bodies; ++++: lysosomal hydrolases and ●●●●: proteinase inhibitor molecules

ming that the lipid mixture was in the solid phase at an experimental temperature of 37 °C.

The examination in the electron microscope showed that only a part of the lipid was transformed into vesicles, whereas the other part had formed large aggregates, which might partly be artifacts of the specimen preparation.

Our results and the vast amount of reported experimental evidences in similar systems are summarized in Fig. 2.

This scheme does not take into account the quite recent finding [3] that a certain amount of the content of positively charged liposomes is discharged immediately into the cytosol by fusion with the plasma membrane. The alterations of lysosomal integrity by stearylamine, that becomes measurable 4 hrs after contact of liver cells with cationic liposomes [3], will not interfere with our conclusions because the hepatocytes were incubated only 2 hrs with the vesicle preparations in our experiments. In addition all possible effects of lipids on protein catabolism were blanked out by control experiments with empty liposomes.

It is well known that the lysosomal membrane has a limited permeability to materials with molecular weights greater than 230 [4]. Thus, the peptide inhibitors once directed into the lysosomal apparatus by their liposomal carriers will be unable to escape from it by diffusion. The molecular weights of leupeptin and pepstatin are 426 and 685, respectively. Therefore, we assume that they develop their inhibitory action within the "hydrolysis bags" of the cell.

References

[1] Poste, G., and D. Papahadjopoulos: Proc. natn. Acad. Sci. U.S.A. **73**, 1603 (1976)
[2] Papahadjopoulos, D., G. Poste, B. E. Schaeffer, and W. J. Vail: Biochim. biophys. Acta **352**, 10 (1974)
[3] Steger, L. D., and R. J. Desnick: Biochim. biophys. Acta **464**, 530 (1977)
[4] Gordon, S., and Z. A. Cohn: Int. Rev. Cytol. **36**, 171 (1973)

Acta. biol. med. germ., Band 36, Seite 1833—1836 (1977)

Department of Clinical Chemistry, Karl-Marx-University, 701 Leipzig, GDR

Turnover of lipogenic enzymes of rat liver in dependence on age

V. Richter

While aging, animal organisms synthesize and metabolize less lipids.
This results in an age-related increase of lipids in tissues and blood [1]. Our studies show an age-dependent reduction of the levels of several lipogenic enzymes of rat liver. Fig. 1 shows the decrease of the levels of glucose-6-phosphate-dehydrogenase, α-glycerophosphate-dehydrogenase, citrate cleavage enzyme and malic enzyme of rat liver in dependence on age.

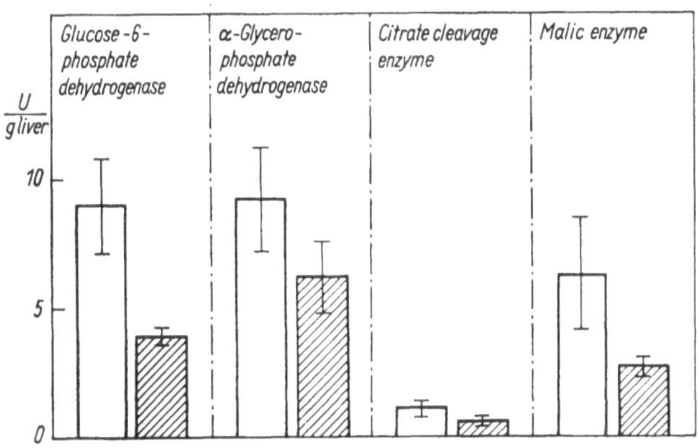

Fig. 1. Glucose-6-phosphate-dehydrogenase, α-glycero-phosphate-dehydrogenase, citrate cleavage enzyme and malic enzyme of rat liver in dependence on age.
Mean values ± standard deviation; □ 3 months, ▨ 18 month-old-rats

The age-dependent reduction of the levels of these lipogenic rat liver enzymes may be the result of an alteration in either the rate of enzyme synthesis, or of enzyme degradation or both. To distinguish between these possibilities, kinetic analyses were performed to obtain measures of the relative rates of synthesis and degradation. The analysis is based on the examination of returning the high enzyme activity from a sucrose diet to a standard diet.
As shown by Haining [2, 3], the change of enzyme levels under various dietary conditions may be thought of in terms of a transition of one steady state level to another. Kinetic analysis of this change enables the determination of the first order rate constant of enzyme degradation by plotting $\ln [E - E_0]$ versus time, where E_t represents the enzyme level at the time t and E_0 represents the new steady state level. The slope of this straight line is the degradation rate constants k_d. Because the enzyme level in the steady state is the quotient of the rate constant of synthesis and degradation, it is possible to calculate the rate constant of enzyme synthesis.

The levels of the measured lipogenic enzymes vary in accordance with the nutritional state; they are suppressed on starvation and restored on refeeding. The increase in enzyme levels that occurs on refeeding starved animals depends on the diet and is largest on diets high in carbohydrate, especially sucrose. Our results show no changes in the nutritional response of these enzymes as a function of age. The time dependence of returning the high enzyme level from a sucrose diet to a standard diet enables the calculation of the half-life time of the measured lipogenic enzymes. The observed enzyme activities, as assayed in the liver cytosol in vitro, reflect the amount of enzyme protein. GIBSON et al. [4] determined the half-life time of isotopically labeled enzymes. There were identical results with the two independent methods and this finding suggests that it is possible to determine the degradation rates of the lipogenic enzymes of rat liver by use of the kinetic analysis.

In Fig. 2 the values of ln $[E_t - E_0]$ of glucose-6-phosphate-dehydrogenase are plotted as a function of time. As can be seen from this figure, the rate constant for glucose-6-phosphate-dehydrogenase destruction of the 3-month-old rats is identical with that of the 18 months old rats. Therefore, the alteration in the rate of enzyme synthesis rather than that of enzyme degradation gives rise to the observed differences between the glucose-6-phosphate-dehydrogenase levels in the liver of 3- and 18-month-old rats.

Similar results were obtained by measuring the kinetics of the degradation rates of the lipogenic rat liver enzymes α-glycerophosphate-dehydrogenase and citrate cleavage enzyme. The degradation rate constants and the half-life time of these enzymes are unaffected by age, whereas the enzyme level decreases. Thus the diminished level of these enzymes in the liver of old rats can be ascribed to a reduced rate of enzyme synthesis.

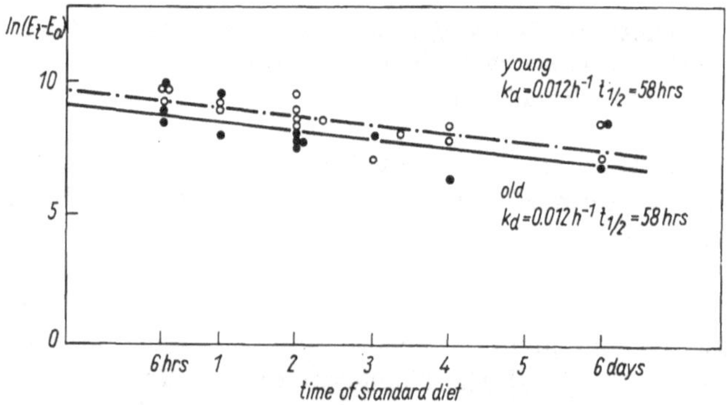

Fig. 2. Kinetics of glucose-6-phosphate-dehydrogenase degradation in vivo in dependence on age.

The slope of the straight lines is equal to k_d, the rate constant for enzyme degradation.*

*E_t: enzyme level at the time t after the change from sucrose diet to standard diet; E_0: the new steady state level under the conditions of standard diet. Each point represents the mean value of the enzyme level of 5 to 7 animals. The straight lines were calculated according to the method of least squares

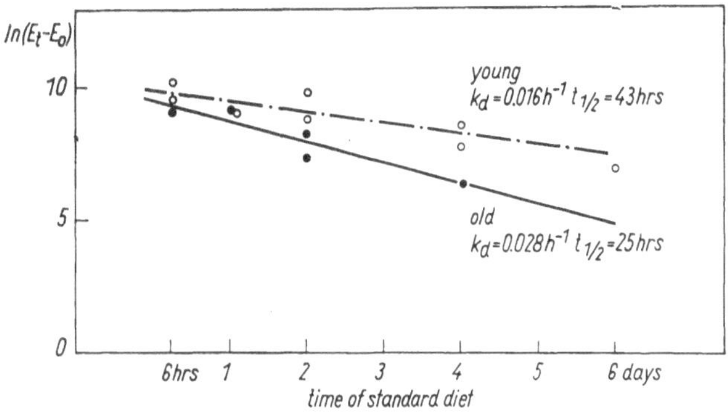

Fig. 3. Kinetics of rat liver malic enzyme degradation in vivo in dependence on age. Each point represents the mean of 5 to 8 rats

In contrast to these observations the half-life time of malic enzyme changes from 43 hrs in young rats to 25 hrs in the liver of old rats. In Fig. 3 the values of $\ln[E_t - E_0]$ of malic enzyme are plotted as a function of time. As can be seen from this figure, the rate constant of degradation of malic enzyme increases in dependence on age. This increased enzyme destruction contributes to the diminished enzyme level of old rat liver.

In Tab. 1 the obtained results are summarized. The diminished level of glucose-6-phosphate-dehydrogenase, α-glycerophosphate-dehydrogenase and citrate cleavage enzyme in old rat liver is the result of a decreased enzyme synthesis. The malic enzyme shows a remarkable difference in half-life between young and old rats and it appears therefore that the decrease of malic enzyme level in old rat liver might be partially due to an increased rate of breakdown of this enzyme. Almost identical results were obtained, if the enzyme levels were expressed on the basis of the liver DNA content instead of the basis of liver fresh weight. These studies on lipogenic enzymes seem to imply that the rate of synthesis, rather than the rate of degradation may be the preferential, although not necessarily the exclusive way to control the levels of the measured lipogenic enzymes in dependence on age.

Table 1
Synthesis and degradation of lipogenic rat liver enzymes

Enzyme	Age	$\frac{U}{g\ liver}$	k_d (h^{-1})	$t_{1/2}$ (h)	k_s $\left(\frac{U}{g\ liver \times h}\right)$
Glucose-6-phosphate-dehydrogenase	3 mo.	8.9 ± 1.8	0.012	58	0.107
	18 mo.	3.9 ± 0.3	0.012	58	0.047
α-glycero-phosphate-dehydrogenase	3 mo.	9.2 ± 2.0	0.018	38	0.166
	18 mo.	6.2 ± 1.4	0.018	38	0.111
Citrate cleavage enzyme	3 mo.	1.1 ± 0.3	0.024	29	0.026
	18 mo.	0.6 ± 0.1	0.024	29	0.014
Malic enzyme	3 mo.	6.3 ± 2.2	0.016	43	0.101
	18 mo.	2.7 ± 0.3	0.028	25	0.076

References

[1] Kritchevsky, D.: Mech. Age Dev. **1**, 275 (1972)
[2] Haining, J. L.: Archs Biochem. Biophys. **144**, 204 (1971)
[3] Haining, J. L., J. S. Legan, and W. J. Lovell: J. Geront. **25**, 205 (1970)
[4] Gibson, D. M., R. T. Lyons, D. F. Scott, and Y. Muto: Adv. Enzyme Regul. **13**, 187 (1972)

Acta biol. med. germ., Band 36, Seite 1837—1841 (1977)

Institute of Physiological Chemistry, Martin-Luther-University Halle/Wittenberg, 402 Halle, DDR

Aging changes in intracellular protein breakdown

B. WIEDERANDERS and I. RÖMER

Summary

Using radioactively labelled cytosol proteins as substrates we were able to exclude the possible accumulation of any specific inhibitor for the lysosomal proteases in rat liver cytosol during the aging process. There were also no gross changes in the molecular weight patterns of these proteins during the aging process. The percentage of more hydrophobic proteins seems to be identical in both the "old" and "young" cytosol proteins. From immunological experiments we suppose a qualitative change in the composition of rat liver cytosol proteins or of their properties during the aging process.

An increasing number of biologists working in the field of experimental gerontology try to explain the phenomenon of aging at the molecular level. In this connection it has been found that most of the metabolic pathways are altered in some way during aging [1]. From these studies it became clear that the protein metabolism is also altered. The kind of this variation is still a matter of discussion: Reports dealing with a diminished protein synthesis in old animals are just as known [2—9] as the counterpart [10, 11]. The same discrepancy can be found in communications on the turnover rates of proteins from animals of different age [8, 12—17]. At least a similar contradiction exists between results concerning the activity of intracellular proteolytic enzymes [14, 15, 18—24]. Despite the fact that in involuting organs and old cell populations the size and the number of lysosomal particles rises [25, 26], we found a weak but significant loss of specific proteolytic activity in liver homogenates of old rats [27, 28]. The smaller proteolytic activity at *p*H 3.0 and 6.0 was especially pronounced in the lysosomal fraction of rat liver homogenate, comparing a young and an old group of animals [27].

Changes in the properties or amount of proteolytic enzymes are not the only possible reason for a change in protein breakdown within the cell. Another reason could be a change in the primary reactions of intracellular protein breakdown, but studies at this level are unfortunately not possible up to now. The third reason could be a change of the digestibility of the substrate proteins. This should be indeed demonstrable experimentally. As we reported two years ago [27] this is in fact the case: Cytosol proteins from old animals are degraded more slowly than those from young animals. This result was very surprising in view of the fact that it was demonstrable only with liver cell derived lysosomal enzyme mixtures. Pepsin, trypsin, papain, pronase but also rat liver cathepsin D degrade "old" and "young" cytosol proteins at a similar rate. But the lysosomal enzyme mixture containing the cathepsins B, L and H [29] showed a proteolysis rate of old cytosol proteins 30% more slowly than those of "young" cytosols. The reason for this behaviour seems to be rather the different substrate concentration necessary for maximal

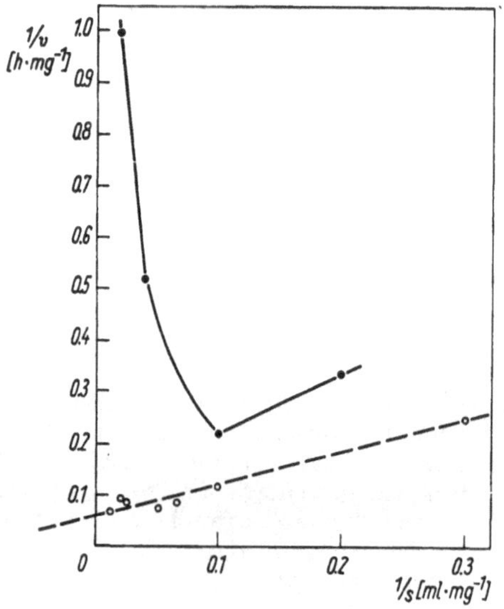

Fig. 1. Degradation of rat liver cytosol proteins by trypsin (o——o) and a soluble lysosomal enzyme mixture, containing the cathepsins H, L and B_1 (●——●). Dependence of the degradation rate on the substrate concentration, Lineweaver-Burk-plot. Incubation conditions for trypsin: 0.2M borate buffer, *p*H 7.5, 0.02% $CaCl_2$; for the lysosomal enzyme mixture: 0.01 M phosphate buffer, *p*H 6.1, 5 mM ethylendiamine tetraacetate, 5 mM dithiothreitol.

degradation rate using various proteinases (see Fig. 1). We found that the lysosomal enzyme mixture shows maximal rate at substrate concentration of about 10 mg/ml. The other enzymes need such high optimum substrate concentrations, which are not attainable due to precipitation of the proteins. We do not therefore believe that the variation of digestibility of the cytosol proteins by lysosomal proteases is rather due to changes in the substrate properties than in the specificity of the proteolytic enzymes.

First of all it was necessary to exclude the accumulation of a specific inhibitor for the cytosol degradation. The information came from mixing experiments: Lysosomal proteases were incubated with radioactively labelled cytosol of young animals in the presence of unlabelled cytosol from old animals and vice versa. The degradation of labelled proteins has been followed. No opposite influence of both kinds of cytosol could be verified in spite of their degradation rate neither by variation of the ratio of old/young cytosol nor by variation of the substrate or enzyme concentrations. Therefore we believe that no such inhibitor is present in the liver cytosol.

Thus it seemed reasonable to us to study such properties of proteins in the cytosol, which are in discussion to influence their own digestibility by proteases: the monomer molecular weight pattern [30], the charge pattern [31], the overall hydrophobicity on the protein surface [32], the percentage of error containing proteins [33]. At first we looked for the molecular weight patterns. It was impossible to find any significant qualitative or quantitative differences between old and young cytosols by means of SDS-polyacrylamide-gel electrophoresis under reducing and nonreducing conditions, as shown in Fig. 2. The only finding visible in the figure is that more protein is precipitated on the top of the gel in the case of the young cytosol, indicating a stronger tendency to aggregate under non reducing conditions. These indications and the results of Bohley et al. [34] lead us to suppose some differences in the hydrophobic character of these two protein groups. But

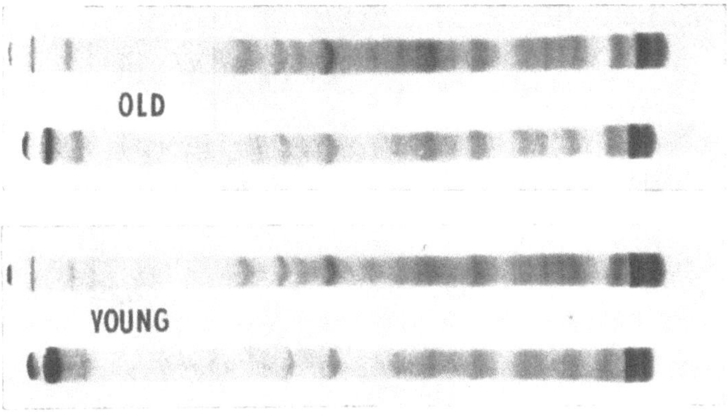

Fig. 2. Sodium dodecylsulfate polyacrylamide gel electrophoresis of 120 μg protein of rat liver cytosol from old and young animals (18 and 3 months, resp.).
11.1% polyacrylamide, containing 1% N,N'-methylene bisacrylamide; running-*p*H 9.2, 8 V/cm, 3 mA/tube, 180 min, staining with Coomassie Brillant Blue G-250. The proteins were denatured before the run in 0.1% sodium dodecylsulfate in the presence (the upper gels) and absence (the lower gels) of 1% β-mercaptoethanol

Table 1
Hydrophobic chromatography of cytosol proteins from livers of old and young rats

% of the total amount of proteins	Octyl-Sepharose		Phenyl-Sepharose	
	old	young	old	young
Non bound	47.4	47.4	42.1	45.3
Eluted with buffer	40.0	41.4	42.1	42.8
Eluted with Triton X 100	10.8	10.9	12.5	11.4
Bound after Triton X 100-treatment	1.8	0.3	3.3	0.5

The age of the animals were 7 and 21 months, resp. 200 μl radioactively labelled protein solution (0.5–1.0 mg/ml) in 0.2 M phosphate buffer, *p*H 7.1, were mixed vigorously with 500 μl Octyl- or Phenyl-Sepharose for 30 s. After sedimentation for 1 min in a centrifuge (TH 12, VEB Zentrifugenbau Engelsdorf) the supernatant was decanted. The Sepharoses were washed 3 times by adding 500 μl buffer of decreasing ionic strength. Then the gels were treated 5 times with 500 μl Triton X100 of increasing concentration (0.1–5%). The radioactivity and the nitrogen were determined in the supernatants. The recovery was between 92% and 105%.

as one can see in Table 1, our hope has been disappointed: the same amounts of proteins both of young and of old cytosols are bound to Octyl- or Phenylsepharose (Pharmacia, Sweden) and are eluted by Triton X100. This experiment has been done only once and has to be repeated. But similar results came from two experiments in which the distribution of the proteins was studied in a water/organic system. The same relative protein amounts were concentrated at the interphase both of the old and young cytosol proteins.

A study of the isoelectric points of the proteins by means of focusing them in *p*H gradients gave no satisfying results due to the precipitation of the proteins before reaching the final position on the gel.

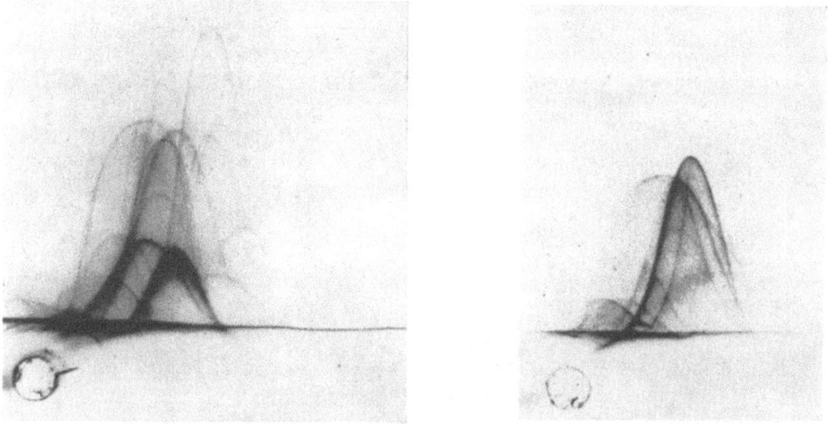

Fig. 3. Two-dimensional immunelectrophoresis in antibody-containing agarose gels. 300 μg rat liver cytosol proteins from a young animal (left) and an old one (right), were separated on a 5 × 5 cm glass sheet, loaded with 4 ml 1% agarose, containing 250 μl antiserum against "young" cytosol. 1st direction: 10 V/cm for 210 min; 2nd direction: 6 V/cm for 18 hrs. The antibodies were produced in rabbits. The ages of the rats were 5 and 20 months

At least a series of experiments was performed to find out immunological differences between the two groups of proteins. We immunized some rabbits with a mixture of three rat cytosols: one group with "old" and the other group with "young" proteins. So we obtained two multispecific antisera against cytosols from old and young rats. Thereafter we analyzed the extent of cross-reactions by means of two-dimensional immunelectrophoresis according to LAURELL [35]. Although we did not try to identify any single protein and although obviously only a very small part of the total mass of proteins in the cytosol is demonstrable by this method, we were able to draw some conclusions: Using antiserum against "young cytosol" we found (a) that the number of precipitation lines is smaller with "old cytosol" as antigen than with cytosol from young rats and (b) that the loss of precipitation lines affects especially the slowly moving proteins, i. e. those with more alkaline isoelectric points.

In the vice versa experiment with antisera against cytosols from old rats the differences were not significant and not so pronounced. Fig. 3 shows two examples for the two-dimensional immuno-electrophoresis with cytosols from young and old rats. How these differences have to be interpreted is a matter of speculation. But because obviously no other distinctions can be drawn between these two groups of proteins, we have to look forward on this way.

References

[1] WILSON, P. D.: Z. Altersforsch. **27**, 353 (1973)
[2] MURTHY, M. R. V., and D. A. RAPPOPORT: Biochim. biophys. Acta **95**, 121 (1965)
[3] BREUER, C. B., and J. R. FLORINI: Biochemistry **4**, 1544 (1965)
[4] MAINWARING, W. I. P.: Biochem. J. **113**, 869 (1969)
[5] HRACHOVEC, J. P.: Gerontologia **17**, 75 (1971)
[6] HELLTHALER, G., D. REIFEGERSTE, R. KÖHLER, and W. ROTZSCH: Z. Alternsforsch. **31**, 457 (1976)
[7] BIELKA, H., I. SCHNEIDER, L. VENKER, and A. HENSKE: Z. Alternsforsch. **31**, 7 (1976)

[8] DELL'ORCO, R. T., and P. L. GUTHRIE: Mech. age. devel. **5**, 399 (1976)
[9] GOLDSPINK, D. F., and G. GOLDSPINK: Biochem. J. **162**, 191 (1977)
[10] BEAUCHENE, R. E., L. M. ROEDER, and C. H. BARROWS Jr.: J. Geront. **25**, 359 (1970)
[11] BEZOOIJEN, C. F. A. van, T. GRELL, and D. L. KNOOK: Biochem. biophys. Res. Commun. **71**, 513 (1976)
[12] FLETCHER, M. J., and D. R. SANADI: J. Geront. **16**, 255 (1961)
[13] HAINING, J. L., J. S. LEGAN, and W. J. LOVELL: J. Geront. **25**, 205 (1970)
[14] COMOLLI, R., M. E. FERIOLI, and S. AZZOLA: Expl Geront. **7**, 369 (1972)
[15] OVE, P., M. OBENRADER, and A. I. LANSING: Biochim. biophys. Acta **277**, 211 (1972)
[16] HAVERBERG, L. N., L. DECKELBAUM, C. BILMAZES, H. N. MUNRO, and V. R. YOUNG: Biochem. J. **152**, 503 (1975)
[17] GOLDSTEIN, S., D. STOTLAND, and R. A. J. CORDEIRO: Mech. age devel. **5**, 221 (1976)
[18] ROSS, M. H., and J. O. ELY: J. Franklin Inst. **285**, 63 (1954)
[19] BARROWS Jr., C. H., and L. M. ROEDER: J. Geront. **16**, 321 (1961)
[20] BARROWS Jr., C. H., L. M. ROEDER, and J. A. FALZONE Jr.: J. Geront. **17**, 144 (1962)
[21] MARKS, N., and A. LAJTHA in: Protein Metabolism in Nervous System. A. LAJTHA (Ed.). Plenum Press, New York and London 1970, p. 39
[22] WATTIAUX, J. M., M. LIBION-MANNAERT, and J. DELCOUR: Gerontologia **17**, 289 (1971)
[23] LUNDHOLM, K., and T. SCHERSTEN: Expl Geront. **10**, 155 (1975)
[24] KNOOK, D. L., and E. C. SLEYSTER: Mech. age devel. **5**, 389 (1976)
[25] CRISTOFALO, V. J. in: Advances in Gerontological Research, **4**, 45. B. STREHLER (Ed.) Academic Press, New York 1972
[26] SCHMUCKER, D. L.: J. Geront. **31**, 135 (1976)
[27] WIEDERANDERS, B., S. ANSORGE, P. BOHLEY, H. KIRSCHKE, J. LANGNER, and H. HANSON in: Intracellular Protein Catabolism II. V. TURK and N. MARKS (Eds). Plenum Press, New York and London 1977, p. 144
[28] WIEDERANDERS, B., S. ANSORGE, P. BOHLEY, H. KIRSCHKE, J. LANGNER, and H. HANSON: Z. Alternsforsch. **31**, 175 (1976)
[29] KIRSCHKE, H., J. LANGNER, B. WIEDERANDERS, S. ANSORGE, P. BOHLEY, and U. BROGHAMMER: Acta biol. med. germ. **35**, 285 (1976)
[30] DEHLINGER, P. J., and R. T. SCHIMKE: Biochem. biophys. Res. Commun. **40**, 1473 (1970)
[31] DICE, J. F., and A. L. GOLDBERG: Proc. natn. Acad. Sci. U.S.A. **72**, 3893 (1975)
[32] BOHLEY, P.: Naturwissenschaften **55**, 211 (1968)
[33] SCHIMKE, R. T., and M. O. BRADLEY in: Proteases and Biological Control. **2**, 515. E. REICH, D. B. RIFKIN and E. SHAW (Eds.). Cold Spring Harbour Laboratories, New York 1975
[34] BOHLEY, P., and S. RIEMANN: Acta biol. med. germ. **36**, 1823 (1977)
[35] LAURELL, C.-B.: Anal. Biochem. **15**, 45 (1966)

Acta biol. med. germ., Band 36, Seite 1843—1853 (1977)

Institute of Physiological Chemistry, Martin-Luther-University Halle-Wittenberg, 402 Halle (Saale), DDR

Cooperation of various subcellular fractions in protein degradation in vitro

E. Schön and P. Bohley

Summary

In order to test the possibilities in protein degradation between cell organelles comparatively, [^{3}H]- and [^{14}C]-leucine short-time labelled subcellular fractions from rat liver were incubated with each other at *p*H 6.9.

All fractions tested were able to degrade short-lived proteins from foreign fractions, whereby the lysosomal supernatant fraction showed the highest proteolytic activity, which declines in the sequence: lysosomes — nuclei — mitochondria — cytosol — microsomes.

Short-lived cytosolic proteins were especially suited as substrate for neutral proteases from all other fractions, but also microsomal, mitochondrial and nuclear proteins were well degraded by foreign fractions in comparison with the substrate autoproteolysis.

Therefore in vivo manyfold cooperations between several organelles in protein catabolism seem to be possible.

Introduction

In elucidating the mechanisms of protein catabolism at the cellular level it is interesting to know whether each organelle is able to degrade its own proteins by itself or needs any cooperation with another organelle. The lysosomes became very fast a main research object in intracellular protein catabolism because of their content of a number of proteolytic enzymes [1—9], but the significance of the extralysosomal proteolytic mechanisms is still widely unclear, because the concerned enzymes in nuclei [10—12], mitochondria [10, 14—16, 18] (compare also Katunuma, Rubio, this symposium) and microsomes [10, 17] (compare also Langner, this symposium) are still insufficiently characterized [8].

Comparing the autoproteolysis of cell organelles in vitro with their in vivo turnover rates it has been stated that all particle fractions of rat liver should be able to degrade their own proteins by themselves and only cytosol proteins must be degraded in other organelles [19—22]. However, detailed investigations with short- and long-lived substrates showed that the short-lived proteins from microsomes, nuclei and mitochondria in vivo must likewise be degraded in cooperation with foreign organelles [23]. Only little information is available in the literature in view

Abbrevations: C = cytosolic fraction, E = enzyme fraction (fraction which proteolytic activity was tested), GSH = reduced glutathion, H = liver homogenate, HI-medium = medium used for homogenisation and incubation, L or LS = lysosomal supernatant fraction, LM = lysosomal membrane fraction, M = mitochondrial fraction, N = nuclear fraction, NMW = nuclear and mitochondrial wash water, PA = proteolytic activity, RSA = relative specific activity (multiple of activity of homogenate), R = microsomal fraction, S = substrate fraction (fraction which protein degradation was tested), $\pm$ s = standard deviation, $\bar{x}$ = mean value, TCA = trichloroacetic acid.

of the cooperation of cell organelles in protein catabolism. Several years ago Sawant et al. [24] studied the breakdown of ribosomal, nuclear and mitochondrial proteins by purified lysosomes, however, the proteolytic activity with the various freeze-thawed substrates were not quantitatively estimated. Bohley et al. reported on the breakdown of cytosolic proteins by lysosomal endopeptidases and other fractions [2, 11, 21, 25—27] (compare also Bohley, this symposium).
We aimed to study to what extent subcellular fractions of rat liver contain:

(1) proteolytic activity for degradation of short-lived proteins from foreign organelles at neutral *p*H and
(2) suitable substrates for neutral proteases from foreign organelles.

Materials and methods

Radioactive labelling and cell fractionation

In 9 experiments two male wistar rats weighing 233—356 g were narcotized by inhalation of ether and following intraperitoneal injection of a 2% sodium-phenobarbital (AWD Dresden). 0.2 mCi[^{3}H]-L-leucine (4, 5) (spec. act. 1.0 mCi/ml, Radiochemical Centre Amersham) or [^{14}C]-L-leucine (U) (spec. act. 0.2 mCi/ml, Radioisotope Institute Prague), resp., were slowly injected into the portal vein. After 30 min the livers were perfused with an ice-cooled Krebs-Henseleit- solution [128] of the following composition: 137.6 mM NaCl, 5.5 mM KCl, 4.125 mM $NaHCO_3$, 1.376 mM KH_2PO_4, 1.376 mM $MgSO_4 \cdot 7\ H_2O$, *p*H 7.3. This solution was proved to produce high incorporation rates in vivo [29]. During these 30 min the labelled amino acids were quickly enriched in the liver cells and mainly incorporated in short-lived proteins with high in vivo turnover rates [30—32]. On the average 17% of injected [^{3}H]-leucine and 15% of [^{14}C]-leucine were found in the liver protein (TCA-precipitable radioactivity).
The livers were removed, cut into pieces, pressed through perlon sieves (mesh diameter 0.8 mm) and homogenized with the equal volume HI-medium of the following composition: 250 mM saccharose, 40 mM KCl, 20 mM NaCl, 10 mM KH_2PO_4/K_2HPO_4 buffer, 5 mM GSH, 1 mM $MgSO_4 \cdot 7\ H_2O$, *p*H 6.9. The cell fractionation was carried out according to De Duve et al. [33] slightly modified [34]. The scheme of differential centrifugation is shown in Fig. 1. The liver homogenate H was centrifuged at $2.3 \cdot 10^3$ g · min (calculation of the integrated values according to [35]) obtaining the first nuclear sediment N', which was washed with four volumes HI-medium to give the nuclear fraction N. The supernatants of

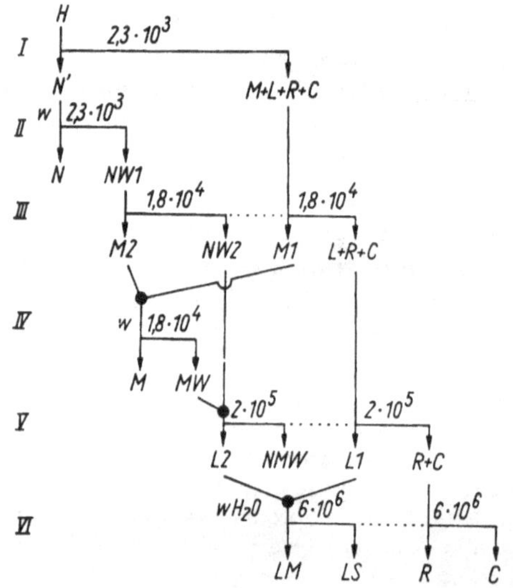

Fig. 1. Scheme of cell fractionation.
The sediment of each centrifugation step is shown below the left arrow, the integrated $g \times$ min — values on the horizontal beam and the supernatant below the right arrow.
w = Washing by homogenisation of the sediment with 4 volumes HI-medium and following centrifugation;
w H_2O = washing by homogenisation of the sediment with 2.5 volumes destilled water and following centrifugation;
● = combination of two fractions before homogenisation or centrifugation;
NW1, NW2, MW = wash fluids of nuclei and mitochondria, resp.; further abbrevations see foot note on the first page of the paper

the first two centrifugation steps were combined and centrifuged at $1.8 \cdot 10^4$ g · min receiving the mitochondrial sediments M1 and M2. These sediments were combined and washed with four volumes HI-medium obtaining the mitochondrial fraction M.
The lysosomes were obtained by sedimenting the supernatants of the steps III and IV at $2 \cdot 10^5$ g · min and after that disrupted by hypotonic lysis with 2.5 volumes destilled water. Centrifugation at $6 \cdot 10^6$ g · min yielded the liberated enzymes in the supernatant LS and the lysosomal membranes in the sediment LM. The supernatant of step V (R+C) was centrifuged to obtain the microsomal fraction R as sediment and cytosol C as supernatant.

Incubations and estimation of radioactivity

In order to determine the autoproteolysis in the fractions before and after incubation, each 100 µl of H, N, M, L, R and C were mixed on ice with 100 µl of HI-medium, incubated 120 and 0 min, resp., at 37 °C and cooled 2 min on ice.
To test the protein degradation of several combinations of different labelled fractions, in six experiments 100 µl of each of the two fractions were mixed. One of them was labelled with [^{3}H]-leucine, the other one with [^{14}C]-leucine. In three experiments we used unlabelled enzyme fractions from earlier cell fractionations.
The samples were incubated as described above; the ten combinations used were L–N, L–M, L–R, L–C, M–N, M–R, M–C, N–R, N–C, R–C.
200 µl 10% TCA were added to each sample and the precipitated protein was sedimented at $3.7 \cdot 10^4$ g · min. 100 µl TCA-supernatant were added to 15 ml scintillation liquid (0.4% 2.5-diphenyloxazolol, 0.03% 1.4-bis-2-(4-methyl-5-phenyloxazolyl)-benzol, 25% isopropanol in toluol p.a.) and counted in narrow channels of a liquid scintillation spectrometer model Packard-tricarb-3375 (yield of ^{14}C = 42%, ^{3}H = 27%, spill over of ^{14}C in the ^{3}H channel = 11%).
The total radioactivity in the fractions was determined by solving 10 µl fraction in 200 µl soluene (Packard) and adding of 5 ml scintillation liquid (composition see above, but without isopropanol). These samples were counted in wide channels (yield of ^{14}C = 66%, ^{3}H = 32%). The cpm-values were converted to dpm-values using the automatic external standardization and calibration curves.

Other methods

The total nitrogen concentration in the fractions was determined using a micro-Kjeldahl-procedure [36].
The activity of β-galactosidase (β-D-galactoside galactohydrolase EC 3.2.1.23) as a lysosomal marker enzyme was determined according to [37].
For all tables the mean values $\bar{x}$ and the standard deviations ± s were calculated. Using *t*-test the differences between ^{3}H- and ^{14}C-values were proved to be not significant.

Results

1. *Results of the cell fractionation*

The distribution of total nitrogen, total radioactivity and activity of β-galactosidase in the fractions are demonstrated in Table 1.
The relatively large deviation of the values may be due to the small amount of starting material (27 ml homogenate from one liver), which gave rise to different separations between sediment and supernatant.
As shown in Table 1 d, the radioactivity was significantly enriched in the fractions R and LM resulting from the distribution of ribosomes with a high content of newly built peptide chains (incorporating the radioactively labelled leucine) [31].
The calculation of the relative specific activity of β-galactosidase produced a fourfold enrichment of lysosomal enzymes in the fraction LS. The lysosomes were distributed among several fractions because of their density and volume hetero-

Table 1
Results of the cell fractionation.
$\bar{x}$ from 18 cell fractionations, $\pm s$ in parenthesis

Fraction	Total nitrogen		Total radioactivity		β-galactosidase	
	a Concentration (μg/ml)	b %	c %	d RSA	e %	f RSA
H	10.27 (2.50)	99.6	99.4	1.00	99.9	1.00
N	5.68 (1.95)	20.5 (9.3)	21.7 (10.3)	1.22 (0.52)	24.1 (2.6)	1.25 (0.36)
M	6.16 (1.64)	18.9 (7.7)	16.0 (5.5)	0.82 (0.12)	33.4 (11.8)	1.86 (0.44)
LM	9.02 (1.37)	11.8 (4.6)	16.6 (4.9)	1.47 (0.25)	9.5 (2.1)	0.86 (0.23)
LS	0.94 (0.28)	4.6 (2.2)	4.3 (1.6)	0.96 (0.18)	17.2 (2.0)	4.11 (1.00)
R	7.44 (2.75)	7.5 (2.8)	12.6 (6.0)	1.64 (0.28)	1.3 (0.6)	0.18 (0.04)
C	4.71 (1.07)	20,4 (3.8)	14.4 (3.1)	0.70 (0.09)	6.2 (2.2)	0.31 (0.08)
NMW	0.86 (0.30)	15.9 (4.4)	13.8 (5.7)	0.85 (0.25)	8.2 (4.4)	0.55 (0.31)

b Calculation of mg N in the fractions and percentage of each fraction on the sum of total N in all fractions.
c Calculation of total radioactivity in the fractions; percentage compare (b).
d RSA = relative specific activity as quotient of the values from columns (c) and (b).
e Calculation of activity of β-galactosidase in the fractions; percentage compare (b).
f RSA = relative specific activity of β-galactosidase as quotient of the values from columns (e) and (b).

geneity [16, 27, 38—42] (compare Rubio, this symposium). Therefore mainly mitochondrial and less nuclear fractions were contaminated by lysosomes.

2. *Protein degradation within the fractions*

The TCA-soluble radioactivity before incubation at 37 °C (so-called zero-minute-values) represents: (1) that part of labelled amino acids which are not yet incorporated into liver protein during 30 min in vivo, and (2) that another part of radioactivity being liberated as TCA-soluble peptides and amino acids resulting from autolysis of labelled proteins during the time span from incorporation in the proteins to TCA-precipitation (about 10 hrs at temperatures below 6 °C).
The sequence of the values in Table 2a (L, C, M, N, R) is in good accord with earlier data [21].
The increase in TCA-soluble radioactivity *after* incubation at 37 °C is shown in Table 2b and represents the proteolytic activity of the fractions degrading their own short-lived proteins. The lysosomal fraction LS produced the highest autoproteolytic values (4%), as expected from the high content of cathepsins. Lower values were obtained for mitochondria (partly produced by lysosomal contamination), nuclei and cytosol. Extremely low autoproteolysis was found in the microsomal fraction.

3. *Protein degradation between the fractions*

a) Proteolytic activity of the enzyme fractions
Determination of proteolytic activity (compare [21]) as

$$PA = \begin{pmatrix}\text{\% protein degradation} \\ \text{during 120 min}\end{pmatrix} \times \frac{\mu g \text{ N in the substrate fraction}}{\mu g \text{ N in the enzyme fraction}}$$

Table 2
Autoproteolysis (TCA-soluble radioactive material before and after incubation). $\bar{x}$ from 18–20 incubations, $\pm s$ in parenthesis

Fraction		a % protein degradation before incubation at 37 °C (zero-min-values)	b Increase of % protein degradation after incubation (120 min at 37 °C)
Homogenate	H	4.11 (1.63)	1.44 (0.67)
Nuclei	N	2.06 (1.12)	1.83 (0.87)
Mitochondria	M	2.39 (1.14)	2.24 (1.10)
Lysosomes	LS	18.24 (4.92)	4.04 (1.22)
Microsomes	R	1.69 (0.79)	0.62 (0.13)
Cytosol	C	15.69 (7.43)	1.15 (0.83)

a Quotient of TCA-soluble and total dpm/µl before incubation.
b Quotient of increase of TCA-soluble (120-min-values minus zero-min-values) and total dpm/µl after incubation.
Incubation conditions and determination of radioactivity see Materials and methods.

Table 3
Proteolytic activity of the fractions for degradation of short-lived proteins $\bar{x}$ from 8–14 incubations, $\pm s$ in parenthesis.

$$PA = \begin{pmatrix}\text{\% protein degradation} \\ \text{during 2 hrs at 37 °C}\end{pmatrix} \times \frac{\mu g\ N\ in\ S}{\mu g\ N\ in\ E}$$

Enzyme fractions (E) in the first line, substrate fractions (S) in the first column, in comparison substrate autolysis values (compare Table 2b) in the diagonal

S	E				
	N	M	LS	R	C
N	1.83 (0.87)	2.52 (1.19)	25.23 (10.74)	1.23 (0.88)	2.86 (2.15)
M	3.86 (1.41)	2.24 (1.10)	31.82 (7.88)	2.04 (0.97)	3.84 (2.24)
LS	1.57 (1.05)	1.20 (0.55)	4.04 (1.22)	0.70 (0.59)	1.79 (1.71)
R	1.40 (0.56)	1.47 (0.90)	14.03 (7.62)	0.62 (0.13)	1.16 (1.04)
C	4.68 (3.58)	3.97 (1.51)	26.37 (18.15)	1.57 (1.11)	1.15 (0.83)

Calculation of PA: TCA-soluble radioactivity after incubation of combination of each two fractions minus substrate autoproteolysis before incubation (zero-min-values, compare Table 2a) as percent from total radioactivity in the substrate fraction yields % protein degradation during 2 hrs (produced by acting of the enzyme fraction). These values were multiplied by the quotient of µg N in the substrate and enzyme fraction obtaining the PA-values.
Determination of radioactivity and incubation conditions see Materials and methods.

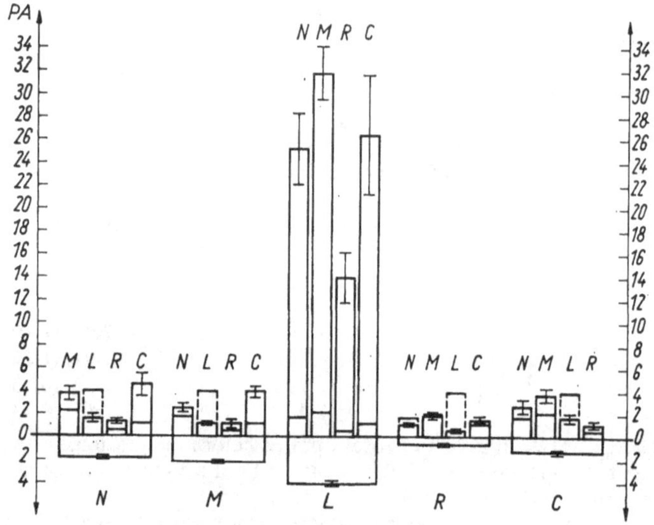

Fig. 2. Proteolytic activity of the enzyme fractions for degradation of short-lived substrate proteins.

Mean values $\bar{x}$ and standard errors of mean values $\pm s_m = \frac{s^2}{n}$.

Below the abscissa: The wide columns represent the autoproteolytic activity of the enzyme fractions (compare Table 2b).

Above the abscissa: The thin columns represent the proteolytic activity (PA) of the enzyme fraction for degradation of the various substrates (compare Table 3). In comparison the substrate autolysis values (compare Table 2b) are shown as horizontal lines within these columns.

Determination of PA see legend to Table 3

allows us to compare directly the protein degradation in combinations of subcellular fractions. These PA-values are shown in Table 3 and Fig. 2.

Under all combinations the lysosomal fraction LS possesses the highest specific activity (about 25%) for degradation of all short-lived substrate proteins, especially from mitochondria, cytosol and nuclei.

The proteolytic activity of the nuclear fraction N was one order lower (about 3%) and declined in the sequence C—M—L—R as substrates. The PA of the mitochondrial fraction M follows nearly the same order and sequence as that of N. The cytosol fraction C showed even less activity declining in the sequence M—N—L—R as substrates. At last the microsomal fraction R yielded the lowest PA. In all cases it did not reach the substrate autolysis values.

b) Suitability of the substrate fractions to degradation by foreign proteases

The other question was: Which fractions of the liver cell contain useful substrates for intracellular proteases and therefore be mainly degraded by foreign organelles in vivo?

In order to demonstrate this, the PA-values were converted to relative specific proteolytic activity (these RSA-values represent the portion of several enzyme

Table 4
Relative specific proteolytic activity of the enzyme fractions for degradation of short-lived substrate proteins.
($\bar{x}$ from 6–8 determinations, $\pm s$ in parenthesis). Enzyme fractions (E) in (the first line; substrate fractions (S) in the first column.

S	E				
	N	M	LS	R	C
N	0.57 (0.33)	1.20 (0.37)	10.21 (3.21)	0.70 (0.28)	1.58 (0.65)
M	1.14 (0.38)	0.47 (0.14)	9.19 (4.12)	0.66 (0.20)	1.62 (0.74)
LS	0.93 (0.48)	0.94 (0.38)	3.60 (2.08)	0.70 (0.32)	1.98 (0.75)
R	1.08 (0.60)	1.22 (0.66)	8.87 (3.46)	0.42 (0.14)	1.34 (0.94)
C	1.16 (0.18)	1.38 (0.59)	6.56 (2.28)	0.79 (0.41)	0.34 (0.12)

RSA = relative specific proteolytic activity

$$= \frac{\text{percentage of the enzyme fraction on the the sum of } (\% \text{ substrate protein degradation} \times \text{volume})}{\text{percentage of the enzyme fraction on total N}}$$

fractions on protein degradation in the substrate fraction), as shown in Table 4, or were related to the substrate autolysis values (equating the latter to 1.0) in Fig. 3. Short-lived cytosolic proteins are evidently suitable as good substrates for all fractions, especially for lysosomal proteinases. But also microsomal, mitochondrial and nuclear proteins are well degraded by foreign neutral PA in comparison with their substrate autoproteolysis.

Lysosomal proteins themselves are relatively unsuitable as substrates because of their high autolysis.

Generally in all fractions short-lived proteins were best degraded by lysosomal, and poorest by microsomal proteases. All fractions degraded foreign proteins better than own substrates.

Discussion

Undoubtedly the lysosomes represent the most important organelles in intracellular protein catabolism because of their high content of proteolytic enzymes and the great activity of lysosomes, lysosomal extracts and highly purified lysosomal endopeptidases for degradation of various extra- and intracellular substrate proteins [1, 2, 6, 20–25, 39, 43–48].

Many papers deal with the degradation of substrate proteins from various organelles by lysosomes. BETZ et al. [49] and BOHLEY et al. [23, 26] found that lysosomal endopeptidases in vitro preferentially degrade short-lived cytosolic and long-lived microsomal proteins. The former phenomenon can be confirmed by our pre-

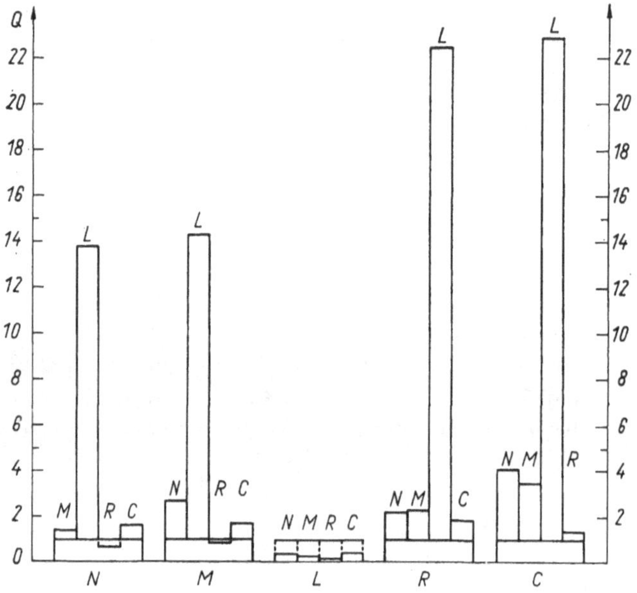

Fig. 3. Suitability of the substrate fractions for degradation by foreign proteases. The letters below the abscissa mark the substrate fractions, the letters of the columns the enzyme fractions.

The hight of the columns represents the quotient from values of proteolytic activity (cf. Table 3) and substrate autoproteolysis (cf. Table 2b), whereby the latter were relative by equated to 1.0

sent results, but the latter one cannot be confirmed, because we labelled mainly short-lived proteins as substrates. In general all efforts to simulate autophagy in vitro have not been successful, although many morphological proofs for the heterophagy of extracellular proteins and autophagy of various intracellular organelles exist. Our results concerning the degradation of microsomal and mitochondrial proteins by the lysosomal fraction are well comparable with the morphometric data about autophagy of microbodies, endoplasmatic reticulum and mitochondria from PFEIFER, presented at this symposium. The proteolytic activity of the lysosomal fraction upon short-lived substrate proteins from all fractions in vitro seems to indicate that the lysosomes in vivo may considerably participate in protein degradation of all organelles.

The relatively high proteolytic activity of our nuclear fraction can be attributed to a true nuclear neutral protease [11, 12] as well as to an insignificant lysosomal contamination [27]. In contrast to our results BROSTROM and JEFFAY [11] found no degradation of cytosol proteins by highly purified nuclei, but it can be supposed that proteolytic enzymes were lost during the purification of nuclei.

Mitochondrial fractions are usually contaminated by lysosomes, and at least it is still unknown whether the proteolytic activity in mitochondria is true or not (compare RUBIO, this symposium and [42]). On the other hand, the results of KATUNUMA (this symposium and [50]) and HAAS et al. [18] confirm the existence of a mitochondrial endopeptidase located in the inner membrane.

Only a small amount of proteolytic activity of the microsomal fraction can be attributed to lysosomal contamination [10, 17]. Our low autoproteolysis values in R correspond well to those reported by LANGNER at this sympsoium; they result from action of a ribosomal endopeptidase upon own ribosomal substrate protein. At the same time BETZ et al. [49, 51] and BOHLEY et al. [23, 25, 26] showed independently that in microsomes in vitro long-lived proteins were better degraded than short-lived ones. Since the lysosomes prefer long-lived microsomal proteins in vitro it was concluded that this system insufficiently simulates the in vivo conditions [52].

The relative low proteolytic activity in the cytosol fraction agrees with comparable data in the literature [2, 19—22, 25, 45], but was higher than in earlier experiments without glutathione [21]. We found that fresh cytosol (up to 24 hrs old) was two to four times more active than an old one (stored for more than 48 hrs at —28 °C). Short-lived cytosol proteins seem to be the best substrates for all fractions. This agrees with their high in vivo turnover rates and their low autolysis in vitro. Comparing the degradation of long- and short-lived cytosolic proteins it was shown [23] that only the lysosomal supernatant fraction degrades short-lived cytosolic proteins better than long-lived ones. This phenomenon may have an important significance in vivo.

We have shown that manifold interactions between cell organelles in protein breakdown seem to be possible, but we cannot directly deduce the physiological significance of these in vitro cooperation phenomena with regard to the following restrictions concerning the differences between in vitro experiments and in vivo conditions:

(1) Homogenates of whole livers were used for the cell fractionation and parenchymal cells were not separated from Kupffer-cells. As shown by KNOOK et al. (this symposium), the nonparenchymal cells have a several times higher lysosomal proteolytic activity than hepatocytes. Therefore considerable differences in the proteolytic behaviour among cell organelles of these various cell types are possible.

(2) Our subcellular fractions were not free of contamination by foreign organelles as shown with the lysosomal marker enzyme. Contaminations other than lysosomal were not checked, but cannot be excluded.

(3) The entireness of the organelles was not controlled, although it was expected that — under our mild conditions — nuclei and mitochondria remained intact and endoplasmatic reticulum was disrupted during the cell fractionation. Lysosomes were treated with destilled water to liberate the enclosed enzymes. On the other hand, it seems to be possible that freeze-thawed substrate organelles facilitate the action of proteolytic enzymes and yield higher PA-values (compare [24]). It is uncertain if this treatment is in better accordance with the in vivo conditions. Furthermore freeze-thawing of the fractions would have damaged the proteolytic enzymes in our experiments, because each fraction in the test tube was regarded as enzyme and substrate fraction as well.

(4) These incubation conditions were chosen to simulate the in vivo surroundings as far as possible. In vitro only two fractions were incubated with each other, however, in vivo a complex system of many different proteases from more than two organelles must participate in normal turnover of cell organelle proteins [41, 52].

To sum up we could show that all liver fractions tested were able to degrade short-lived proteins from foreign organelles at neutral *p*H, the lysosomes showing the highest specific proteolytic activity and cytosol proteins being the best suited substrates.

We confirm the importance of the lysosomes in protein degradation in the cell, but there is no reason to underestimate the extralysosomal proteolytic mechanisms. Their biological significance is worth to be further investigated.

References

[1] Coffey, J. W., and C. de Duve: J. biol. Chem. **243**, 3255 (1968)

[2] Kirschke, H., J. Langner, B. Wiederanders, S. Ansorge, and P. Bohley: Acta biol. med. germ. **28**, 305 (1972)

[3] Kirschke, H., J. Langner, B. Wiederanders, P. Bohley, and U. Broghammer: Acta biol. med. germ. **35**, 285 (1976)

[4] Wiederanders, B., S. Ansorge, P. Bohley, U. Broghammer, H. Kirschke, and J. Langner: Acta biol. med. germ. **35**, 269 (1976)

[5] Wiederanders, B., S. Ansorge, P. Bohley, H. Kirschke, J. Langner, and H. Hanson in: Intracellular protein catabolism. H. Hanson and P. Bohley (Eds.). Barth, Leipzig 1975, p. 221

[6] Barrett, A. J.: Biochem. J. **104**, 601 (1967)

[7] Bohley, P., H. Kirschke, J. Langner, and S. Ansorge: FEBS Lett. **5**, 233 (1969)

[8] Poole, B., and C. de Duve in: Intracellular protein catabolism. H. Hanson and P. Bohley (Eds). Barth, Leipzig 1975, p. 13

[9] Towatari, T., K. Tanaka, D. Yoshikawa, and N. Katunuma: FEBS Lett. **67**, 284 (1976)

[10] Umaña, R.: Archs Biochem. Biophys. **119**, 526 (1967)

[11] Brostrom, C. O., and H. Jeffay: Biochim. biophys. Acta **278**, 15 (1972)

[12] Siebert, G.: in: Comprehensive biochemistry. **23**, 1. M. Florkin and E. H. Stotz (Eds). Elsevier Publishing Company, Amsterdam 1968

[13] Alberti, K. G. M. M., and W. Bartley: Biochem. J. **95**, 641 (1965)

[14] Alberti, K. G. M. M., and W. Bartley: Biochem. J. **87**, 104 (1963)

[15] Alberti, K. G. M. M., and W. Bartley: Biochem. J. **111**, 763 (1969)

[16] Fitzpatrick, K., and R. J. Pennington: Biochem. J. **111**, 29p (1969)

[17] Nagel, W., and F. Willig: Z. Vitam.-Horm.-Fermentforsch. **14**, 89 (1965/1966)

[18] Haas, R., T. Nagasawa, and P. C. Heinrich: Hoppe-Seyler's Z. physiol. Chem. **358**, 241 (1977)

[19] Bohley, P.: Naturwissenschaften **55**, 211 (1968)

[20] Bohley, P., H. Kirschke, J. Langner, S. Ansorge, B. Wiederanders, and H. Hanson in: Tissue Proteinases. A. J. Barrett and J. T. Dingle (Eds). North-Holland, Amsterdam and London 1971, p. 187

[21] Bohley, P., H. Kirschke, J. Langner, S. Ansorge, and H. Hanson: Acta biol. med. germ. **27**, 229 (1971)

[22] Huisman, W.: Dissertation, Rijksuniversiteit te Groningen, 1974

[23] Bohley, P., H. Kirschke, J. Langner, B. Wiederanders, and S. Ansorge: Acta biol. med. germ. **35**, 301 (1976)

[24] Sawant, P. L., J. D. Desai, and A. L. Tappel: Biochim. biophys. Acta **85**, 93 (1964)

[25] Bohley, P., C. Miehe, M. Miehe, S. Ansorge, H. Kirschke, J. Langner, and B. Wiederanders: Acta biol. med. germ. **28**, 323 (1972)

[26] Bohley, P., H. Kirschke, J. Langner, B. Wiederanders, S. Ansorge, and H. Hanson in: Intracellular protein catabolism. H. Hanson and P. Bohley (Eds). Barth, Leipzig 1975, p. 201

[27] Gray, R. W., C. Arsenis, and H. Jeffay: Biochim. biophys. Acta **222**, 627 (1970)

[28] Krebs, H. H., and K. Henseleit: Hoppe-Seyler's Z. physiol. Chem. **210**, 33 (1932)

[29] Löffler, E.: Unpublished results

[30] Miehe, M., C. Miehe, and P. Bohley: Acta biol. med. germ. **28**, 299 (1972)

[31] MIEHE, M. in: Intracellular protein catabolism. H. HANSON and P. BOHLEY (Eds). Barth, Leipzig 1975, p. 142
[32] PIHA, R. S., M. CUÈNOD, and H. WAELSCH: J. biol. Chem. **241**, 2397 (1966)
[33] DE DUVE, C., B. C. PRESSMANN, R. GIANETTO, R. WATTIAUX, and F. APPELMANS: Biochem. J. **60**, 604 (1955)
[34] MIEHE, M.: Dissertation, Martin-Luther-Universität Halle-Wittenberg, Medizinische Fakultät 1974
[35] KEIL, D. S., and D. S. ŠORMOVÁ: Laboratoriumstechnik für Biochemiker. Akademische Verlagsgesellschaft Geest und Portig KG, Leipzig 1965, p. 50
[36] BOHLEY, P.: Hoppe-Seyler's Z. physiol. Chem. **348**, 100 (1967)
[37] CAYGILL, J. C., C. P. J. ROSTON, and F. R. JEVONS: Biochem. J. **98**, 405 (1966)
[38] NOVIKOFF, A. B. in: The Cell. **2**, 433. J. BRACHET and A. E. MIRSKY (Eds). Academic Press, New York, London 1961
[39] TAPPEL, A. L. in: Comprehensive Biochemistry. **23**, 77. M. FLORKIN and E. H. STOTZ (Eds). Elsevier Publishing Company, Amsterdam 1968
[40] DE DUVE, C., and R. WATTIAUX: A. Rev. Physiol. **28**, 435 (1966)
[41] POOLE, B., and M. WIBO in: Intracellular protein catabolism. H. HANSON and P. BOHLEY (Eds). Barth, Leipzig 1975, p. 130
[42] RUBIO, V., and S. GRISOLIA: FEBS Lett. **75**, 281 (1977)
[43] KAZAKOVA, O. V., V. N. ORECHOVIČ, and K. F. FIRFAROVA: Biochimia **35**, 721 (1970)
[44] LOGUNOV, A. J., and V. N. ORECHOVIČ: Biochimia **37**, 1061 (1972)
[45] ANSORGE, S., P. BOHLEY, H. KIRSCHKE, J. LANGNER, and H. HANSON: Acta biol. med. germ. **26**, 953 (1971)
[46] MEGO, J. L. in: Intracellular protein catabolism. H. HANSON and P. BOHLEY (Eds). Barth, Leipzig 1975, p. 30
[47] GROSS, N. J., G. S. GETZ, and M. RABINOWITZ: J. biol. Chem. **244**, 1552 (1969)
[48] FOWLER, S., and C. DE DUVE: J. biol. Chem. **244**, 471 (1969)
[49] BETZ, H., M. GRATZL, and H. REMMER: Hoppe-Seyler's Z. physiol. Chem. **354**, 567 (1973)
[50] KATUNUMA, N., E. KOMINAMI, K. KOBAYASHI, Y. BANNO, K. SUZUKI, K. CHICHIBU, Y. HAMAGUCHI, and T. KATSUNUMA: Eur. J. Biochem. **52**, 37 (1975)
[51] BETZ, H. in: Intracellular protein catabolism. H. HANSON and P. BOHLEY (Eds). Barth, Leipzig 1975, p. 209
[52] HANSON, H., H. KIRSCHKE, J. LANGNER, B. WIEDERANDERS, S. ANSORGE, and P. BOHLEY in: Intracellular protein catabolism II. V. TURK and N. MARKS (Eds). Plenum Press, New York and London 1977, p. 1

Acta biol. med. germ., Band 36, Seite 1855—1861 (1977)

Institute of Pharmacology and Toxicology, Medical Academy Erfurt, Erfurt, GDR

Pharmacological control of hyperproteolytic states in blood by enzyme inhibitors

F. MARKWARDT

Proteolytic enzymes are not only required for cleavage of alimentary proteins, but they participate also extensively in the mobilization of tissue proteins and in the liberation of pharmacologically active biogenic peptides and peptide hormones. Modern biochemistry has shown that a number of biological processes in blood, such as coagulation, fibrinolysis, kininogenesis, and complement activity, occur through substantially analogous chains of reaction which are governed through specific proteolytic enzymes. The reaction principle consists of an activation of proenzymes in blood to the active enzymes thrombin, plasmin, kallikrein, and C$\bar{1}$-esterase, which cause the formation or liberation of the final products during the next following reaction step on the basis of their specific proteolytic activity. These proteolytic systems are related to each other, either directly or indirectly, so that the activation of one of the proteases in the blood will often also cause an activation of the other. Thus, factor XII (Hageman factor) activated by surface contact, will not only result in formation of the prothrombin activator, but will also cause the activation of kallikreinogen and plasminogen. If one considers that plasmin can also activate kallikreinogen and the complement system, one will realize that the reactions in these examples go beyond a simple analogy (Fig. 1). Errors in one of these normally well balanced systems through excessive activation may lead to serious disorders such as thromboembolism, haemorrhage, inflammatory reaction and shock. After the pathogenic importance of such hyperproteolytic processes was clarified, the chemical control of these enzyme systems assumed great interest. The use of inhibitors that react with the active centre of enzymes — and thus complement the biological regulation of enzyme activity such as the repression of genetically controlled protein synthesis — opened great opportunities.

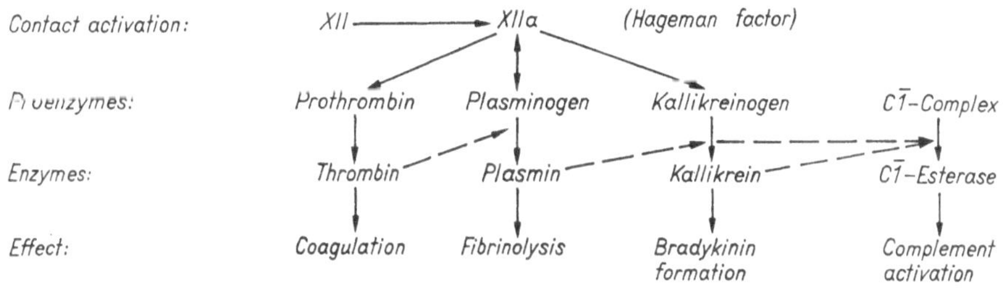

Fig. 1. Activation of the proteolytic enzyme system of the blood

The resulting pharmacological problem was seen in the development of inhibitors that block the enzymes which participate in the reactions in the organism, thus controlling the underlying pathogenetic processes. We attempted initially to solve this problem by isolation and pharmacological characterization of naturally occurring inhibitors, such as the specific thrombin inhibitor from medicinal leeches (hirudin) [6, 7] or the polyvalent inhibitor of beef organs (aprotinin) [15, 20, 24]. Owing to difficulties in production and the necessity of parenteral administration, the use of these high-molecular-weight polypeptides as well as the organic inhibitors was limited.

A decisive progress, therefore, was the development of synthetic low-molecular-weight inhibitors of proteolytic enzymes [10, 18, 22]. A condition for the development of such antiproteolytics was the demonstration of the structure and mode of action of proteinases, which are the receptors for inhibitory drugs.

Eventually important enzymes in blood belong to the group of trypsin-like serine proteinases. These are estero-proteolytically active endopeptidases that exhibit their catalytic activity by means of a specific serine residue whose β-hydroxyl group enters into an intermediary covalent bond with the substrate molecule. The enzyme specificity is determined by the structural conformation of the substrate-binding centre. This consists of a hydrophobic pocket which is formed by non-polar amino acid side chains, and which has at its bottom a dissociated carboxyl group of aspartic acid residue. This carboxyl group reacts with the protonated basic groups of lysine or arginine residues of the protein substrate, accompanied by ion binding. The fixation of the substrate is further supported by hydrophobic interactions of the non-polar side chain of the substrate with the hydrophobic slit, as well as by hydrogen bridge formation with other areas of the active enzyme surface. In this way the enzyme is enabled to fix its substrate in such a manner that the cleavable bond achieves contact with the reactive serine residue. From the intermediary enzyme-substrate complex an acyl enzyme is formed by liberation of the first cleavage product, and after hydrolysis (deacylation) the enzyme is again free to react anew with the substrate (Fig. 2a).

Inhibitors can be produced which enter into a covalent or non-covalent bond with the active centre of the enzyme by imitating the acylating component of enzyme substrates. The examination of homologous series of such compounds has shown

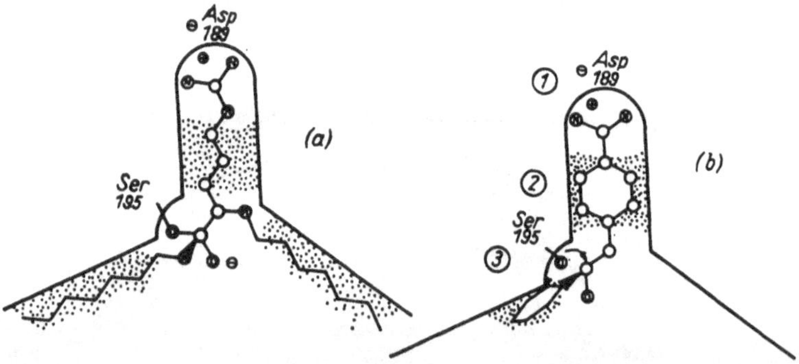

Fig. 2. Interaction of serine proteinases with substrates (a) and synthetic inhibitors (b)

that, in order to be effective, the following structural conditions must be met in addition to the required steric conformation (Fig. 2b):

(1) A basic group for the formation of ionic relationships.

(2) Structural fragments that allow hydrophobic interactions with the substrate-binding pocket of the enzyme.

(3) Other structural elements that increase the affinity as well as the specificity of inhibitors by additional bond formation and interactions with areas of the enzyme other than the substrate-binding pocket.

In this way, biochemical investigations allowed the identification of highly active inhibitors.

Estimating the different types of inhibitors investigated it could be shown that competitive inhibitors, especially aromatic amidino compounds, were most suitable for the chemical control of the activity of serine proteinases in blood. Investigations on the pharmacodynamics and pharmacokinetics of the most effective inhibitors had shown that 4-amidinophenylpyruvic acid (APPA) is a suitable tool for studying the antiproteolytic effect of such inhibitors in vivo. The activity of the inhibitor towards several enzyme systems is characterized by the K_i-values (Table 1).

Table 1
Serine proteinases of the blood.
Physiological and pathogenetic role as well as pharmacological relevance of their inhibitors

System	Enzymes	Physiology	Pathology	Pharmacology
Blood coagulation	Thrombin Clotting factors VIIa, IXa, Xa and XIIIa	Haemostasis	Hypercoagulation Thrombosis	Anticoagulants Antithrombotics
Fibrinolysis	Plasmin and activators	Thrombolysis	Hyper-fibrinolysis Bleeding	Antifibrinolytics Haemostyptics
Plasmakinin formation	Kallikrein	Supply of blood to tissue	Shock Inflammation	Treatment of shock Antiphlogistics
Complement	C1-Esterase	Mediation of immune reactions	Immune complex diseases	Anticomplement action; Immun-supressive drugs

Already at this time, the inhibitor can serve as a useful pharmacological model for compounds of this nature and allows an estimate for the potential therapeutic effect of this class of drugs.

Inhibitors of blood coagulation

Since intravascular coagulation in cardiovascular disease is a life-threatening complication, or in many cases even the cause of the disease, proteinase inhibitors were first developed for their anticoagulant effect, which was caused by inhibition of serine proteinases that participate in coagulation [2, 8, 9, 11].

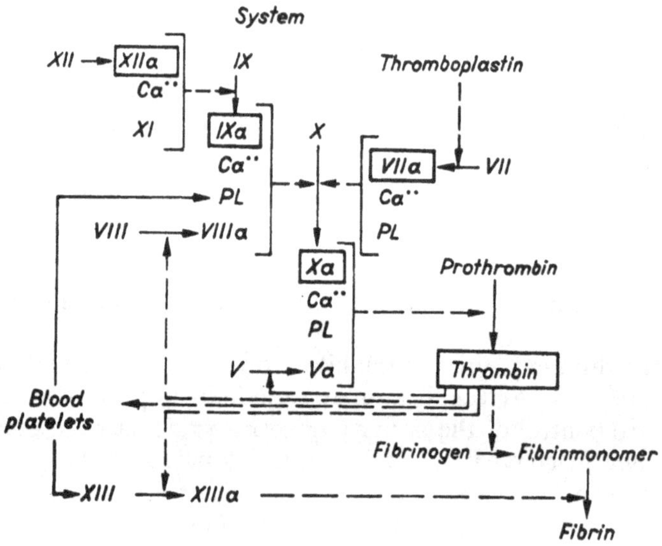

Fig. 3. Scheme of the coagulation system.
(Marginated area = serine proteinases inhibited by benzamidine derivatives)

For the analysis of the anticoagulant effect it remains to be seen if the benzamidine derivative is a separate inhibitor for thrombin, or whether it is a broad spectrum inhibitor which inhibits a number of clotting factors. This is not unlikely, since the activated factors are considered to be proteolytic enzymes (Fig. 3). Besides thrombin and factor Xa further four ones (VII, IX, XI and XII) possess a reactive serine residue. Furthermore, the anticoagulant effect of the inhibitor is not only based on its inhibitory effect on the thrombin-fibrinogen reaction, but also on its inhibitory influence on the other thrombin-catalyzed reactions involved in haemostasis and thrombosis, such as thrombin-induced platelet aggregation, the prothrombin activation step, and fibrin stabilization.
The objective was to obtain an anticoagulant that may be administered orally and that had a rapid action. This was thought to have a number of advantages over conventional anticoagulants. Some of these inhibitors are already under investigation, both experimentally and clinico-pharmacologically, and they have been used successfully in the prophylaxis of intravascular thrombus formation, such as APPA [14, 17].

Inhibitors of fibrinolysis

Ten or more years ago, increasing insight into the importance of fibrinolytic processes in the development of life-threatening haemorrhagic conditions had led to a systematic search for synthetic inhibitors that might interfere with fibrinolytic reactions [19]. This problem of therapeutic interference with fibrinolysis was solved satisfactorily with the development of synthetic antifibrinolytics, such as ε-aminocaproic acid (EACA), aminomethylcyclohexane carboxylic acid (AMCA) [23] and p-aminomethyl-benzoic acid (PAMBA) [5, 16]. Points of attack for the synthetic inhibitors are plaminogen activation and plasmin action (Fig. 4).

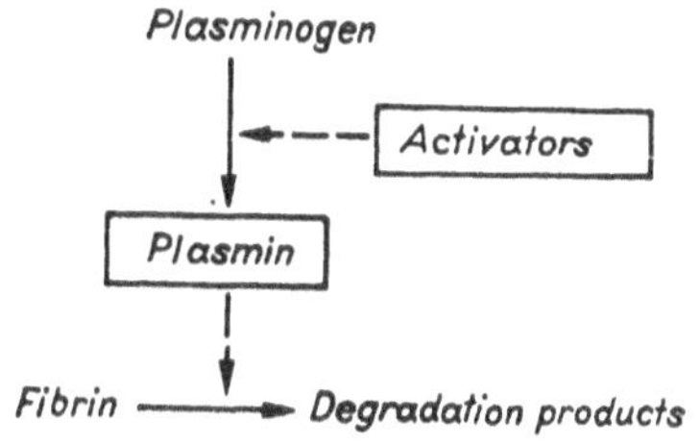

Fig. 4

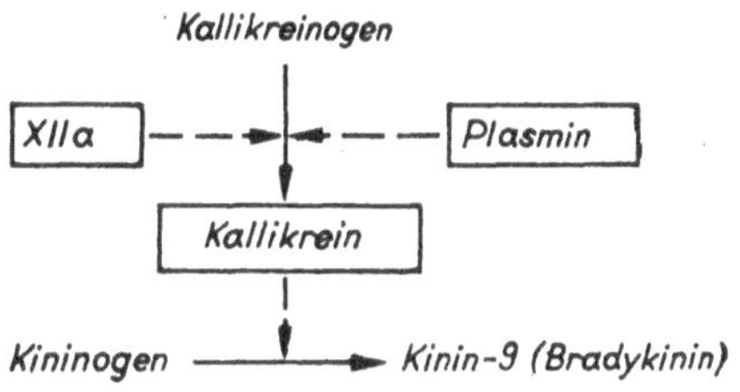

Fig. 5

Fig. 4. Scheme of the fibrinolytic system.
(Marginated area = serine proteinases inhibited by benzamidine derivatives)

Fig. 5. Scheme of the kinin system.
(Marginated area = serine proteinases inhibited by benzamidine derivatives)

The inhibition of plasmin activity prevents the resolution of wound-covering fibrin and the appearance of coagulation-inhibitory split products so that the disease, which is caused by hyperfibrinolysis, can be controlled.

Inhibitors of the kinin system

Even without a clear understanding of the physiological role of the kinin-system, it is known that the uncontrolled liberation of plasma kinins may participate in the development of pathological processes. It is therefore necessary to subject kinin systems to pharmacological control. Since specific antagonists of kinins have not yet been found, the chemical regulation of kinin liberation has become important. Investigations of recent years have shown that the effects of kallikrein may be prevented in vivo with synthetic inhibitors of serine proteinases [12, 13]. This allowed a regulatory manipulation of the pathogenesis of certain diseases as well as some states of shock and inflammation in which the liberation of plasma kinins by kallikrein appeared to be of causative importance. Possibilities of interference with the kinin system are shown in Fig. 5.

Inhibitors of the complement system

The complement system represents an extracellular effector and modulator of biological membranes. It is the primary mediator of antigen-antibody reactions, moreover, its many membrane-oriented functions may operate in various pathological conditions. The complement system shows analogies in its elements and the activation mechanism to the clotting, fibrinolytic and kinin forming systems (Fig. 6). It consists of eleven distinct components representing proteins or glycoproteins. Three functional parts may be differentiated:

- the recognition unit with the three subcomponents of the C1-complex C1 q, C1 r, and C1 s;
- the activation unit with the components C2, C3, and C4;
- the membrane attack unit with the components C5 to C9.

The three proenzymes C1r, C1s, and C2 are activated by specific limited proteolysis. The active subcomponent C1r activates C1s to the active estero-proteolytic

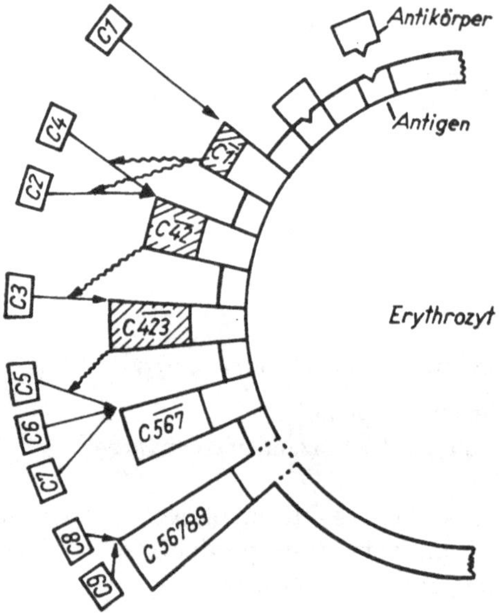

Fig. 6. Scheme of the complement system

enzyme C1s̄, the so-called C1̄-esterase, which shares features with some other serine proteinases. At least four peptides are released during complement activation, two of them are anaphylatoxins. Activation is also initiated by trypsin, plasmin and kallikrein. Such interrelationships between different enzyme systems in blood let one suppose that pathological activation of one of the particular systems brings about activation of the complement system, and therefore the complement system may be influenced pharmacologically by chemical regulation of its activity with inhibitors of serine proteinases. For example, initial investigations have shown that complement-dependent haemolysis of sensitized erythrocytes can be prevented with synthetic inhibitors [3].

The development of this class of antiproteolytics was primarily directed towards the control of proteolytic events in the blood, since they allow a clear formulation of objectives for a pharmacological interference through knowledge of their pathogenetic importance. This work may be extended also to other serine proteinases of the organism. For example, one may think of a blockade of trypsin activity, which can be activated in the pancreas during pathological conditions of that organ [21]. One may further consider an inhibition of the enzyme acrosin in sperm, which allows its penetration of the ovum by means of proteolytic activity [1].

Final remarks

Synthetic inhibitors may become therapeutic tools, and the specificity of their activity may be enhanced, as their safety is improved and their pharmacokinetic behaviour is adapted to the therapeutic objective. They may become a new class of drugs which may be defined by the collective term antiproteolytics or synthetic low-molecular-weight inhibitors of serine proteinases.

It is important to consider that these examples demonstrate the possibilities of a goal-oriented development of new drugs whose conception differs from the conventional procedures. Thus, the pharmacological problem arises from the disease condition and the clarification of its pathogenesis, in particular the patho-biochemistry. The problem extends from the molecular-biological level under elucidation of structure-effect relationships to the animal experiment with specific investigation of pharmacodynamics. The study of pharmacokinetics and compatibility in man eventually allows the introduction into clinical medicine.

Summary

Modern biochemistry has shown that a number of biological processes in blood, such as coagulation, fibrinolysis, kininogenesis, and complement activity, occur through substantially analogous chains of reaction which are governed through specific proteolytic enzymes. Errors in one of these normally well balanced systems through excessive activation may lead to serious disorders such as thromboembolism, haemorrhage, inflammatory reaction and shock. The resulting pharmacological problem was seen in the development of inhibitors that block the enzymes which participate in the reactions in the organism, thus controlling the underlying pathogenetic processes. Biochemical investigations allowed the identification of highly active inhibitors whose pharmacodynamic and pharmacokinetic properties and antiproteolytic activity were then investigated in animal experiments. As a result, some of these inhibitors were clinically evaluated, and others have already been used therapeutically. They may become a new class of drugs which may be defined by the collective term antiproteolytics or synthetic low-molecular-weight inhibitors of serine proteinases.

References

[1] Markwardt, F.: Blutgerinnungshemmende Wirkstoffe aus blutsaugenden Tieren. Fischer, Jena 1963

[2] Markwardt, F.: Meth. Enzymol. **19**, 924 (1970)

[3] Markwardt, F., H.-P. Klöcking, K.-O. Haustein, and J. Perlewitz: Acta biol. med. germ. **16**, 15 (1966)

[4] Markwardt, F., and M. Richter: Pharmazie **23**, 620 (1969)

[5] Trautschold, I., E. Werle, and G. Zickgraf-Rüdel: Biochem. Pharmac. **16**, 59 (1967)

[6] Werle, E., I. Trautschold, H. Haendle, and H. Fritz: Ann. N.Y. Acad. Sci. **146**, 464 (1968)

[7] Markwardt, F.: Folia haemat. **98**, 381 (1972)

[8] Markwardt, F., and H. Landmann: Ergebn. exp. Med. **9**, 125 (1972)

[9] Okamoto, S., and A. Hijikata: Drug Design **6**, 143 (1975)

[10] Glusa, E., F. Markwardt, and J. Perlewitz: Farmak. Toks. **37**, 70 (1974)

[11] Markwardt, F.: Nova Acta Leopoldina (N. F. 202) **36**, 47 (1971)

[12] Markwardt, F.: Thromb. Diath. haemorrh. **27**, 99 (1972)

[13] Markwardt, F.: Haemostasis **3**, 185 (1974)

[14] Markwardt, F., and H.-P. Klöcking: Thrombos. Res. **1**, 243 (1972)

[15] Markwardt, F., H.-P. Klöcking, and G. Nowak: Thromb. Diath. haemorrh. **24**, 240 (1970)

[16] Markwardt, F., H. Landmann, and H.-P. Klöcking: Fibrinolytika und Antifibrinolytika. Fischer, Jena 1972

[17] Okamoto, S., and U. Okamoto: Keio J. Med. **11**, 105 (1962)

[18] Lohmann, K., F. Markwardt, and H. Landmann: Thromb. Diath. haemorrh. **10**, 424 (1964)

[19] Markwardt, F., H.-P. Klöcking, and H. Landmann: Thromb. Diath. haemorrh. **15**, 561 (1966)

[20] Markwardt, F., J. Drawert, and P. Walsmann: Acta biol. med. germ. **26**, 123 (1971)

[21] Markwardt, F., J. Drawert, and P. Walsmann: Biochem. Pharmac. **23**, 2247 (1974)

[22] Hauptmann, J., and F. Markwardt: Biochem. Pharmac. **26**, 325 (1977)

[23] Markwardt, F., P. Walsmann, and J. Hoffmann: Acta biol. med. germ. **32**, 433 (1974)

[24] Bhattacharyya, A. K., L. J. D. Zaneveld, B. M. Dragoje, G. F. B. Schumacher, and J. Travis: J. Reprod. Fert. **47**, 97 (1976)

Acta biol. med. germ., Band 36, Seite 1863—1871 (1977)

Department of Biochemistry, J. Stefan Institute, University of Ljubljana, Ljubljana, Yugoslavia
*Istituto di Pharmacologia, Università degli Studi di Trieste, Trieste, Italy

Biochemical and biological properties of cell and tissue neutral proteinases and inhibitors

M. Kopitar, A. Suhar, T. Giraldi*, and V. Turk

Introduction

Recent studies in many laboratories indicate that cells and tissues contain besides acid also neutral proteinases [1—6]. It was also found that inhibitors of neutral proteinases exist inside the cell [7—10]. Stable and active samples of these enzymes could be obtained only after removal or inactivation of these inhibitors. In our previous study [8] on the neutral proteinases and inhibitors from leucocytes we found that these inhibitors are unstable at *p*H 3—5, whereas they are stable in the physiological *p*H region. Based upon this finding we succeeded in isolating the elastase and chymotrypsin-like neutral proteinases from spleen homogenate.

Material and methods

Fresh bovine spleens were cut to the pieces and frozen overnight at −20 °C. Frozen spleen was homogenized in two volumes of cold (4 °C) 0.9% NaCl. The homogenate was immediately acidified with 6.37 N H_2SO_4 to *p*H 3.5. The acidified homogenate was then centrifuged (for 20 min at 5000 × *g* at 0 °C) and the pellet was discarded. The supernatant was then dialyzed against water, during next 36 hrs. The precipitate formed during the dialysis was removed by centrifugation and the supernatant was concentrated by ultrafiltration (Amicon H1DP 10). The *p*H was adjusted again to 3.5. The protein was precipitated with ethanol. The alcohol precipitates were dissolved in buffer, *p*H 5.5 (0.1 M Na acetate + 0.9% NaCl). These samples were used for further purification of enzymes. The described extraction procedure represents the modified extraction method published previously [11]. Leucocytes were isolated from fresh heparinized pig blood and subjected to subcellular fractionation. From the post granular supernatant fraction the inhibitors were isolated. Proteinase activity and the inhibition tests were performed. This was all reported previously [8]. The amidase activity of cathepsin B1 was determined using N-benzoyl-DL-arginine-2-naphthylamide (BANA) according to Barrett [12].
Polyacrylamide gel electrophoreses at *p*H 8.5 (13] and at *p*H 4.3 SDS [14] were performed. Protein was determined by the method of Lowry et al. Histones and hemoglobin were prepared in our laboratory. Fluorescein-labelled polymeric collagen was gift from Dr. F. Steven from Manchester university. $Ac(Ala)_3$-Ala-CH_2Cl and $Ac(Ala)_2$Pro-AlaCH_2Cl were gift from Dr. J. C. Powers (USA), p-carbamido phenyl-3,3 dimethyl thiazene was gift from Dr. K. Nisi from Trieste, Italia and $beta_1$AC was gift of Dr. D. Wooley from Manchester University. All other compounds and reagents were high purity preparations obtained from commercial sources.

Results and discussion

Proteolytic activity of alcohol extracts measured on hemoglobin *p*H 3.5 and *p*H 7.5 are shown in Table 1. In these experiments was used alcohol extract 40% a. This extract was dialyzed against 0.05 M Tris/HCl buffer, at *p*H 8.0. The dialyzed extract was purified on DEAE cellulose equilibrated with the same buffer. The elution pattern is shown in Fig. 1. Elution with a gradient to 0.5 M NaCl in the

Table 1
Proteolytic activity of alcohol precipitates of bovine spleen extracts

Alcohol concentration %	0.1 ml enz. Hb 3.5/10 min	0.4 ml enz. Hb 7.5/120 min	mg prot./ml
20*	0.430	0.230	9.42
20**	0.300	0.150	6.72
40*	0.770	0.650	10.68
40**	0.492	0.539	9.05
60*	1.000	0.341	5.04
60**	0.820	0.240	2.68

* First extraction in buffer *p*H 5.5;
** second extraction in buffer *p*H 5.5

same buffer yielded 3 separated peaks of neutral proteinase activity. In the first protein peak appeared cationic proteins that did not bind to DEAE cellulose. In this peak elastase was eluted before cathepsin D and B1. In the second peak chymotrypsin-like neutral proteinase together with cathepsins appeared. The neutral proteinase activity of the third peak is not subject of this paper. The elastase was pooled and concentrated by lyophilization. It was further separated on Sephadex G-75 in 0.05 M Tris buffer, *p*H 8.0. The elution pattern is shown in Fig. 2. The elastase fractions, free of cathepsins were concentrated by ultrafiltration (Amicon UM-10) and used as the source of pure spleen elastase (controlled by acrylamide gel electrophoresis) in all subsequent experiments. Concentrated chymotrypsin-like neutral proteinase was dialyzed against 0.1 M Na acetate containing 0.9% NaCl, *p*H 5.5 and separated on Bio-gel P-100 as shown in Fig. 3. The neutral

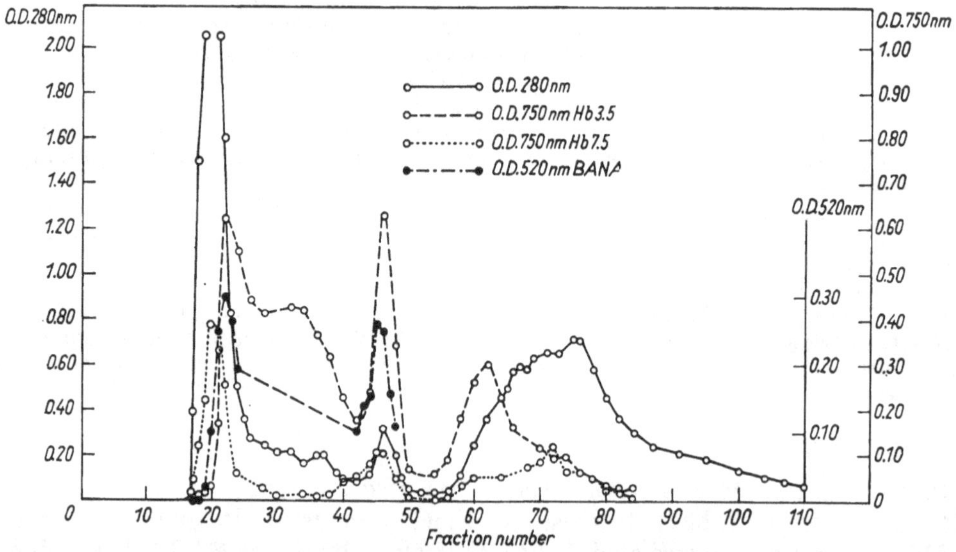

Fig. 1. Elution profile of acid spleen extract (40% a) on a DEAE – cellulose column (2.8 × 60 cm)

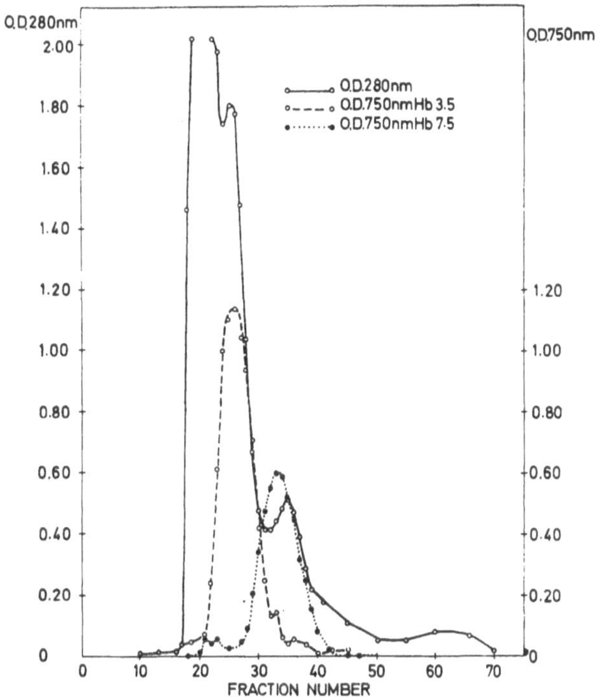

Fig. 2. Elution profile of pooled fractions 16–20, from DEAE-cellulose on a Sephadex G 75 column (2 × 55 cm)

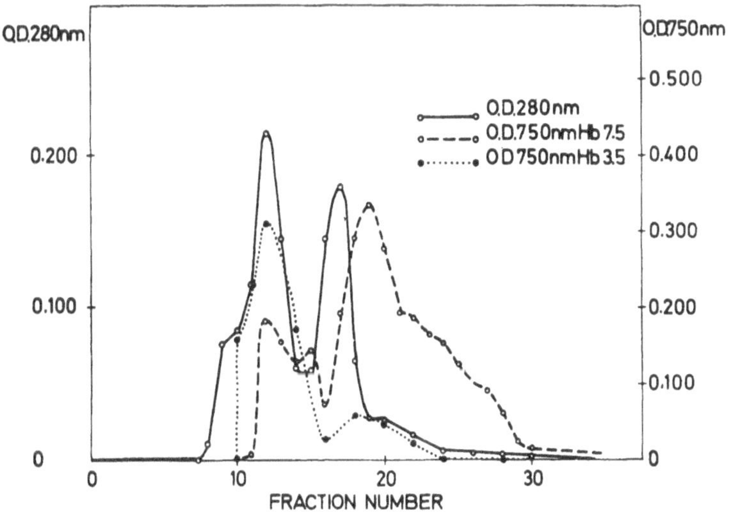

Fig. 3. Elution profile of pooled fractions 42–48 from DEAE-cellulose on a BioGel P-loo column (1.8 × 50 cm)

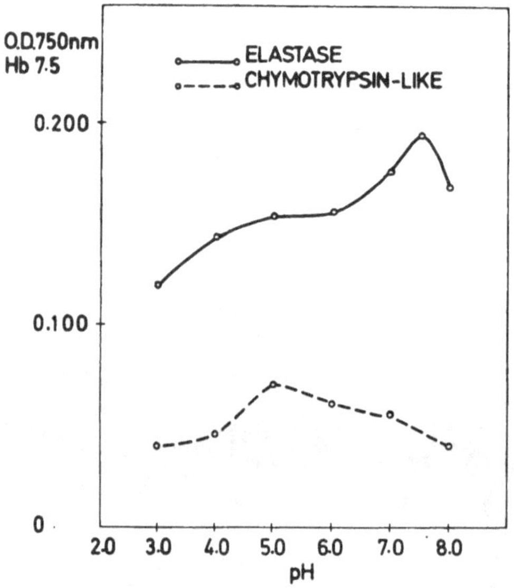

Fig. 4. Effects of *p*H on elestase and chymotrypsin-like neutral proteinase.
Buffer and enzymes were maintained for 10 min at 37 °C, in volume ratio 1:1. The residual acitivities were determined using hemoglobin *p*H 7,5, as substrate. Time of hydrolysis was 2 hrs

proteinase activity was eluted in two peaks and chymotrypsin-like neutral proteinase was eluted in the second peak.

*p*H stability of elastase and chymotrypsin-like neutral proteinase is shown in Fig. 4. Elastase is most stable in the *p*H range 7—8, whereas chymotrypsin-like neutral proteinase between *p*H range 5—6.

When comparing hydrolysis of various proteins at *p*H 7.5 further differences in enzymatic activity were detected (Table 2). Elastase degraded besides elastin (detected on elastin-agar-plates) all the tested substrates, whereas chymotrypsin-like neutral proteinase did not degrade albumin and fibrinogen. This enzyme exhibits high ability for the degradation of histones.

STEVEN et al. [15] reported that F-Pc was degraded in telopeptide region of tropocollagen molecule also by a neutral proteinase, that was presented in polymorphonuclears of synovial fluid. We used the same substrate to test both neutral proteinases. Elastase showed great ability for the degradation of this substrate (Fig. 5),

Table 2
Degradation rates of various proteins by purified bovine spleen elastase and chymotrypsin-like neutral proteinase

	Elastase		Chymotrypsin-like neutral proteinase	
Substrate	O. D. 750 *p*H 7.5/2 hrs	Relative activity	O. D. 750 *p*H 7.5/2 hrs	Relative activity
Hemoglobin	0.096	100	0.070	100
Casein	0.130	135	0.070	100
Fibrinogen plasminogen r.	0.170	177	0.000	
Fibrinogen plasminogen free	0.130	135	0.000	
Albumin	0.055	57	0.000	
Histone	0.240	250	0.690	985

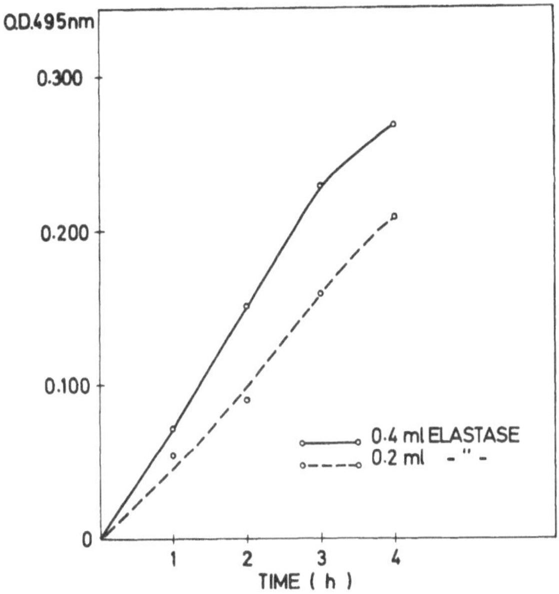

Fig. 5. Solubilization of fluorescein-labelled peptides over a period of 4 hrs at 37 °C by 0.2 ml and 0.4 ml of bovine spleen elastase.

Solubilized fluorescein-labelled peptides were measured spectrophotometrically at 495 nm

whereas no degradation was found with chymotrypsin-like neutral proteinase. Both enzymes were free of cathepsin B1 and both did not degrade fibrous tendon collagen.

The results of inhibition studies on both enzymes are presented in Table 3. Both enzymes were completely inhibited by Dip-F and by leucocyte und spleen intracellular inhibitors of molecular weight 40000. TPCK completely inhibited chymotrypsin-like neutral proteinase. Woolley inhibitor $beta_1AC$ inhibited only chymotrypsin-like neutral proteinase, but did not inhibit elastase. The intracellular inhibitors of molecular weight of 15—20000 exhibit very similar effect.

The change in proteolytic activity on hemoglobin and fibrinogen at *p*H 7.5, after 1 hr digestion, with an increasing range of elastase concentration demonstrated linearity over the whole range of enzyme used (Fig. 6).

In Fig. 7 is shown the elution profile of leucocyte post granule supernatant on CM cellulose column. Two regions of enzyme inhibition were observed. Time dependence of elastase inhibition by the second inhibitor was detected. Results on elastase are shown in Fig. 8. Inhibitor of the first peak showed a very small inhibition of elastase, whereas inhibitor from the second peak inhibited elastase up to 80% and no reversibility was observed. The first inhibitor peak, from CM cellulose, was further purified on Sephadex G-100. After this purification we obtained the inhibitor only in one elution peak, of molecular weight about 20000. This inhibitor now showed no inhibition of the elastase, whereas the inhibition of chymotrypsin-like neutral proteinase was 100%.

Table 3
Effect of potential inhibitors on bovine elastase and chymotrypsin-like neutral proteinase

	Compound	Final con. (mM)	% of residual activity	
			elastase	chym. LNP
a	Dip-F	5.0	5	8
b	$Ac(Ala)_3$-$AlaCH_2Cl$	0.15	81	n. d.
b	$Ac(Ala)_2$-Pro-$AlaCH_2Cl$	0.5	78	n. 1.
b	p-carboxamido phenyl-3,3 dimethylthiazene	5.0	55	n. d.
	4-chloromercuribenzoate	0.5	100	82
	JAA	0.5	100	100
	Cysteine	0.5	79	100
	DTE	0.5	100	n. d.
	EDTA	0.5	100	100
a	TPCK	0.5	100	0
c	Woolley inhibitor	1 mg/ml	100	45
c	Leu. inh. (40000)	0.4 mg/ml	9	0
c	Leu. inh. (20000)	0.6 mg/ml	92	7
c	B. s. inh. (40000)	3 mg/ml	5	0
c	B. s. inh. (20000)	0.7 mg/ml	100	0
	$alpha_1$ AT	3 mg/ml	5	0

Enzymatic activity is expressed as a percentage of residual enzyme activity according to enzyme without inhibitor. Inhibitors marked *a* were made up as stock solution in propan-2-ol. Inhibitors marked *b* were made in dimethyl sulphoxide. Assays were of proteolytic activity – O. D. 750 Hb 7.5 except for those marked *c* in case of chymotrypsin-like proteinase which were histones as substrate. n. d. – not determined. Preincubation time for all inhibitors were 15 min, except for TPCK (2 hrs) and for Power's and Nisi's inhibitors (30 min).

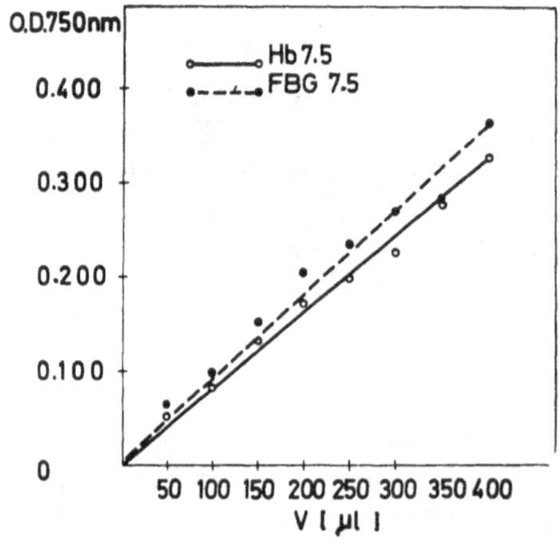

Fig. 6. Degradation of hemoglobin and fibrinogen by elastase with increasing range of elastase, after 1 h incubation

Gel filtration of the second inhibitor from CM cellulose is shown in Fig. 9. In this case four inhibiting peaks were obtained, 3 of them having molecular weights of about 70000, 40000 and about 15000; the fourth seems to be of low molecular weight. In this paper only the specificity of the main inhibitor (m. wt. 40000) was studied. This inhibitor completely inhibited both tested enzymes, as already shown in Table 3.

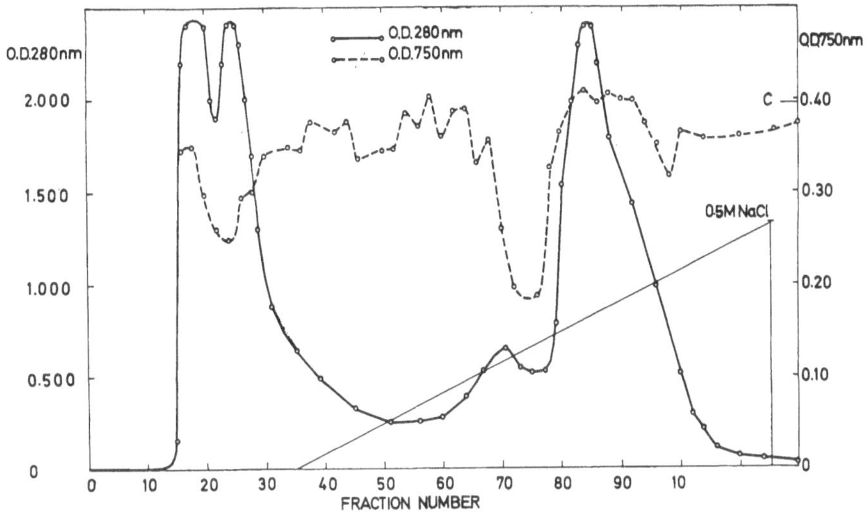

Fig. 7. Profile of ion exchange chromatography of a post granule supernatant sample on a 2.5 × 40 cm CM-cellulose column, equilibrated with 0.05 M Na-acetate, *p*H 5.6.

After elution of the first protein peak the buffer was changed to 0.05 M Tris/HCl buffer, *p*H 7.5, with linear NaCl gradient up to 0.5 M. The inhibitory effect of eluted fractions was tested on neutral proteinase sample (40% b) with casein at *p*H 7.5. Time of hydrolysis was 2 hrs

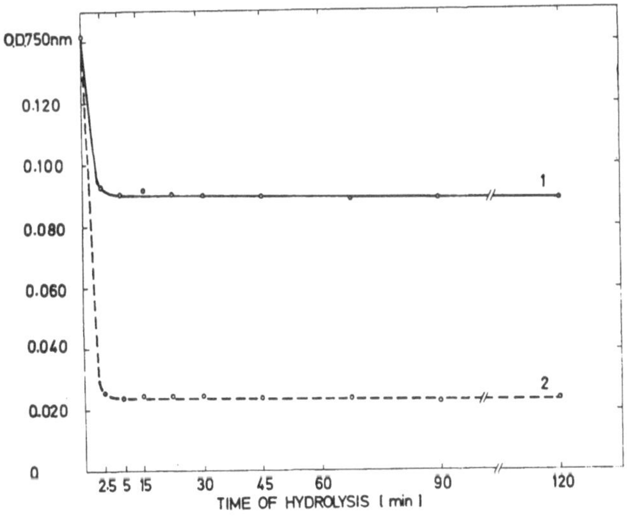

Fig. 8. Time dependence of elastase inhibition by the first (1) and the second (2) inhibitor from CM-cellulose.

2 ml of each inhibitor was treated with 2 ml of elastase at 22 °C. At intervals, as indicated in the graph, 0.4 ml portions of each mixture were withdrawn and assayed with 2 ml of hemoglobin, *p*H 7.5. Neutral proteinase activity is expressed in the figure in absorbance change, after 2 hrs of hydrolysis

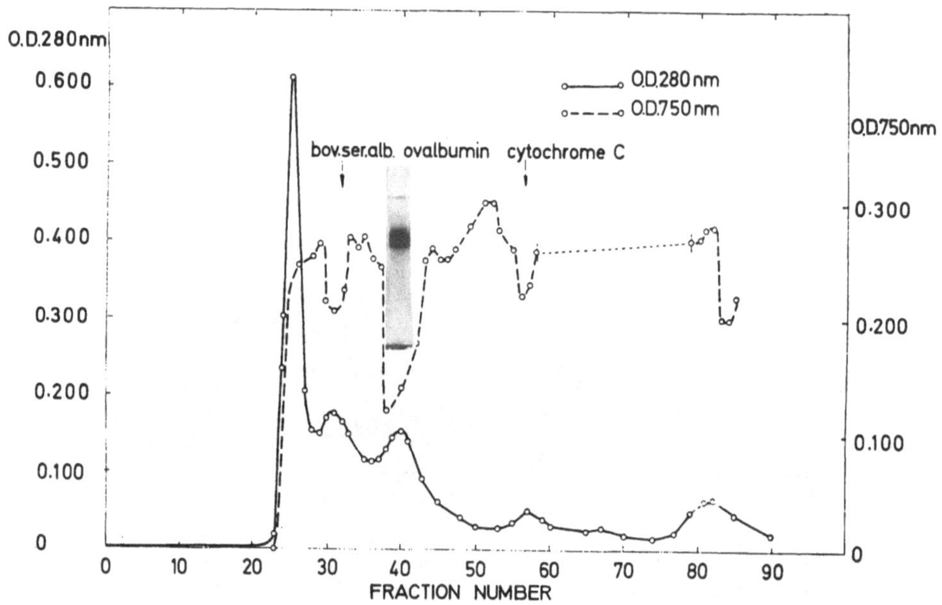

Fig. 9. Profile of gel filtration of the concentrated fractions 69—77 from CM-cellulose, on a 2× 80 cm Sephadex G-100 column, equilibrated with 0.05 M Tris/HCl buffer, *p*H 7.5. The inhibitory effect of eluted fractions was tested on neutral proteinase sample (40% b) with casein at *p*H 7.5. Time of hydrolysis was 2 hrs

The effect of the mixture of these inhibitors on the growth of the Lewis lung carcinoma in mice and the development of lung metastases was studied. It was observed that leucocyte neutral proteinase inhibitors caused the regression of primary tumour and the lowering of lung metastases. The effects of inhibitors are less pronounced on a tumour line of higher malignancy.

The elastase isolated from the beef spleen is similar in its enzymatic properties to the elastase from leucocytes [1—3, 8] and to the elastase isolated from the human spleen [5].

The properties of chymotrypsin-like neutral proteinase strongly suggest that it is identical with the chymotrypsin-like neutral proteinase of human neutrophils that has been described by RINDLER-LUDWIG et al. [4] and SCHMIDT and HAVEMANN [16]. Chymotrypsin-like neutral proteinase isolated from bovine spleen was completely inhibited by TPCK and is most stable at *p*H range 5—6.

In contrast to elastase this enzyme did not degrade fibrinogen, albumin and F-Pc.

Presented experiments clearly demonstrate the presence of two specific inhibitors of neutral proteinases in leucocyte cells, one with the m.wt. of about 20000 inhibited only chymotrypsin-like neutral proteinase, whereas the second with the m.wt. of 40000 inhibits both the tested enzymes.

Acknowledgement

The authors thank Mrs. M. BOŽIĆ for her excellent technical assistance during neutral proteinase isolation and characterization, as well as Mrs. J. KOMAR and Mr. K. LINDIČ. Supported by the research grant from the Research Council of Slovenia and in part by the NSF, USA.

References

[1] JANOFF, A., and J. SCHERER: J. exp. Med. **128**, 1137 (1968)
[2] OHLSON, K., and I. OLSSON: Eur. J. Biochem. **42**, 519 (1974)
[3] KOJ, A., J. CHUDZIK, and A. DUBIN: Biochem. J. **153**, 397 (1976)
[4] RINDLER-LUDWIG, R., F. SCHMALZL, and H. BRAUNSTEINER: Br. J. Hemat. **27**, 57 (1974)
[5] STARKEY, P. M., and A. J. BARRETT: Biochem. J. **155**, 255 (1976)
[6] KIRSCHKE, H., J. LANGNER, B. WIEDERANDERS, S. ANSORGE, P. BOHLEY, and U. BROGHAMMER: Acta biol. med. germ. **35**, 285 (1976)
[7] DAVIES, P., A. G. RITA, K. KRAKAUER, and G. WEISSMANN: Biochem. J. **123**, 559 (1971)
[8] KOPITAR, M., and D. LEBEZ: Eur. J. Biochem. **56**, 571 (1975)
[9] STEVEN, F. S., D. W. MILSOM, and J. A. A. HUNTER: Eur. J. Biochem. **67**, 165 (1976)
[10] DUBIN, A.: Eur. J. Biochem. **73**, 429 (1977)
[11] SUHAR, A., and D. LEBEZ in: Intracellular Protein Catabolism II. V. TURK and N. MARKS (Eds). Plenum Press, New York and London 1977, p.343
[12] BARRETT, A. J.: Anal. Biochem. **47**, 280 (1972)
[13] DAVIES, B. J.: Ann. N.Y. Acad. Sci. **121**, 404 (1964)
[14] WEBER, K., and OSBORN, M.: J. biol. Chem. **244**, 4406 (1969)
[15] STEVEN, F. S., A. TORRE-BLANCO and J. A. A. HUNTER: Biochim. biophys. Acta **405**, 188 (1975)
[16] SCHMIDT, W., and K. HAVEMANN: Hoppe Seyler's Z. physiol. Chem. **355**, 1077 (1974)

Acta biol. med. germ., Band 36, Seite 1873—1881 (1977)

Institute of Organic Chemistry and Biochemistry
Czechoslovak Academy of Sciences, 166 10 Prague 6,
Czechoslovakia

Naturally occurring inhibitors of intracellular proteinases

H. Keilová and V. Tomášek

Summary

The papain inhibitor isolated from chicken egg white inhibits the enzymatic activity of cathepsin B_1 and cathepsin C. The inhibitor bears two nonoverlapping reactive sites: one binds cathepsin B_1, papain, ficin, and bromelain, the other one cathepsin C. The inhibitor decreases the degree of an immunologic hypersensitive reaction, the so-called Arthus reaction. A statistically significant inhibition of this immunologically developed inflammation occurs only if the inhibitor is applied intradermally and simultaneously with the provoking dose of the antigen to rabbits sensitized to the same antigen.
The pepsin inhibitor from the body walls of the roundworm Ascaris lumbricoides inhibits the proteolytic activity of cathepsin E. This inhibitor covalently bound to Sepharose 4B was used for affininity chromatography of cathepsin E.
A cathepsin D inhibitor was isolated from potato tubers and its inhibitory and chemical characteristics were studied. The inhibitor does not inhibit either cathepsin E or pepsin yet inhibits trypsin in the alkaline *p*H-range. The molecular weight of the inhibitor is 21 790 and its molecule consists of 199 amino acid residues. The sequence of 17 amino acid residues was determined by Edman degradation of the inhibitor molecule.

Introduction

Still more attention has been focused on naturally occurring inhibitors of proteolytic enzymes. These studies have primarily been designed to examine the possibilities of using these inhibitors for therapy in medical practice. From the theoretical viewpoint the reactions of these inhibitors with enzymes represent an excellent model for studies of interactions of macromolecules in the general sense. So far attention has been directed mostly to naturally occurring inhibitors of extracellular proteinases whereas data on natural inhibitors of intracellular proteinases are relatively meagre. The presence of inhibitors of cathepsin B and C has been detected in liver homogenate [1]. An inhibitor of brain acid proteinase has been detected in brain tissue homogenate [2]. From skin, an inhibitor has been isolated and partly characterized, which inhibits the activity of an SH-dermoproteinase playing an important role in inflammatory processes [3, 4]. Intracellular proteinases like almost all proteinases are inhibited by the α_2 macroglobulin isolated from blood plasma [5]. Numerous inhibitors of peptidic character and molecular weight < 1000 which inhibit the proteolytic activity of enzymes of different type and origin have been isolated from the culture media of various Streptomyces strains. These inhibitors inhibit also the proteolytic activity of tissue proteinases [6].
The aim of the present study is to summarize the results of our earlier experiments with naturally occurring inhibitors of tissue proteinases and to provide additional

data on the cathepsin D inhibitor from potatoes and on the practical application of naturally occurring inhibitors of cathepsin B_1 and cathepsin E.

Materials and methods

All cathepsins used were isolated in our laboratory. Cathepsin B_1, C and D were prepared from bovine spleen [7, 8], cathepsin E from bone marrow [9].
All naturally occurring inhibitors used in our experiments were prepared in our laboratory. The papain inhibitor from chicken egg white was isolated according to FOSSUM and WHITAKER [10], the pepsin inhibitor from the body walls of Ascaris lumbricoides according to PEANASKY and ABU-ERREISH [11]. The purification of cathepsin D inhibitor from potatoes was described in our preceeding paper [12, 13]. Papain, ficin, and bromelain were commercial products of Calbiochem, USA. Trypsin was purchased from LÉČIVA, Prague; chicken pepsin was prepared in our laboratory [14]. Human serum albumin was purchased from the Institute of Sera and Vaccines, Prague, the trypsin inhibitor from cow colostrum was a generous gift of Dr. ČECHOVA of our institute.
Sepharose 4B was a product of Pharmacia Fine Chemicals, Sweden.

Assay of enzymatic activity

The assay of the enzymatic activity of cathepsin B_1, thiol plant proteases, cathepsin C, and of the inhibition of these activities were described in our preceeding papers [15].
The assay of the enzymatic activity of cathepsin D, E, trypsin, and of the inhibition of these activities were described earlier [16].

Ascaris inhibitor Sepharose column

Sepharose 4B, activated by cyanogen bromide [17], was washed exhaustedly with cold 0.1 M $NaHCO_3$, *p*H 9, and subsequently with cold 0.01 M phosphate buffer, *p*H 6.8. The suspension (10 ml) was treated dropwise with 20 ml of the inhibitor solution (pH 6.8). The mixture was stirred overnight at 4 °C, packed into a column, and washed with phosphate buffer, *p*H 6.8, till the effluent was free of inhibitory activity (tested with chicken pepsin). The column was then equilibrated with acetic acid, *p*H 3.5. The capacity of the column was tested also with chicken pepsin: 1 ml of Ascaris inhibitor Sepharose was capable of binding 2 mg of chicken pepsin [14].
A sample of partly purified cathepsin E in acetic acid, *p*H 3.5, was placed onto this column. Specifically bound cathepsin E was displaced from the column by 0.01 M phosphate buffer, *p*H 6.8.

Amino acid analyses were performed on Beckman Spinco, Model 120B amino acid analyzer according to BENSON and PATTERSON [18].

Automatic sequential degradation

The native cathepsin D inhibitor from potatoes (6 mg) and the performic acid oxidized sample were subjected to Edman degradation [19] in Beckman Sequencer, Model 890 C. The degradation proceeded according to the Fast Quadrol Program. The phenylthiohydantoins were identified by thin layer chromatography or by gas chromatography.

The determination of the sedimentation constant was effected by schlieren optics in Beckman-Spinco Model E ultracentrifuge.

Development and inhibition of Arthus reaction

Male albino rabbits weighing about 2 kg were sensitized by 5 doses of 150 mg of human serum albumin applied subcutaneously at intervals of 2 days. The presence of antibodies in the serum was tested by the precipitin test. The dermal test was carried out 13 days after the last antigen dose. Arthus reaction was induced by intradermal injection of 5 mg of human serum albumin in 100 µl of physiological saline on 16 spots located symmetrically to the spine in the shaved dorsal area. The inhibitor (25 μg/in 100 μl of physiological saline) or controls containing 100 μl of physiological saline only were injected intradermally to identical spots as serum albumin at different time intervals after application of the antigen. The size of the edema formed was measured by a caliper rule after 2, 4, and 24 hrs. The data obtained were evaluated statistically by the *t*-test.

Results and discussion

Most of intracellular proteinases belong with respect to the character of their active sites either to thiol proteinases or to carboxyl proteinases. Only few of them are serine proteinases. The naturally occurring inhibitors are classified according to the classification of enzymes which they inhibit.

Naturally occurring inhibitors of SH-dependent tissue proteinases

We have examined both the chemical and enzymatic characteristics of cathepsin B_1 in detail in our laboratory and found that these characteristics are very similar to those of vegetal thiol proteinases [20], even as regards the N-terminal amino acids (isoleucine in papain and leucine in cathepsin B_1). The second amino acid from the N-terminus in both proteins is proline. Therefore, it is not surprising that the papain inhibitor from chicken egg white [10] inhibited also cathepsin B_1 [15]. The molecular weight of this inhibitor is 12500; it reacts with cathepsin B_1 at a 1:1 molar ratio. Similarly to papain the free thiol group in the active center, which is essential for enzymatic activity, is not required for the interaction with the inhibitor. The interaction takes place even if the enzymes are in inactive mercury form.

The papain inhibitor from chicken egg white inhibits also the activity of cathepsin C [21]. Cathepsin C is an SH-dependent dipeptidyl aminopeptidase, an enzyme which both in its enzymatic specificity and chemical structure diametrally differs both from cathepsin B_1 and papain. We found that this enzyme forms a complex with its inhibitor even after the thiol group of the active center has been blocked by mercury, i. e., even if the enzyme is inactive. On the other hand the binding of this inhibitor by cathepsin C requires — similarly to the binding of the substrate — the presence of halogen ions. We are lacking therefore an explanation why this inhibitor specifically interacts with thiol proteinases only if the thiol group is not essential for the reaction.

Since cathepsin B_1 and C are two considerably different enzymes, we were interested in finding whether these two enzymes act with the inhibitor at a common site on the surface of the inhibitor molecule or whether two different reactive sites are involved. Therefore we prepared the complex of cathepsin B_1 with this inhibitor and examined the inhibition of enzymic activity of different thiol-dependent enzymes like papain, ficin, bromelain and cathepsin C by this complex. In these experiments the enzymatic activity of cathepsin C only was inhibited by the complex of cathepsin B_1 with the inhibitor; the enzymatic activity of all the plant proteinases tested remained unaltered. Our results show that there are two independent nonoverlapping reactive sites on the molecule of this inhibitor: one for the binding of cathepsin B_1, papain, ficin, and bromelain, and the other one for the binding of cathepsin C.

Hayashi et al. [3] observed that the Arthus type of hypersensitivity reaction was paralleled by increased activity of an SH-dependent protease and that the activity of this enzyme was decreased at the later stage of this inflammation by a specific inhibitor. Both the enzyme and the inhibitor were partly purified [4]. It was shown that this thiol proteinase has certain enzymatic characteristics similar to those of papain and that the purified inhibitor inhibits in vitro not only the activity of this proteinase but also the activity of papain. In vivo this inhibitor inhibited the extent of Arthus reaction. In view of this observation we endeavored to affect the extent of Arthus reaction by another inhibitor of SH-proteinases, namely by the papain and cathepsin B_1 inhibitor from chicken egg white [22]. Human serum albumin was used as antigen for the sensibilization of rabbits; Arthus reaction was induced by intradermal application of the same antigen to sensitized rabbits. In control experiments 100 μl of physiological saline was applied to identical spots as the antigen at different time intervals, in other experiments 100 μl of physiological saline containing 25 μg of inhibitor was applied in the same manner. With controls a marked erythema and edema can be observed as soon as 2 hrs after the intradermal application of the antigen. The reaction achieved a maximum 4 to 5 hrs after the application of the antigen. Hemorrhages and even necroses were observed later on but the size of the edema no longer increased. As can be seen in Fig. 1, the inhibitor from chicken egg white significantly decreases the size of the edema. A statistically significant inhibition takes place, however, only if the inhibitor has been injected simultaneously with the antigen. Under these conditions the edema did not even develop in several cases. If the inhibitor was applied as late as 30 min after the antigen the decrease of the reaction was only little evident. When a 25 μg dose of inhibitor was added twice, i. e., the first simultaneously with the antigen and the second 30 min later, the blockade was the same as after a single dose of inhibitor. The intradermal application of the inhibitor in the absence of the antigen did not cause any local reaction on the skin. Our results are similar to those described for the inhibitor isolated from the skin by Japanese authors. It is most probable that the inhibitor from the skin and the in-

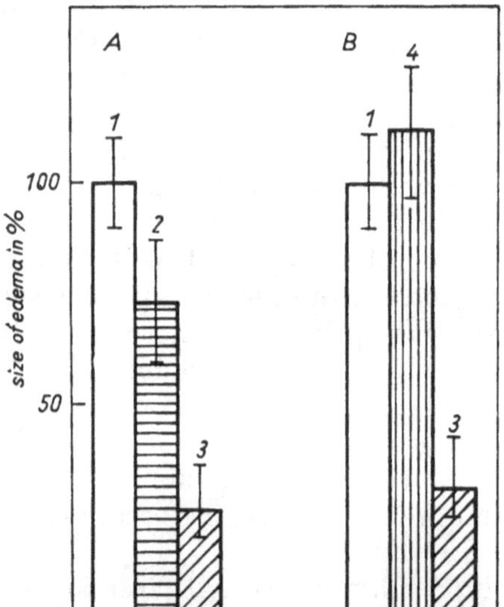

Fig. 1 Effect of papain inhibitor from chicken egg wihite on size of edema in Arthus inflammation.

Size of edema in cm ^{3}/4 hrs after intradermal application of the antigen.

A. Inducing antigen: 20 μg of HSA; B. inducing antigen: 5 mg of HSA.

1) Control (without inhibitor); 2) 25 μg of inhibitor 30 min after antigen; 3) 25 μg of inhibitor simultaneously with antigen; 4) 100 μg of inhibitor from cow colostrum simultaneously with antigen

hibitor of papain and cathepsin B_1 from chicken egg white interact with the same enzyme.

To verify the specificity of this effect we carried out one series of experiments with a trypsin inhibitor from cow colostrum, which inhibits many proteinases of the serine type. Even though this inhibitor was applied in relatively high doses (100 μg) the extent of the skin reaction was not inhibited.

Naturally occurring inhibitors of carboxyl tissue proteinases

A pepsin inhibitor of mol. wt. of 7000 has been isolated from the body walls of the roundworm Ascaris lumbricoides. It was observed in our laboratory that this inhibitor inhibits besides hog and chicken pepsin also the proteolytic activity of cathepsin E; it does not inhibit, however, the activity of cathepsin D, another proteinase of the same type [23]. The interaction of this inhibitor with cathepsin E has been exploited for the purification of cathepsin E by affinity chromatography on Sepharose 4B to which the inhibitor was covalently bound. The course of the affinity chromatography of cathepsin E is shown in Fig. 2. The partly purified fraction of cathepsin E was applied to the column of inhibitor-Sepharose equilibrated with acetic acid, *p*H 3.5. The inactive protein and the quantity of cathepsin E which exceeded the capacity of the column emerged in the first fraction. Cathepsin E which had interacted with the inhibitor attached remained adsorbed in the column and was displaced by 0.01 M phosphate buffer at *p*H 6.8.

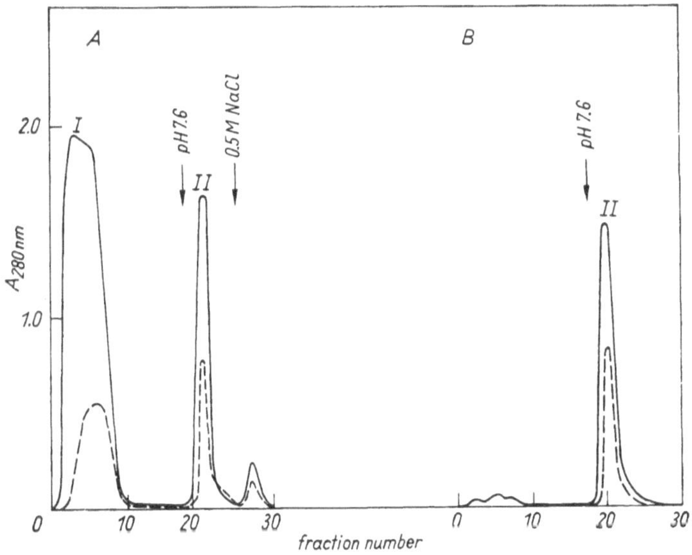

Fig. 2. Affinity chromatography of cathepsin E on Sepharose 4 B with covalently bound pepsin inhibitor from Ascaris lumbricoides.

A) 10 ml of partly purified cathepsin E was applied onto the 1 × 6 cm column at *p*H 3.5. The flow rate was 60 ml/h. The start elution by 0.01 M phosphate buffer, *p*H 6.8, is marked by an arrow.

B) Rechromatography of peak II-material on the same column under identical conditions
——— A_{280} nm; – – – proteolytic activity

The enzyme solution was dialyzed and rechromatographed on the same column under identical conditions. As can be seen in Fig. 2b all of cathepsin E was retained in the column and was displaced only after the *p*H had been raised to 6.8. We have been able to isolate a naturally occurring inhibitor of another carboxyl tissue proteinase — of cathepsin D — from potato tubers [12, 13, 16]. Potato tubers are a well known rich source of various inhibitors [24]. Potato inhibitors have been reported of trypsin and chymotrypsin, kallikrein, carboxypeptidase, and of some bacterial proteinases. Some of these inhibitors have been isolated in homogenous state. In spite of the fact that many inhibitors have been isolated from potatoes, none of them is known to inhibit proteinases of the carboxyl type. The process of preparation of the cathepsin D inhibitor is illustrated schematically in Fig. 3. By this procedure we were able to obtain 25—30 mg of this inhibitor from 1 kg of potato tubers. The homogeneity of the preparation was examined by sedimentation analysis in the ultracentrifuge, by N-terminal end group analysis, and by discontinouus electrophoresis in polyacrylamide gel at *p*H 4 and 8.3. One peak only was observed upon sedimentation analysis in 0.1 M phosphate buffer at *p*H 7.7 and one N-terminal amino acid, glutamic acid, was determined by the phenylisothiocyanate method. One discrete zone only was observed when the preparation was subjected to discontinuous electrophoresis at *p*H 4 and 1—2 weak zones in addition to the main zone were detected at *p*H 8.3.

It has been shown above that the fraction inhibiting cathepsin D at acid *p*H also inhibited trypsin in the alkaline *p*H-region. This phenomenon can be accounted for either by contamination of the preparation by traces of a very active trypsin inhibitor or by assuming a broad specificity of the inhibitor. We endeavored to elucidate this problem in two different ways: (a) by specific affinity chromatography and (b) by preparing the inhibitor by dissociation of the corresponding enzyme-inhibitor complex. The affinity chromatography was carried out both on Sepharose with attached cathepsin D and on Sepharose with covalently attached trypsin. In experiments with cathepsin D-Sepharose the sample was applied at *p*H 4 and the inhibitor adsorbed was displaced by buffer at *p*H 7.6. In experiments with trypsin-Sepharose the sample was applied at *p*H 7.6 and the inhibitor adsorbed eluted by a buffer at *p*H 3.8. In both cases the inhibitor liberated inhibited both cathepsin D and trypsin.

In another series of experiments a complex of the inhibitor with cathepsin D was prepared at *p*H 4.0 and with trypsin at *p*H 7.6. An excess of inhibitor was used in both cases. The latter was carefully removed after the interaction by gel filtration. Both complexes were subsequently dissociated by proper change in *p*H and the inhibitors liberated were examined for the inhibition of cathepsin D and trypsin. We observed that the inhibitor released from both complexes again inhibits cathepsin D at acid *p*H and trypsin at alkaline *p*H. We concluded from our observations thath both inhibitory activities are inseparable and represent an intrinsic characteristics of the inhibitor molecule.

The inhibitor was shown to be stable in the *p*H range 2—10.5. It could be heated without loss of activity at 60 °C for 30 min, lost, however, its activity after 1-min heating at 85 °C. Its isoelectric point measured by isoelectric focusing was 7.9. The inhibitor was not hydrolyzed by pepsin. It inhibits cathepsin D in acid media,

Potatoe tubers homogenate
↓
Extraction
(0.1 M acetate, *p*H 4.0)
↓
Ammonium sulphate precipitation
(0.3 saturation)
↓
Chromatography on Sephadex G 50
↓
Chromatography on DEAE-Sephadex A 25
(0.01 M Tris-HCl, *p*H 7.6)
↓
Chromatography on SE-Sephadex C25
(0.01 M formate buffer, *p*H 3.0
lin. gradient 0—0.5 M NaCl
↓
Affinity chromatography on Cathepsin D-Sepharose 4B | Affinity chromatography on Trypsin-Sepharose 4B

Fig. 3. Isolation of cathepsin D inhibitor from potatoes

does not inhibit hog or chicken pepsin and cathepsin E. In alkaline media it inhibits trypsin. The inhibition of both enzmes, i. e., of cathepsin D and trypsin, is reversible and competitive. The molecular weight determined by gel-chromatography is 27000, the value obtained by sedimentation analysis in the ultracentrifuge is 20880 ± 420, and the value calculated from amino acid composition is 21790.

The molecular weights of most inhibitors from potatoes were originally reported as 20000—25000. Many inhibitors were later observed to consist of subunits of lower molecular weight. The problem of subunits of the cathepsin D inhibitor has not been elucidated in detail; its molecule may also consist of subunits of lower molecular weight. This seems to be supported by the fact that the value of sedimentation coefficient, which is 2.9 S in buffer without urea, dropped to 1.5 S in the presence of 6 M urea. This drop could be caused, among others, by a degradation of the molecule to subunits in urea-containing media.

The amino acid composition of the entire inhibitor molecule is shown in Table 1. The molecule contains 199 amino acid residues and three disulfide bonds; it lacks histidine and contains one methionine only. The presence of one methionine residue is advantageous from the viewpoint of cyanogen bromide cleavage in sequential studies on the inhibitor which will begin in near future in our laboratory.

Since N-terminal end group analysis by the phenylisothiocyanate method showed the presence of one N-terminal amino acid only, the inhibitor was subjected to automatic Edman degradation and the following 17-residue N-terminal sequence was determined:

Glu-Ser-Pro-Leu-Pro-Lys-Pro-Val-Leu-Asp-X-Asn-Gly-Lys-Glu-Leu-Gln.

The inhibitor was subjected to sequential analysis both native and oxidized by performic acid. The results obtained with both preparations were identical. Un-

Table 1
Amino acid composition
of cathepsin D inhibitor from potatoes

Lysine	10	Alanine	7
Histidine	0	1/2 Cystine	6
Arginine	8	Valine	16
Aspartic acid	26	Methionine	1
Threonine	9	Isoleucine	12
Serine	14	Leucine	22
Glutamic acid	12	Tyrosine	8
Proline	16	Phenylalanine	12
Glycine	19	Tryptophan	1
		Total	199

fortunately, the sequence determined could not be extended even when the oxidized preparation was used because the reaction products were very little soluble and the results were not reliable.

If we compare the amino acid composition of our cathepsin D inhibitor with the amino acid composition of other inhibitors from potatoes, our cathepsin D inhibitor is not identical with any of the latter. It resembles somes of them, e. g., by lacking histidine, yet differs in its N-terminal amino acid or disulfide content. It has the same N-terminal amino acid as other inhibitors, yet differs in other characteristics. It appears that it is therefore a new inhibitor and not merely an inhibitor discovered earlier and showing additional specificity.

Studies on the interaction of high molecular weight inhibitors with cathepsin D and E showed interesting differences in the behavior of these enzymes. The pepsin inhibitor from Ascaris inhibits cathepsin E but not cathepsin D. The cathepsin D inhibitor from potatoes does not inhibit either cathepsin E or pepsin. Hence judging by the interaction with the high molecular weight inhibitors studied, cathepsin E is more similar to pepsin than to cathepsin D.

References

[1] FINKENSTAEDT, J.: Proc. Soc. exp. Biol. Med. **95**, 302 (1957)
[2] D'MONTE, B., N. MARKS, A. LAJTHA, and P. MELA: Trans. Am. Soc. Neurochem. **1**, 37 (1970)
[3] HAYASHI, A., K. UDAKA, H. MYIOSHI, and S. KUDO: Lab. Invest. **14**, 665 (1965)
[4] UDAKA, K., and H. HAYASHI: Biochim. biophys. Acta **97**, 251 (1965)
[5] STARKEY, P. M., and A. J. BARRETT: Biochem. J. **131**, 823 (1973)
[6] UMEZAWA, H.: Enzyme Inhibitors of Microbial Origin. University Park Press, Baltimore, London, Tokyo 1972
[7] KEILOVÁ, H., and V. TOMÁŠEK: FEBS Lett. **29**, 335 (1973)
[8] KEILOVÁ, H. in: Tissue Proteinases. A. J. BARRETT and T. J. DINGLE (Eds). North-Holland Publishing Co., Amsterdam 1971 p. 45
[9] LAPRESLE, C. in: Tissue Proteinases. A. J. BARRETT and T. J. DINGLE (Eds). North-Holland Publishing Co., Amsterdam 1971, p. 135
[10] FOSSUM, K., and J. WHITAKER: Archs Biochem. Biophys. **125**, 367 (1968)
[11] PEANASKY, R. J., and GHALEB, M. ABU-ERREISH: Proceedings of the International Resarch Conference on Proteinases Inhibitors, Munich 1970. De Gruyter, Berlin, New York 1971, p. 289
[12] KEILOVÁ, H., and V. TOMÁŠEK: Coll. Czech. chem. Commun. **41**, 489 (1976)
[13] RUPOVÁ, L., H. KEILOVÁ, and V. TOMÁŠEK: Coll. Czech. chem. Commun. (in press)

[14] KEILOVÁ, H., A. SALVETOVÁ, and V. KOSTKA: Coll. Czech. chem. Commun. **40**, 580 (1975)
[15] KEILOVÁ, H., and V. TOMÁŠEK: Biochim. biophys. Acta **334**, 179 (1974)
[16] KEILOVÁ, H., and V. TOMÁŠEK: Coll. Czech. chem. Commun. **41**, 2440 (1976)
[17] PORATH, J., K. ASPBERG, H. DREVIN, and R. AXEN: J. Chromat. **86**, 53 (1973)
[18] BENSON, Jr. J. V., and J. A. PATTERSON: Anal. Chem. **37**, 1108 (1965)
[19] EDMAN, P., and A. HENSCHEN: Protein Sequence Determination. 2nd Edit. Springer, Berlin, Heidelberg, New York 1975, p. 232
[20] KEILOVÁ, H., and V. TOMÁŠEK: Intracellular Protein Catabolism, Reinhardsbrunn 1973. Wissensch. Beiträge der Martin-Luther Universität Halle-Wittenberg 1974/76, p. 237
[21] KEILOVÁ, H., and V. TOMÁŠEK: Coll. Czech. chem. Commun. **40**, 218 (1975)
[22] KEILOVÁ, H., and J. CHUTNÁ: Unpublished results
[23] KEILOVÁ, H., and V. TOMÁŠEK: Biochim. biophys. Acta **284**, 461 (1972)
[24] VOGEL, R., I. TRAUTSCHOLD, and E. WERLE: Natural Proteinase Inhibitors. Academic Press, New York, London 1968, p. 33

Acta biol. med. germ., Band 36, Seite 1883—1886 (1977)

Department of Biochemistry, J. Stefan Institute,
University of Ljubljana, Ljubljana, Yugoslàvia

Isolation and characterization of inhibitors of neutral proteinases from spleen

J. Brzin, M. Kopitar, and V. Turk

Summary

Two different types of neutral proteinase inhibitors were isolated from postmicrosomal supernatant of bovine spleen. Inhibitor A with molecular weight 40,000 inhibits elastases and chymotrypsin-like neutral proteinases from bovine spleen, whereas inhibitor B with estimated molecular weight 20000 inhibits only chymotrypsin-like neutral proteinase.

Introduction

The last investigations in the field of neutral proteinases have shown that their action is extracellulary [1] and intracellularly [2—5] regulated by inhibitors. The extracellular inhibitors were much more studied than intracellular inhibitors. There are only a few studies regarding their existence inside the leucocytes. Even less was reported on their separation and specificity.
The successful isolation of neutral proteinases from bovine spleen following acid inactivation of intracellular inhibitors lead us to their isolation.

Materials and methods

Fresh spleen was cut to pieces and cells squeezed out to avoid their excessive damage. A 1:5 w/v suspension of the cells in Hank's solution was prepared and centrifuged at low speed to remove serum proteins. This procedure was repeated 3 times, followed by gentle homogenization of the cells with teflon-glass homogenizer. The homogenate was diluted with Hank's solution to final ratio 1:8 w/v and centrifuged at 7000 x *g* for 30 min, to remove unbroken cells and cell debris together with nuclei, mitochondria and granules. Supernatant was further centrifuged at 100000 x *g* for 60 min to remove the remaining microsomal particles. The resulting supernatant was concentrated by lyophilization and used for the further isolation of inhibitors.
Purification was carried out on a Sephadex G-200 column in 1 mM Na_2HPO_4 and 0.1 M NaCl, *p*H 7.0. Sephadex G-150 and G-100 with the same eluent were also used in subsequent isolation steps. Protein content of eluted fractions was estimated from absorbance at 280 nm. The inhibitor was determined in the effluent by measuring the inhibition of neutral proteinase activity. The substances used for column calibration were blue dextran, bovine albumin, chymotrypsinogen and cytochrome c, all from Sigma (USA).
Inhibition tests were performed as described previously [4]. The following substrates were used: 1% casein, 2% hemoglobin, 1% histones in 0.2 N phosphate buffer, *p*H 7.5. Hemoglobin and histones were prepared in our laboratory, casein was from BDH (England). We tested the inhibition of the following enzyme preparations: spleen elastase and chymotrypsin-like neutral proteinase and the highly active mixture of neutral proteinases extracted from bovine spleen.

Results and discussion

Gel chromatography on Sephadex G-200 revealed three protein peaks (Fig. 1). Two inhibitors could be detected. They were marked A and B. The fractions con-

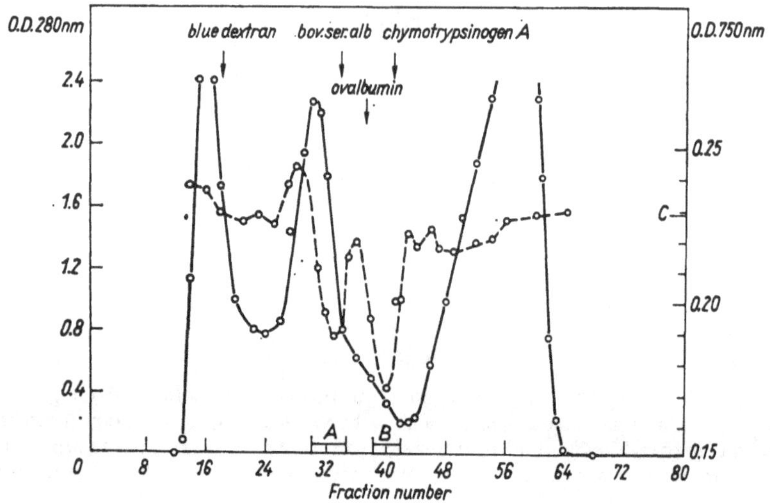

Fig. 1. Elution profile of spleen supernatant on a Sephadex G-200 column (4.0 × 100 cm)

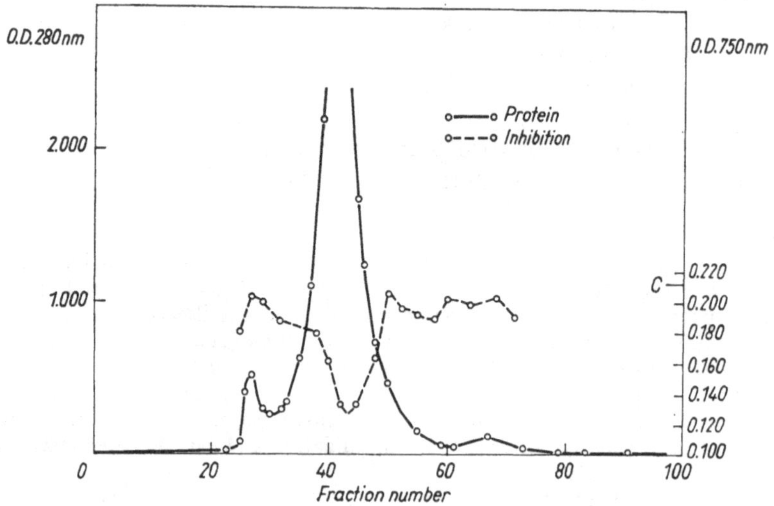

Fig. 2. Elution profile of pooled fractions of inhibitor A from Sephadex G-200 on a Sephadex G-150 column. (1.7 × 100 cm)

taining inhibitors were pooled. Peak A was concentrated by ultrafiltration and applied to the column of Sephadex G-150. The elution profile is shown in Fig. 2. The small amount of low molecular weight inhibitor (peak B) was well separated on this column. Fractions containing high molecular weight inhibitor A were pooled and concentrated by ultrafiltration.

The low molecular weight inhibitor B was further purified on Sephadex G-100 (Fig. 3). Four protein peaks were found. A small amount of inhibitor A was present in the first peak. Inhibitor B was found in tail of the second peak. The molecular weights of both inhibitors were estimated in this experiment. It was found that inhibitor A has molecular weight of 40000 and inhibitor B of 15—20000.

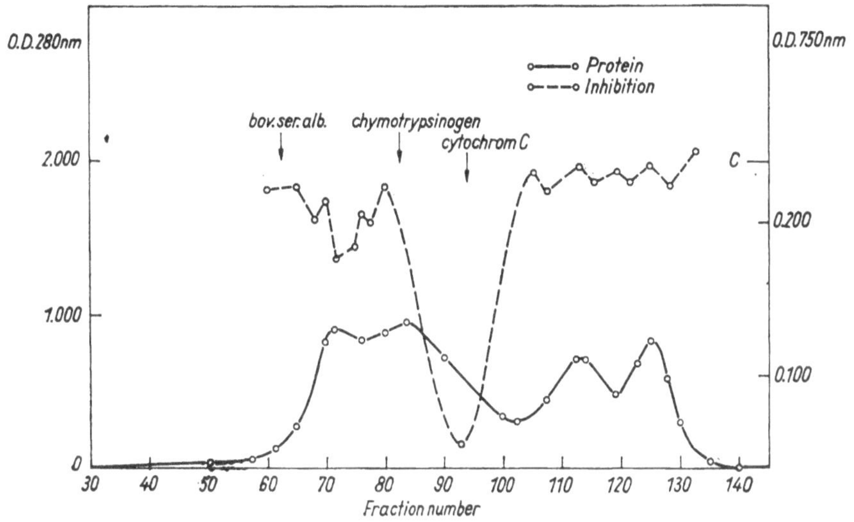

Fig. 3. Elution profile of pooled fractions of inhibitor B from Sephadex G-200 on a column of Sephadex G-100 (1.7 × × 100 cm)

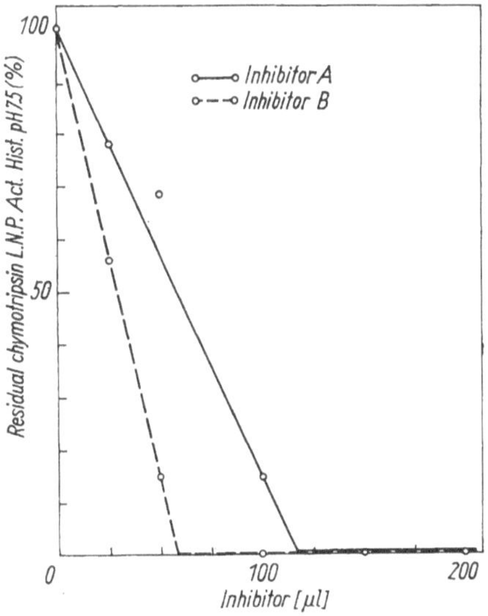

Fig. 4

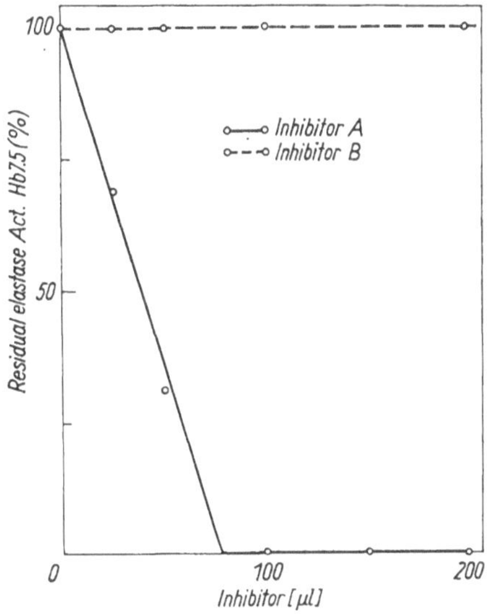

Fig. 5

Fig. 4. Inhibition of spleen chymotrypsin-like neutral proteinase by inhibitors A and B by different concentration of inhibitors

Fig. 5. Inhibition of spleen elastase by different concentrations of inhibitor A and B

Fig. 4 shows inhibition of chymotrypsin-like neutral proteinase from bovine spleen with increasing amounts of inhibitors A and B. Both inhibitors were able to inhibit this neutral proteinase. Fig. 5 demonstrates the effect of both inhibitors on elastase. It is evident that inhibitor B does not inhibit elastase even at highest concentration, whereas inhibitor A abolished elastase activity completely. The effect

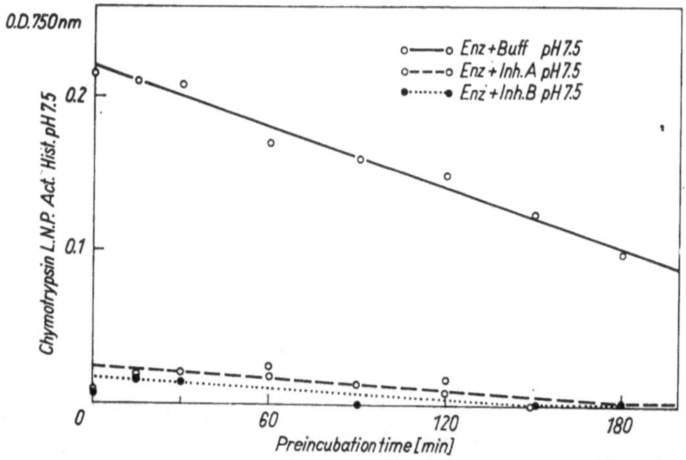

Fig. 6. Time dependence of chymotrypsin-like neutral proteinase on inhibitor effect of inhibitors A and B.

2 ml of each inhibitor was treated with 2 ml of enzyme, at 22 °C. At intervals as indicated in the graph, 0.4 ml portions of each mixture were withdrawn and assayed with 2 ml of histones at *p*H 7.5. Neutral proteinase activity is expressed in the figure in the absorbance change, after 2 hrs of hydrolysis. Upper line represents the inactivation of chymotrypsin-like neutral proteinase in buffer solution at *p*H 7.5 and 22 °C

of preincubation time on the extent of inhibition of chymotrypsin-like neutral proteinase is shown in Fig. 6. Both inhibitors are of the fast reacting type and no preincubation is needed to reach the full inhibition. It is also evident that even after 3 hrs of preincubation the enzyme remained inactive, and no reversibility of inhibition could be detected.

The presented data have shown that bovine spleen contains two specific inhibitors of neutral proteinases.

Acknowledgements

We thank Mrs. M. Božič, Mrs. M. Pregelj and Mr. K. Lindič for their skillful technical assistance. This investigation was supported by a grant from the Research Council of Slovenia and in part from NSF, USA

References

[1] Fritz, H., H. Tschesche, L. J. Greene, and E. Truscheit (Eds): Proteinase inhibitors. Springer, Berlin, Heidelberg, New York 1974
[2] Davies, P., A. G. Rita, K. Krakauer, and G. Weissmann: Biochem. J. **123**, 559 (1971)
[3] Janoff, A., and J. Blondin: Proc. Soc. exp. Biol. Med. **136**, 1050 (1971)
[4] Kopitar, M., and D. Lebez: Eur. J. Biochem. **56**, 571 (1975)
[5] Steven, F. S., P. M. Milsom, and J. A. Hunter: Eur. J. Biochem. **67**, 165 (1976)

Acta biol. med. germ., Band 36, Seite 1887—1891 (1977)

Université Catholique de Louvain, Laboratoire de Chimie Physiologique,
and International Institute of Cellular and Molecular Pathology, B-1200 Bruxelles, Belgium

Production of rabbit antibodies against active rat cathepsin B

M. PIERART-GALLOIS, A. TROUET, and P. TULKENS*

Introduction

Antisera directed against lysosomal hydrolases and constituents are powerful tools to investigate the role of lysosomes in cell and tissue physiopathology (see e. g. [1—5]). No investigator however has reported successful obtention of antisera against native cathepsin B, although this enzyme can be obtained highly purified from liver extract [6]. This is unfortunate in view of the key roles ascribed to cathepsin B in intra- and extracellular proteolytic processes [7—9], and we accordingly decided to reappraise the question.

Materials and methods

Enzymatic assays

Cathepsin B activity was assayed using α-N-benzoyl-DL-arginine-β-2-naphtyl amide (BANA) as substrate, by the method of BARRETT [10]. Proteins were measured by the Lowry's technique.

Preparation of soluble fraction of lysosomes

Lysosomes were purified from livers of rats injected with the non-ionic detergent Triton WR-1339, following the procedure described by TROUET [11]. Lysosomes were ruptured by hypotonic shock and the soluble extract was separated from the insoluble material by centrifugation; the pellet was washed once with 0.15 M NaCl and the supernatants were pooled.

Gel chromatography

All gel chromatography experiments were performed with Sephadex G-100, using 0.15 M NaCl-3 mM, imidazole, *p*H 7.0, as eluant.

Preparation of IgG

Purified IgG was obtained from rabbit sera by ion exchange chromatography on DEAE-Sephadex [12], followed by precipitation with half-saturated $(NH_4)_2SO_4$ IgG was resuspended in 0.15 M NaCl-3 mM Na/K-phosphate buffer, *p*H 7.4, and made free of ammonium sulfate by gel chromatography on Sephadex G-25.

Immunization of animals

Rabbits were immunized by two successive series of 3 injections of antigen preparation (10 mg of protein) at weekly intervals, and separated by a 3 weeks rest. For the first injection of each series, the antigen preparation was mixed with Freund's complete adjuvant. Rabbits were bled one week after the last injection.

* Chargé de Recherches of the Belgian Fonds National de la Recherche Scientifique

Results

Preparation of partially purified cathepsin B

The soluble extract of lysosomes was subjected to gel filtration on Sephadex G-100. We separated by this process a fraction of proteins of low molecular weight (between 20—30.000 daltons), that contained more than 80% of the BANAase activity of the original soluble lysosomal preparation. The purification of this enzymatic activity from the original homogenate was about 500fold on a protein basis with a yield of circa 20%. No further purification of this material was attempted and we will refer at it as paritially purified cathepsin B.

Conjugation of cathepsin B to bovine serum albumin

The preparation of partially purified cathepsin B, obtained as described above, was injected to several rabbits, but we could not detect the formation of antibodies against cathepsin B in any of their sera, even after prolonged injection periods. We therefore decided to increase the immunogenicity of cathepsin B by polymerization. Direct action of glutaraldehyde, as a coupling agent, on the cathepsin B preparation resulted however in the complete loss of the enzymatic activity. We accordingly attempted to couple cathepsin B to albumin, avoiding direct contact of the enzyme with large concentrations of glutaraldehyde. This was achieved as follows: Bovine serum albumin was exposed to an excess of glutaraldehyde and thereafter filtered through Sephadex G-100, to remove unreacted glutaraldehyde. Cathepsin B preparation was immediately mixed with the "activated" serum albumin, and the mixture was then filtered again through Sephadex G-100. We obtained a preparation of proteins of an apparent molecular weight larger than 150.000 daltons, and displaying good hydrolytic activity towards BANA, suggesting the coupling of cathepsin B with dimers or polymers of albumin. This preparation will be referred henceforth as conjugated cathepsin B.

Characterization of antibodies against cathepsin B

IgG obtained from rabbits, immunized with conjugated cathepsin B was found to inhibit the enzymatic activity of unconjugated cathepsin B, either from the partially purified cathepsin B preparation, from the complete lysosomal soluble fraction, or from the supernatant of a lyzed liver homogenate. The enzyme preparations were incubated with purified IgG for 1 hr at 37 °C at *p*H 7.0; the enzymatic activity was thereafter assayed by addition of BANA, buffered at *p*H 6.0, in presence of cysteine and EDTA. Results are presented in Table 1. IgG from control rabbits, or rabbits immunized with bovine serum albumin did not affect the activity of cathepsin B. By contrast, IgG from rabbits immunized with conjugated cathepsin B strongly inhibited the activity of cathepsin B from all preparations tested.

No precipitation of the cathepsin B activity could however be evidenced, in presence of IgG from rabbits immunized with conjugated cathepsin B, even after overnight incubation at 0 °C. Indirect precipitation of an immune complex, by means of goat (anti-rabbit) IgG could not be satisfactorily evidenced, because the large amount of goat IgG, necessary to precipitate all rabbit IgG present in the

Table 1
Inhibitory action of IgG on the hydrolysis of BANA by rat liver fractions

Source of enzyme	Activity[1] measured in presence of IgG (0.9 mg/ml)		
	from control rabbits	from rabbits immunized with serum albumin	from rabbits immunized with conjugated cathepsin B
Partially purified cathepsin B[2]	96	94	25
Complete soluble lysosomal fractions	99	—	36
Supernatant[3] from rat liver homogenate	99	—	47

[1] In % of the activity measured in absence of IgG (35 m Units/ml);
[2] see Results §1;
[3] from rat liver homogenate prepared in distilled water; this preparation contained 70% of the total BANA activity of the liver.

incubation mixture, exerted an important inhibition on the cathepsin B activity of the samples.

We therefore attempted to evidence directly the formation of immune complexes between cathepsin B and rabbit IgG. A preparation of partially purified cathepsin B was mixed with IgG from control animals or animals immunized with conjugated cathepsin B. These mixtures were passed through a Sephadex G-100 column. Results are shown in Fig. 1. In presence of control IgG, the elution profile of the BANAase activity dissociated markedly from that of the proteins, as could be expected from the differences of molecular weight between IgG and the proteins constituting the partially purified cathepsin B preparation and their relative concentrations in the mixture. In presence of IgG from immunized rabbits, the BANAase activity was largely inhibited, but he bulk of the remaining enzymatic activity eluted short before the proteins; less than 10% of the original activity was eluted as in the control experiment.

Discussion

The experiments reported in this paper show that purified IgG obtained from rabbits immunized with a preparation of cathepsin B partially purified and conjugated to serum albumin, inhibits strongly the BANAase activity 1) of lysosomal proteins of low molecular weight, 2) of a complete soluble extract from lysosomes and 3) of the supernatant of a lyzed liver homogenate. Moreover, incubation of a preparation of partially purified cathepsin B with this IgG results in an apparent increase of the molecular weight of the lysosomal enzyme(s) responsible of the hydrolysis of BANA. As these results are only observed with IgG from immunized animals, it is likely that they are the consequence of the reaction of specific antibodies against the protein(s) responsible of the BANAase activity.

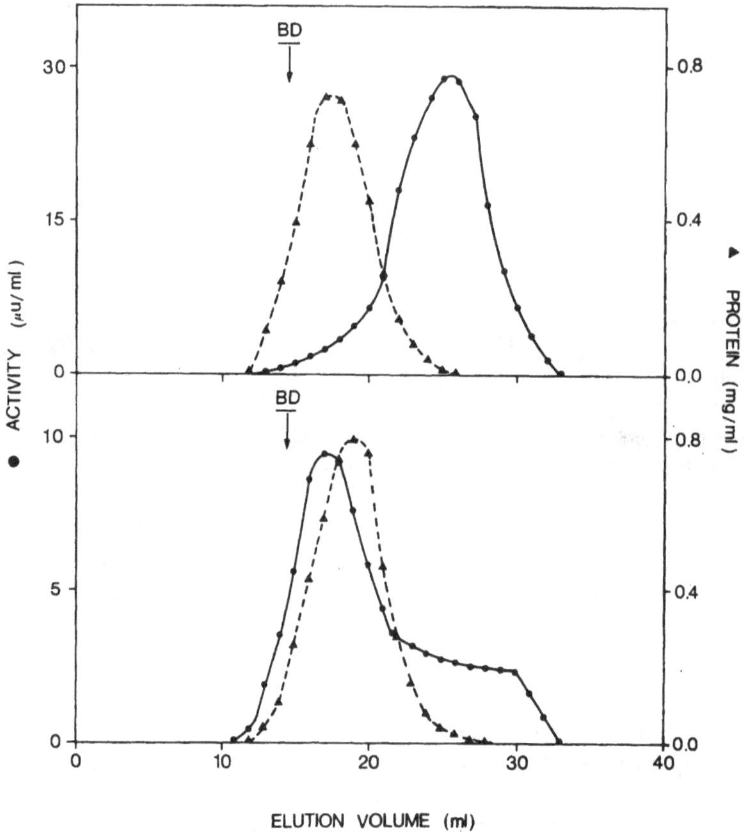

Fig. 1. Gel chromatography of a mixture of partially purified cathepsin B and rabbit IgG. 0.05 mg of enzyme preparation was mixed with 0.9 mg of IgG, incubated 1 hr at 37 °C and 24 hrs at 0 °C; the mixture was applied to column of Sephadex G-100. ▲— — —▲: elution profile of protein; ●———●: elution profile of BANAase activity. Upper part of the diagram: in presence of IgG from control rabbits; lower part: in presence of IgG from rabbit immunized with conjugated cathepsin B. Note the inhibitory acition exerted by these last IgG on the total BANAase activity. Recoveries of enzymatic activities in the chromatography were 87% and 90%, respectively.
The arrows marked ,,BD" refer to the median elution volume of blue dextran (av. m.w.t 2×10^6 daltons)

Antibodies raised against enzymes have usually been shown to inhibit their catalytic activities, probably by steric hindrance [13]; although this effect is most often observed with substrates of large molecular weight, inhibition of enzymatic activity towards small molecules by antibodies has also been reported [14]. The lack of precipitation of the enzyme by the specific IgG could be explained by the existence of a unique antigenic site on the enzyme molecules. which would therefore be unable to form precipitates with IgG; this hypothesis would easily be understandable, in view of the relatively low molecular weight of the proteins responsible of the hydrolysis of BANA. The results of Fig. 1 show clearly that there is an association between IgG from immunized rabbits and the enzyme(s) hydrolyzing BANA.

It has been clearly demonstrated that most, if not all enzymatic activity of rat liver towards BANA is found in lysosomes [15] and this activity has long been ascribed to a single enzyme, cathepsin B, formerly called cathepsin B 1 [16]. Recent data however have disclosed that lysosomes contain at least two distinct enzymes that hydrolize BANA, in presence of cystein and EDTA [17, 18]. Those enzymes have been named cathepsin B and cathepsin H (or cathepsin B 1') respectively. Both enzymes have similar molecular weights (24—28.000) and are therefore collected together in our preparation of partially purified cathepsin B.
Our experiments show that IgG from immune sera react with the bulk of the proteins responsible for the hydrolysis of BANA in liver. This suggests that we could have actually antibodies directed against both cathepsin B and cathepsin H. Separation of the two enzymes, or differential assay using other substrates or inhibition by leupeptin are however necessary to establish the precise specificity of our antiserum. As such, and in association with antibodies against other lysosomal proteases our antiserum should already be useful in the unraveling of the functions of lysosomes in intracellular and extracellular protein catabolism.

Acknowledgements

This work was supported by the Belgian Fonds de la Recherche Scientifique Médicale. The skilful help of Mrs. F. Renoird-Andries and Mr. J. Demeyere is greatly appreciated.

References

[1] Tulkens, P., A. Trouet, and F. van Hoof: Nature, Lond. **228**, 1282 (1970)
[2] Dingle, J. T., A. R. Poole, G. S. Lazarus, and A. J. Barrett: J. exp. Med. **137**, 1124 (1973)
[3] Weston, P. D., and A. R. Poole in: Lysosomes in Biology and Pathology. J. T. Dingle (Ed.). **3**, 425. North-Holland Publ. Co., Amsterdam 1973
[4] Tulkens, P. in: Methodological Developments in Biochemistry. E. Reid (Ed.), **4**, 327. Longman, London 1974
[5] Szego, C. M., M. B. Nazareno, and D. D. Porter: J. Cell Biol. **73**, 354 (1977)
[6] Barrett, A. J.: Biochem. J. **131**, 809 (1973)
[7] Huisman, W., J. M. W. Bouma, and M. Gruber: Biochim. biophys. Acta **297**, 93 (1973)
[8] Huisman, W., J. M. W. Bouma, and M. Gruber: Biochim. biophys. Acta **297**, 98 (1973)
[9] Werb, Z., and J. T. Dingle in: Lysosomes in Biology and Pathology. J. T. Dingle and R. T. Dean (Eds) **5**, 127. North-Holland Publ. Co., Amsterdam 1976
[10] Barrett, A. J.: Anal. Biochem. **47**, 280 (1972)
[11] Trouet, A.: Meth. Enymol. **31**, 323 (1974)
[12] Sober, M., M. J. Gutter, M. M. Wyckoff, and E. A. Peterson: J. Am. chem. Soc. **78** 756 (1956)
[13] Cinader, B., and K. J. Lafferty: Immunology **7**, 342 (1963)
[14] Kaplan, N. O., and S. White: Ann. N.Y. Acad. Sci. **103**, 835 (1963)
[15] Bouma, J. M. W., and M. Gruber: Biochim. biophys. Acta **113**, 350 (1966)
[16] Barrell, A. J., and R. Dean in: Cell Biology. P. L. Altman and D. D. Katz (Eds). FASEB Biological Handbook, Bethesda, Md., 1976, p. 317
[17] Kirschke, H., J. Langner, B. Wiederanders, S. Ansorge, P. Bohley, and U. Broghammer: Acta biol. med. germ. **35**, 285 (1976)
[18] Davison, E., and B. Poole: Biochim. biophys. Acta **397**, 437 (1975)

Acta biol. med. germ., Band 36, Seite 1893—1897 (1977)

Institute of Pharmacology and Toxicology, Medical Academy Erfurt, 50 Erfurt, DDR

Role of heparin in the interaction of serine proteinases with antithrombin III

J. Stürzebecher

Summary

To characterize the mode of action of heparin, the kinetics of inhibition of thrombin, factor Xa, and plasmin by antithrombin III was studied without and in the presence of heparin. Following the concentration dependence of inactivation a linear dependence was found between the apparent first-order inactivation rate constant and the antithrombin III concentration. This behaviour is typical of enzyme-activator interaction. Values of kinetic constants of the inactivation reaction could be determined. Thus, heparin acts obviously as an activator of the enzymes and enhances their affinity for antithrombin III.

Introduction

At the present time, the acidic mucopolysaccharide heparin is the most important drug for prophylaxis of thrombin-induced thrombotic processes. The anticoagulant effect of heparin occurs only when it interacts with a cofactor, that is antithrombin III (AT). AT is an α-glycoprotein with a molecular weight of 65.000 present in mammalian plasma. As early as 1959, Markwardt and Walsmann [1] demonstrated that heparin accelerates the slowly proceeding reaction between thrombin and AT. Heparin acts as a catalyst and is not consumed. It has been assumed that the affinity of thrombin for AT is enhanced by the binding of heparin to the enzyme, whereby the rate of inactivation of thrombin by AT is accelerated. Studies on the binding of heparin to thrombin confirmed this conception of the mechanism of action [2—4].

In subsequent years, AT was found to inhibit several other serine proteinases of the blood; these are factors IXa [5—8], Xa [7—9], XIa [10], XIIa [11], as well as plasmin [10, 12] and kallikrein [13]. In all cases, heparin speeds up the inactivation. The fact that these serine proteinases are rapidly inactivated by AT and heparin and the recent demonstration of tight binding of heparin to AT [14—16] suggest the alternative mechanism that heparin acts by rendering AT more sensitive to the enzymes [17, 18]. These mechanisms are difficult to describe, since due to its polyanionic character heparin possesses high affinity for numerous proteins [19]. In order to distinguish between these mechanisms, attempts have been made to analyse the kinetics of the reaction between thrombin and AT and heparin. Also the clotting factor Xa (FXa) and plasmin were investigated. FXa is an enzyme acting in the reaction chain of the coagulation system earlier than thrombin and whose inhibition could have a stronger anticoagulant effect than the inhibition of thrombin [20]. In constrast, plasmin is an enzyme which does not participate directly in the coagulation mechanism. Since the investigations revealed an unusual example of a proteinase-inhibitor-activator system, the procedure of analysis is briefly described.

Kinetic studies

The reaction between the enzymes and AT is commonly believed to proceed accord-ng to equation (1)

$$E + I \underset{}{\overset{K_i}{\rightleftharpoons}} EI \xrightarrow{k_2} E{-}I \tag{1}$$

First between the enzyme (E) and AT as inhibitor (I) an intermediate complex (EI) is formed which is converted into the $E{-}I$ compound. The covalent bond between thrombin and AT is a carboxylic ester [21]. To clarify whether an intermediate complex was formed and to determine the constants k_2 and K_i, the concentration dependence of the inactivation was studied as described by KITZ and WILSON [22]. First, under the conditions $I > E$ the apparent first-order inactivation rate constant k_{app} is determined. The dependence of the pseudo first-order rate constant on the concentration of AT (I) is given by equation (2):

$$\frac{1}{k_{app}} = \frac{1}{k_2} + \frac{K_i}{k_2} \cdot \frac{1}{I} \tag{2}$$

The inactivation of thrombin, FXa, and plasmin at pH 8.0 and 25 °C by AT was observed to obey first-order kinetics. By the use of specific peptide substrates for thrombin, FXa, and plasmin (Bz-Phe-Val-Arg-pNA, Bz-Ile-Glu-Gly-Arg-pNA, H-D-Val-Leu-Lys-pNA) the loss of amidase activity was measured. The methods are described in detail elsewhere [23]. Fig. 1 shows an example of the inhibition of thrombin by three AT concentrations. From the slope $\left(= -\frac{k_{app}}{2.303}\right)$ the apparent inactivation rate constants k_{app} were determined. The reciprocal plots of k_{app} vs inhibitor concentrations yield straight lines with a positive intercept on the ordinate (Fig. 2—4). According to the equation (2) from the slope ($= K_i/k_2$) and the intercept ($= 1/k_2$), the values of k_2 and K_i were calculated (Table 1). Of special

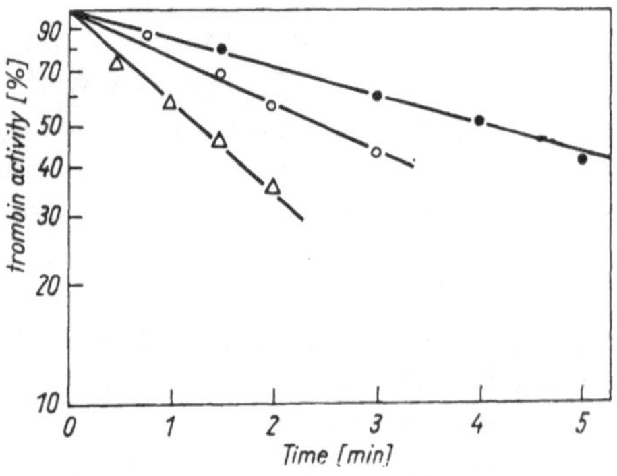

Fig. 1

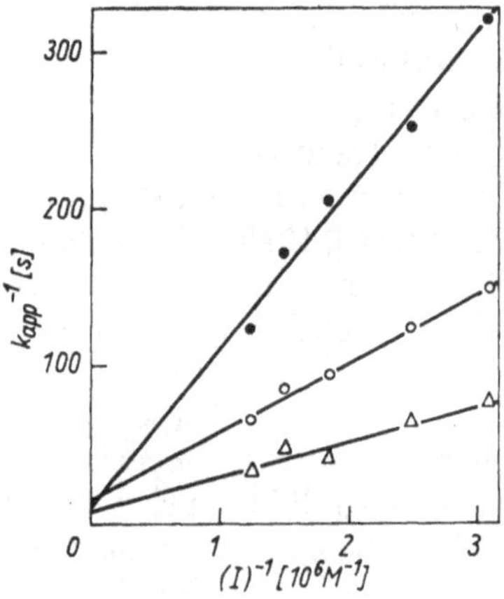

Fig. 2

Fig. 1. Inactivation of thrombin ($1.3 \cdot 10^{-7}$ M) by $3.2 \cdot 10^{-7}$ M (●), $5.4 \cdot 10^{-7}$ M (○) and $8.1 \cdot 10^{-7}$ M (△) antithrombin III

Fig. 2. Dependence of k_{app} on the concentration of antithrombin III (I) by the inhibition of thrombin ($1.3 \cdot 10^{-7}$ M) by antithrombin III; without heparin (●), with $1.8 \cdot 10^{-8}$ M (○) and $3.6 \cdot 10^{-8}$ M (△) heparin interest is the result that the rate constant k_2 for the thrombin-AT reaction is greater than the constants for the reaction with FXa or plasmin, resp. Thus, in case of thrombin, the undissociated inactive compound forms very rapidly from the non-covalent complex.

During the reaction between AT and the enzymes in the presence of heparin, the rate of inactivation increases in all three enzymes. The reactions obey first-order kinetics so that the rate constants k_{app} could be determined. The reciprocal plots of k_{app} vs AT concentration revealed also straight lines for the inhibition of thrombin, FXa, and plasmin by AT in the presence of heparin (Fig. 2—4). The slope of the straight lines declines considerably with increasing heparin concentration. For the discussion of these results equation (1) must be extended. Two possible mechanisms can be presupposed. Either heparin makes the proteinases more sensitive to inhibition by AT, or heparin activates AT to make it more effective inhibitor.

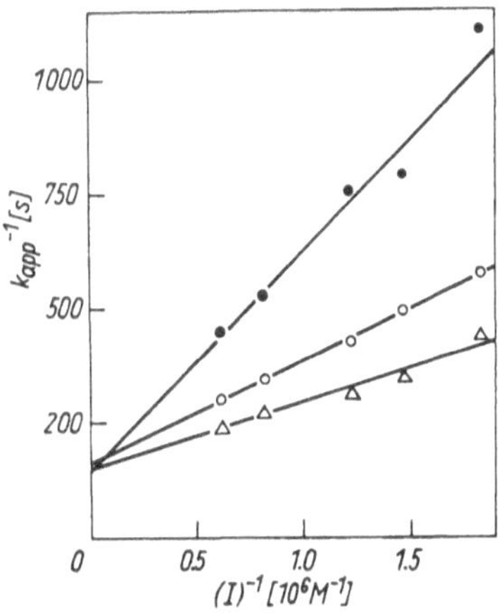

Fig. 3

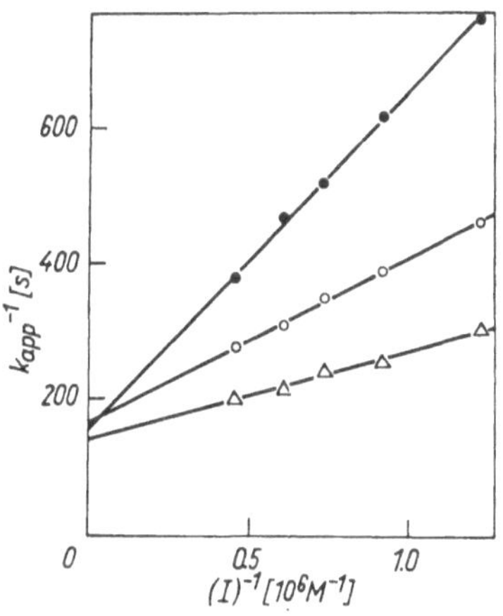

Fig. 4

Fig. 3. Dependence of k_{app} on the concentration of antithrombin III (I) by the inhibition of factor Xa ($2.2 \cdot 10^{-8}$ M) by antithrombin III; without heparin (●), with $0.9 \cdot 10^{-8}$ M (○) and $1.8 \cdot 10^{-8}$ M (△) heparin

Fig. 4. Dependence of k_{app} on the concentration of antithrombin III (I) by the inhibition of plasmin ($7.8 \cdot 10^{-8}$ M) by antithrombin III; without heparin (●), with $1,8 \cdot 10^{-8}$ M (○) and $3.6 \cdot 10^{-8}$ M (△) heparin

Table 1

Kinetic constants for the inhibition of thrombin, factor Xa, and plasmin by antithrombin III.

The values were calculated according to equations (2) and (4)

Enzyme	k_2 (s^{-1})	K_i (10^{-6} M)	K'_i (10^{-6} M)	K_a (10^{-6} M)
Thrombin	0.1	10	0.1	0.8
Factor Xa	0.007	3	0.5	0.02
Plasmin	0.007	3	0.1	0.2

According to the first mechanism, heparin acts as a reversible activator (A) of the enzymes; the mechanism is described by

$$\mathrm{E} + A \overset{K_a}{\rightleftharpoons} EA$$
$$EA + I \overset{K_i'}{\rightleftharpoons} EAI \overset{k_2}{\longrightarrow} E{-}I + A \tag{3}$$

Equation (4) predicts a linear dependence of the apparent first-order inactivation rate constant on the concentration of AT

$$\frac{1}{k_{\mathrm{app}}} = \frac{1}{k_2} + \frac{K_i'}{k_2} \cdot \left(1 + \frac{K_a}{A}\right) \cdot \frac{1}{I} \tag{4}$$

For the second mechanism, heparin activates AT to make it more effective for interaction with enzymes, the reaction equations are

$$I + \mathrm{A} \overset{K_a}{\rightleftharpoons} AI$$
$$E + AI \overset{K_i'}{\rightleftharpoons} EAI \overset{k_2}{\longrightarrow} E{-}I + A \tag{5}$$

The dependence of the apparent first-order inactivation rate constant on the concentration of AT is not linear, for only that amount of AT (I) and heparin (A) reacts with the enzyme which is bound in the complex (AI):

$$\frac{1}{k_{\mathrm{app}}} = \frac{1}{k_2} + \frac{K_i'}{k_2} \cdot \frac{1}{I + A + K_a \pm \sqrt{(I + A + K_a)^2 - 4A \cdot I}} \tag{6}$$

In deriving equations (4) and (6) the formation of the (EI) complex according to equation (1) was neglected.

Discussion

The reciprocal plots of the apparent first-order inactivation rate constants vs inhibitor concentrations (Fig. 2—4) yielded straight lines and positive intercepts in all cases for the inhibition of the enzymes by AT also in the presence of heparin. The regression analysis gives a good linear correlation ($r > 0.9$). The intercepts do not differ significantly from each other, when the reactions were carried out either with or without heparin. This behaviour corresponds to the mechanism described by equations (3). Thus, heparin acts obviously as an activator of the enzymes and make them more sensitive to AT. Equation (4) was used in order to determine the dissociation constants K_a and K_i' from the slope (Table 1). The different values of the dissociation constant K_a show that heparin possesses high affinity especially for FXa. This high affinity has, however, only a weak effect on the dissociation constant of the FXa-AT complex. Despite the lower affinity of heparin for thrombin, the dissociation constant of the thrombin-AT complex is changed most significantly by heparin. Since the rate of inactivation is the highest one in case of thrombin, it is believed that the anticoagulant effect of heparin is caused primarily by thrombin inactivation.

References

[1] Markwardt, F., and P. Walsmann: Hoppe-Seyler's Z. physiol. Chem. **317**, 64 (1959)
[2] Li, E. H. H., C. Orton, and R. D. Feinman: Biochemistry **13**, 5012 (1974)
[3] Machovich, R.: Thromb. Diath. haemorrh. **34**, 867 (1975)

[4] MACHOVICH, R.: Biochim. biophys. Acta **412**, 13 (1975)
[5] DAMUS, P. S., M. HICKS, and R. D. ROSENBERG: Nature, Lond. **246**, 355 (1973)
[6] ROSENBERG, J. S., P. W. MCKENNA, and R. D. ROSENBERG: J. biol. Chem. **250**, 8883 (1975)
[7] KURACHI, K., K. FUJIKAWA, G. SCHMER, and E. W. DAVIE: Biochemistry **15**, 373 (1976)
[8] ØSTERRUD, B., M. MILLER-ANDERSSON, U. ABILDGAARD, and H. PRYDZ: Thromb. Haemost. **35**, 295 (1976)
[9] YIN, E. T., S. WESSLER, and P. STOLL: J. biol. Chem. **246**, 3703 (1971)
[10] ROSENBERG, R. D.: Thromb. Diath. haemorrh. **33**, 51 (1974)
[11] STEAD, N., A. P. KAPLAN, and R. D. ROSENBERG: J. biol. Chem. **251**, 6481 (1976)
[12] HIGHSMITH, R. F., and R. D. ROSENBERG: J. biol. Chem. **249**, 4335 (1974)
[13] LAHIRI, B., A. BAGDASARIAN, B. MITCHELL, R. C. TALAMO, R. W. COLMAN, and R. D. ROSENBERG: Archs Biochem. Biophys. **175**, 737 (1976)
[14] LI, E. H. H., J. W. FENTON II., and R. D. FEINMAN: Archs Biochem. Biophys. **175**, 153 (1976)
[15] HOPWOOD, J., M. HÖÖK, A. LINKER, and U. LINDAHL: FEBS Lett. **69**, 51 (1976)
[16] EINARSON, R., and L.-O. ANDERSSON: Biochim. biophys. Acta **490**, 104 (1977)
[17] ROSENBERG, R. D., and P. S. DAMUS: J. biol. Chem. **248**, 6490 (1973)
[18] ABILDGAARD, U.: Thromb. Diath. haemorrh. **33**, 38 (1974)
[19] KOBAYASHI, N., T. MAEKAWA, and Y. TAKEDA: Abstracts 16th Congress of Hematology, Kyoto 1976, p. 314
[20] WESSLER, S.: Thromb. Diath. haemorrh. **34**, 718 (1975)
[21] OWEN, W. G., G. D. PENICK, E. YODER, and B. L. POOL: Thromb. Haemost. **35**, 87 (1976)
[22] KITZ, R., and I. B. WILSON: J. biol. Chem. **237**, 3245 (1962)
[23] STÜRZEBECHER, J., and F. MARKWARDT: Thromb. Res. **11**, 835 (1977)

Acta biol. med. germ., Band 36, Seite 1899—1915 (1977)

Institute of Microbial Chemistry, Kamiosaki 3-Chome, Shinagawa-ku, Tokyo, and Department of Antibiotics,
National Institute of Health, Tokyo

Protease inhibitors produced by microorganisms

Hamao Umezawa

Introduction

Micoorganisms produce limitless number of organic compounds which have no obvious function in growth of microbial cells and these compounds are called microbial secondary metabolites. This structure of the microbial world where microorganisms producing limitless number of various compounds are distributed has been revealed by studies of antibiotics and enzyme inhibitors. Experimental data indicating involvement of plasmids in production of secondary metabolites are increasing [1—3]. A molecular change in a chromosomal genetic unit for production of a primary metabolite causes the death of cells, while a molecular change in plasmid or in a genetic unit involved in production of secondary metabolites does not cause cell death and the surviving cells produce different secondary metabolites. It is possible that in the natural environment, molecular changes have occurred in plasmids or genetic units for production of secondary metabolites and limitless number of different genetic units for production of secondary metabolites have been distributed in microbial world [4, 5].
Since 1944, the author has continued the study of antibiotics, finding new compounds, elucidating their structures, studying their activities, their biosyntheses, mechanisms of actions and their utility. It is felt that a most valuable contribution to antibiotic research would be to extend this research to a new and potentially fruitful area. In around 1965, NMR, mass spectroscopy and X-ray crystallography had already been introduced into natural product chemistry and the structural determination had become far easier than before that time. On the basis of this development in natural product chemistry, during 1965 the author initiated the study of enzyme inhibitors found in microbial culture filtrates [6, 7]. The author thought that enzyme inhibitors would be useful in analysis of biological functions and disease processes and have potential utility in the treatment of diseases. After initiating this study, in the last 10 years, the author could find nearly 40 enzyme inhibitors of small molecular size. Their structures were rapidly elucidated, revealed new types of inhibitor structures which had never been imagined and stimulated the study of the mechanism of inhibition and structure-activity relationships.
In this study, inhibitors of various proteases such as serine proteases, thiol proteases, acid proteases, metalloendopeptidases and aminopeptidases have been found in culture filtrates of actinomycetes [8, 9], and used for identification of types of proteases in various tissues or cells, as ligands for affinity chromatography of proteases, for analysis of mechanisms of protease reactions, and for analysis of func-

tions of various proteases in vivo. It has also been found that inhibitors of proteases on the surface of animal cells affect immune response.
In this paper, the studies of the last eleven years on protease inhibitors found in actinomycetes culture filtrates will be reviewed.

Results

Inhibitors of serine and thiol proteases

Considering a possible utility of a plasmin inhibitor as an antiinflammatory agent, the author and AOYAGI first screened for the activity of actinomycetes culture filtrates to inhibit the hydrolysis of fibrinogen by human plasmin [8]. Then, many strains of streptomyces which could be classified to more than 18 species were found to produce active agents of a same type. The active agent was isolated and named leupeptin [10—19]. Leupeptin is the name of a group of compounds, propionyl (or acetyl)-L-leucyl-L-leuzyl-L-argininal and their analogs which contain L-isoleucine or L-valine instead of L-leucine. In a thin layer chromatography developed with butanol-butyl acetate-acetic acid-water 4:2:1:1, even a single pure leupeptin produces two spots. N$^{\alpha}$-acetylargininal also shows two spots in this thin layer chromatography. Leupeptin dibutyl acetal shows one spot and is easily converted to the original leupeptin. NMR of leupeptin aqueous solution indicates that most of leupeptin exists as the hydrated and the hydroxypiperidine forms.

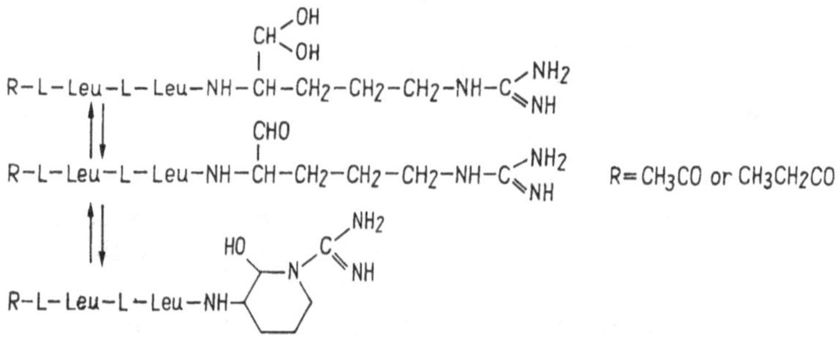

Leupeptins

Leupeptin which was extracted by cation exchange resin process was found to be a mixture of diastereomers containing L or D argininal. Acetyl-L-leucyl-L-leucyl-L-argininal and acetyl-L-leucyl-L-leucyl-D-argininal were chemically synthesized and only the former was confirmed to be active. The racemization of the asymmetric center in the argininal moiety of leupeptin easily occurs: after 4 days in *p*H 8.0 aqueous solution at room temperature, this asymmetric center is completely racemized and the activity decreases to 50% of the original. By a new extraction process without using a cation exchange resin, leupeptin which is not contaminated with inactive isomers has been obtained from fermented broths. Leupeptin inhibits plasmin, trypsin, papain and cathepsin B but not chymotrypsin. The aldehyde group in the argininal moiety is the absolute requirement for the activity. If it is oxidized to acid or reduced to alcohol, the activity disappears. L-argininal or N$^{\alpha}$-acetylargininal shows no activity. Acetyl-L-leucyl-L-argininal shows the same degree of the activity as leupeptin.

Leupeptin prolongs the blood coagulation time of rabbit and human. However, this inhibition by leupeptin is temporary and is recovered after 30 to 60 min. Inhibition of blood coagulation is not seen in the blood of mice, rats and dogs. LD50 value by intravenous injection to rabbits is smaller compared with those to mice and rats as follows:

Mice: i. v. = 118 mg/kg; s. c. = 1450 mg/kg; oral > 1550 mg/kg
Rats: i. v. = 125 mg/kg; s. c. > 4000 mg/kg; oral > 4000 mg/kg
Rabbits: i. v. = 35 mg/kg; s. c. = > 4000 mg/kg; oral > 1500 mg/kg

The smaller LD50 value by intravenous injection to rabbits may correlate with the inhibition of blood coagulation. 10 mg/kg by intravenous injection showed a temporary hypotensive effect against rabbits. Oral application of 500 mg/kg daily for 180 days caused no toxicity in rabbits.
Leupeptin inhibits carrageenin edema. Leupeptin ointment (1%) applied to a burn immediately suppresses pain and blister formation and has been used in the author's laboratories.

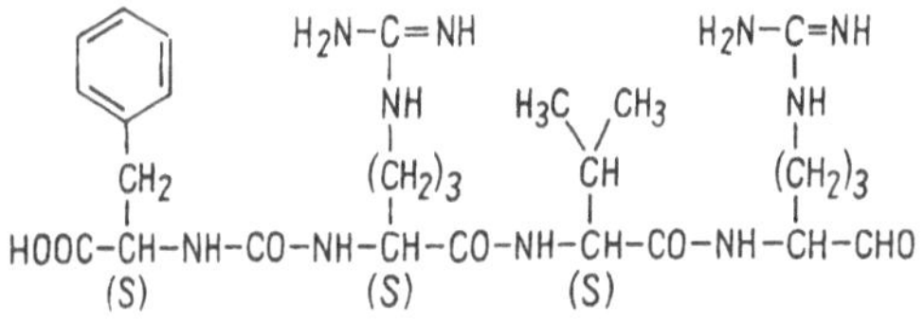

Antipain

Testing the activity of actinomycetes culture filtrates to inhibit papain [8] another active agent was found and named antipain [20—23]. As shown by the structure formulae, it also contains C-terminal L-argininal and its N-terminal amino group is covered by [(1S)-carboxyphenethyl]-carbamoyl group. This type of the structure, that is, the binding of the N-terminal amino group to the amino group of an amino acid forming an ureid bond, was first found in protease inhibitors produced by streptomyces. As minor components, other antipains containing L-leucine or L-isoleucine instead of L-valine have been found in the same culture filtrate. The dibutyl acetal of antipain and the permanganate oxidation product (antipain acid) undergo trypsin action and are hydrolyzed to [(1S)-carboxyphenethyl]-carbamoyl-L-arginine and L-valyl-argininal dibutyl acetal of L-valyl-arginine. The racemization of the argininal moiety occurs during extraction. Antipain which contains L-argininal shows an antiprotease spectrum resembling to that of leupeptin. Antipain inhibits papain, trypsin, cathepsin A, cathepsin B. The action on plasmin is very much weaker than that of leupeptin. It shows inhibition of carrageenin edema and prolongs the blood coagulation time of human and rabbit.
Intravenous injection of 250 mg/kg and intraperitoneal injection of 1000 mg/kg of antipain caused no death of mice. Absorption of antipain by rabbits has been studied comparatively with leupeptin. Blood level of antipain after oral administration to rabbits is lower than leupeptin and the amount extracted in urine is less than that for leupeptin. In the case of leupeptin, after 500 mg/kg of oral administration, blood level reached 220 μg/ml in 1—2 hrs after the administration, and

in 24 hrs 27% was excreted in urine. However, in the case of antipain, after 500 mg/kg of oral administration, the highest blood level was about 30 μg/ml after 0.5—1 and only 1.8% was excreted in the urine during 24 hrs after administration. The amount excreted in faeces was much lower than that expected: 0.5% of the administered leupeptin and 9.4% of the administered antipain. In a rabbit liver homogenate, the activity of antipain decreased rapidly.

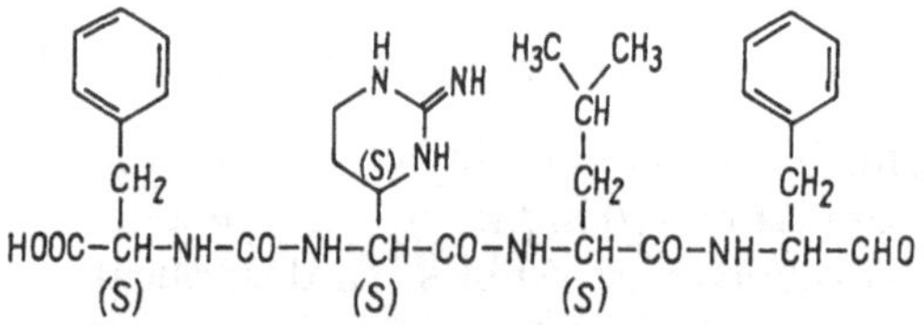

Chymostatin A

Chymotrypsin inhibitors named chymostatins A, B and C [24—26] have been found in culture filtrates of actinomycetes. As shown by the structural formula, they are different in one amino acid moiety: leucine in A, valine in B and isoleucine in C. All chymostatins contain an unusual amino acid: 2-[2-iminohexahydro-(4S)-pyrimidyl]-(S)-glycine which is a diastereomer of capreomycidine. Capreomycidine is one of the amino acid components in capreomycin and has the 2S, 3R configuration. The permanganate oxidation product of chymostatin A undergoes the reaction of carboxypeptidase, and the C-terminal L-phenylalanine and L-leucine are liberated successively. The residual molecular part, [(1S)-carboxyphenethyl]carbamoyl-2-[2-iminohexahydro-(4S)-pyrimidyl]-(S)-glycine, has been synthesized chemically and the total structures of chymostatins have been elucidated. Chymostatin inhibits all chymotrypsins but not trypsin. It inhibits also papain, but this action is much weaker than that against chymotrypsins. Chymotrypsin is known to inhibit carrageenin edema. Intraperitoneal injection of chymostatin also inhibits this edema.

TORSTENSSON [27] reported isolation of a trypsin inhibitor and a chymotrypsin inhibitor from Streptomyces violaceus. The latter may be identical with chymostatin.

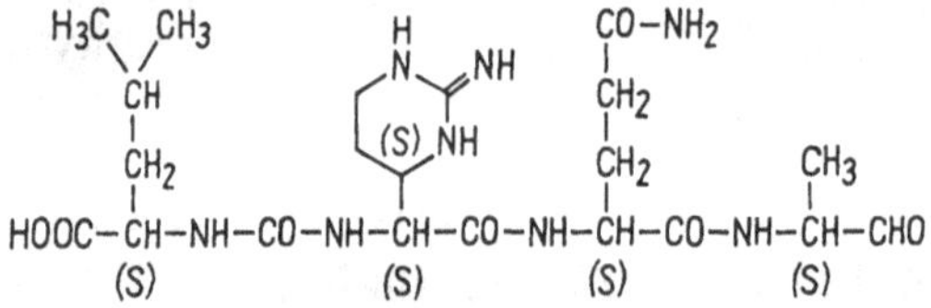

Elastatinal

Testing the activity of actionomycetes culture filtrates to inhibit hydrolysis of elastin-congored by elastase, an inhibitor was found and named elastatinal [28, 29]. Acid hydrolysis of elastatinic acid which is obtained by permanganate oxidation of elastatinal gives L-alanine, L-glutamic acid, 2-[2-iminohexahydro-(4S)-pyrimidyl]-(S)-glycine which is also contained in chymostatin, L-leucine and a mixture of hydantoins formed from [(1S)-carboxyisopentyl]carbamoyl-2-[2-iminohexahydro-(4S)-pyrimidyl]-(S)-glycine. Carboxypeptidase digestion of elastatinic acid gives L-alanine. The structure of the main hydantoin has been confirmed by chemical synthesis. The presence of a glutamine moiety was elucidated by conversion of the amide group to an amino methyl group. Hydrolysis after this conversion gives ornithine instead of glutamic acid.

Elastatinal inhibits elastase but not the other proteases and its inhibition is competitive with the substrate. K_i observed was $2.4 \cdot 10^{-7}$ M with acetyl-alanyl-alanyl-alanine p-nitroanilide and $2.1 \cdot 10^{-7}$ M with acetyl-alanyl-alanyl-alanine methyl ester. The intravenous injection of 250 mg/kg caused no toxicity in mice. Elastatinal also inhibits carrageenine edema.

As described above, leupeptin, antipain, chymostatin and elastatinal, all contain C-terminal aldehyde groups, and if these aldehyde groups are oxidized to acids, they lose activity. Trypsin cleaves the carboxyl side of arginine and lysine and is inhibited by the inhibitors containing the C-terminal L-argininal. This aldehyde structure for inhibition of serine proteases was first found in leupeptin. Thereafter, SHIMIZU et al. [15] who collaborated with the author for the chemical synthesis of leupeptin synthesized acetyl-leucyl-leucyl-phenylalaninal and confirmed that this compound inhibits chymotrypsin although its effect was much weaker than chymostatin. Chymotrypsin hydrolyzes the carboxyl side of L-phenylalanine in peptides. After leupeptin had been reported, THOMPSON synthesized acetyl-prolyl-alanyl-prolyl-alaninal and confirmed its action to inhibit elastase. Elastase hydrolyzes the carboxyl side of L-alanine. Thus, inhibitors of microbial origin revealed the active structures for inhibition of serine proteases.

If a leupeptin-producing strain is cultured in an acriflavine-containing medium and spread on an agar plate, then the strains thus obtained lose the ability to produce leupeptin in a high frequency. It suggests the involvement of a plasmid in the biosynthesis of leupeptin. HORI et al. succeeded in extraction of a multienzyme from a leupeptin-producing strain (Streptomyces roseus) by DEAE cellulose chromatography of a fraction obtained by Sephadex G-200 chromatography of the cell homogenate. In the reaction mixture containing acetate, L-leucine, [^{14}C]-L arginine and ATP, this enzyme fraction catalyzes the reaction to produce acetyl-L-leucyl-L-leucyl-L-arginine (leupeptin acid). The homogenate of this leupeptin-producing strain contains an enzyme which reduces leupeptin acid to leupeptin. This enzyme is very labile. It has been suggested that a plasmid is involved in the biosynthesis of a multienzyme on which leupeptin acid is produced. This leupeptin study suggests that plasmids would be involved in other protease inhibitors, and antipain, chymostatin and elastatinal might be produced by reduction of their corresponding acids.

Inhibitors of acid proteases [30—49]: *Pepstatin, Pepstanone, Hydroxypepstatin*

Besides inhibitors of serine proteases, inhibitors of other various proteases have been found in actinomycetes culture filtrates.

Strains of streptomyces belonging to various species have been found to produce pepstatins by testing the activity to inhibit pepsin [8].

As shown by the structure formula, various pepstatins are different from one another in the fatty acid moiety, and the pepstatin containing an isovaleryl group has been most widely used for biological and biochemical studies. This pepstatin and the other containing a *n*-caproyl group are the main components of the active

RCO-L-Val-L-Val-AHMHA-L-Ala-AHMHA

AHMHA =

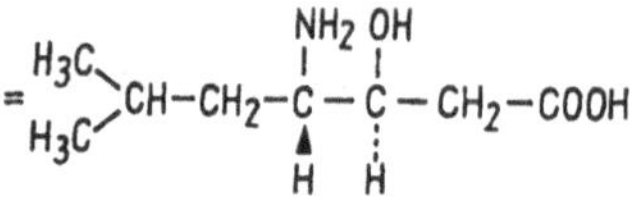

R = $CH_3(CH_2)_n$–, n = 0–20; $(CH_3)_2CH(CH_2)_n$–, n = 1–17

Pepstatins

RCO-L-Val-L-Val-AHMHA-L-Ala-AMHN

AMHN =

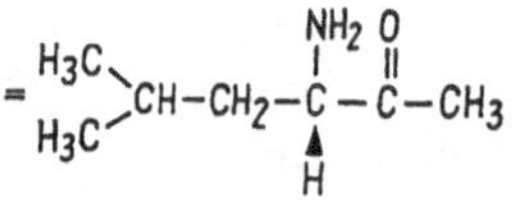

R = $CH_3(CH_2)_n$–, n = 0–20; $(CH_3)_2CH(CH_2)_n$–, n = 1–17

Pepstanones

RCO-L-Val-L-Val-AHMHA-L-Ser-AHMHA

R = $CH_3(CH_2)_n$–, n = 0–20; $(CH_3)_2CH(CH_2)_n$–, n = 1–17

Hydroxypepstatins

agents produced by a strain belonging to Streptomyces testaceus. As minor components, other pepstatins, pepstanones and hydroxypepstatins have been found in the culture filtrates of the same strain.

Pepstatins containing acetyl, propionyl or butyryl groups have been found in strains belonging to other species such as Streptomyces parvisporogenes. A pepstatin containing an isobutyl group has also been found.

As well known, peptide antibiotics are biosynthesized on multienzyme systems specific for each of them, but not on the ribosome system. As described above, leupeptin acid is biosynthesized on a multienzyme system. Pepstatins also seem to be biosynthesized by similar means. [^{14}C]-labeled AHMHA is not incorporated into pepstatin during fermentation, but [^{14}C]-L-leucine and [^{14}C]-acetate are incorporated into this amino acid moiety in pepstatin. Production of pepstatins is eliminated by treatment of its producing strain with acriflavine and the involvement of plasmids in their biosyntheses has been suggested.

Acid hydrolysis of a pepstatin gives a fatty acid, 2 moles of L-valine, 1 mole of alanine and 2 moles of an unusual amino acid (AHMHA). The structure of this unusual amino acid, (3S, 4S)-4-amino-3-hydroxy-6-methylheptanoic acid has been determined by X-ray analysis of its N-p-bromo-benzoyl derivative. The sequence of the fatty acid and amino acids in the pepstatin molecule can be shown by mass spectroscopy.

As shown by the structure of pepstanone, the terminal carboxyl group is not involved in the activity. Esters and amide of pepstatin, pepstatinal and pepstatinol in which the carboxyl is reduced to aldehyde or alcohol show a similar activity as pepstatin against pepsin. The inner 4-amino-3-hydroxy-6-methylheptanoic acid moiety is necessary for the activity. (3S, 4S)-4-amino-3-hydroxy-6-methylheptanoic acid (AHMHA) or its N-acyl derivative has no activity. Its N-valyl derivative shows no activity. However, the N-acetylvalyl derivative shows activity and the addition of another valine between the acetyl and valyl groups does not increase its activity. Addition of L-alanine to the C-terminal group increases the activity about 100 times. It suggests that the acyl-valyl-AHMHA-L-alanine moiety may be involved in binding with pepsin and cathepsin D. KINOSHITA et al. [38] have synthesized acetyl-L-valyl-L-valyl-[(3S, 4R)-4-amino-3-hydroxy-6-methyl]-heptanoic acid. It shows no activity. It suggests that the 4S-configuration of AHMHA is the requirement for the activity.

Pepstatins, pepstanones and hydroxypepstatins are active against pepsin and cathepsin D, but pepstatins are more active against renin than pepstanones and hydroxypepstatins. Activity of pepstatin against renin increases with an increase in the number of carbon atoms in the fatty acid moiety (Table 1). An enzyme which hydrolyzes pepstatins to the fatty acid, L-valine and the residual tetrapeptide has been found in Bacillus sphaericus. From this tetrapeptide, water-soluble pepstatin analogs (benzoyl-L-valyl-AHMHA-L-alanyl-AHMHA etc.) have been synthesized. They show a similar activity as pepstatin to inhibit pepsin and cathepsin D, but almost no effect on renin. Addition of another valine may be necessary for inhibition of renin. Therefore, it is possible to prepare water-soluble pepstatin analogs exhibiting strong inhibition against pepsin and cathepsin D, but it seems to be a difficult work to develop water-soluble analogs exhibiting strong inhibition against renin.

Table 1
Inhibition of pepsin, cathepsin D and renin by pepstatins

RCO	50% inhibition concentration		
	Pepsin ($\cdot 10^{-8}$ M)	Cathepsin D ($\cdot 10^{-9}$ M)	Renin ($\cdot 10^{-10}$ M)
Acetyl	1.5	9.3	24.9
Propionyl	1.5	9.1	15.2
n-Butyryl	1.4	8.9	9.7
**iso*-Valeryl	1.4	8.8	6.6
n-Caproyl	1.4	9.3	4.3
iso-Heptanoyl	1.4	9.1	2.5
n-Capryl	1.4	8.9	1.7
Pepstanone A (R=*iso*-valeryl)	2.0	17	39
Hydroxypepstatin A (R=*iso*-valeryl)	1.7	11.4	20

* Competitive with Phe-Gly-His-Phe(NO_2)-Phe-Ala-PheOMe
$K_i = 9.7 \cdot 10^{-11}$ M

As shown by the extremely small K_i value, that is, 10^{-10} M, the tight binding with pepsin and cathepsin D is strong enough to use pepstatin for titration of these enzymes. The equimolar pepsin-pepstatin complex can be shown by Sephadex chromatography.

Pepstatin has very low toxicity: LD50 by intravenous injection is: 1000 mg/kg to mice, 820 mg/kg to rabbits, 450 mg/kg to dogs; LD50 by oral administration is larger than 2000 mg/kg. Daily oral administration of 200 mg/kg and 1000 mg/kg for 180 days caused no toxicity in rats. Daily oral administration of 1000 mg/kg to monkeys also caused no toxicity. It has been shown by oral administration of [^{3}H]-pepstatin that pepstatin given orally is practically not absorbed. Intraperitoneal injection of 500 mg/kg of pepstatin suspended in 0.5% carboxymethylcellulose caused the death of 3 rats, and in these lethal cases blood levels exceeded 30 µg/ml. The data suggest that pepstatin levels higher than 30 µg/ml would be lethal to rats. Intraperitoneal injection of 500 mg/kg to dogs caused death, and in this case also pepstatin levels in the blood went up to 30 µg/ml. Oral administration of pepstatin has never caused any toxic effects to pregnant mice and rats or their embryos.

Pepstatin is very effective in Shay rat ulcer, that is, ulcer caused by pylorus ligation. It suggests that the excreted pepsin is the main cause of this ulcer. The effect of pepstatin on stomach ulcers in man has been observed during clinical studies. Intraperitoneal injection of pepstatin shows inhibition of carrageenine edema.

Inhibitor of metalloendopeptidases: *Phosphoramidon* [50—53]

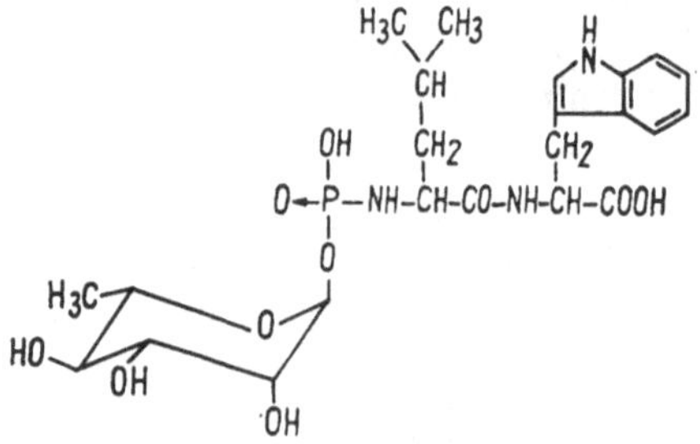

Phosphoramidon

After inhibitors of serine, thiol and acid proteases had been found, the study was extended to find inhibitors of all other proteases. Thermolysin is a zinc enzyme, and its inhibitor has been found in streptomyces. The structure of this inhibitor was elucidated to be N-(α-L-rhamnopyranosyloxyhydroxyphosphinyl)-L-leucyl-L-tryptophan and named phosphoramidon. It inhibits thermolysin ($K_i = 2.8 \cdot 10^{-9}$ M) and related enzymes. It inhibits a thermolysin type enzyme which has been called an elastase of Pseudomonas aeruginosa, causing pneumonia in minks. Boiling of phosphoramidon with baryta splits the rhamnose moiety and the barium salt of phosphoryl-L-leucyl-L-tryptophan precipitates. This partially hydrolyzed product exhibits a 10 times higher activity to inhibit thermolysin ($K_i = 2.0 \cdot 10^{-9}$ M). Thermolysin hydrolyzes the amino side of the hydrophobic aminoacyl group in the peptides. It suggests that the N-phosphate of a hydrophobic amino acid would be the active structure. N-(α-L-rhamnopyranosyloxyhydroxyphosphinyl)-L-leucyl methyl ester shows almost no activity and N-(α-L-rhamnopyranosyloxyhydroxyphosphinyl)-L-leucyl-L-histidine shows less activity than phosphoramidon. It indicates that addition of tryptophan or another amino acid to C-terminal group of phosphoryl-L-leucine is necessary for the activity. Phosphoramidon has a low toxicity and the LD50 is higher than 1.0 g/kg in mice by intravenous injection.

Use of inhibitors for identification of types of enzyme [54—60]

After the author reported the inhibitors described above, he received many proposals for their use and these inhibitors have been used widely for various purposes. They have been utilized as ligands for affinity chromatography of proteases, to protect cellular proteins from proteases during their extraction and to identify types of proteases.

Leupeptin inhibits cathepsin B, antipain inhibits cathepsins A and B, and pepstatin inhibits cathepsin D. These anticathepsin spectra of these inhibitors have been utilized for identification of cathepsins in macrophages. URATA et al. has used elastatinal for typing of an enzyme which inactivates apo-δ-aminolevulinate synthetase. This enzyme was inhibited by diispropylfluorophosphate and suggested to be a member of serine proteases. It was found that hydrolysis of acetyl-alanyl-alanyl-alanine methyl ester by this enzyme was inhibited by elastatinal but hydrolysis of acetyl-alanyl-alanyl-alanine amide was not inhibited.

Inhibitors of aminopeptidases and their effect on immune response [61—67]

The compounds described above are inhibitors of endopeptidases. Aminopeptidase B is an exopeptidase and hydrolyzes N-terminal peptide bonds containing N-terminal arginine or lysine. In the study of an inhibitor of this enzyme prepared from rat liver, a new compound was obtained and named bestatin.

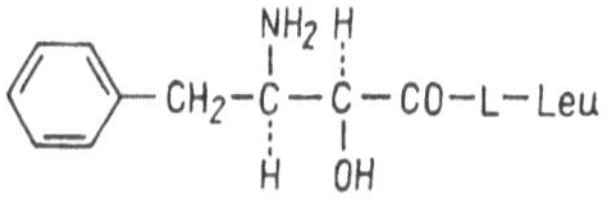

Bestatin

Bestatin inhibits not only aminopeptidase B but also leucine aminopeptidase. But it inhibits neither aminopeptidase A nor endopeptidases. The type of inhibition is competitive with substrates such as L-arginine-2-naphthylamide for aminopeptidase B and L-leucine-2-naphthylamide for leucine aminopeptidase and K_i values are $6.0 \cdot 10^{-8}$ M and $2.0 \cdot 10^{-8}$ M, respectively.

Bestatin has three asymmetric centers and eight stereoisomers have been synthesized. The S-configuration of the C-2 of the (2S, 3R)-3-amino-2-hydroxy-4-phenylbutanoyl moiety is the key stereochemistry for the activity (Table 2). All four bestatin stereoisomers of the 2S-configuration have the activity to inhibit aminopeptidase B and leucine aminopeptidase. But all four other stereoisomers, that is, those of the 2R-configuration, have no or slight activity.

Bestatin analogs which contain various amino acids instead of leucine have been synthesized. Among them, those containing proline or lysine have no or slight activity. An analog containing isoleucine shows a similar activity as bestatin to inhibit aminopeptidase B. The other containing norleucine has a slightly weaker activity. Analogs which contain p-methylbenzyl or p-nitrobenzyl group instead of benzyl group in bestatin have almost the same activity as bestatin. AOYAGI et al. [10] found that intact animal cells liberate N-terminal amino acids or N-terminal di or tripeptides from synthetic peptides without release of the enzymes into the medium. This study indicates the presence of aminopeptidases such as leucine aminopeptidase, aminopeptidase B etc. on the cellular surface (Fig. 1). As shown

Table 2
Inhibition of aminopeptidase B and leucine aminopeptidase by stereoisomers of bestatin

Stereoisomers*	I_{50} (μM)	
	Aminopeptidase B	Leucine aminopeptidase
(2S, 3R)-AHPA-(S)-Leu	0.16	0.032
(2S, 3R)-AHPA-(R)-Leu	1.8	11
(2S, 3S)-AHPA-(S)-Leu	4.1	0.23
(2S, 3S)-AHPA-(R)-Leu	0.081	8.8
(2R, 3R)-AHPA-(S)-Leu	320	24
(2R, 3R)-AHPA-(R)-Leu	>800	>800
(2R, 3S)-AHPA-(S)-Leu	>800	>800
(2R, 3S)-AHPA-(R)-Leu	440	>800

* The inhibition of aminopeptidase B and leucine amino-peptidase by bestatin, (2S, 3R)-AHPA-(S)-Leu, and its stereoisomers was determined at various concentrations to estimate each I_{50} value.

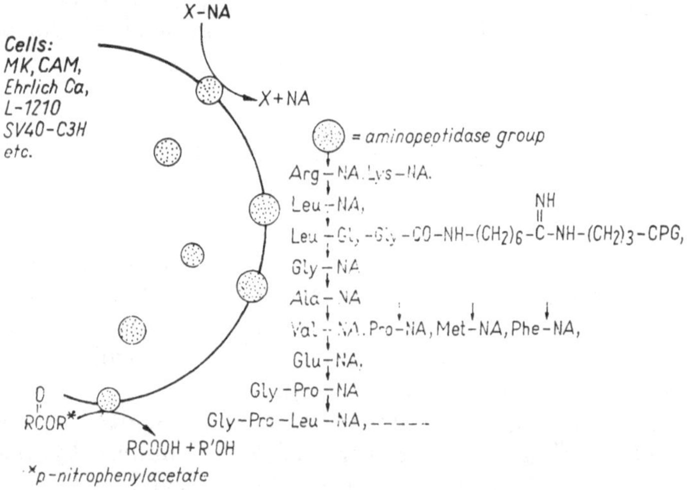

Fig. 1. Hydrolysis of N-terminal amino acids from peptides by aminopeptidases on surface of mammalian cells

in Table 3, aminopeptidase B and leucine aminopeptidase activities of cells are inhibited by bestatin. It indicates that bestatin binds to these enzymes on the cellular surface. This binding has been confirmed by the binding of the radioactivity of [^{125}I]-p-hydroxybestatin to cultured FMSA cells (established from a mammary tumor of mouse strain C3H-He): after exposure to bestatin for 20 min, the binding of $2.2 \cdot 10^7$ molecules of this radioactive bestatin analog per cell was calculated. Based on these findings, the author proposed that inhibitors of such enzymes might inhibit hydrolysis of proteins which are involved in communication between cells, especially between those involved in immunity, or these inhibitors might bind with these enzymes on the cellular surface and decrease or increase the activity of cells involved in immunity. The author, ISHIZUKA and TAKEUCHI found that bestatin enhanced delayed-type hypersensitivity. Intraperitoneal injection of 0.1 to 1,000 µg/mouse at the time of immunization, that is, at the time of the injection of sheep red blood cells into the footpad, enhances the reaction elicited by a second injection of the same cells into the footpad of the other side. The greatest effect was shown by 1.0 to 100 µg/mouse. Injection of bestatin at the time of eliciting the reaction does not show any influence. A large dose such as 1.000 µg/mouse of bestatin at the time of immunization or 24 hrs before or after immunization increases the number of antibody-forming cells, but lower doses which show a marked action in increasing delayed-type hypersensitivity do not increase the number of antibody-forming cells. Bestatin does not influence the reaction of mice immunized by sheep red blood cells and the reaction is elicited by human red blood cells or vice versa. As already described, stereoisomers which have the 2S-configuration have strong activities to inhibit aminopeptidase B and leucine aminopeptidase as well as bestatin but other isomers which have the 2R-configuration have not or only slight activity to inhibit these enzymes. Intraperitoneal injection of 0.1 µg/mouse of the isomers which inhibit these enzymes strongly increases delayed-type hypersensitivity, but injection of 10 µg of other isomers does not show a significant effect. It suggests that the action of bestatin to enhance immune response is due to its interaction with aminopeptidases.

If Ehrlich carcinoma cells are inoculated into the footpad of mice, then tumor growth in this location is resistant to treatment with antitumor compounds

Table 3

Effect of bestatin against aminopeptidase B and leucine aminopeptidase on various cells

Enzymes	Final conc. of inhibitor (µg/ml)	% Inhibition						
		Rat liver	MK	MDCK	L	Ehrlich	L-1210	Yoshida
Aminopeptidase B	10	76.8	84.5	71.2	66.7	90.4	51.0	84.8
	2	61.0	71.0	47.6	47.1	73.6	44.8	63.1
	0.5	44.9	52.3	26.8	30.2	53.6	30.5	30.4
	0.1	24.4	34.0	11.5	14.6	26.8	18.7	10.2
Leucine aminopeptidase	50	48.2	56.0	60.9	43.6	40.7	26.5	65.4
	10	31.6	38.8	42.2	32.3	18.5	22.2	55.8
	2.5	23.8	24.8	28.3	23.7	6.5	17.6	37.5
	1.0	18.4	17.5	20.6	18.0	2.8	7.8	29.0

Bestatin is a specific inhibitor of aminopeptidase B and leucine aminopeptidase isolated from the culture filtrate of Streptomyces olivoreticulli. The structure of bestatin is [(2S, 3R)-3-amino-2-hydroxy-4-phenylbutanoyl]-L-leucine.

such as bleomycin, mitomycin C, adriamycin, etc. Using this experimental system, the effect of bestatin on immunity to this tumor has been studied and bestatin has been confirmed to yield immune resistance and to enhance the therapeutic effect of bleomycin on this tumor. For instance, in an experiment, 10^6 tumor cells were inoculated into the right footpad and the treatment was started 24 hrs later and continued for 6 days. On the day after the last treatment 10^6 cells were inoculated into the left footpad. The size of tumors produced by the first inoculation was measured on the 14th day after the first inoculation and the size of tumors produced by the second inoculation was measured on the 14th day after the second inoculation. Bestatin alone (10 μg/mouse daily for 6 days) produced resistance to the second inoculation and the combination of bleomycin with bestatin (10 μg/mouse) produced complete resistance to the second inoculation.

The oral or intraperitoneal administration of 1—100 μg of bestatin to mice after inoculation of Ehrlich carcinoma cells into footpad enhanced the effect of bleomycin. But the high dose (1 mg/mouse) which did not enhance delayed-type hypersensitivity did not enhance the bleomycin effect. The dosis of bestatin to enhance delayed-type hypersensitivity also enhanced the therapeutic effect of adriamycin on Ehrlich carcinoma and L-1210 mouse leukemia.

Treatment with bestatin alone exhibited a strong inhibition against Gardner lymphosarcoma and IMC-carcinoma. As shown in Table 4, when 10^5 cells of Gardner lymphosarcoma obtained from the ascites form were subcutaneously inoculated to C3H-He mice and the weight of each tumor was measured on day 30, oral administration of 10 μg/mouse/day of bestatin (8 mice for each dose group) for 5 days on day 1—5 showed a strong inhibition: 77.9% inhibition by 10 μg/mouse/day; 59.9% inhibition by 100 μg/mouse/day, although as shown in Table 4 the degree of inhibition fluctuated in each mouse of each dose group: 52—92% inhibition in 10 μg/mouse/day group; 31—93% inhibition in 100 μg/mouse/day group.

Table 4
Effect of bestatin on Gardner lymphorsarcoma

Bestatin (μg/mouse/day)	Tumor weight on day 30 (mg) (mean ± (range)	% Inhibition
0	1375.3 (570—2174)	—
10	303.3 (105—561)	77.9
100	551.8 (93—947)	59.9

Cells were collected from the ascites form, and washed with physiological saline and 10^5 cells were subcutaneously inoculated into the inguinal area of C3H-He mice. 8 mice for each dose. Bestatin was orally administered daily on day 1—5

IMC-carcinoma is the carcinoma which appeared spontaneously in CDF_1 mice in my laboratories. Intraperitoneal inoculation of 10^6 cells of this ascites tumor cells caused death of mice after 8—10 days. But in the case the cells are subcutaneously inoculated, the subcutaneous tumor continues the growth and the weight of tumor increases to more than 10 g. As shown in Table 5, treatment with 1, 10, 100 μg/mouse/day of bestatin orally for 5 days on day 1—5, on day 8—12, or day 14—18 showed strong inhibition. The size of tumor in the control on day 30 of the inocula-

Table 5
Effect of bestatin on IMC-carcinoma

Bestatin (μg/mouse/day)	Treatment days and % inhibitions mean (range)			
	−7−1	1−5	8−12	14−18
1	—	43.1 (52−27)	48.7 (89− 0)	55.0 (76− 3)
10	—	41.7 (75−26)	82.0 (89−76)	71.0 (84−58)
100	42.3 (91−0)	36.3 (63− 0)	71.6 (82−61)	71.3 (81−62)

Bestatin was orally administered: −7 means daily for 7 days before inoculation of the tumor cells; 1−5 means daily for 5 days on day 1−5 of the inoculation. 10^6 tumor cells collected from the ascites form were washed with saline and inoculated on day 0. Tumors were weighed on day 30.
Mean weight of tumors in non-treated mice was 10.31 g ± 0.74 g (13.3−7.0 g).

tion was relatively even (13.3 g—7.0 g in 8 mice), but as shown in Table 5, the size of tumor of treated groups more fluctuated. It should be emphasized that even if treatment was started from day 8 or day 14 of the inoculation, a marked inhibition occurred. A stronger inhibition was observed in the treatment on day 8—14 than in the treatment on day 1—5. It suggests that the tumor on day 8—12 might provide more useful antigens than the tumor on day 1—5 of the inoculation. Although bestatin alone was effective on IMC-carcinoma, the effect was the suppression of rate of growth of tumors. We thought that bestatin treatment combined with tumor antigens might cause the shrinking of existed tumors.

Macromomycin [68] which was discovered by the author has been found to produce a resistance to a second inoculation of the same tumor cells. However, the author and Ishizuka confirmed that macromomycin neither enhanced delayed-type hypersensitivity nor increased the number of antibody-forming cells. It seems that macromomycin does not affect immune system but may affect on tumor cells and provide tumor antigens to immune system. Therefore, we examined the effect of bestatin in combination of inoculation of macromomycin-treated IMC-carcinoma cells. 10^6 cells of IMC-carcinoma were subcutaneously inoculated to the inguinal area of CDF_1 mice and on day 21, 10^7 cells mixed with 10 μg of macromomycin were subcutaneously injected to the opposite inguinal area and at the same time bestatin treatment (10 μg/mouse/day) was started and continued daily up to day 40 of the first cell inoculation. Then, tumors which had been found by other experiments to have grown up to about 6 g on day 21 increased the size up to about day 25—30 and thereafter shrinked gradually with light necrosis and on day 40, the mice gained the weight and looked completely healthy except for a small tumor in the inoculated place. Without bestatin treatment, after inoculation of the mixture of the tumor cells with macromomycin, strong necrosis and bleeding occurred in the tumor and on day 40 mice were in the state of strong cachexia. In the control, the tumor continued to grow and mice with strong cachexia died 35—40 days after the inoculation.

The results suggest that combination of a cell-immunity-enhancing agent with tumor antigens may be useful in treatment of cancer.

An inhibitor of aminopeptidase A has been found by the author et al. to increase the number of antibody-forming cells.

The study on inhibitors of aminopeptidases on the cellular surface has been continued and extended to inhibitors of other enzymes on the cellular surface. The study on inhibitors of enzymes on the cellular surface will contribute to develop useful agents in enhancing or decreasing immune reactions. Moreover, these inhibitors will be useful in analysis of functions and structures of cell membrane.

Conclusions

The author initiated the study of protease inhibitors produced by microorganisms and has found small molecular inhibitors of serine proteases, thiol proteases, acid proteases, metalloendopeptidases and aminopeptidases in actinomycetes culture filtrates. They were peptides and revealed new types of structures for inhibition of each group of proteases. Based on their specific activity, they have been used in analysis of roles of proteases in growth [69], various biological functions and disease processes [70—77] and as ligands for affinity chromatography of proteases [78—80]. They have been used for identification of types of tissue proteases. Their possible utility in treatment of diseases has been studied. There are papers which report the action of serine protease inhibitors to suppress chemical carcinogenesis or chemical mutation [81—85]. These small molecular inhibitors of proteases have been utilized to protect tissue proteins from proteases during their extraction and purification [86].

Inhibitors of aminopeptidases have been shown to enhance immune response. This is the first finding of small molecular microbial compounds enhancing immune response. Based on this finding a method to find compounds with such activities has been established and will contribute to the progress in immunotherapy.

As shown by the study of leupeptin biosynthesis, all inhibitor peptides seem to be biosynthesized on multienzyme systems specific for each of them. Moreover, such multienzyme systems have been suggested to be produced on the basis of genetic information contained in plasmids.

In the natural environment, molecular changes have occurred in plasmids and limitless number of different plasmids have been distributed in the microbial world. On the basis of the possible presence of a great variety of plasmids, more and more various compounds which have various bioactivities will be found in microbial culture filtrates.

References

[1] OKANISHI, M., T. OHTA, and H. UMEZAWA: J. Antibiot. **23**, 45 (1970)
[2] AKAGAWA, H., M. OKANISHI, and H. UMEZAWA: J. gen. Microbiol. **90**, 336 (1975)
[3] KIRBY, R., L. F. WRIGHT, and D. A. HOPWOOD: Nature, Lond. **254**, 265 (1975)
[4] UMEZAWA, H.: Advances in microbial secondary metabolites: Enzyme inhibitors: Symposium on horizons in medicinal chemistry: Elli Lilly Centennial Lectures, Centennial Lectures, Centennial Meeting of American Chemical Society, New York, April, 5, 1976
[5] UMEZAWA, H.: Kagaku (Science) **46**, 130 (1976) (in Japanese)
[6] UMEZAWA, H.: Enzyme inhibitors of microbial origin. University of Tokyo Press 1972
[7] UMEZAWA, H.: Pure appl. Chem. **33**, 129 (1973)
[8] UMEZAWA, H.: Meth. Enzymol. **45**, Part B, 678 (1976)
[9] AOYAGI, T., and H. UMEZAWA: Structures and activities of protease inhibitors of microbial origin. Proteases and Biological Controls. Cold Spring Harbor Laboratory, New York 1975, p. 429

[10] Aoyagi, T., T. Takeuchi, A. Matsuzaki, K. Kawamura, S. Kondo, M. Hamada, K. Maeda, and H. Umezawa: J. Antibiot. **22**, 283 (1969)
[11] Kondo, S., K. Kawamura, J. Iwanaga, M. Hamada, T. Aoyagi, K. Maeda, T. Takeuchi, and H. Umezawa: Chem. pharm. Bull. **17**, 1896 (1969)
[12] Kawamura, K., S. Kondo, K. Maeda, and H. Umezawa: Chem. pharm. Bull. **17**, 1902 (1969)
[13] Aoyagi, T., S. Miyata, M. Nanbo, F. Kojima, M. Matsuzaki, M. Ishizuka, T. Takeuchi, and H. Umezawa: J. Antibiot. **22**, 558 (1969)
[14] Maeda, K., K. Kawamura, S. Kondo, T. Aoyagi, T. Takeuchi, and H. Umezawa: J. Antibiot. **24**, 402 (1971)
[15] Shimizu, B., A. Saito, A. Ito, K. Tokawa, K. Maeda, and H. Umezawa: J. Antibiot. **25**, 515 (1972)
[16] Saeki, H., Y. Shimada, N. Kawakita, B. Shimizu, E. Ohki, K. Maeda, and H. Umezawa: Chem. pharm. Bull. **21**, 163 (1973)
[17] Ikezawa, H., T. Aoyagi, T. Takeuchi, and H. Umezawa: J. Antibiot. **24**, 488 (1971)
[18] Fritz, H., B. Förg-Brey, and H. Umezawa: Hoppe-Seyler's Z. physiol. Chem. **354**, 1304 (1973)
[19] Saito, M., T. Hagiwara, T. Aoyagi, and Y. Nagai: Jap. J. exp. Med. **42**, 509 (1972)
[20] Suda, H., T. Aoyagi, M. Hamada, T. Takeuchi, and H. Umezawa: J. Antibiot. **25**, 263 (1972)
[21] Umezawa, S., K. Tatsuta, K. Fujimoto, T. Tsuchiya, H. Umezawa and H. Naganawa: J. Antibiot. **25**, 267 (1972)
[22] Fujimoto, K., K. Tatsuta, T. Tsuchiya, S. Umezawa, and H. Umezawa: J. Antibiot. **27**, 685 (1974)
[23] Ikezawa, H., K. Yamada, T. Aoyagi, T. Takeuchi, and H. Umezawa: J. Antibiot. **25**, 738 (1972)
[24] Umezawa, H., T. Aoyagi, H. Morishima, S. Kunimoto, M. Matsuzaki, M. Hamada, and T. Takeuchi: J. Antibiot. **23**, 425 (1970)
[25] Tatsuta, K., N. Mikami, K. Fujimito, S. Umezawa, H. Umezawa, and T. Aoyagi: J. Antibiot. **26**, 625 (1973)
[26] Ito, A., K. Tokawa, and B. Shimizu: Biochem. biophys. Res. Commun. **49**, 343 (1972)
[27] Torstensson, N. T. L.: Archs Microbiol. **91**, 11 (1973)
[28] Umezawa, H., T. Aoyagi, A. Okura, H. Morishima, T. Takeuchi, and Y. Okami: J. Antibiot. **26**, 787 (1973)
[29] Okura, A., H. Morishima, T. Takita, T. Aoyagi, T. Takeuchi, and H. Umezawa: J. Antibiot. **28**, 337 (1975)
[30] Umezawa, H., T. Aoyagi, H. Morishima, M. Matsuzaki, H. Hamada, and T. Takeuchi: J. Antibiot. **23**, 259 (1970)
[31] Morishima, H., T. Takita, T. Aoyagi, T. Takeuchi, and H. Umezawa: J. Antibiot. **23**, 263 (1970)
[32] Nakamura, H., H. Morishima, T. Takita, H. Umezawa, and Y. Iitaka: J. Antibiot. **26**, 255 (1973)
[33] Aoyagi, T., S. Kunimoto, H. Morishima, T. Takeuchi, and H. Umezawa: J. Antibiot. **24**, 687 (1971)
[34] Kunimoto, S., T. Aoyagi, H. Morishima, T. Takeuchi, and H. Umezawa: J. Antibiot. **25**, 251 (1972)
[35] Kunimoto, S., T. Aoyagi, R. Nishizawa, T. Komai, T. Takeuchi, and H. Umezawa: J. Antibiot. **27**, 413 (1974)
[36] Morishima, H., T. Takita, and H. Umezawa: J. Antibiot. **26**, 115 (1973)
[37] Morishima, H., T. Takita, and H. Umezawa: J. Antibiot. **25**, 551 (1972)
[38] Kinoshita, M., S. Aburaki, A. Hagiwara, and J. Imai: J. Antibiot. **26**, 249 (1973)

[39] UMEZAWA, H., T. MIYANO, T. MURAKAMI, T. TAKITA, T. AOYAGI, T. TAKEUCHI, H. NAGANAWA, and H. MORISHIMA: J. Antibiot. **26**, 615 (1973)

[40] MIYANO, T., M. TOMIYASU, H. IIZUKA, S. TOMISAKA, T. TAKITA, T. AOYAGI, and H. UMEZAWA: J. Antibiot. **25**, 489 (1972)

[41] AOYAGI, T., Y. YAGISAWA, M. KUMAGAI, M. HAMADA, H. MORISHIMA, T. TAKEUCHI, and H. UMEZAWA: J. Antibiot. **26**. 539 (1973)

[42] MORISHIMA, H., T. SAWA, T. TAKITA, T. AOYAGI, T. TAKEUCHI, and H. UMEZAWA: J. Antibiot. **27**, 267 (1974)

[43] AOYAGI, T., H. MORISHIMA, R. NISHIZAWA, S. KUNIMOTO, T. TAKEUCHI, H. UMEZAWA, and H. IKIZAWA: J. Antibiot. **25**, 689 (1972)

[44] TONE, H., N. SHIBAMOTO, Y. MATSUSHITA, T. INUI, A. TAKAMATSU, T. AOYAGI, T. TAKEUCHI, and H. UMEZAWA: J. Antibiot. **28**, 1009 (1975)

[45] TONE, H., Y. MATSUSHITA, Y. YAGI, A. TAKAMATSU, T. AOYAGI, T. TAKEUCHI, and H. UMEZAWA: J. Antibiot. **28**, 1012 (1975)

[46] MATSUSHITA, Y., H. TONE, S. HORI, Y. YAGI, A. TAKAMATSU, H. MORISHIMA, T. AOYAGI, T. TAKEUCHI, and H. UMEZAWA: J. Antibiot. **28**, 1016 (1975)

[47] KNIGHT, C. G., and A. J. BARRETT: Biochem. J. **155**, 117 (1976)

[48] CHANG, W., and K. TAKAHASHI: J. Biochem., Tokyo **74**, 231 (1973)

[49] TAKAHASHI, K., W. CHANG, and J. KO: J. Biochem., Tokyo **76**, 897 (1974)

[50] SUDA, H., T. AOYAGI, T. TAKEUCHI, and H. UMEZAWA: J. Antibiot. **26**, 621 (1973)

[51] UMEZAWA, S., K. TATSUTA, O. IZAWA, T. TSUCHIYA, and H. UMEZAWA: Tetrahed. Lett. **97**, (1972)

[52] KOMIYAMA, T., H. SUDA, T. AOYAGI, T. TAKEUCHI, H. UMEZAWA, K. FUJIMOTO, and S. UMEZAWA: Archs Biochem. Biophys. **171**, 727 (1975)

[53] KOMIYAMA, T., T. AOYAGI, T. TAKEUCHI, and H. UMEZAWA: Biochem. biophys. Res. Commun. **65**, 325 (1975)

[54] TÖKÉS, Z. A., and S. M. CHAMBERS: Biochim. biophys. Acta **389**, 325 (1975)

[55] BARRETT, A. J.: Biochem. J. **131**, 809 (1973)

[56] BARRETT, A. J., and P. M. STARKEY: Biochem. J. **133**, 709 (1973)

[57] HAYASAKA, S., S. HARA, and K. MIZUNO: J. Biochem., Tokyo **78**, 1365 (1975)

[58] KREGAR, I., V. TURK, F. GUBENŠEK, and R. W. SMITH: Croat. chem. Acta **46**, 129 (1974)

[59] YAGO, N., and W. E. BOWERS: J. biol. Chem. **250**, 4749 (1975)

[60] SAHEKI, T., and H. HOLZER: Biochim. biophys. Acta **384**, 203 (1975)

[61] UMEZAWA, H., T. AOYAGI, H. SUDA, M. HAMADA, and T. TAKEUCHI: J. Antibiot. **29**, 97 (1976)

[62] SUDA, H., T. TAKITA, T. AOYAGI, and H. UMEZAWA: J. Antibiot. **29**, 100 (1976)

[63] NAKAMURA, H., H. SUDA, T. TAKITA, T. AOYAGI, H. UMEZAWA, and Y. IITAKA: J. Antibiot. **29**, 102 (1976)

[64] SUDA, H., T. TAKITA, T. AOKAGI, and H. UMEZAWA: J. Antibiot. **29**, 600 (1976)

[65] AOYAGI, T., H. SUDA, M. NAGAI, K. OGAWA, J. SUZUKI, T. TAKEUCHI, and H. UMEZAWA: Biochim. biophys. Acta **452**, 131 (1976)

[66] UMEZAWA, H., M. ISHIZUKA, T. AOYAGI, and T. TAKEUCHI: J. Antibiot. **29**, 857 (1976)

[67] SUDA, H., T. AOYAGI, T. TAKEUCHI, and H. UMEZAWA: Archs Biochem. Biophys. **177**, 196 (1976)

[68] ISHIZUKA, M., M. HAMADA, S. HORI, K. KIMURA, J. IWANAGA, T. TAKEUCHI, and H. UMEZAWA: J. Antibiot. **21**, 44 (1968)

[69] LEVY, M. R., and S. CHOU: Experientia **31**, 52 (1975)

[70] MCKOWN, M. M., R. J. WORKMAN, and R. I. GREGERMAN: J. biol. Chem. **249**, 7770 (1974)

[71] SCHÖLKENS, B. A., and W. JUNG: Archs int. Pharmacodyn. Ther. **208**, 24 (1974)

[72] Orth, H., E. Hackenthal, J. Lazar, U. Miksche, and F. Gross: Circulation Res. **35**, 52 (1974)
[73] Lazar, J., P. Oster, F. Gross, and E. Hackenthal: Biochem. Pharmac. **23**, 2776 (1974)
[74] Miyamoto, M., H. Terayama, and T. Ohnishi: Biochem. biophys. Res. Commun. **55**, 84 (1973)
[75] Lin, T., and H. R. Williams: Experientia **31**, 209 (1975)
[76] Greenbaum, L. M., P. Grebow, M. Johnston, A. Prekash, and G. Semente: Cancer Res. **35**, 706 (1975)
[77] Lockshin, R. A.: Life Sci. **17**, 403 (1975)
[78] Devaux, C., P. Corvol, C., Auzan, J. Ducloux, and J. Menard: C. r. Acad. Sci., Paris. **277**, 2561 (1973)
[79] Devaux, C., P. Corvol, and J. Menard: Biochim. biophys. Acta **359**, 421 (1974)
[80] Murakami, K., and T. Inagami: Biochem. biophys. Res. Commun. **62**, 757 (1975)
[81] Hozumi, M., M. Ogawa, T. Sugimura, T. Takeuchi, and H. Umezawa: Cancer Res. **32**, 1725 (1972)
[82] Yuasa, Y., H. Shimojo, T. Aoyagi, and H. Umezawa: J. natn. Cancer Inst. **54**, 1255 (1975)
[83] McIlhinney, A., and B. L. M. Hogan: Biochem. biophys. Res. Commun. **60**, 348 (1974)
[84] Collard, J. G., and L. A. Smets: Expl Cell Res. **86**, 75 (1974)
[85] Umezawa, K., T. Matsushima, and T. Sugimura: Proc. Jap. Acad. **53**, Ser. B, 30 (1977)
[86] Huisman, W., L. Lanting, H. J. Doddema, J. M. W. Bouma, and M. Gruber: Biochim. biophys. Acta **370**, 297 (1974)

Acta biol. med. germ., Band 36, Seite 1917—1921 (1977)

Department of Biochemistry and Biophysics,
The Pennsylvania State University,
University Park, PA 16802, U.S.A.

Inhibition of glycoprotein catabolism in vivo and in the perfused rat liver

W. A. DUNN and N. N. ARONSON, JR.

Summary

Leupeptin is a peptide which inhibits several of the lysosomal proteases. When this compound was added in low concentrations to a perfused liver, the degradation of ^{125}I-asialo-fetuin by the liver was dramatically slowed. When 5 mg leupeptin were added to the perfusate 1 h prior to the radioactive glycoprotein, the liver retained from 70 to 90% or the radioisotope 60 min after infusing ^{125}I-asialo-fetuin. However, untreated livers contained less than 20% of the radioactivity at that time. Subcellular fractionation experiments showed that the radioactivity accumulated in the heavy and light mitochondrial fractions (ML) of the homogenate. At 80 min after the glycoprotein was added, almost 40% of the radioactivity was still located with these fractions. Very similar inhibitory effects were seen upon treating rats intravenously with 5 mg of leupeptin 60 min prior to injection of ^{125}I-labelled asialo-fetuin. A 7fold increase in liver radioactivity was observed 6 hrs after the glycoprotein had been given to the treated animals. Purified human liver cathepsin B digested fetuin to about 3% of total hydrolysis and the major peptide fragment produced had an SDS-electrophoretic mobility equivalent to that of ovalbumin.

Introduction

Our laboratory has previously characterized the very effective manner by which rat liver digests intravenously injected ^{125}I-labelled asialo-fetuin [1]. The metabolism of this glycoprotein derivative can be divided into at least five separate events upon its entrance to the circulation. The metabolic steps which the glycoprotein undergoes are: (1) a specific binding by a lectin-like molecule present on the hepatocyte plasma membrane [2], (2) phagocytic uptake into the liver cells, (3) accumulation within lysosomes after phagosome-lysosome fusion, (4) complete digestion by the lysosomal hydrolases, and (5) release from the lysosomes of the final digestion products and their reutilization by the liver or peripheral tissues. This same heterophagic processing of ^{125}I-asialo-fetuin takes place in a perfused rat liver, and we have been using such an experimental system in conjunction with experiments done in vivo in order to characterize each portion of the above degradative pathway.

The compound which has been found to interfere the most effectively with ^{125}I-asialo-fetuin heterophagy is the protease inhibitor, leupeptin. Leupeptin is known to be a potent inhibitor of cathepsin B, and therefore we have studied as well the pattern of digestive products caused by this enzyme when acting on fetuin as a substrate. This paper describes the inhibitory effects of leupeptin on ^{125}I-asialo-fetuin metabolism when the peptide has been added both to rats in vivo and to perfused rat livers.

Materials and methods

The preparation of ^{125}I-asialo-fetuin, intravenous injection of this glycoprotein, fractionation of liver homogenates, perfusion of livers, and analyses of radioactivity were done by methods as previously reported [1, 3]. Leupeptin was kindly provided by Dr. H. UMEZAWA and cathepsin B purified from human liver [4] was generously given to us by Dr. ALAN BARRETT. Cathepsin B was assayed in the presence of 1 mM 1.2 dithioglycerol (BAL) purchased from Sigma Chemical Co.

Results and discussion

Initially experiments were tried using drugs which modify microtubule function in order to perturb the normal metabolism of ^{125}I-asialo-fetuin by the liver. Addition of vinblastine (2 μM) to the perfusate 30 min prior to the input of radioactive glycoprotein resulted in the $T\frac{1}{2}$ for removal of the latter substance from the perfusate being raised from 4.1 min for an untreated liver to 7.8 min. The release of radioactive products from the liver was dramatically slowed as well. The treated liver retained over 80% of the added isotope at 35 min after the glycoprotein was added, while a control liver contained only 30% at this same time. In the treated liver there was a shift in the subcellular location of the ^{125}I-containing material to the microsomal fraction. This possibly indicates there was an accumulation of phagosomes in the cells or a build-up of glycoprotein on the plasma membrane upon stoppage of phagocytosis.

Colchicine (22 μM) caused similar changes in the liver metabolism of asialo-fetuin. Treatment of the perfused liver with the latter compound resulted in 57% of the ^{125}I-radioactivity being retained by the tissue 90 min after addition of the labelled glycoprotein. This represents a 5 fold increase in isotope retention by the liver when compared to the behavior of untreated tissue. Although the general effect of such microtubule poisons was to reduce the overall ability of the liver to process the glycoprotein, the quantitative level of the inhibition was not experimentally reproducible.

The effects of leupeptin on the metabolism of asialo-glycoprotein by the perfused liver are shown in Fig. 1. This protease inhibitor at low concentrations (71 μM) did not alter the rate of removal of ^{125}I-asialo-fetuin from the perfusing medium when added 60 min prior to the glycoprotein. The $T\frac{1}{2}$ was 3.8 ± 0.5 min in the presence of leupeptin and 3.6 ± 0.4 min in its absence. However, the treatment with leupeptin dramatically slowed down the degradation of the protein. Such experimentally tested organs retained from 70 to 90% of the radioactivity 1 h after glycoprotein infusion while less than 20% of the isotope was left in untreated livers at that time. At 90 min the inhibited tissue still contained 65—80% of the initially added radioisotope.

Examination of homogenates of these livers by subcellular fractionation showed that after normal enrichment in the microsomal fraction (containing plasma membrane fragments and phagosomes [1]) the radioactivity had accumulated in the ML fraction (Fig. 2). From 30 to 40% of the injected isotope was present there between 30 and 80 min after addition of the glycoprotein to the perfusate. The heavy mitochondrial fraction (M) contained more than half of this amount of radioactivity and this indicates that leupeptin caused an increase in lysosomal size. This fact was substantiated by the observed shift in β-D-hexosaminidase activity from the L to the M fraction (data not shown).

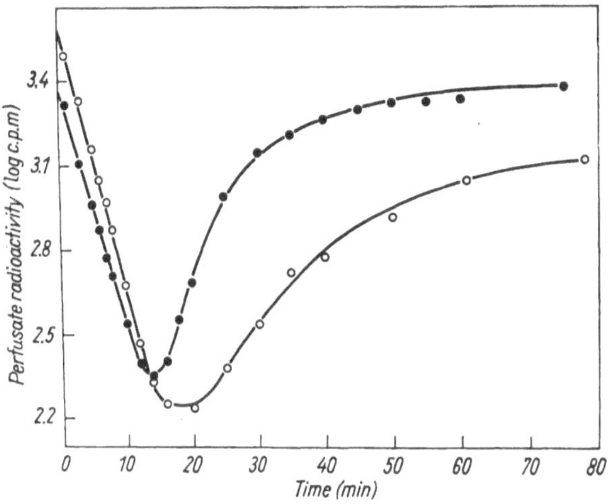

Fig. 1. Effect of leupeptin on ^{125}I-asialo-fetuin metabolism.
The liver of an anaesthetized rat (225 g body weight) was excised and placed in a perfusion apparatus as previously described [3]. Either 1 ml of water (●) or 1 ml of water plus 2.5 mg leupeptin (○) was added to the 70 ml of recirculating perfusate medium followed 60 min later by the input of 0.1 mg of ^{125}I-asialo-fetuin (1.2 × 10 cpm). Samples of 0.2 ml were removed periodically from the perfusate and their content of radioactivity was measured with an automatic gamma radiation counter

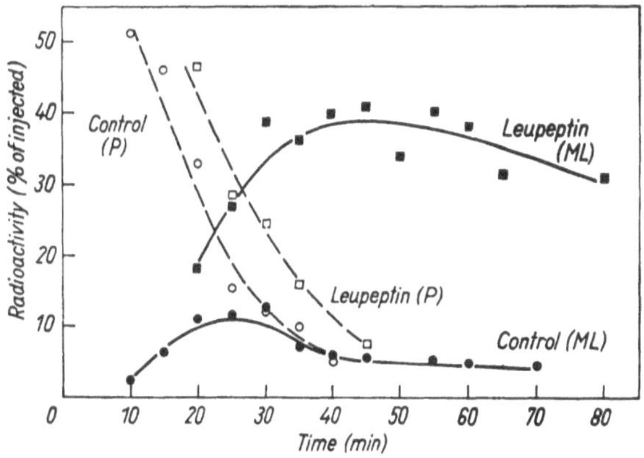

Fig. 2. Subcellular localization of radioactivity.
Livers from animals were experimentally treated with radioactive glycoprotein either in the presence (■, □) or the absence (●, ○) of leupeptin (2.5 mg) exactly as described in the legend to Fig. 1. At various times after ^{125}I-asialo-fetuin addition to the perfusate medium the livers were removed from perfusion, perfused with cold 0.25 M sucrose, and homogenized in the latter medium. The homogenates were subjected to subcellular fractionation [1, 3] and the distribution of ^{125}I-radioactivity was measured in the microsomal fraction (P) □, ○, and in the combined heavy plus light mitochondrial fractions (ML) ■, ●

Table 1
Effect of leupeptin on glycoprotein degradation in vivo

Treatment	Time of leupeptin injection (hrs before ^{125}I-asiolo-fetuin injection)	Liver radioactivity 6 hrs after injection ^{125}I-asialo-fetuin (% of injected dosage)
None (control)	—	3.4
Leupeptin (5 mg)	1	23.2
Leupeptin (5 mg)	24	3.4
Leupeptin (3 × 5 mg)	25, 18, 1	48.6

Rats weighing 200—250 g received intravenous injections of leupeptin (5 mg) at different times prior to an injection of ^{125}I-asialo-fetuin (0.09—0.15 mg, 1.2—3.0 × 10^6 cpm). After 6 hrs the animals were killed and their livers were removed, perfused with cold 0.25 M sucrose and then homogenized in the same medium. Samples of the homogenate were analyzed for their content of radioactivity and the remainder was subjected to subcellular fractions (data not shown) by methods previously described [1, 3].

A similar inhibition of glycoprotein degradation by leupeptin occurred in vivo (Table 1). Intravenous injection of 5 mg of inhibitor 1 h prior to the glycoprotein being injected caused a 7 fold increase in the liver radioactivity 6 hrs later when compared to the radioactivity found in the liver of untreated animals. If 3 similar injections of leupeptin were given over a 24 hrs period, then almost 50% of the ^{125}I-isotope was still present in the liver 6 hrs after the animal received the radioactive glycoprotein. Again the subcellular distribution of radioactivity corresponded to the ML fraction of the liver homogenate.

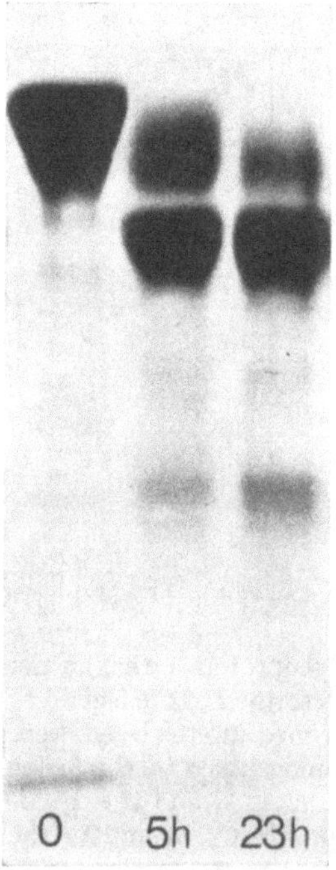

Fig. 3. Digestion of fetuin by cathepsin B.
4 mg fetuin in a volume of 1 ml which contained 1 mM BAL and 0.05 N acetic acid were incubated at 37 °C with 50 μg of purified human liver cathepsin B [4]. At several times 0.1 ml samples were removed and their cathepsin B was inactivated by adding iodoacetic acid to a final concentration of 0.1 mM. Portions (20 μl) of this were either assayed for ninhydrin reactivity (data not shown) or subjected to SDS-gel electrophoresis in the presence of mercaptoethanol [7]. Each sample represents 12 μg original fetuin and the direction of migration was downward towards the cathode

The digestion of fetuin by cathepsin B was studied both by measuring the increase in ninhydrin reactivity of the products and by analyzing the digest with SDS-gel electrophoresis under reducing conditions. The final digest at 23 hrs contained ninhydrin reactive material which represented only 2.5% of that which would have been present if the fetuin had been completely broken down to free amino acids. Fig. 3 shows the peptide pattern obtained after electrophoresis of 0, 5 and 23 hrs samples from the reaction. The original fetuin had a mobility equivalent to that of serum albumin (m.wt. 67,000) while the major peptide product present at both 5 and 23 hrs migrated the same as ovalbumin (m.wt. 40,000). The actual m.wt. of fetuin is 48,000 so that its mobility (and possibly that of its fragments) is anomalous. This is most probably due to the high carbohydrate content of the glycoprotein.
Several reports have shown leupeptin to be a potent inhibitor of cathepsins B, L and H using either purified enzymes or extracts of purified lysosomes in vitro [4—6]. The results of this present work are the first to describe the efficient inhibitory action of leupeptin in the perfused rat liver and in rats in vivo. Such a use of leupeptin in vivo will hopefully provide a means for investigating the function lysosomes have in overall protein degradation within cells. Although it is not yet known which of the leupeptin-inhibitable cathepsins is most critical for the digestion of ^{125}I-asialo-fetuin, the endo-hydrolytic action of cathepsin B on fetuin is the type of reaction step which would tend to be rate limiting for complete breakdown of a protein. In order to stop completely the concerted digestion of hyaluronic acid by the lysosomal mixture of glycosidases: hyaluronidase, β-D-hexosaminidase and β-D-glucuronidase, it was necessary to inhibit only hyaluronidase, the single endoglycosidase among the three enzymes [8].

This work was supported by grant AM-15465 from the National Institute of Arthritis Metabolism and Digestive Diseases of the U.S. Public Health Service. A portion of the work was done at The Strangeways Research Laboratory, Cambridge, England, while N.N.A. was a Fellow of the British and American Heart Associations.

References

[1] LABADIE, J. H., K. PETERSON, and N. N. ARONSON: Biochem. J. **152**, 271—279 (1975)
[2] ASHWELL, G., and A. G. MORELL.: Trends biochem. Sci. **2**, 76—78 (1977)
[3] LABADIE, J. H., W. A. DUNN, and N. N. ARONSON.: Biochem. J. **160**, 85—95 (1976)
[4] BARRETT, A. J.: Biochem. J. **131**, 809—822 (1973)
[5] KIRSCHKE, H., J. LANGNER, B. WIEDERANDERS, S. ANSORGE, and P. BOHLEY: Eur. J. Biochem. **74**, 293—302 (1977)
[6] HUISMAN, W., L. LANTING, H. J. DODDEMA, and M. GRUBER.: Biochim. J. M. W. BOUMA, biophys. Acta **370**, 297—307 (1974)
[7] STARKEY, P. M., and A. J. BARRETT.: Biochem. J. **155**, 255—263 (1976)
[8] ARONSON, N. N., and C. de DUVE.: J. biol. Chem. **243**, 4564—4573 (1968)

Acta biol. med. germ., Band 36, Seite 1923—1925 (1977)

Bereich Tierernährung der Sektion Tierproduktion und
Veterinärmedizin der Humboldt-Universität zu Berlin,
104 Berlin, DDR
Physiologisch-chemisches Institut der Martin-Luther-Universität Halle Wittenberg,
402 Halle (Saale), DDR

Studies on the in vivo-action of leupeptin on the nitrogen retention in rats

O. Simon, P. Bohley, R. Münchmeyer, H. Bergner, and C. Hückel

Summary

A daily s.c. injection of 0.5 mg leupeptin for 7 days does not influence the digestibility of food-N but seems to improve the N-retention. A daily injection of 1.0 mg leupeptin for 14 days is without influence on the digestibility of N, too, but the N-retention was decreased. At this leupeptin level the half-lives of intestinal proteins were prolonged. The data indicate the possibility to influence the N-retention using leupeptin.

Hitherto, there have been published some papers concerning the improvement of nitrogen balance in animals. Emphasis was laid on increasing synthetic rates of proteins. Nitrogen retention, however, depends on the relation between synthesis and degradation of proteins. Therefore, our study was aimed at decreasing the intracellular degradation of proteins.

For this purpose it was necessary to use an inhibitor acting on the main part of intracellular proteinases. Because leupeptin is rapidly taken up by tissues after injection [2] and seems to enter the cells, it was chosen as an inhibitor of lysosomal proteinases in our experiments. Leupeptin is a peptide aldehyde (N-acetyl-leucyl-leucyl-argininal) which inhibits the most important lysosomal proteinases cathepsin L and B in very low concentrations (less than 1 μM) very effectively [1]. Cathepsin H is inhibited, too, but at higher concentrations of leupeptin (10 μM) in vitro.

Two series of experiments have been carried out. As shown in Table 1 the food intake was limited in the first experiment, therefore the daily gain was low. The daily dose of leupeptin was 0.5 mg (injected s.c.) for a period of 7 days. In the second experiment the animals were fed ad libitum, therefore the daily gain was high. The dose of leupeptine was increased to 1 mg per day and the experimental period was extended to 15 days.

Because leupeptin is a very effective inhibitor of trypsin, too, it seemed possible that the digestibility of proteins in the alimentary tract could be decreased by leupeptin. Therefore, wee looked for any effects of leupeptin on the true digestibility of food nitrogen.

The most interesting effect of our study was the influence of leupeptin on the nitrogen balance. As can be seen from Tables 2 and 3, this value will be always positive if any net nitrogen retention takes place. Because of the restricted food intake in experiment 1 (Table 2), there were similar intakes of nitrogen in both groups. Furthermore leupeptin had not any effect on the true digestibility of

Table 1
General characterization of the experiments

	Experiment 1	Experiment 2
Food intake	limited	ad libitum
Daily gain	low	high
Leupeptin (mg/day)	0.5	1.0
Experimental period	7	15

Table 2
Influence of leupeptin on the true digestibility of food nitrogen and on the nitrogen balance (experiment 1)

Leupeptin (mg/day)	Gain (g/day)	N-Intake during the balance period (mg)	True digestibility of nitrogen (%)	Nitrogen balance (% of intake)
0.0	1.5 ± 0.41	961 ± 56	90.9 ± 0.84	18.6 ± 4.77
0.5	2.0 ± 0.24	922 ± 27	91.3 ± 0.42	21.1 ± 2.35

Table 3
Influence of leupeptin on the true digestibility of food nitrogen and on the nitrogen balance (experiment 2)

Leupeptin (mg/day)	Gain (g/day)	N-Intake during the balance period (mg)	True digestibility of nitrogen (%)	Nitrogen balance (% of intake)
1. Balance period (day 1–6)				
0.0	4.92 ± 0.24	890 ± 18.1	87.0 ± 0.25	68.1 ± 0.63
1.0	4.10 ± 0.16	815 ± 18.7	86.7 ± 0.33	64.8 ± 0.76
2. Balance period (day 10–15)				
0.0	5.14 ± 0,21	1005 ± 27.4	86.5 ± 0.24	67.0 ± 0.76
1.0	3.28 ± 0.12	846 ± 18.4	86.7 ± 0.31	62.5 ± 0.99

proteins. On the other hand, the daily gain and the nitrogen balance were somewhat increased under the influence of leupeptin. In the second series of experiments (Table 3) two balance periods were used. Again we found no differences in the true digestibility of nitrogen. Under the conditions of ad libitum food intake and a high growth rate, however, the daily gain as well as the nitrogen balance were decreased by leupeptin. It should be noted, however, that the nitrogen intake in the control group was higher.

These data indicate the possibility to influence the nitrogen retention in rats using leupeptin. However, it remains to find optimal conditions for a high nitrogen retention (dose and mode of application of leupeptin, feeding scheme, period of treatment).

Furthermore we tried to get some informtiaon on the influence of leupeptin on the half-lives of proteins in tissues of the same rats. For this reason we injected [C^{14}]-guanidino-arginine and estimated the decay of the radioactivity in proteins 6, 24, 48 and 96 hrs after the application of the tracer amino acid. This method of pulse labelling is not suitable for estimations of half-lives of muscle proteins. Moreover, our values for radioactivity in liver proteins showed too large variations for any exact determinations of half-lives in this tissue.

Thus, we are in the bad position to present here the values for intestinal proteins only (Table 4 and 5). A dose of 0.5 mg leupeptin injected daily for 7 days did not influence the half-lives of intestinal proteins at all. In both cases the proteins of the large intestine turn over more slowly than proteins of the small intestine. However, using 1 mg leupeptin daily for 15 days the treated animals showed prolonged half-lives in both parts of the intestine. Furthermore, in this experiment we investigated the possibility of reutilization of labelled amino acids using simultaneously[^{3}H]-4,5-leucine. In all cases we found longer half-lives estimated by use of [^{3}H]-leucine. This effect was extremly high in the leupeptin treated animals, especially in the large intestine. From these results it can be concluded that an increased reutilization of amino acids unter the influence of leupeptin may be possible.

Leupeptin was kindly provided by Prof. Dr. H. UMEZAWA.

Table 4
Half-lives of intestinal proteins measured after labelling with [^{14}C]-guanidino-L-arginine (experiment 1)

Leupeptin (mg/day)	Small intestine (hrs)	Large intestine (hrs)
0.0	37	64
0.5	38	63

Table 5
Half-lives of intestinal proteins measured after labelling with [^{14}C]-guanidino-L-arginine and simultaneously with [^{3}H]-L-leucine (values in brackets) (experiment 2)

Leupeptin (mg/day)	Small intestine (hrs)	Large intestine (hrs)
0.0	43 (56)	63 (78)
1.0	49 (108)	75 (276)

References

[1] KIRSCHKE, H., J. LANGNER, B. WIEDERANDERS, S. ANSORGE, and P. BOHLEY: Eur. J. Biochem. **74**, 293 (1977)
[2] MIYAMOTO, M. H. TERAYAMA, and O. OKNISKI: biochim. Biophys. Res. Commun. **55**, 84 (1973)
[3] SIMON, O., P. BOHLEY, C. HÜCKEL, R. MÜNCHMEYER, and H. BERGNER: Arch. Tierernähr. **26**, 307 (1976)

Acta biol. med. germ., Band 36, Seite 1927—1930 (1977)

Department of Biochemistry, J. Stefan Institute, [1] Department of Chemistry, University of Ljubljana, Ljubljana, Yugoslavia
[2] Institute of Pharmaceutical Chemistry, University of Trieste, Trieste, Italy.

Inactivation studies of cathepsin D with diazo compounds

I. KREGAR, B. STANOVNIK[1], M. TIŠLER[1], C. NISI[2], F. GUBENŠEK, and V. TURK

Summary

Cathepsin D was inactivated with various diazo compounds at very high concentration. Reaction proceeded maximally at *p*H 4.5 in the presence of cupric ions. With 3-diazoindazole and triazene the inactivation was noted also in the absence of cupric ions what indicates that the mechanism is mediated through triazene. CD-spectrum of partially inactivated enzyme shows that conformational changes occurred after treatment with diazo compound.

Introduction

Diazo compounds have been known for a long time as inactivators and modificators of enzymes. They have been used particularly in studies of carboxyl proteinases. Many authors observed complete stoichiometric inactivation of pepsin with diazo compounds in the presence of cupric ions [1—3]. They have shown that the loss of activity is due to the specific esterification af carboxyl group with diazo compound in the active site of pepsin. The peptide containing the modified carboxyl group was isolated and its sequence was determined [4]. Now the complete structure of pepsin is known and the aspartic acid-215 is identified as one of the catalytic residues. Similarly, the inactivation of various acid proteinases of microbial origin with diazo compounds was also found. The effect of these inactivators on cathepsin D was studied by KEILOVA [5, 6] and FERGUSSON et al. [7]. They found that much higher concentrations of diazo compounds were required for the inactivation of cathepsin D than for pepsin. In our work we investigated the inactivation process of cathepsin D using various diazo compounds.

Materials and methods

Cathepsin D was prepared in our laboratory from bovine spleen by the method of SMITH and TURK [8]. Electrophoretically pure form was used in the experiments.

The following diazo compounds were tested: diazoacetyl glycinamide, diazoacetyl-L-leucine ethyl ester, diazoacetyl-L-phenylalanine ethyl ester, diazoacetyl-DL-norleucine methylester, 3-diazoindazole, 4-diazo-3,5-dimethylpyrazole and l(indazolyl-3′)-3-phenyl triazene.

Inactivation studies: cathepsin D in acetate buffer, *p*H 4.5, (5 μM solution) was preincubated at room temperature with cupric acetate for 15 min followed by the addition of diazo compound dissolved in methanol. At different time intervals aliquotes were withdrawn for

Abbreviations: DAG = diazoacetyl-glycinamide, DAL = diazoacetyl-L-leucine ethyl ester, DAP = diazoacetyl-L-phenylalanineethylester, DAN = diazoacetyl-D,L-norleucine methylester, DDP = 4-diazo-3,5-dimethylpyrazole, DI = 3-diazo-indazole.

determination of proteolytic activity against hemoglobin by the method of ANSON [9]. CD measurements were performed on Jobin-Yvon Dichrograph III using 0.2 Å band pass which enables the best resolution.

Results and discussion

The effect of *p*H on the inactivation of cathepsin D was studied with DAG. It was found that maximal inactivation took place at *p*H 4.5.

The inactivation of cathepsin D with diazo compounds at three different concentrations in the presence of 1000 fold molar excess of cupric ions is presented in Table 1. It is evident that after 1 h even at very high concentration of inactivator 6—20% of initial activity is still present. In some cases the loss of activity was smaller. The most pronounced effects were obtained with DAL, DAP and DAN. Without addition of cupric ions the enzyme activity remained unchanged. DI proved to be a strong inactivator but caused the loss of activity by 40% also in the absence of Cu(II)acetate. Similar effect had also triazene what is shown in Table 2.

Time dependence of inactivation with DAP and DAN is shown in Figs. 1 and 2 for DDP, DI and triazene, respectively. The major part of activity is lost after 20 min, afterwards inactivation proceeds more slowly.

Table 1

Inactivation of cathepsin D with various diazo compounds (enzyme, Cu(II)az etate and inactivator were incubated for 60 min at room temperature)

Diazo compound	Molar ratio E:I:Cu % of initial activity			
	1:2500:1000	1:5000:1000	1:10000:1000	1:10000:—
DGA	80	65	60	90
DAL	40	30	10	98
DAP	72	34	22	93
DAN	40	27	23	90
DDP	80	80	76	70
DI	46	21	6	62

Table 2

Inactivation of cathepsin D with indazolyl phenyl triazene

Molar excess of triazene	% of initial activity
170	96
340	96
850	86
1700	84
3400	64
8500	43

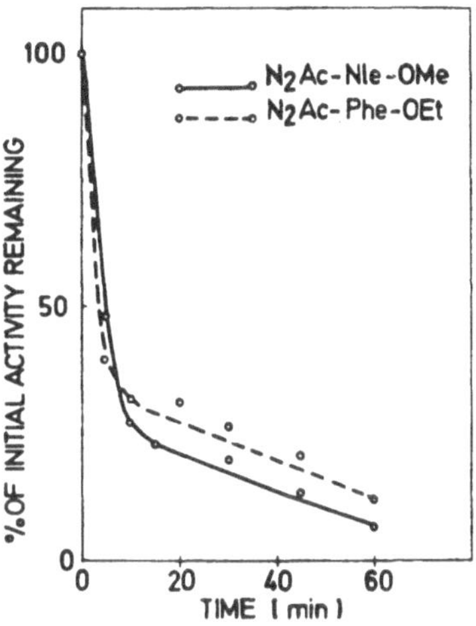

Fig. 1

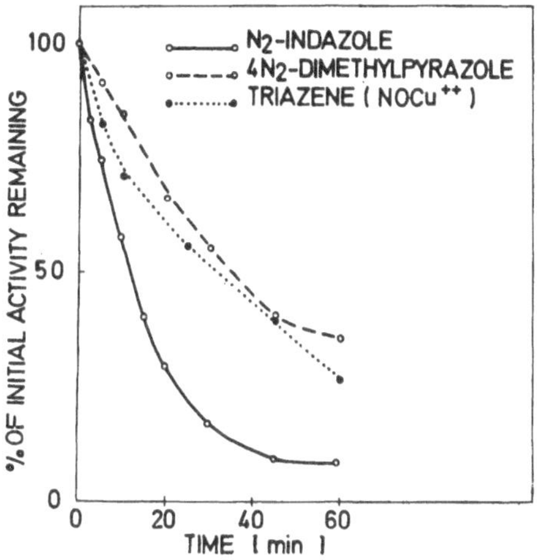

Fig. 2

Fig. 1. Time dependence of cathepsin D inactivation with 8000fold molar excess of DAP and 9000fold molar excess of DAN. The molar excess of cupric ions over enzyme was 10000fold. The reaction was performed at room temperature

Fig. 2. Time dependence of cathepsin D inactivation with 20000-fold molar excess of DDP, 14000-fold excess of DI and 8500-fold excess of triazene. The molar excess of Cu(II)ions over enzyme was 10000-fold except in the case of triazene, where the reaction was performed in the absence of Cu(II)acetate

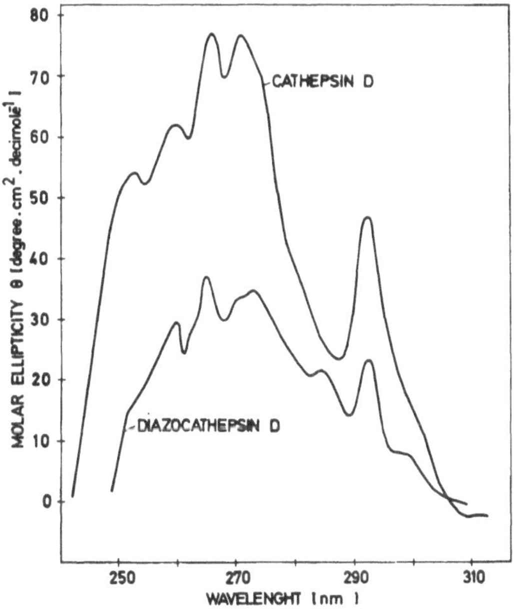

Fig. 3. CD-spectrum of native and DAN treated cathepsin D

In order to see if inactivation caused any conformational changes, we prepared cathepsin D partially inactivated with DAN. After gel chromatography on Sephadex G-25 CD spectrum of DAN treated cathepsin D was recorded. Fig. 3 shows that binding of norleucine causes pronounced change in the near UV CD spectrum. Although the enzyme remained partly active the spectrum was changed considerably. Comparison with the spectrum of pepstatin inhibited cathepsin D shows essentially the same feature. This indicates that aromatic side chains are involved in binding of inhibitor or substrate. Apparently, the observed conformational changes hinder the interaction between enzyme and substrate.

The obtained results are in agreement with those of FERGUSSON et al. [7]. They explained the requirement of high concentrations of diazo compounds for the inactivation to the weaker binding of inactivator to the active site of cathepsin D. In our opinion the loss of cathepsin D activity at 10000 fold molar excess of diazo compound in the presence of Cu(II)ions makes the specific interaction with carboxyl group as the only process questionable. The inactivation with DI and triazene in the absence of Cu(II)ions can be explained by a mechanism in which carbene is formed from triazene intermediate through interaction of diazo compound with amino groups in protein. Metal-complexed carbene intermediates were also proposed by LUNDBLAD and STEIN [3] in the inactivation of pepsin.

The investigation on the stoichiometry of the reaction which will contribute to the explanation of the mechanism of cathepsin D inactivation are in progress.

The authors thank Mrs. M. PREGELJ and Mrs. K. LEONARDIS for their excellent technical assistance. The work was supported by the research grant from the Research Council of Slovenia and in part by the NSF, USA.

References

[1] DELPIERRE, G. R., and J. S. FRUTON: Proc. natn. Acad. Sci. U.S.A. **54**, 1161 (1965)
[2] RAJAGOPALAN, T. G., W. H. STEIN, and S. MOORE: J. biol. Chem. **241**, 4295 (1966)
[3] LUNDBLAD, R. L., and W. STEIN: J. biol. Chem. **244**, 154 (1969)
[4] BAYLLISS, R. S., J. R. KNOWLESS, and G. B. WYBRANDT: Biochem. J. **113**, 377 (1969)
[5] KEILOVA, H.: FEBS Lett. **6**, 312 (1970)
[6] KEILOVA, H., and V. TOMAŠEK: Intracellular Protein Catabolism. H. HANSON and P. BOHLEY (Eds). Barth, Leipzig 1976, p. 237
[7] FERGUSSON, J. B., J. R. ANDREWS, I. M. VOYNICK, and J. S. FRUTON: J. biol. Chem. **248**, 6701 (1973)
[8] SMITH, R., and V. TURK: Eur. J. Biochem. **48**, 245 (1974)
[9] ANSON, M. L.: J. gen. Physiol. **22**, 79 (1939)

Acta biol. med. germ., Band 36, Seite 1931—1937 (1977)

Institute of Pharmacology and Toxicology, Medical Academy, 50 Erfurt, DDR

Inhibition of serine proteinases by benzamidine derivatives

P. Walsmann

Summary

Derivatives of benzamidine inhibit competitively the activity of the serine proteinases trypsin, plasmin, thrombin, and of the clotting factor Xa. The inhibitor activities (K_i-values) of various benzamidine derivatives against the several enzymes were compared. Besides parallels, deviations in the corresponding structure-activity relationships were found.

From these results it is concluded that the similar enzymes exhibit certain differences in the structure of the primary and secondary binding sites.

Introduction

Factor Xa and thrombin are key enzymes in the mechanism of blood coagulation, whereas plasmin is responsible for the dissolution of fibrin clots. In these enzymes, large tracts of the amino acid sequence, including the catalytically important residues, show extensive homology with the pancreatic endopeptidase trypsin [1—6]. Their catalytic sites contain residues homologous with Ser-195, His-57, and Asp-102 in trypsin and form the "charge-relay system" typical of serine proteinases. Close to the catalytic sites is a deeply invaginated hydrophobic pocket which is responsible for substrate binding. At its bottom is an aspartic acid corresponding to Asp-189 in trypsin. The primary specificity of trypsin and trypsin-like serine proteinases of the blood is directed towards bonds of arginine and lysine, because the positively charged guanidyl and ε-amino groups are attracted by the negative charge of this aspartate. All these proteinases hydrolyse the synthetic substrate tosyl-L-arginine methyl ester, however, their specificity towards natural substrates differs considerably. Thrombin cleaves only four arginyl-glycyl bonds when clotting fibrinogen. In contrast, trypsin cleaves about 300 peptide bonds C-terminal to arginine and lysine in fibrinogen [7, 8]. Between these extremes is plasmin. Factor Xa cleaves only two arginyl bonds in prothrombin, and thrombin another one.

In the last few years, low-molecular-weight inhibitors have received increasing attention for investigations on the nature and specificity of the active sites of particular enzymes towards their natural substrates. Moreover, these inhibitors may be useful as antiproteolytic agents, for example as potential drugs.

Like trypsin, also the trypsin-like enzymes are competitively inhibited by benzamidine. As demonstrated by X-ray diffraction data, benzamidine is fixed in the substrate-binding pocket [10, 11].

Materials and methods

The antitrypsin, antiplasmin, and antithrombin activity of the substances was determined by measuring the inhibition of hydrolysis of N^{α}-benzoyl-D,L-arginine-4-nitroanilide catalyzed by these enzymes at *p*H 8.0 and 25 °C. In case of factor Xa, N^{α}-tosyl-L-arginine methyl ester was used as substrate. Inhibitor constants (K_i) were estimated graphically according to DIXON [9]. The precise description of methods, the origin and purification of enzymes as well as synthesis of inhibitors were published previously.

Results and discussion

The influence of a series of derivatives of benzamidine on the activity of trypsin, plasmin, thrombin, and factor Xa was investigated. The K_i-values were determined as a measure of the inhibitor strength.

Table 1

Inhibition of serine proteinases by derivatives of benzamidine

Electron-donating substituents ←— H —→ Electron-accepting substituents	
NH_2, OH, CH_3	*Br, NO_2*

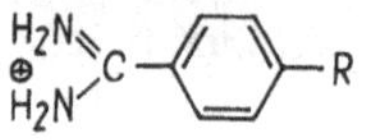

Potency ranking of benzamidine derivatives for:

Trypsin	*NH_2 (K_i: 12 µM) < CH_3 < H (K_i: 35 µM) < Br < OH < NO_2 (K_i: 330 µM)*
Plasmin	*NH_2 (K_i: 130 µM) < Br < CH_3 < H (K_i: 350 µM) < OH < NO_2 (K_i: >2000 µM)*
Thrombin	*NH_2 (K_i: 80 µM) < OH = H (K_i: 220 µM) = Br < CH_3 < NO_2 (K_i: >2000 µM)*
Factor Xa	*NH_2 (K_i: 54 µM) < OH < H (K_i: 410 µM) < Br < CH_3 < NO_2 (K_i: >2000 µM)*

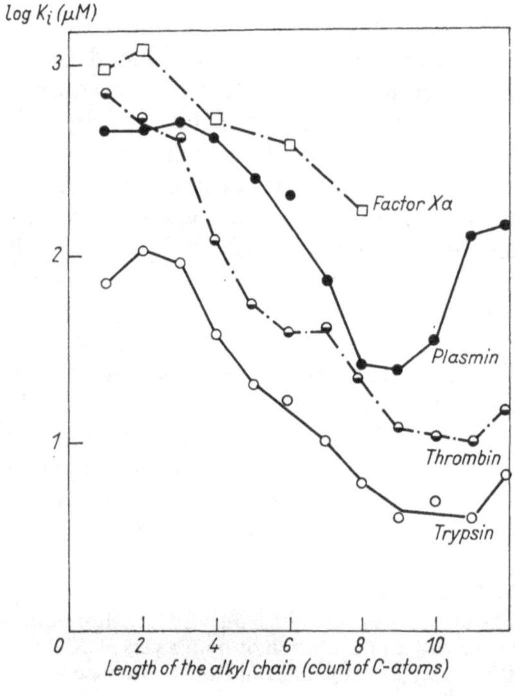

Fig. 1. Inhibition of serine proteinases by 4-amidinophenyl alkyl ethers

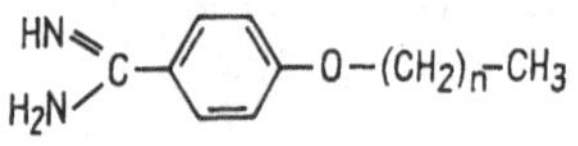

n = 0,1,2,3,4,5,6,7,8,9,10,11,

Inhibition of: factor Xa □—·—□; plasmin ●——●; thrombin ◒—·—◒; trypsin ○——○

Substitution of benzamidine with the electron-donating amino group led to an increase in the inhibitory activity against all enzymes tested (Table 1) [12, 13]. In contrast, nitrobenzamidine possessed only an extremely low percentage of the inhibitor strength of benzamidine. The affinity of "simple" benzamidine derivatives for trypsin is ten times higher than for the other enzymes. The lowest affinity was found for factor Xa [14]. The inhibitor strength against the various enzymes differs as well as the potency ranking of inhibitors for a particular enzyme.

Inhibitor molecules with longer side chains could be bound additionally to other areas of the enzyme surface outside the substrate-binding pocket.

The study of alkyl and alkoxybenzamidines led to the assumption that the alkyl chains of these compounds may interact with a second hydrophobic site [15, 16]. This assumption was confirmed by quantitative structure-activity correlations describing the antitrypsin, antithrombin, and antiplasmin activities of 4-amidinophenyl derivatives with lipophilic and electronic substituent constants [17]. The enhancement of the inhibitor strength with increasing chain length differed in the individual enzymes (Fig. 1).

The slightest increase in affinity was observed in factor Xa [14]. In contrast, the investigation of the 3-amidinoalkoxy derivatives revealed that with increasing length of the alkyl chain the antifactor Xa activity surpassed the inhibitory activity against the other enzymes. A comparison between the inhibitory activities of 3- and 4-isomers showed clearly differences in specificity of the proteinases (Table 2). This comparison reveals a higher affinity of the 4-amidinophenyl ethers for trypsin and of the 3-isomers for factor Xa.

The aralkoxy derivatives exerted stronger inhibitory effects than the alkoxy derivatives (Table 3) [18]. Naphthyl derivatives and bisamidine compounds were

Table 2

Relationships of inhibitor activity of 3- and 4-alkoxybenzamidines to factor Xa and trypsin

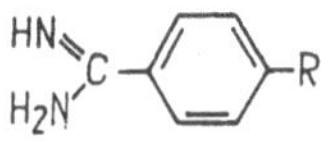	K_i 3-isomer / K_i 4-isomer	
R	Factor Xa	Trypsin
O CH_3	0.12	3.14
O C_2H_5	0.16	1.8
O C_4H_9	0.096	2.5
O C_6H_{13}	0.076	3.41
O C_7H_{15}		7.1

Table 3

Inhibition of serine proteinases by amidinophenyl and amidinobenzyl ethers

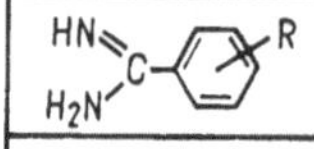	K_i (μM) 3-isomers				4-isomers			
R	Trypsin	Plasmin	Thrombin	Factor Xa	Trypsin	Plasmin	Thrombin	Factor Xa
OC_6H_{13} (n)	58	80	58	29	17	200	39	380
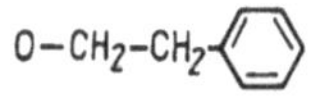	38	40	18	6.2	14	300	100	260
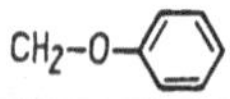	9	100	60	6.8	9	400	58	380
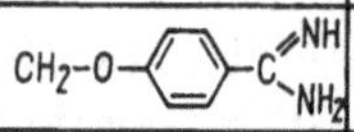	3.9	40	33	23	4.8	27	140	580
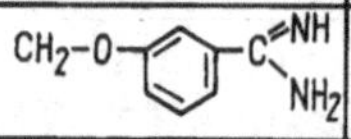	6.1	54	60	44	5.6	33	26	32
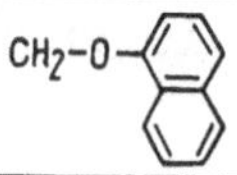	1.5	220	24	7.8	2.6	100	6.6	35
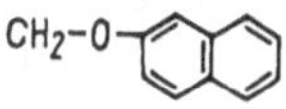	3.8	180	39	3.9	3.8	100	62	150

found to be the most potent trypsin inhibitors. The antithrombin activity of one of these derivatives was in the same order of magnitude as its antitrypsin activity. In contrast, the inhibitory effects against plasmin and factor Xa were relatively weak. According to the results obtained with aliphatic ethers, in the 3-isomers a weaker antitrypsin activity could be expected than in the corresponding 4-derivatives. The results listed in Table 4 show that the 3-amidinobenzyl ethers are, however, also very potent trypsin inhibitors. As in case of the alkoxy derivatives, the 3-amidinobenzyl ethers are more effective inhibitors of factor Xa than the corresponding 4-isomers [14].

Thus, the affinity of these inhibitors for factor Xa is comparable with that for trypsin. This result is remarkable in as much as the above-mentioned compounds are strong trypsin inhibitors but weak inhibitors of factor Xa.
Compared with other amidinophenylalkylcarboxylic acids exerting only minimal inhibitory effects, 4-amidinophenylpyruvic acid exhibited high affinity especially for trypsin and thrombin (Table 5) [19]. From the marked deviation from the structure-activity correlations ascertained by Coats [17], additional bonds resulting from the carbonyl function were concluded.

This assumption led us to investigate a group of amidinophenyl derivatives containing aliphatic and araliphatic side chains with ketone structure (Table 6) [20—23]. It was found that a carbonyl function at β-position of the amidinophenyl ring increased significantly the affinity of the compounds for thrombin and trypsin.

Table 4

Relationships of inhibitor activity of 3-and 4-aralkoxybenzamidines to factor Xa and trypsin

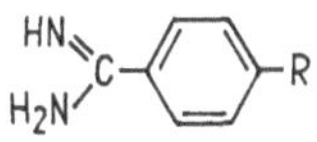	$\frac{K_i \text{ 3-isomer}}{K_i \text{ 4-isomer}}$	
R	*Factor Xa*	*Trypsin*
OC_6H_{13} (n)	*0.076*	*3.41*
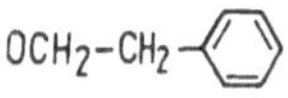	*0.024*	*2.71*
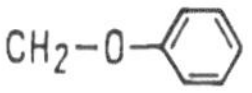	*0.018*	*1.0*
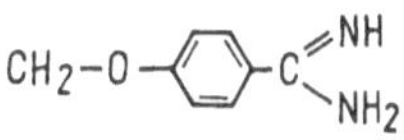	*0.04*	*0.81*
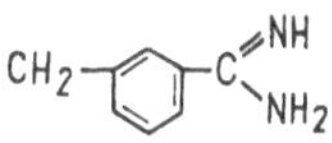	*(1.38)*	*1.09*
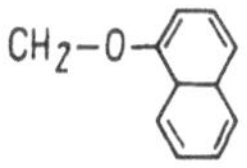	*0.22*	*0.58*
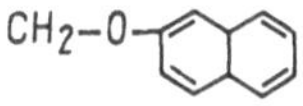	*0.025*	*1.0*

Quantitative structure-activity correlations revealed that electron-accepting substituents of the carbonyl carbon favoured binding to the enzymes (Table 7) [24]. Accordingly, affinity-increasing interactions could possibly occur via polarization of the carbonyl group. As seen from the positive sign of the electronic term σ_I in the correlations, the affinity becomes higher with increasing electrophilic character of the carbonyl carbon. As for the enzyme-substrate reaction, the hydroxyl group of serine 195 of the active centre could be considered the nucleophilic partner. The interaction between carbonyl carbon and serine hydroxyl can be considered as a type of transition state comparable with the tetrahedral intermediate supposed to form during substrate hydrolysis. From structure-activity correlations as well as from the K_i-values of the inhibitors it can be concluded that besides parallels there exist also differences in the structure of the various serine proteinases. The different affinity of the inhibitors for trypsin and the trypsin-like enzymes may be due to structural differences of the primary as well as of the secondary binding sites. Inhibitors with longer side chains are additionally fixed on areas of the enzyme surface outsite the binding pocket by hydrophobic bonds. The different adaption of definite constituents of inhibitor molecules to the enzyme surface is mainly due to steric differences of the secondary binding sites. These sites may be responsible for the specificity of proteinases towards their natural substrates.

X-ray diffraction data of the enzyme-inhibitor complexes may contribute to an exact localization of secondary binding sites, to an estimation of their distances to the active centres and their steric conformation.

Table 5

Inhibition of serine proteinases by amidinophenylalkylcarboxylic acids

Substance	K_i (µM)	
	Trypsin	Thrombin
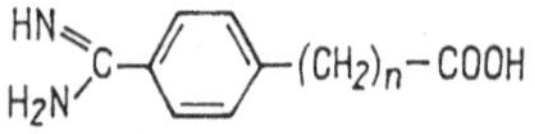 n = 0,1,2	~ 500	7 - 10 000
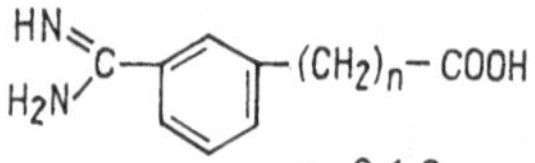 n = 0,1,2	50 - 170	2900 - 6400
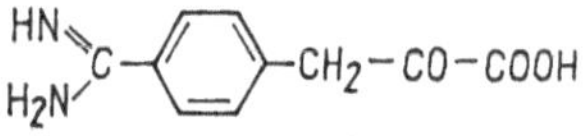	1.6	6.5
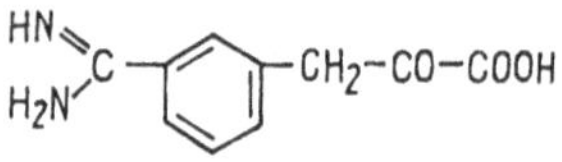	30	790

Table 6

Structure of the 4-amidinophenyl compounds with keto group

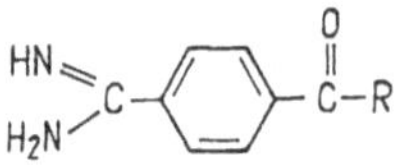

(I) α-Ketones

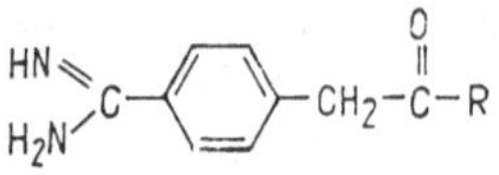

(II) β-Ketones

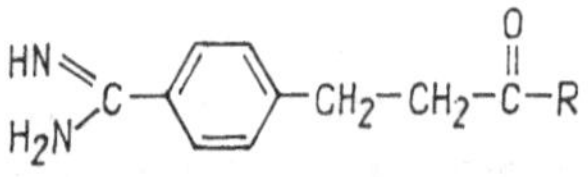

(III) γ-Ketones

Table 7

Comparison between the different quantitative structure-activity relationships of 4-amidinobenzyl ketones

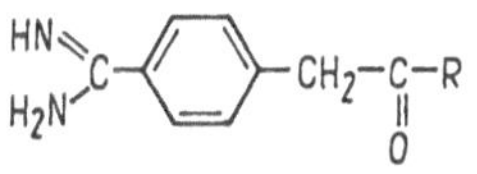

π = Lipophilic parameters
σ_I = Electronic parameters
n = Count of compounds
r = Correlation coefficients

$$\log 1/K_i = a + b\sigma_I + c\pi$$

Enzyme	a	b	c	n	r
Thrombin	0.882	4.003	0.329	16	0.771
Plasmin	0.584	2.239	–	16	0.630
Trypsin	1.441	3.798	0.381	16	0.886

References

[1] HARTLEY, B. S.: Phil. Trans. R. Soc. Ser. B **257**, 77 (1970)
[2] MAGNUSSON, S., L. SOTTRUP-JENSEN. T. E. PETERSEN, and H. CLEAYS in: Prothrombin and Related Coagulation Factors. H. C. HEMKER and J. J. VELTKAMP (Eds). University Press, Leiden 1975, p. 25
[3] TITANI, K., M. A. HERMODSON, K. FUJIKAWA, L. H. ERICSSON, K. A. WALSH, H. NEURATH, and E. W. DAVIE: Biochemistry **11**, 4899 (1972)
[4] GROSKOPF, W. R., L. SUMMARIA, and K. C. ROBBINS: J. biol. Chem. **244**, 3590 (1969)
[5] ROBBINS, K. C., P. BERNABE, L. ARZADON, and L. SUMMARIA: J. biol. Chem. **247**, 6757 (1972)
[6] ROBBINS, K. C., P. BERNABE, L. ARZADON, and L. SUMMARIA: J. biol. Chem. **248**, 1631 (1973)
[7] PECHET, L., and B. ALEXANDER: Biochemistry **1**, 875 (1962)
[8] MIHALYI, E., and J. E. GODFREY: Biochim. biophys. Acta **67**, 73 (1963)
[9] DIXON, M.: Biochem. J. **55**, 170 (1953)
[10] KRIEGER, M., L. M. KAY, and R. M. STROUD: J. molec. Biol. **83**, 209 (1974)
[11] BODE, W., and P. SCHWAGER: J. molec. Biol. **98**, 693 (1975)
[12] MARKWARDT, F., H. LANDMANN, and P. WALSMANN: Eur. J. Biochem. **6**, 502 (1968)
[13] MARKWARDT, F., P. WALSMANN, and H. G. KAZMIROWSKI: Pharmazie **24**, 400 (1969)
[14] STÜRZEBECHER, J., F. MARKWARDT, and P. WALSMANN: Thrombos. Res. **9**, 637 (1976)
[15] MARKWARDT, F., P. WALSMANN, and H. LANDMANN: Pharmazie **25**, 551 (1970)
[16] WALSMANN, P.: Folia haemat. **98**, 471 (1972)
[17] COATS, E. A.: J. med. Chem. **16**, 1102 (1973)
[18] WALSMANN, P., H. HORN, H. LANDMANN, F. MARKWARDT, J. STÜRZEBECHER, and G. WAGNER: Pharmazie **30**, 386 (1975)
[19] WALSMANN, P., F. MARKWARDT, P. RICHTER, J. STÜRZEBECHER, G. WAGNER, and H. LANDMANN: Pharmazie **29**, 333 (1974)
[20] STÜRZEBECHER, J., F. MARKWARDT, P. RICHTER, B. VOIGT, G. WAGNER, and P. WALSMANN: Pharmazie **31**, 459 (1976)
[21] WALSMANN, P., R. GRIESSMANN, H. HORN, F. MARKWARDT, P. RICHTER, J. STÜRZEBECHER, and G. WAGNER: Pharmazie **31**, 410 (1976)
[22] WALSMANN, P., F. MARKWARDT, J. STÜRZEBECHER, B. VOIGT, and G. WAGNER: Pharmazie **31**, 733 (1976)
[23] STÜRZEBECHER, J., F. MARKWARDT, B. VOIGT, P. WALSMANN, and G. WAGNER: Pharmazie **31**, 886 (1976)
[24] STÜRZEBECHER, J., F. MARKWARDT, G. WAGNER, and P. WALSMANN: Acta biol. med. germ. **35**, 1665 (1976)

Acta biol. med. germ., Band 36, Seite 1939—1944 (1977)

Institute of Physiological Chemistry,
Martin Luther University Halle-Wittenberg, 402 Halle, DDR

Studies on some effectors of lysosomal proteinases from rat liver

Z. B. SALAMA and P. BOHLEY

Introduction

The main interest of this study is the attempt to find out specifically new effectors which may activate or inhibit the thiolproteinases of lysosomes in rat liver. The objective is to characterize and assign the enzymes present in the lysosomal supernatant (LS), the subfractions and isolated enzymes according to the various catalytic classes of proteinases such as thiol-, serine-, carboxyl-, and metallo-proteinases.

Materials and methods

The cell centrifugation procedure and the preparation of LS, L20, L60 und L120 was described in [1—4].
The investigations were first carried out with the lysosomal supernatant (LS) and azocaseine as substrate; then the percentage of inhibition or activation were determined [4]; finally the effectors which showed a certain influence on the activity of LS were tested regarding their effect on the subfractions L20, L60 and L120.
It is aimed through the above procedure to find out whether these effects are caused by proteinases with different molecular weights, namely with 20000 (L20), 60000 (L60) or 120000 (L120) molecular weights. For example, with L20, it is concerned with a fraction of thiolproteinases (cathepsin L, cathepsin B1, cathepsin H as well as other proteinases) [5, 6]. In the same sense serves the application of double labelled cytosol proteins as a physiological substrate and LS, cathepsin L and L20C12 as sources of enzymes for the further characterization of the above mentioned effectors.
The selective labelling of long-lived (^{14}C-labelled) and short-lived (tritium labelled) rat liver cytosol proteins in vivo [7] and their subsequent use as substrates for unlabelled enzymes of lysosomes rat liver (incubations at *p*H 6 in $5 \cdot 10^{-3}$ M reduced glutathione, determination of trichloracetic acid soluble radioactivity by liquid scintillation counting in a tricarb 3375) enable us to distinguish the different influences of the effectors on the degradation of these long-lived and short-lived cytosol proteins.
From the radioactivity in the supernatant of the trichloroacetic acid the percentage of the degradation of the long- and short-lived proteins was calculated [4].

Results and discussion

Fraction LS

From the obtained results the following can be stated:
65 to 80% of the activities of the soluble lysosomal proteinases in LS can be attributed to thiol proteinases. These activities can be inhibited by leupeptin, p-chloromercuribenzoate and iodoacetamide.
About 70 to 85% of the activity for the degradation of long-lived and short-lived proteins in LS belong to thiol proteinases.

The observed inhibitions in LS which are caused by trypsin-inhibitors or the serine-proteinase inhibitors are either inhibitions of a part of thiol proteinases that are present in LS and can be inhibited by these inhibitors or the soluble lysosomal proteinases in LS contain a part of trypsin-like proteinases (or other serine proteinases) which can also be inhibited by these inhibitors. This part, however, cannot possibly amount to more than 20% of the total activity.
The metallo-proteinases hardly take part in the total activity of soluble lysosomal proteinases.
Less than 10% of the activities in LS are carboxyl proteinasas at *p*H 6.1, because the carboxyl proteinases inhibitor pepstatin shows a negligible inhibiting effect on LS also in high concentrations.

Fraction L20

The investigations regarding the characterization of proteinases of this fraction allow to make the following statements:
It is known that the most important enzymes of this fraction are the thiol proteinases cathepsin L, cathepsin B1 and cathepsin H as well as other thiol proteinases of the fraction L20C1; the main part of the activities of this fraction can be attributed to cathepsin L [5, 6].
The investigations in L20 up to now indicate that this fraction is composed nearly exclusively of thiol proteinases. The results of our investigations in L20 with leupeptin, p-chloromercuribenzoate and iodacetamide confirm this statement.

Table 1

The influence of some effectors on the activity of the proteinases in the lysosomal supernatant LS and in the subfractions L20, L60 and L120 with azocaseine as substrate

Effector	Percentage residual activity							
	LS		L20		L60		L120	
	10^{-3}	10^{-6}	10^{-3}	10^{-6}	10^{-3}	10^{-6}	10^{-3}	10^{-6}
Phenyl-3-guanidinobenzoate nitrate	72	100	84	100	83	100	85	100
Thiophenyl-3-guanidinobenzoate nitrate	71	100	83	100	61	100	72	100
Benzyl-3-guanidinobenzoate nitrate	66	100	89	100	75	100	74	100
4-Nitrobenzyl-4′-guanidinobenzoate nitrate	51	100	69	100	45	100	40	100
n-Octyl-4-guanidinobenzoate nitrate	70	100	94	100	73	100	66	100
3-Amidinophenyl-4′-methylbenzene-sulfonate · HCl	77	100	85	100	89	100	82	100
3-Amidinophenyl-β′-naphthalene-sulfonate · HCl	61	100	82	100	56	100	51	100
4-Aminobenzamidine dihydrochloride	130	100	100	100	117	100	116	100
Leupeptin	35	35	0	9	—	92	—	96
p-Chloromercuribenzoate (pCMB)	28	97	0	68	58	100	85	100
Iodoacetamide	55	100	58	100	68	100	83	100
Phenylmethane-sulphonyl fluoride (PMSF)	78	100	—	—	—	—	—	—
Reduced glutathione	163	100	258	100	161	100	137	100

Our investigations with trypsin- and serine proteinase inhibitors show that the thiol proteinases of this fraction could be inactivated in different degrees only at high concentrations of inhibitors.

Fraction L60

The activity of the proteinases in L60 is very weakly influenced by leupeptin. The activity of L60 could be raised to about 80% by addition of reduced glutathione ($6 \cdot 10^{-3}$ M). This can be considered as a further proof for the presence of some thiol proteinase activity in this enzyme fraction, although L60 mainly contains carboxyl proteinases.

Without reduced glutathione and by an increase of the concentration of p-chloromercuribenzoate higher than $3.3 \cdot 10^{-5}$ M a considerable part (50—60%) of the measured activity remains non-inhibited. The non-inhibited part of the activity is composed of other proteinases which cannot be inactivated by the inhibitors of thiol proteinases.

Fraction L120

Our investigations regarding the influence of leupeptin on the activity of L120 show hardly any inhibition.

The fraction L120 contains a very small part of thiol proteinases which can be activated by reduced glutathione and inhibited by the inhibitors of thiol proteinases such as leupeptin, p-chloromercuribenzoate and iodoacetamide.

The main part of proteinases in this fraction is composed of serine-proteinases. Our systematic investigation with the serine proteinase inhibitors and the use of azocaseine as substrate shows that the proteinases with high molecular weights in L60 and 120 could be more effectively inactivated by these inhibitors than the proteinases of the lysosomal supernatant LS and L20.

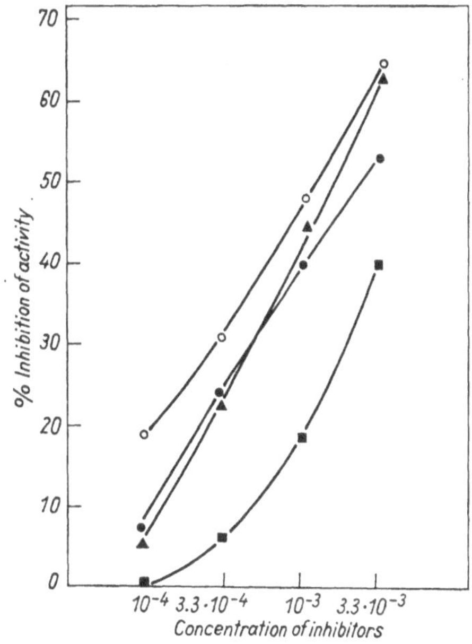

Fig. 1. The influence of 3-amidinophenyl-β'-naphthalene-sulfonate · HCl on the activity of lysosomal proteinases from rat liver. LS (●): Lysosomal supernatant; L120 (○), L60 (▲), and L20 (■): Subfractions of LS with molecular weights from about 120000, 60000 and 20000

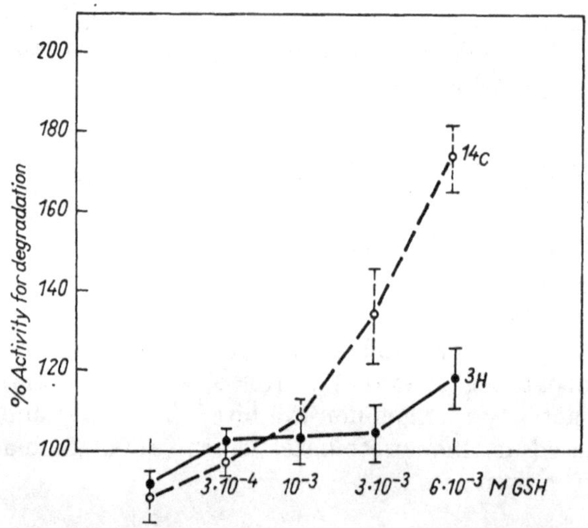

Fig. 2. The influence of reduced glutathione on the degradation of double labelled cytosol proteins by lysosomal supernatant LS.
^{3}H = Short-lived cytosol proteins; ^{14}C = Long-lived cytosol proteins. GSH = Reduced glutathione

This can be clearly shown in Fig. 1 which illustrates the influence of 3-amidino-phenyl-β'-naphthalenesulfonate · HCl as a representative of the tested serine proteinase inhibitors on the activity of lysosomal proteinases in LS and the sub-fractions L20, L60 and L120.

The other tested serine-proteinase inhibitors show similar pictures [4].

Activation of the lysosomal proteinases by reduced glutathione was also investigated.

We found that reduced glutathione acts as an effective activator for all tested enzyme fractions, the effect increasing in the following order: L20 $>$ cathepsin L $>$ LS $>$ L60 $>$ L120.

Also, our investigations have shown that reduced glutathione activated the degradation of long lived cytosol proteins by LS preferentially. This is indicated in Fig. 2. Where could the reasons for this strongly rising degradation of the long-lived cytosol proteins be looked for? Probably this is a result of splitting of the disulphide bonds of the long-lived cytosol proteins by the reduced glutathione under the formation of free SH-groups. So, perhaps, through the destruction of the -S-S-bonds and the concomitant structural changes the long-lived cytosol proteins are better degraded by the proteinases in LS than those have the disulphide bonds intact. Neither the content of disulphide bonds in both long-lived and short-lived cytosol proteins nor the role in preserving the structure of the double labelled cytosol proteins is known up to now.

A comparison of the results obtained by studying the influence of some effectors on the degradation of the short-lived and long-lived cytosol proteins by proteinases of lysosomal supernatant LS, subfraction L20C12 and cathepsin L is shown in Table 2.

Table 2

Comparison of the results obtained by studying the influence of some effectors on the degradation of the short-lived and long-lived cytosol proteins by proteinases of the lysosomal supernatant LS, L20C12 and cathepsin L

Effector	Concentration of the effector (M)	Residual activity for the degradation of short-lived cytosol proteins	Residual activity for the degradation of long-lived cytosol proteins
Leupeptin	$3 \cdot 10^{-4}$	15	15
LS	10^{-5}	18	21
	10^{-6}	30	31
p-Chloromercuribenzoate	$3 \cdot 10^{-3}$	16	20
LS	10^{-3}	57	70
	$3 \cdot 10^{-4}$	79	81
	10^{-4}	88	89
Iodoacetamide	$3 \cdot 10^{-3}$	38	38
LS	10^{-3}	58	64
	$3 \cdot 10^{-4}$	70	84
	10^{-4}	83	89
Phenyl-3-guanidinobenzoate			
L20 C12	10^{-3}	73	82
Cathepsin L	10^{-3}	73	87
Thiophenyl-3-guanidinobenzoate			
L20 C12	10^{-3}	75	85
Cathepsin L	10^{-3}	83	99
Benzyl-3-guanidinobenzoate			
L20 C12	10^{-3}	77	81
Cathepsin L	10^{-3}	76	84
4-Nitrobenzyl-4′-guanidinobenzoate			
L20 C12	10^{-3}	76	81
Cathepsin L	10^{-3}	71	80
n-Octyl-4-guanidinobenzoate			
L20 C12	$3 \cdot 10^{-3}$	86	88
Cathepsin L	$3 \cdot 10^{-3}$	67	74
3-Amidinophenyl-4′-methyl-benzene-sulfonate			
L20 C12	10^{-3}	64	73
	10^{-4}	87	94
	10^{-5}	96	100
Cathepsin L	10^{-3}	56	68
	10^{-4}	87	97
	10^{-5}	84	92
3-Amidinophenyl-β′-naphthalene-sulfonate			
L20 C12	10^{-3}	59	62
	10^{-4}	92	92
	10^{-5}	100	100
Cathepsin L	10^{-3}	44	56
	10^{-4}	101	93
	10^{-5}	102	98
Reduced glutathione			
LS	$1.1 \cdot 10^{-2}$	117	172
	$8 \cdot 10^{-3}$	103	133
	$6 \cdot 10^{-3}$	103	107
	$5.3 \cdot 10^{-3}$	100	99
	$5.1 \cdot 10^{-3}$	90	89

We found that the influence of the tested serine-proteinase inhibitors on the degradation of the double labelled cytosol proteins by cathepsin L and L20C12 was not specific. For example about 40 to 50% of the activity of cathepsin L for the degradation of short-lived and long-lived cytosol proteins could be inhibited only at the very high concentration of $3 \cdot 10^{-3}$ M of some of these inhibitors such as 3-amidinophenyl-4'-methylbenzene-sulfonate · HCl and 3-amidinophenyl-β'-naphthalene-sulfonate · HCl. In the presence of the tested inhibitors the difference between the inhibition of the degradation of the short-lived and long-lived cytosol proteins by the proteinases in LS, L20C12 and cathepsin L was very small.

Acknowledgements

We wish to thank Prof. Dr. H. UMEZAWA (Tokyo), Prof. Dr. G. WAGNER (Leipzig) and Prof. Dr. Dr. F. MARKWARDT (Erfurt) for their kind gifts of inhibitors.

References

[1] BOHLEY, P., H. KIRSCHKE, J. LANGNER, and S. ANSORGE: FEBS Lett. 5, 233–235 (1969)
[2] BOHLEY, P., H. KIRSCHKE, J. LANGNER, S. ANSORGE and H. HANSON: Acta biol. med. germ. 27, 229–243 (1971)
[3] KIRSCKHE, H., J. LANGNER, B. WIEDERANDERS, S. ANSORGE, and P. BOHLEY: Acta biol. med. germ. 28, 305–322 (1972)
[4] SALAMA, Z. B.: Promotion A. Fakultät für Naturwissenschaften der Martin-Luther-Universität, Halle-Wittenberg 1977
[5] KIRSCHKE, H., J. LANGNER, B. WIEDERANDERS, S. ANSORGE, P. BOHLEY, and H. BROGHAMMER: Acta biol. med. germ. 35, 285–299 (1976)
[6] KIRSCHKE, H., J. LANGNER, B. WIEDERANDERS, S. ANSORGE, and P. BOHLEY: Eur. J. Biochem. 74, 293–301 (1977)
[7] BOHLEY, P., H. KIRSCHKE, J. LANGNER, B. WIEDERANDERS, and S. ANSORGE: Acta biol. med. germ. 35, 300–307 (1976)

Acta biol. med. germ., Band 36, Seite 1945—1950 (1977)

Institute of Biochemistry, Bulgarian Academy of Sciences, 1113-Sofia, Bulgaria

Endogenous proteolytic activity of chromatin

B. Anachkova and G. Russev

Summary

Chromatin from rat liver and Ehrlich ascites tumor (EAT) was isolated by two different procedures and the chromatin preparations were incubated at 37 °C. To follow the proteolysis at 0, 4, 8, and 24 hrs, aliquots were taken and analysed by SDS polyacrylamide gel electrophoresis. Although there were some differences in the proteolytic activity of the different chromatins, in general they were found to sustain a several hours incubation without appreciable degradation to occur. However, when prior to incubation the chromatins were dissociated, a rapid proteolysis took place. This shows that there are specific, chromatin bound proteinases that are inactive while immobilized in the chromatin structure and become activated on dissociation.

Introduction

In the course of chromatin isolation a considerable degradation of chromosomal proteins may take place. The isolated chromatin is further subjected to treatments including incubation, dissociation or digestion which gives additional opportunity for the activation of proteinases. Thus the final product might significantly differ from its native state. Some authors underestimate the rate of proteolysis occurring in chromatin during its isolation and further manipulations and take no measures to restrict the proteinase activity. Others exaggerate the danger of proteolysis and use at all experimental steps high concentrations of proteinase inhibitors, which, however, might cause significant changes in the properties of the product. This situation often leads to contradictory results and hinders the comparison of the experimental data.

In the present paper we tried to estimate the contribution of several general factors to the proteolysis of the chromosomal proteins. As such factors the isolation procedure, the source, and the degree of nativeness of chromatin were considered. It was shown that the critical factor for the degradation of the chromosomal proteins was the dissociation of the chromatin.

A second point of interest is the origin of the chromatin proteinases. There are some data that proteolytic enzymes are normally present in chromatin [1—4], but these data are strongly doubted by other investigators claiming that the chromosomal proteinases were of cytoplasmic origin [5, 6]. Some evidence is presented here favouring rather the first case.

Materials and methods

Animals and EAT cells

3-month-old albino rats weighing 160—170 g were used. The animals were killed by cervical dislocation and the livers were immediately used for isolation of chromatin. NE-chromatin was isolated from livers extensively perfused with 0.25 M sucrose, 5 mM EDTA, *p*H 8.

Albino mice strain Agnes-Blum were injected i. p. with 0.3 ml ($1.5-2 \cdot 10^8$ cells per ml) of undiluted ascites of Ehrlich-Lettré hyperdiploid ascites tumor cells (EAT). 7 days after inoculation the mice were killed and the ascites cells collected by centrifugation.

Isolation of chromatin

Two general procedures for isolation of chromatin from rat liver and EAT were applied and in each case two detergents, either Nonidet P40 or Triton X100 were used in final concentration of 0.2% to prepare the nuclei. The first procedure included successive extractions by means of homogenization and centrifugation of the nuclei with solutions of increasing up to 0.35 M NaCl salt concentration and yield "salt extracted" (SE) chromatin [7]. According to the second procedure, resulting in "nonextracted" (NE) chromatin, EAT cells or hepatocytes from perfused rat liver were extensively washed with 0.25 M sucrose of very low ionic strength, *p*H 8, by means of gentle suspending and low-speed centrifugation. Then the cells were disrupted with detergent and the nuclei were washed by centrifugation through 0.25 M sucrose, *p*H 8.5 [8].
All isolation procedures were carried out in duplicate, one in the absence and one in the presence of 1 mM phenylmethylsulphonyl fluoride (PMSF, Serva). After dialysis against deionized water overnight the chromatin preparation was suspended in deionized water to make 10 A_{260} per ml.

Dissociation and digestion of chromatin

Rat liver SE-chromatin was dissociated in 0.4 M guanidinium chloride, 6 M urea, 0.01 M Tris-HCl, 0.002 M EDTA, *p*H 7, by gentle shaking at 4 °C for 2 hrs.
Rat liver NE-chromatin was digested in 0.1 mM $CaCl_2$ 1 mM Tris-HCl, pH 8, at 37 °C for 10 min and 1 h with 2 μg per ml of micrococcal nuclease EC 3.1.4.7 (Worthington) to give about 10% and 50% acid soluble material, respectively. The reaction was stopped by adding EDTA to a final concentration of 1 mM EDTA.

Analytical procedures

Protein was determined by the method of LOWRY et al. [9], and DNA by the method of BURTON [10]. SDS polyacrylamide gel electrophoresis in 8.75% polycrylamide gel was carried out according to LAEMMLI [11] as previously described [12]. The samples were dissociated by boiling in 1% SDS, 1% 2-mercaptoethanol, 0.06 M Tris-HCl, *p*H 6.5, for 3 min and were directly applied onto the gels without removing DNA.

Results

All chromatin preparations exhibited histone to DNA ratios close to 1. The non-histone chromosomal protein (NHP) to DNA ratio for liver and EAT SE-chromatins was 1.2 and 0.8, respectively, and for the corresponding NE-chromatins 1.9 and 1.2, respectively. Chromatin solutions in deionized water with concentration of about 10 A_{260} per ml were incubated at 37 °C for 4, 8, and 24 hrs and aliquots were taken and analysed by SDS-polyacrylamide gel electrophoresis. Fig. 1 shows the electrophoretic profile of rat liver SE-chromatin isolated with Nonidet P40 and incubated as specified above. It is seen that no proteolysis has taken place in the course of the incubation and that no preferential degradation of some of the fraction has occurred. The same picture was obtained with rat liver SE-chromatin isolated in the presence of PMSF which shows that in the case of SE-chromatins the isolation procedure alone is sufficient to prevent the cellular proteinases from degrading the chromosomal proteins. The same results were obtained with EAT-SE chromatin (Fig. 2). None of the fractions with the exception of a markedly dense band with apparent molecular weight of 60000 daltons were degraded in the

Fig. 1

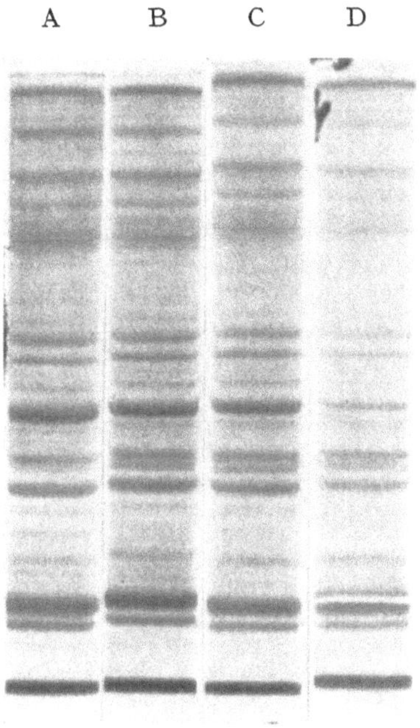

Fig. 2

Fig. 1. SDS polyacrylamide gel electrophoresis of chromosomal proteins of rat liver SE-chromatin isolated in the absence of PMSF and incubated at 37 °C for 0(A), 4(B), 8(C), and 24 hrs(D)

Fig. 2. SDS polyacrylamide gel electrophoresis of chromosomal proteins of EAT SE-chromatin isolated in the absence of PMSF and incubated at 37 °C for 0(A), 4(B), 8(C), and 24 hrs (D)

course of the 24 hrs incubation. Why this particular fraction was preferentially degraded is not clear, but since it is far less dense in the corresponding NE-chromatin, it cannot be ruled out that it was a contamination and not really embedded in the chromatin.

Fig. 3 illustrates the course of proteolysis of rat liver NE-chromatin isolated with Nonidet P40. It can be seen that incubation at 37 °C for 24 hrs causes some non-specific degradation evidenced by loss of resolution and increased background staining. However, it can be judged that although higher than in the corresponding SE-chromatins, the rate of endogenous proteolytic activity of the NE-chromatins was also very low. The same holds true with EAT NE-chromatin as well (Fig. 4). The presence of PMSF during the isolation procedure improved the performance of the NE-chromatin preparations on incubation and in these cases practically no degradation was detected (Fig. 3E). The comparison of the electrophoretic profiles of rat liver and EAT SE- and NE-chromatins isolated either with Nonidet P40 or Triton X100 revealed no differences both in the patterns and in the proteolytic activity of the preparations isolated with Nonidet P40 and Triton X100. The results obtained so far show that the adopted isolation procedures and especially that resulting in SE-chromatin, yield undegraded chromatin preparations of very low endogenous proteolytic activity. These chromatins can be incubated

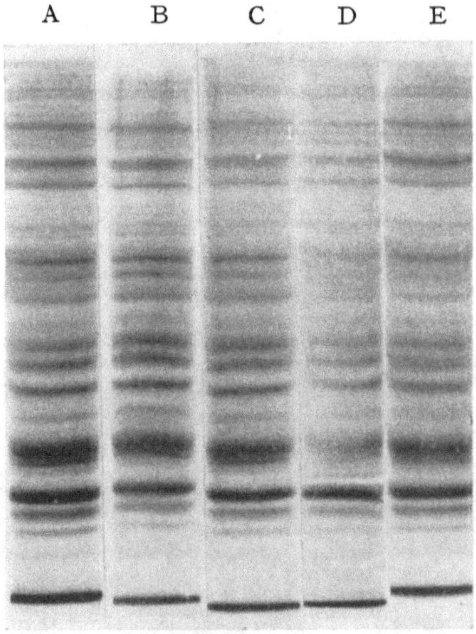

Fig. 3

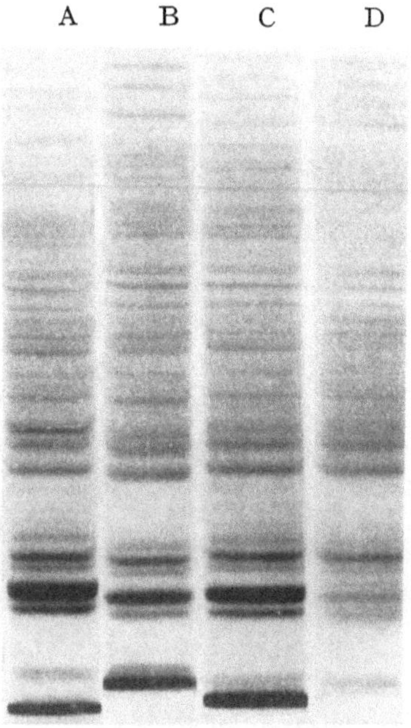

Fig. 4

Fig. 3. SDS polyacrylamide gel electrophoresis of chromosomal proteins of rat liver NE-chromatin isolated in the absence of PMSF and incubated at 37 °C for 0(A), 4(B), 8(C), and 24 hrs (D). The profile of rat liver NE-chromatin isolated in the presence of 1 mM PMSF and incubated at 37 °C for 24 hrs (E) is also shown

Fig. 4. SDS polyacrylamide gel electrophoresis of chromosomal proteins of EAT NE-chromtin isolated in the absence of PMSF and incubated at 37 °C for 0(A), 4(B), 8(C), and 24 hrs (D)

at moderately high temperatures for many hours without any degradation of the chromosomal proteins. This, however, is only true with chromatin preparations whose structure has not been previously affected. To study the effect of destroying the chromatin structure on the degradation of the NHP, the following experiments were carried out. Rat liver SE-chromatin was dissociated in 0.4 M guanidinium chloride/6 M urea and the course of proteolysis was followed as above. In spite of the fact that under such conditions the enzyme activity is, as a rule, manifold reduced, the chromosomal proteins, and especially the NHP, were considerably degraded and even the presence of 1 mM PMSF was not sufficient to completely restrict this process (Fig. 5).

Similarly, when rat liver NE-chromatin was digested with micrococcal nuclease, a rapid degradation of the chromosomal proteins took place during incubation (Fig. 6).

In order to understand whether the increased rate of proteolysis was due to dissociation of some of the chromosomal proteins or was simply due to the fragmentation of chromatin, rat liver SE-chromatin was extensively sonicated with a MSE ultrasonic unit and then incubated at 37 °C. Just as in the case with the corresponding untreated chromatin, no proteolytic degradation was detected in the sonicated chromatin in the course of the 24 hrs incubation.

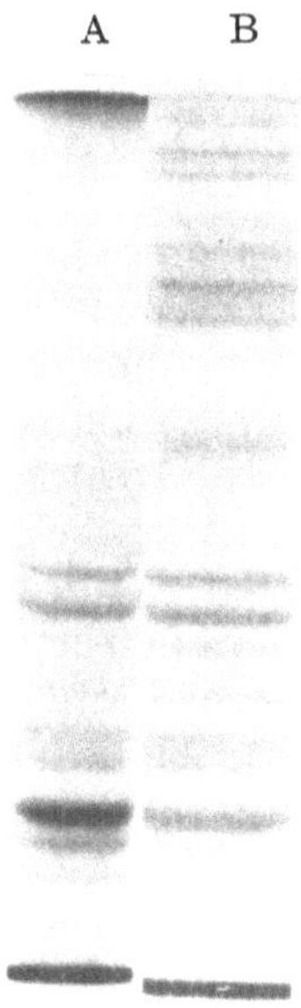

Fig. 5

Fig. 6

Fig. 5. SDS polyacrylamide gel electrophoresis of chromosomal proteins of rat liver SE-chromatin dissociated in 0.4 M guanidinium chloride/6 M urea and incubated at 2 °C for 4 hrs in the absence (A), and in the presence (B) of 1 mM PMSF

Fig. 6. SDS polyacrylamide gel electrophoresis of chromosomal proteins of rat liver NE-chromatin digested with micrococcal nuclease for 0(A), 10(B) and 60 min (C) and incubated at 37 °C for 4 hrs

Discussion

Two major groups of procedures for the isolation of chromatin are generally used at present. According to the first, total homogenates or isolated nuclei are extracted with solutions of high ionic strength. The chromatin obtained in this way is referred to as "salt extracted" (SE) chromatin. Although its structure is disturbed to some extent by the extractions, it is believed to be free from cytoplasmic contaminations [13, 14] and for this reason is mainly used to study the none histone proteins. The second group of procedures requires isolation of nuclei and of chromatin using only solutions of very low ionic strength. Although the presence of some cytoplasmic contaminations in this chromatin (referred to as "nonextracted" — NE) cannot be completely ruled out, it preserves its native structure and is used for studies on the organization of chromatin [8, 15].

The experiments described under Results show that these two procedures used in the present study for the isolation of SE-, and NE-chromatin, respectively, give nondegraded chromatin preparations of very low endogenous proteolytic activity both with normal rat liver and EAT cells as starting material. In addition the endogenous proteolytic activity of the NE-chromatin was always somewhat higher than that of the corresponding SE-chromatin, which has obvious relevance to the higher content of NHP of the former. This activity, however, was found possible to be completely suppressed in the presence of PMSF. On the other hand, the destruction of the structure of these apparently lacking proteinase activity chromatins by dissociation or digestion with micrococcal nuclease brought about a rapid degradation of the chromosomal proteins which was not possible to completely restrict even in the presence of PMSF.

It can be suggested that although the adopted isolation procedures efficiently remove most of the cellular proteinases, some proteinases remain fixed in chromatin, most probably being its normal constituents. While immobilized in the chromatin structure they remain inactive thus giving an illusion for absence of proteolytic activity in the native chromatin. However, any treatment resulting in liberation of these proteinases causes a rapid degradation of the chromosomal proteins regardless of whether the latter are also dissociated, as it is the case with the dissociated chromatin, or remain fixed in the chromatin structure as in the case of micrococcal nuclease treated chromatin. This second situation offers a plausible explanation of the fact that some authors have found no NHP in micrococcal nuclease produced nucleosomes [16], while recently the presence of NHP in the nucleosomes of native chromatin was undoubtedly demonstrated [17].

It was also reported that the chromatin proteinases degraded histones preferentially than NHP [1, 2]. However, our results show that the proteinases which remain fixed in the chromatin structure exhibited no such selectivity. They degraded all proteins, the rate of degradation being more or less straightly dependent on the molecular weight of the polypeptides.

References

[1] Garrels, J. I., S. R. Elgin, and J. Bonner: Biochem. biophys. Res. Commun. **46**, 545 (1972)
[2] Chong, M. T., W. T. Garrard, and J. Bonner: Biochemistry **13**, 5128 (1974)
[3] Carter, D. E., and C.-B. Chae: Biochemistry **15**, 180 (1976)
[4] Carter, D. B., P. H. Efrid, and C.-B. Chae: Biochemistry **15**, 2603 (1976)
[5] Destree, O. J., H. A. D'Adelhart-Toorop, and R. Charles: Biochim. biophys. Acta **368**, 5 (1975)
[5] Destree, O. J., H. A. D'Adelhart-Toorop, ane Charles: Biochim. biophys. Acta **378**, 450 (1075)
[6] Heinrich, C., G. Raydt, B. Puschendorf, and M. Jusic: Eur. J. Biochem. **62**, 37 (1976)
[7] Tsanev, R., and G. Russev: Eur. J. Biochem. **43**, 253 (1974)
[8] Yaneva, M., and G. Dessev: Eur. J. Biochem. **66**, 535 (1976)
[9] Lowry, O. H., N. J. Rosebrough, A. L. Farr, and R. J. Randall: J. biol. Chem. **193**, 265 (1951)
[10] Burton, K.: Biochem. J. **62**, 315 (1956)
[11] Laemmli, U. K.: Nature, Lond. **227** (1970)
[12] Russev, G., B. Anachkova, and R. Tsanev: Eur. J. Biochem. **58**. 253 (1975)
[13] Johns, E. W., and S. Forrester: Eur. J. Biochem. **8**, 547 (1969)
[14] Anachkova, B., G. Russev, and R. Tsanev: Int. J. Biochem. **8**, 135 (1977)
[15] Hancock, R.: J. molec. Biol. **86**, 649 (1974)
[16] Augenlicht, L. H., and M. Lipkin: Biochem. biophys. Res. Commun. **70**, 540 (1976)
[17] Bustin, M., D. Goldblatt, and R. Sperling: Cell **7**, 297 (1976)

Acta biol. med. germ., Band 36, Seite 1951—1954 (1977)

Central Institute of Molecular Biology of the Academy of Sciences of the GDR, Department of Cell Regulation, 1115 Berlin-Buch, GDR

Degradation of phosphorylated chromosomal nonhistone proteins

G. SCHMIDT and R. LINDIGKEIT

Summary

In experiments with in vivo ^{32}P-labelled nonhistone proteins of rat liver nuclei it was shown that these components are more sensitive against degradation than the mass of the nonhistone proteins. In the presence of 0.1 mM phenylmethylsulfonylfluoride and 1 mM sodium molybdate, however, they are protected against degradation.

Introduction

Phosphorylated chromosomal nonhistone proteins are of great importance for eukaryotic gene control [1—3]. In order to study the function of phosphorylated nonhistone proteins in reconstructed chromatin, it is necessary to retain these components in an undegraded state during the reconstruction procedure. Reconstruction of chromatin is usually accomplished with 5 M urea and 2 M sodium chloride. Unfortunately, under these conditions chromatin proteases are strongly activated [4]. Therefore we have developed a method which allows isolation of phosphorylated nonhistone proteins in an undegraded state.

Material and methods

The phosphorylated nonhistone proteins were labelled in vivo by intraperitoneal injection of ca. 15 mC [^{32}P]-orthophosphate per rat, 50 days old. 90 min later the rats were killed and the liver nuclei were isolated by a modification of CHAVEAUS method [5, 6].
From the pure nuclei the nonhistone proteins were either obtained by extraction with 2% SDS or 5 M urea/2 M NaCl. For control purposes, the RNA was labelled with [^{3}H]-orotic acid in vivo in parallel experiments.

Results and discussion

The typical pattern of nonhistone proteins in the SDS-gel electrophoresis [7] is shown in Fig. 1. The highest peak of ^{32}P-radioactivity is found in the nonhistone protein band of 30—40000 dalton, but also the other bands are significantly labelled with ^{32}P. The contamination with ^{32}P-labelled RNA is restricted to the regions of low molecular weights as can be seen from Fig. 1. In order to separate the proteins completely from RNA, the SDS-extracts were treated with phenol. After that the ^{3}H-labelled RNA is found in the aqueous phase (see Fig. 2). Also ^{32}P-orthophosphate and some high molecular weight proteins remain in this phase. As can be seen from Fig. 3 the nonhistone proteins of the phenol phase yield a similar pattern as the proteins of the SDS-extract but in the 12000 dalton region the protein peak is enhanced. The phosphorylation pattern, however, is strongly changed.
From the fact that now the 12000 band is highly labelled we suggest that preferentially the ^{32}P-labelled proteins are degraded to 12000 dalton components.

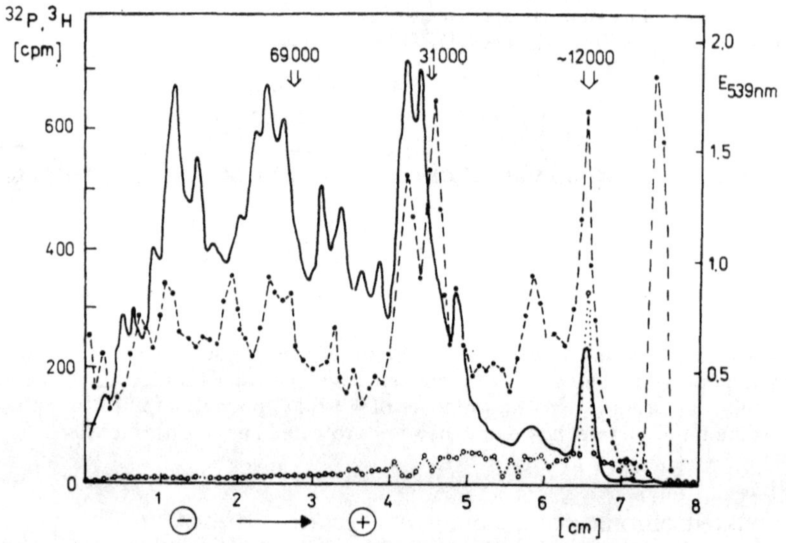

Fig. 1. SDS-gel-electrophoretic pattern of chromosomal nonhistone proteins. The proteins were extracted by 2% SDS, 10 mM Tris, 1% mercaptoethanol, *p*H 8.2, from in vivo ^{32}P-labelled rat liver nuclei which were freed before of the soluble proteins and the histones with 0.15 M NaCl and 0.25 M HCl, respectively.

—— E = 539 nm (Coomassie staining); - - - - - ^{32}P-activity, ... [^{3}H]-orotic acid (RNA labelling).

Marker proteins: bovine serum albumin, DNase I, cytochrome c

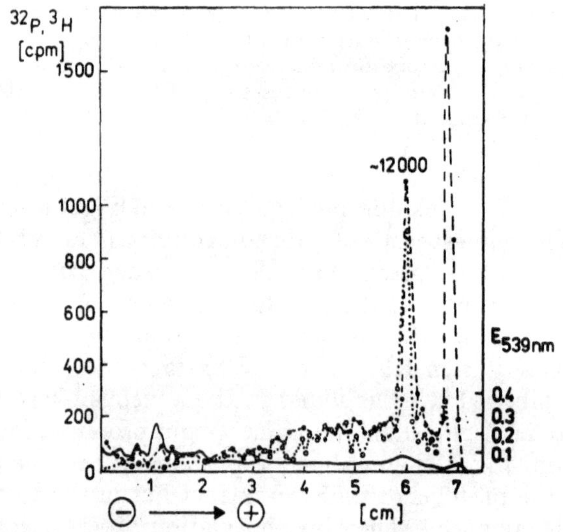

Fig. 2. SDS-gel electrophoretic pattern of the aqueous phase obtained by treatment of the SDS-nonhistone protein extract with phenol for 5 min at 65 °C.

—— E = 539 nm (Coomassie staining), - - - - - ^{32}P-activity, ... [^{3}H]-orotic acid activity

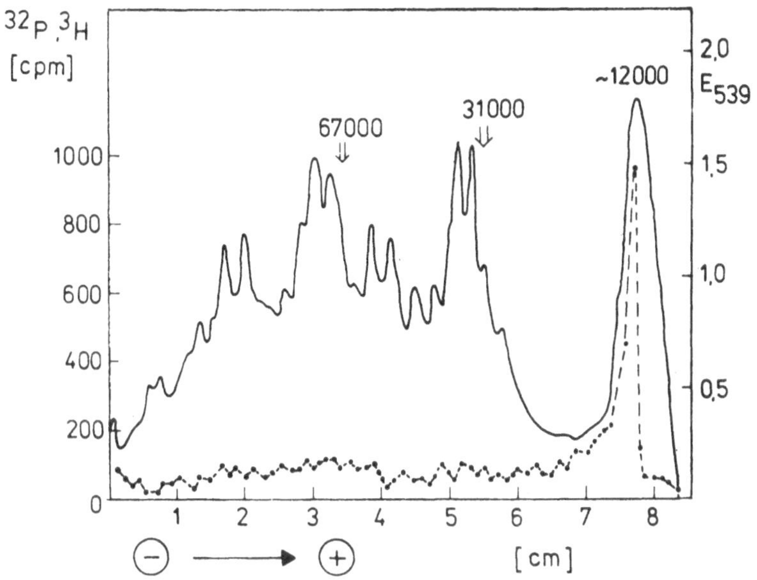

Fig. 3. SDS-gel-electrophoretic pattern of the phenol phase obtained by treatment of the SDS-nonhistone protein extract.

——— E = 539 nm; - - - - - ^{32}P-activity

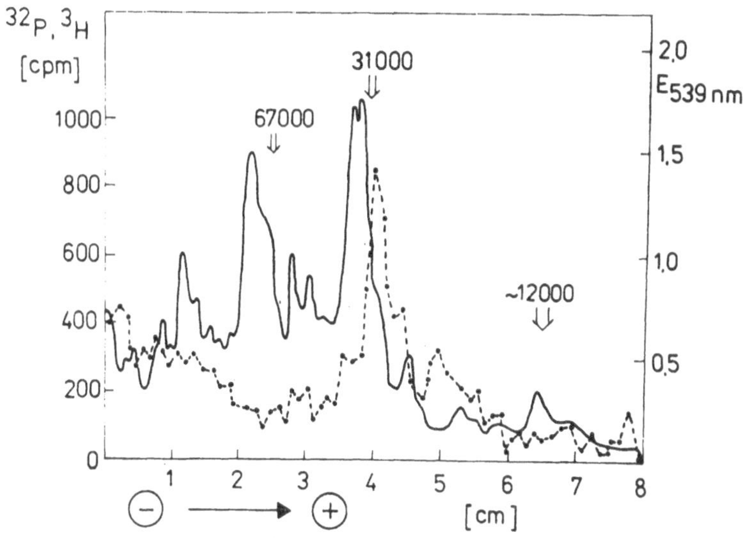

Fig. 4. SDS-gel-electrophoretic pattern of the phenol phase obtained by treatment of the SDS-nonhistone extract.

All procedures were performed in the presence of 0.1 mM PMSF and 1 mM sodium molybdate.

——— E = 539 nm; - - - - - ^{32}P-activity

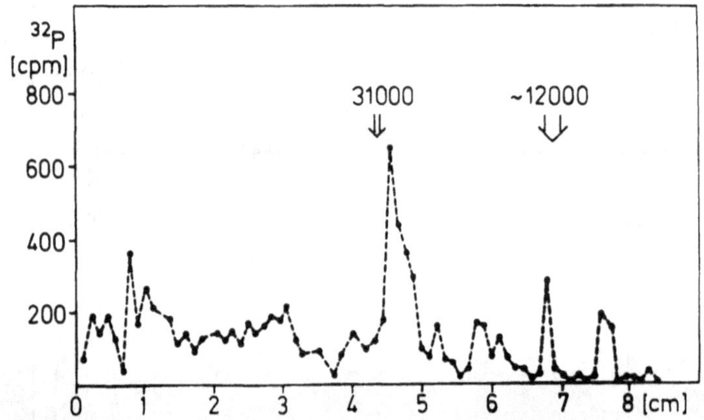

Fig. 5. SDS-gel-electrophoretic pattern of the phenol phase obtained by treatment of the nonhistone proteins which were isolated from the nuclei with 5 M urea/2 M NaCl, in the presence of 0.1 mM PMSF and 1 mM sodium molybdate.
----- ^{32}P-activity

The possible contamination of the nuclei with proteases was checked by the azocasein method [8].
By this procedure no protease activity was found. To inactivate specific endoproteases as well as phosphatases in our nonhistone protein extracts, in the further experiments 0.1 M phenylmethylsulfonylfluoride (PMSF) and 1 mM sodium molybdate were added to all extraction media. These inhibitors protect effectively the SDS extracted nonhistone proteins against degradation. Even after phenol extraction the ^{32}P-labelled proteins of more than 30000 dalton are preserved as shown in Fig. 4. This comes also true if the nonhistone proteins are first extracted by a solution of 5 M urea/2 M NaCl before being treated with phenol (Fig. 5).
The gel electrophoretic pattern of the proteins occur unchanged even under conditions under which the ^{32}P-labelled proteins are degraded to 12000 dalton fragments. Therefore we suggest that the phosphorylated nonhistone proteins are especially susceptible to endoproteases of the nuclei.

We are indebted to Dr. D. I. STOTT (Glasgow) for his advice to use sodium molybdate as phosphatase inhibitor and to Dr. P. BOHLEY (Halle) for the investigation of protease activity in the rat liver nuclei.

References

[1] STEIN, G. S., T. C. SPELSBERG, and L. J. KLEINSMITH: Science, N.Y. **183**, 817 (1974)
[2] CAMERON, I. L., and J. R. JETER, jr.: Acidic Proteins of the Nucleus. Academic Press, New York 1974
[3] STEIN, G. S., and L. J. KLEINSMITH: Chromosomal Proteins and their Role in the Regulation of Gene Expression. Academic Press, New York 1975
[4] CARTER, D. B., P. H. EFIRD, and C. B. CHAE: Biochemistry **15**, 2603 (1976)
[5] CHAUVEAU, J., Y. MOULÉ, and C. ROUILLER: Expl Cell Res. **11**, 317 (1956)
[6] FENSKE, H., I. EICHHORN, and R. LINDIGKEIT: Acta biol. med. germ. **34**, 303 (1975)
[7] LAEMMLI, U. K.: Nature, Lond. **227**, 650 (1970)
[8] BOHLEY, P.: Unpublished data

Acta biol. med. germ., Band 36, Seite 1955—1958 (1977)

Department of Medical Microbiology and Immunology, School of Medicine, Comenius University, 801 00 Bratislava, Czechoslovakia

Interaction of intracellular proteases and immune mechanisms

J. Štefanovič, M. Ferenčik, D. Kotulová, and I. Murgašová

Summary

Intracellular proteases play an important role both in nonspecific and specific immune reactions. Results concerning the interaction of these enzymes with phagocytic factors responsible for killing microorganisms are presented. In inflammatory foci, proteases released from destroyed leukocytes have been found to modify the function of antibodies present. They particularly reduce their complement fixation activity. Macrophages with differing proteolytic activity demonstrated diverse effects on the formation of antibodies tested by Jerne's plaque technique in young rabbits immunized with sheep erythrocytes. Whereas alveolar macrophages diminished antigen immunogenicity, peritoneal macrophages enhanced it.

Introduction

Studies concerning the role of intracellular proteases in immune mechanisms can be traced relatively far back in history. The distinguished immunologist I. Mečnikov as well as the outstanding biochemist E. Abderhalden were intrigued by this problem. Presently available information confirms that intracellular proteases are significantly involved both in the mechanisms of nonspecific and specific acquired immunity, as well as in immunopathologic processes [1—4]. The purpose of the presented paper has been to summarize the results of investigations on the role of acid intracellular proteinases, represented mainly by cathepsin D, in mechanisms of phagocytosis, in inflammatory processes, and also in inducing immune response. Out of the whole complex of mechanisms of phagocytosis, most effort has been devoted to the study of interaction of intracellular proteases and antibacterial factors, aiming at prevention, further the effect of intracellular proteases on agglutinative and complement fixation activity of antibodies has been studied, and finally results of investigations dealing with the role of macrophages with diverse proteolytic activity in inducing immune response are presented.

Material and methods

The following cells were obtained from rabbits and chickens used in the experiments: Polymorphonuclear leukocytes by injecting saline solution with glycogen [5]; macrophages, obtained only from rabbits by rinsing pulmonary alveoli with saline solution [6] or by rinsing the peritoneum on the 5th day following i.p. injection of paraffin oil [5].

Extracts from cells were prepared after their disintegration on using saponin at low temperatures (for enzymatic activity determination), or by repeated six-fold freezing and thawing (for bactericidal activity determination). Cathepsin D was prepared from rabbit [5] and chicken [7] spleens. Cathepsin D activity was either assessed by using human serum albumin [5] or bovine haemoglobin [8], as substrates. Acid phosphatase was determined according to Jacob and Weir [9].

Anticathepsin serum to chicken cathepsin D was prepared by immunizing rabbits, and to rabbit cathepsin D by immunizing sheep on using the method according to Dingle et al. [10].

The agglutination reaction was performed both in test tubes and on Takatsy microtitrator. In the complement fixation reaction (CFR), the serum was diluted in logarithmic order. Dilution resulting in 50% haemolysis in the given system (2% suspension of erythrocytes and complement) was considered to be the final point of reaction.
The production of haemolytic complement-fixing antibodies IgM was assayed on applying JERNE's plaque method [11] modified by ŠTERZL and MANDEL [12] by using sheep red blood cells (SRBC).

Results and discussion

The series of studies [13—17] lead to the finding that following irradiation of animals, the activity of acid proteases is increasing with a simultaneous decrease in the total antibacterial activity and in the activity of individual components responsible for the killing of microbes. This has been established both in rabbits and chickens. Adding cathepsin D to extracts from PMN is accompanied by decreased antibacterial, myeloperoxidase, and catalase activity, whereas lysozyme activity is not affected at *p*H 3.5. Cathepsin D inhibitors, including anticathepsin D IgG, inhibit the process of inactivation. Before irradiation, chickens and rabbits were administered anticathepsin D IgG that reduced the variations in the parameters under study, extending simultaneously the average survival rate of irradiated animals (Fig. 1). Extracts from PMN leukocytes added to the serum with antibodies after incubation at *p*H 3.5—4.0, failed to affect the results of the agglutination reaction, but they diminished the capacity of antibodies for complement fixation. This property is determined by the ability of acid proteases, and particularly of cathepsin D, to degrade IgG molecules both in allogenous and xeno-

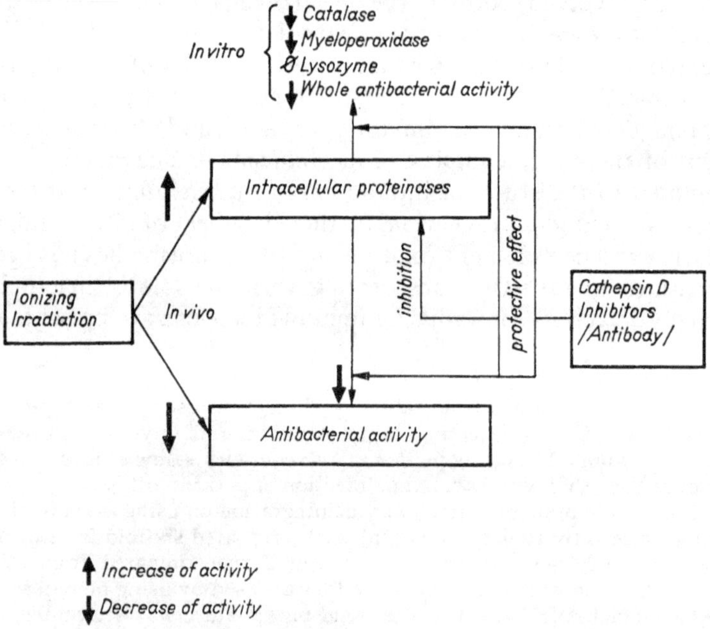

Fig. 1. The effect of ionizing irradiation on proteolytic and antibacterial activities of leukocytes

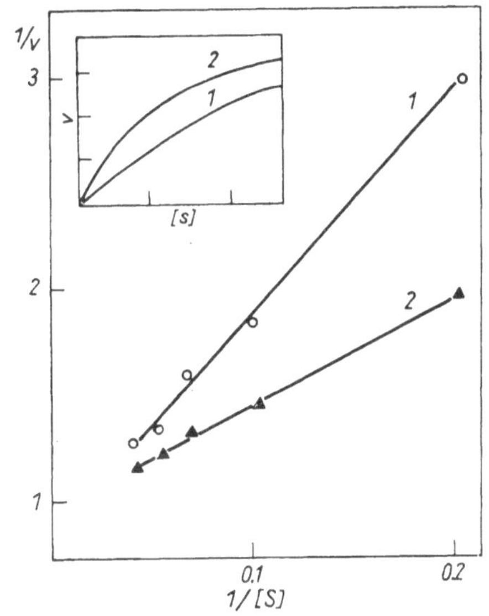

Fig. 2

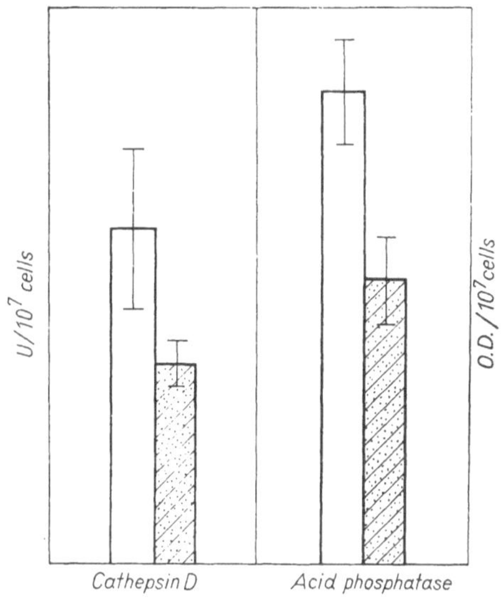

Fig. 3

Fig. 2. The degradation of human (1) and rabbit (2) IgG by rabbit cathepsin D

Fig. 3. Enzymatic activity of rabbit alveolar (empty columns) and peritoneal (hatched columns) macrophages

genous relations [18, 19]. Rabbit cathepsin D was efficient in degrading both rabbit and human IgG (Fig. 2). This finding suggests that in the focus of inflammation, with an acid *p*H and substances released from PMN leukocytes present, a decrease in antibody function might also take place. In comparing the enzymatic activity of alveolar and peritoneal macrophages, the former were found to have a significantly higher activity due to their continuous stimulation by inspired antigens (Fig. 3). Further the relationship between the activity of macrophages and the formation of antibodies to SRBC was studied in young rabbits. The antigen concerned is thymus-dependent and requires the presence of macrophages for inducing antibody production. Young rabbits present the model of choice for following up antibody production since their ability to produce antibodies is reduced in their early postnatal period. Erythrocytes were administered to three- to four-day-old rabbits, and that either unaccompanied or along with alveolar or peritoneal macrophages. Five days after immunization, the number of IgM antibodies producing cells was evaluted by Jerne's plaque technique. Administration of erythrocytes in combination with macrophages was seen to affect antigen immunogenicity. It is deranged by the effect of the more active alveolar macrophages, which results in a lowered antibody response, whereas peritoneal macrophages were found to enhance immunogenicity (Table 1).

The results lead to the conclusion that the properties of those macrophages that come into contact with the antigen determine its immunogenicity. Although macrophages are derived from a common precursor, after having settled in the tissues, their functional and biochemical characteristics undergo changes induced

Table 1

Number of plaque forming cells (PFC) in the spleen in young rabbits, i. p. immunized with SRBC, and alveolar or peritoneal macrophages of adult animals

I. p. immunization of 3–4 days old rabbits	Number of PFC in 10^8 spleen cells (M $\pm$ SE) of 9–10 days old rabbit
10^9 SRBC	194 $\pm$ 14
10^9 SRBC + 10^7 peritoneal macrophages	243 $\pm$ 23
10^9 SRBC + 10^7 alveolar macrophages	142 $\pm$ 14

by local conditions [20]. Owing to the high activity of lysosomal enzymes, degradation of the antigen and loss of its immunogenicity are effected, as has been observed in the case of alveolar macrophages. Though cells of the peritoneal exudate also decompose the major part of erythrocytes, a certain part, and that with increased immunogenicity, remains there and participates in the induction of the specific immune response of antibody production.

The interaction of intracellular proteases and immune mechanisms is an important problem for the study and understanding of several immunologic phenomena with favourable or adverse consequences for the host.

References

[1] WEISSMANN, G., and P. DUKOR: Adv. Immun. **12**, 283 (1970)
[2] GOLDSTEIN, I.: Prog. Allergy **20**, 301 (1976)
[3] VISCHER, T. L., U. BRETZ, and M. BAGGIOLINI: J. exp. Med. **144**, 863 (1976)
[4] MOREAU, P., J. DORNAND, and J. G. KAPLAN: Can. J. Biochem. **53**, 1337 (1975)
[5] ŠTEFANOVIČ, J., T. WEBB, and C. LAPRESLE: Ann. Inst. Pasteur **103**, 276 (1962)
[6] MYRVIK, Q. N., E. S. LEAKE, and B. FARRIS: J. Immun. **86**, 128 (1961)
[7] FERENČÍK, M., and J. ŠTEFANOVIČ: Biológia, Bratisl. **29**, 453 (1974)
[8] ANSON, M. L.: J. gen. Physiol. **22**, 79 (1938)
[9] JACOB, K. H. A., and D. M. WEIR: Immunology **21**, 419 (1971)
[10] DINGLE, J. T., A. J. BARRETT, and P. D. WESTON: Biochem. J. **123**, 1 (1971)
[11] JERNE, N. K., and A. A. NORDIN: Science, N.Y. **140**, 405 (1963)
[12] ŠTERZL, J., and L. MANDEL: Folia microbiol. **9**, 173 (1964)
[13] ŠTEFANOVIČ, J., Š. KIŠON, and O. ABSOLONOVÁ: Folia microbiol. **13**, 424 (1968)
[14] ŠTEFANOVIČ, J. in: "Non-Specific" Factors Influencing Host Resistance, W. BRAUN and J. UNGAR (Eds). Karger, Basel 1973, p. 62
[15] FERENČÍK, M., and J. ŠTEFANOVIČ: Folia microbiol. **18**, 402 (1973)
[16] ŠTEFANOVIČ, J., M. FERENČIK, O. ABSOLONOVÁ in: Intracellular Protein Catabolism II. V. TURK and N. MARKS (Eds). Plenum Press, New York, London 1977, p. 270
[17] FERENČÍK, M., and J. ŠTEFANOVIČ in: Intracellular Protein Catabolism II. V. TURK and N. MARKS (Eds). Plenum Press, New York, London 1977, p. 275
[18] LO SPALLUTTO, J., K. FAHR, and M. ZIFF in: Proceedings of the International Symposium on Immune Complex Diseases. L. BONOMO, and J. L. TURK (Eds). Carlo Erba Found., Milan 1970, p. 62
[19] GHETIE, V., and S. MIHAESCU: Immunochemistry **10**, 251 (1973)
[20] VAN FURTH, R. in: Progress in Immunology II. **4**, p. 73. L. BRENT and J. HOLBOROW (Eds). North-Holland Publ. Co., Amsterdam, Oxford, American Elsevier Publ. Co., Inc. New York 1974

Acta biol. med. germ., Band 36, Seite 1959—1968 (1977)

Molecular Pathology Department, Strangeways Research Laboratory, Cambridge, CB1 4RN. England

The diversity of cellular proteinases in physiology and pathology

ALAN J. BARRETT

Summary

1. It is suggested that the functions of cellular proteinases are far more diverse than has usually been realized. 2. A scheme is proposed in which isolation of a pure proteinase leads to a rather detailed exploration of its biological significance. 3. Representative proteinases from the serine, thiol, carboxyl and metallo-classes are briefly reviewed with emphasis on the relationship between improved understanding at the molecular level and eventual progress in the understanding of some important physiological and pathological processes. 4. An attempt is made to forsee future developments in this area of biochemistry, in terms of both new trends in research, and the eventual application of knowledge of the proteinases to medical problems.

It is not long since most biochemists considered the major function of the cellular proteinases to be the intracellular turnover of proteins, probably after spontaneous denaturation. Some of the endopeptidases must indeed be concerned primarily with the complete digestion of proteins, but we now know that the available enzymes are far more numerous and diverse than this process would seem to require, and have good reason to believe that they serve many other vital functions.

Before we come to consider a few of the exciting recent developments concerning the individual enzymes, it might be worthwhile to take stock of the general procedures which are contributing to our progress in understanding the molecular biology of the cellular proteinases. As is illustrated in Fig. 1, the isolation of each enzyme in pure form can be seen as a key step. This can lead directly to experiments in which one will discover whether the enzyme has the capacity to act on particular physiologically significant proteins; also, one can recognize and investigate the naturally occurring inhibitors of the proteinase that may regulate its functions. Equally important, one can provide oneself with new tools for the study of the enzyme, by raising specific antisera, and by exploring the specificity of the enzyme with a view to discovering new synthetic substrates and inhibitors. The availability of these new tools allows one to enter into a third stage of the investigation in which the enzyme is detected and assayed in cells and tissues with new sensitivity and specificity, by use of the new substrates, active-site titration with inhibitors, or immuno-assay. Moreover, one can begin to obtain direct evidence of the biological activities of the proteinase by inhibiting it selectively (with chemical or immunological reagents) in appropriate tissue culture or whole animal systems. The precise localization of the enzyme in cells or tissue sections should be possible with chromogenic substrates, which see activity, or with labelled antibodies, which recognize zymogens and enzyme-inhibitor complexes as well as active enzyme. To complete the investigation of the biology of the enzyme one

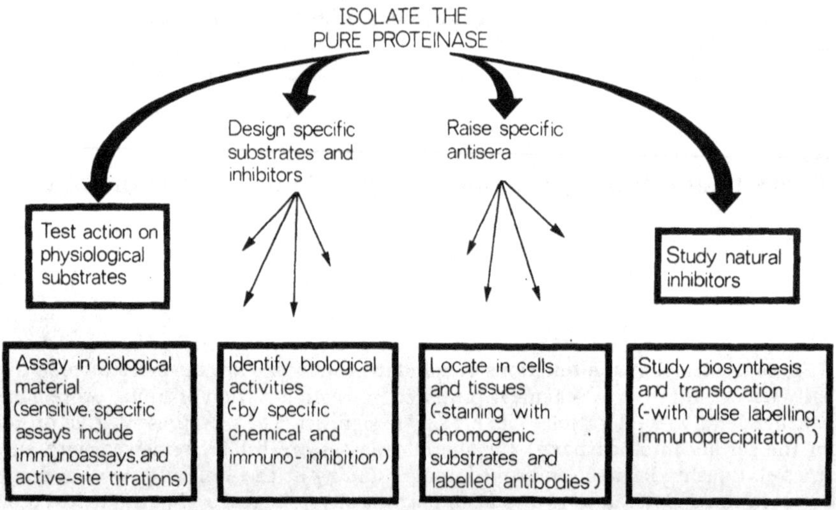

Fig. 1. An approach to the molecular biology of tissue proteinases.
The scheme is intended to show how the initial purification of a proteinase can lead to the development of a comprehensive approach to the study of its functions and regulation. The attainment of the ultimate objectives of the fundamental part of the study (boxed in the diagram) should provide a basis for work directly applied to human health and disease

may study its biosynthesis and translocation by means of pulse-labelling, with specific immuno-precipitation of the labelled protein from separated tissue fractions.

This then is an indication of the sort of general approach by which work on the proteinases starting at the molecular level can be extended progressively into more complex systems. Much of the fundamental work can be done with human tissues from health and disease, and this is appropriate since the ultimate practical justification of our work is the relief of human illness.

At present it would have to be admitted that work on the tissue proteinases has contributed little to the treatment of disease, but there are sound reasons for thinking that this situation may soon change. Evidence implicating proteinases in a new, important area of physiology or pathology is now appearing almost monthly, and the extent of our fundamental knowledge and technical competence is just sufficient to give us reasonable hopes of answering some of the fascinating questions raised.

Some of these questions, and the emerging beginnings of their answers can now be considered in the framework of the enzymologists' classification of the proteinases. Representatives of each of the four recognized catalytic groups of proteinase, the serine, thiol, carboxyl and metallo-proteinases have been the subject of investigations along the sort of lines indicated above.

Progress with the cellular serine proteinases has been relatively recent. Amongst the better known of these are the lysosomal elastase of human neutrophil leucocytes, and the chymotrypsin-like cathepsin G from the same source. Purification from peripheral blood leucocytes [1] and whole spleen [2] has been followed by the raising of specific antisera [3, 4], the design of selective, active-site directed inhibitors [5], elucidation of the specificity of action on the B chain of insulin [6, 7], and the design of new substrates [8]. This progress at the fundamental level (reviewed by STARKEY, ref. [9]) has provided a firm basis for work aimed at understanding the functions of the enzymes in leucocytic digestion of bacteria [10, 11] and their contribution to the apparently undesirable degradation of the structural elements of articular cartilage-proteoglycan [12, 13] and collagen [14]. Studies of the inhibition of the enzymes by α_1-proteinase inhibitor, α_2-macroglobulin and other physiological inhibitors [15] further contribute to a framework of knowledge that should soon validate or disprove the suggestion that these enzymes make an important contribution to crippling tissue damage in pulmonary emphysema [5] glomerulonephritis [16] and arthritis [17].

The plasminogen activators secreted by some cells, or carried on the cell membrane, are themselves serine proteinases that have been the subject of intense interest because there is an impressive correlation between the production of the enzyme by cells in culture and viral or other transformation of the cells to a state of less regulated "malignant" growth [18, 19]. Amongst the major contributions to this topic have been the isolation of the activator from sarcoma virus-transformed cells [20] and the raising of a specific antiserum against it, with which it is possible to investigate its relationship to the activators of normal tissues such as vascular endothelium and kidney [21].

The discovery of intracellular serine proteinases with selectivity for the apo-forms of pyridoxal enzymes, and certain other particular classes of protein (reviewed in refs. [22, 23]) indicated that alternatives may exist to the lysosomal route of intracellular protein catabolism. This idea is gaining support from work such as that on a mitochondrial serine proteinase [24], and a trypsin-like enzyme in nuclear chromatin [25]. Interest in the nuclear enzyme has been stimulated by reports of work with leupeptin and related inhibitors which suggest that trypsin-like enzymes might be essential for lymphocyte transformation [26] and for aspects of tumour formation [27].

Another of the serine proteinases that is receiving much attention at the moment is acrosin, the trypsin-like enzyme of the acrosome of spermatozoa. It has been proposed that this enzyme may play a key role at that stage of fertilization in which the spermatozoon penetrates the zona pellucida, and that contraception might be achieved by chemical or immunological inhibition of the enzyme [28, 29]. MORTON [30] has recently reviewed our knowledge of acrosin and other proteinases of the reproductive system. Acrosin seems to have a higher molecular weight zymogen precursor, like the pancreatic serine proteinases, but unlike most cellular proteinases.

Interest in thiol-dependent proteinases goes far back in the literature of the proteolytic enzymes [31], but it is only in the last decade that any full characterization of the enzymes has been attained. OTTO [32] showed that the thiol-dependent hydrolysis of Bz-Arg-NH_2 previously attributed to "cathepsin B" included a contribution from a carboxypeptidase, cathepsin B2 [33], later termed lysosomal carboxypeptidase, B [34]. Still further heterogeneity has now been revealed in the thiol proteinase activity of rat liver lysosomes, and cathepsin H and L have been defined [35, 36]. A "collagenolytic cathepsin" somewhat like cathepsin L has also been described [37]. The use of inhibitors for the thiol proteinases as a group (e.g. iodoacetate, antipain, leupeptin) with mixtures of lysosomal enzymes or living tissue systems [38—40] point to an important role for this group of enzymes in intracellular protein catabolism. The intracellular environment, in which glutathione may provide a thiol concentration as high as 5 mM [41], and regions of low *p*H are created, seems ideally suited to the thiol proteinases. It has been suggested that cathepsin B secreted by tumour cells is a factor contributing to the processes of invasion and metastasis, although the properties of the enzyme do not seem to suit it well for an extracellular function.

There are strong indications that cathepsin B may also participate in specific, limited proteolytic steps. The important work of Otto cited above arose from the discovery of the inactivation of glucokinase and aldolase by the enzyme, and inactivation of tyrosine aminotransferase was reported a little later [42]. In contrast, the limited proteolysis of hexosediphosphatase by cathepsin B is seen as activation in some assay systems, because it involves substantial changes in kinetic parameters, including *p*H optimum [43]. The limited proteolytic steps seen in the generation of insulin and other hormones, as well as serum albumin, from their higher molecular weight precursors [44, 45] also may be attributable to cathepsin B. This is suggested especially by the high activity of cathepsin B in the cleavage of bonds on the carboxyl side of pairs of basic residues [34], but there is a need for more substrates and inhibitors showing selectivity within the group of thiol proteinases to facilitate investigation of their individual physiological functions.

Amongst the carboxyl proteinases cathepsin D is by far the best characterized; it was the first recognized of the tissue proteinases, the original "cathepsin", and is arguably the most fully studied, and yet its biological functions remain somewhat obscure [46], and this despite the availability of the pure enzyme, of specific antisera and of an excellent inhibitor, pepstatin. The inhibitors have provided evidence for a role of cathepsin D in the lysosomal digestion of endocytosed proteins by macrophages [47] and of cellular proteins in perfused liver [48], although the enzyme appears to contribute little to proteolysis by lysosomal components in vitro [38, 39].

The best known cellular metallo-endopeptidases are undoubtedly the collagenases-enzymes so specific that there has been a tendency not to think of them as proteinases at all. Although a great deal has been learnt about the collagenases [49] they still hold several secrets. The molecular basis of the "latency" of the enzyme as it is frequently encountered has been the subject of an intensive controversy between the proponents of the "zymogen" and "enzyme-inhibitor complex" theories. At the time of writing the inhibitor theory seems to be gaining ground [50]. The impressive body of circumstantial evidence for a contribution of collagenase to many forms of pathological tissue damage has been reviewed [49].

The metallo-proteinase of rabbit kidney brush border has been thoroughly purified and characterized [51—53], and seems to make an important contribution to the degradation of glucagon in rat kidney preparations also [54]. Potent inhibition of this enzyme by phosphoramidon offers the promise of facilitated purification by use of affinity chromatography, and new insights into the biological functions of the enzyme.

The "waiting list" of proteinases well recognized but not conclusively assigned to a catalytic class always has interest. These enzymes are the exceptions that question the general applicability of the group-specific reagents used for the classification of proteinases. Moreover, each enzyme in the list holds the potential of revealing a truly new hydrolytic mechanism, and thus founding a fifth class of proteinases to be explored. A particular interesting group of the proteinases that do not fit neatly into HARTLEY's [55] classes are the enzymes that are activated by Ca^{2+}, and also activated or markedly stabilized by thiol compounds; accordingly, they are inhibited by EDTA and by N-ethylmaleimide. These enzymes seem to include the neutral endopeptidases of the lens [56], muscle [57] and brain [58], as well as the "Pz-peptidase" [59]. There is no evidence that these enzymes are metallo-proteins, or that zinc is involved in their activity, but they may well be of great importance in the normal protein catabolism of their various tissues.

What trends can one perceive for the immediate future of research into the cellular proteinases? Interest in the role of proteinases in control processes in cells and tissues continues to increase. Such processes seem to include aspects of cell growth, division and locomotion, and cell to cell communication. Many of the enzymes that we should like to study in this area will be available in very small quantities, from particular subfractions of small numbers of cells. In order to take advantage of the various research strategies that depend on purification of the enzyme we shall need to develop a new range of ultra-micro-methods. These must include alternatives to the conventional methods for staining and assay of proteins, and radiochemical methods show obvious promise.

The switching on and switching off of biological activities by cleavage of one or a few peptide bonds is seen in the generation and subsequent inactivation of the active forms of hormones (thyroxin [60], angiotensin, oxytocin, bradykinin [61], ACTH, insulin, glucagon [53]), of enzymes (plasmin [19]; acrosin [62]) and of structural proteins (collagen [63, 49]). Study of the systems involving strictly limited proteolysis requires detection of the cleavage of single peptide bonds, rather than the formation of substantial quantities of trichloroacetic acid-soluble fragments, which has been so important in the past. Fortunately, the necessary technique, SDS gel electrophoresis, is already highly developed, and a recent study [56] clearly underlines the usefulness of the technique in our area of work.

In response to the widespread social pressures for scientific research to supplement its academic excellence with short or medium term practical objectives we may expect to see greater attention being given to the increasing number of areas wherein a convincing case can be made for a proteinase being a mediator of an important disease process. This trend will be associated with the increasing use of physiologically significant protein substrates in assays; amongst these will be procollagen (for the procollagen endopeptidases), prohormones, histones, membrane proteins, viral proteins and many others. The substrates will often be required in radiochemically labelled form, and since they should ideally be of human origin, methods of labelling in vitro may be emphasized.

Most of us would agree that the longer term objectives of the study of cellular proteinases must include a contribution to human medicine, but what specific applications would we envisage?

The simplest type of disease process that we might think of trying to modify is that in which the physical structure of a tissue is degraded by the excessive activity of extracellular proteinases against the structural macromolecules. This is illustrated by damage to the articular cartilage in inflammatory joint disease [14, 49], to the ulcerated cornea [49, 65], to the emphysematous lung [5, 66] and to the kidney in glomerulonephritis [16]. Anti-inflammatory steroids already used in these conditions probably inhibit the synthesis and secretion of proteinases by cells [67], but they have the disadvantage of inhibiting the resynthesis of structural components also [68]. Development of methods by which to deliver the drugs specifically to the right cells should be useful [69], but there is a need for more work at the cellular level on the mechanisms of control of production of the proteinases. The problems of handling this kind of situation should not be underestimated, however. The tissue damage may often be due to the concerted action of several proteinases, so that inhibition of one alone will be ineffective. It is also necessary to remember that the same enzymes may be serving a very valuable function elsewhere in the organism, so that general inhibition would be unacceptable. Thus the neutrophil elastase that may degrade elastin and collagen in the emphysematous lung also participates in the digestion of bacteria by the leucocytes in their defence of the lung against infection [10, 11]. The possibility of using inhibitors that will not enter cells obviously deserves consideration, and the evidence that at least one form of the lung disease arises as a result of the genetic lack of α_1-proteinase inhibitor [66] gives support to the validity of the principle of treatment by inhibitors.

The activities of extracellular proteinases do not concern only structural elements of the tissues. The idea that chronic inflammation may be maintained by a positive feedback loop in which proteinases secreted by macrophages activate complement factors which further stimulate the cells [70] clearly invites intervention by inhibitors. The action of cathepsin D on the basic protein of myelin releases a peptide that causes allergic encephalomyelitis, a disease with resemblances to multiple sclerosis, in experimental primates [71]. Also fragments generated by the action of lysosomal proteinases on immunoglobulin G may be significant autoantigens in rheumatoid arthritis [72].

The usefulness of inhibitors in modifying the metabolism of polypeptide hormones is illustrated by the clinical potential of the synthetic inhibitor of the angiotensin converting enzyme, peptidyl-dipeptidase [73], and the potentiating activity of Trasylol for subcutaneously injected parathyroid hormone in the chick [74].

No sharp line can be drawn between the physiological situations in which extracellular proteins are modified by enzymes secreted from cells in soluble form, and those in which the enzymes remain on the exterior of the cell membrane. The latter may include processes of cellular attachment, penetration (as by spermatozoa) and invasion (as by the trophoblast in implantation [30] and by malignant tumours [75]). Again, extracellular inhibitors may be effective, although some of the cells will have the capacity rapidly to replace the enzyme on their surface.

Inhibition of intracellular proteolysis within the lysosomal system gives rise to morphological changes reminiscent of the lysosomal storage diseases [47], and may not have therapeutic possibilities.

It is not established that any of the recognized lysosomal storage diseases involves deficiency of a proteinase, but it is perfectly possible that functional deficiencies occur. Thus, it has been suggested that a primary defect in cystic fibrosis may be the lack of a proteinase that normally destroys the basic polypeptides that inhibit ciliary motion [76], and a deficiency of proteolytic activity could be involved in pulmonary alveolar proteinosis [77]. In contrast, DANNENBERG et al. [78] have discussed the desirability of inhibiting proteolytic liquefaction of the caseous deposits of tuberculosis. If specific deficiencies of proteinases can be pinpointed, it may be possible to repair them, at least temporarily, by use of exogenous proteinases. The feasibility of this is illustrated by the current clinical use of urokinase [79], and the fibrin-degrading enzymes of snake venoms [80].

It is clear then that many possible applications exist for the new knowledge of cellular proteinases that is rapidly being acquired. Most of these present technical difficulties which must not be underemphasized, but the diseases concerned are of such importance that eventual improvements in treatment would be of the greatest value to medicine.

Addendum: Nomenclature and classification of the cellular proteinases*

The proteolytic enzymes of cells consist of exopeptidases, endopeptidases, and a few enzymes with characteristics of both groups. The exopeptidases can usually be named and classified in terms of their specificity, according to the principles that are applied to enzymes in general [81]. For this reason we agreed, in our previous discussions at the First International Symposium on Intracellular Pro-

Table 1
The present status of the "cathepsin" nomenclature.
More detailed information on the nomenclature of the cathepsins, with a summary of the properties of each enzyme can be found in ref. [31]

Obsolete name	Current name (abbreviation)	Comment	References
Cathepsin A	Lysosomal carboxypeptidase A (LC-A)	Exopeptidase	[83]
Cathepsin B1	Cathepsin B	Only one cathepsin B is now recognized	[34, 83, 84]
Cathepsin B2	Lysosomal carboxypeptidase B (LC-B)	Exopeptidase	[33, 34, 83]
Cathepsin B3	Cathepsin H	Endo-exopeptidase	[85]
Cathepsin C	Dipeptidylpeptidase I (DPP I)	Exopeptidase	[81]
–	Cathepsin D	–	[46]
–	Cathepsin E	–	[46]
–	Cathepsin F	–	[86]
"Chymotrypsin-like enzyme"	Cathepsin G	Neutral optimum	[4]
–	Cathepsin L	–	[36]
–	Cathepsin M	Neutral optimum	[61]
–	Cathepsin S	–	[87]

* A summary of the concensus expressed during the discussions at Reinhardsbrunn Castle on June 4th, 1977.

tein Catabolism [82], that exopeptidases should cease to be named "cathepsins", but should receive names more specific to their catalytic activities. In consistency with this it has been generally agreed that cathepsins A, B2 and C should be renamed (Table 1).

It is well recognized that the usual system of naming and classification of enzymes by specificity is not applicable in any simple way to the endopeptidases. The idea of classification by catalytic mechanism [55] was accepted for purposes of the Enzyme Commission list [81], but does not automatically suggest a system for naming the enzymes. The present system, wherein a new cellular proteinase is to be named a "cathepsin", with a distinguishing letter of the alphabet, regardless of *p*H optimum [82], suffers the disadvantages that the word "cathepsin" has previously been used differently, and that a limited number of letters remains to be used [31]. There is no doubt, therefore, that the introduction of a satisfactory new system would be welcomed by scientists working with the cellular proteinases. One possibility would be for the discoverer of a new proteinase to give it a completely trivial name, preferably consisting of one short word, analogous to the current, and perfectly adequate "trypsin", "pepsin" and "papain". A second system, more cumbersome but potentially more informative, would use names such as "serine proteinase A" (abbreviated "SP-A"). The name of an endopeptidase probably can indicate the catalytic class of the enzyme without serious risk of subsequently being found erroneous, but naming in terms of a particular substrate, or source, has proved very unsatisfactory in the past [31]. It is suggested that these and any alternative systems be given serious consideration, pending the time in the not too distant future when a new system will have to be agreed.

References

[1] SCHMIDT, W., and K. HAVEMANN: Hoppe-Seyler's Z. physiol. Chem. **355**, 1077–1082 (1974)
[2] STARKEY, P. M., and A. J. BARRETT: Biochem. J. **155**, 255–263 (1976)
[3] STARKEY, P. M., and A. J. BARRETT: Biochem. J. **155**, 265–271 (1976)
[4] STARKEY, P. M., and A. J. BARRETT: Biochem. J. **155**, 273–278 (1976)
[5] POWERS, J. C.: Trends biochem. Sci. **1**, 211–214 (1976)
[6] BLOW, A. M. J.: Biochem. J. **161**, 13–16 (1977)
[7] BLOW, A. M. J., and A. J. BARRETT: Biochem. J. **161**, 17–19 (1977)
[8] KNIGHT, C. G.: J. Chromat. **123**, 429–433 (1976)
[9] STARKEY, P. M. in: Proteinases in Mammalian Cells and Tissues. A. J. BARRETT (Ed.). North-Holland, Amsterdam 1977, pp. 57–89
[10] THORNE, K. J. I., R. C. OLIVER, and A. J. BARRETT: Infect. Immun. **14**, 555–563 (1976)
[11] BLONDIN, J., and A. JANOFF: J. clin. Invest. **58**, 971–979 (1976)
[12] KEISER, H., R. A. GREENWALD, G. FEINSTEIN, and A. JANOFF: J. clin. Invest. **57**, 625–632 (1976)
[13] ROUGHLEY, P. J., and A. J. BARRETT: Biochem. J. (in press)
[14] STARKEY, P. M., A. J. BARRETT, and P. M. BURLEIGH: Biochim. biophys. Acta (in press)
[15] OHLSSON, K., and U. ÅKESSON: Clinica chim. Acta **73**, 285–291 (1976)
[16] DAVIES, M., A. J. BARRETT, J. TRAVIS, E. SANDERS, and G. A. COLES: Clin. Sci. molec. Med. (in press)
[17] BARRETT, A. J., and P. M. STARKEY in: Rheumatoid Arthritis. Cellular Pathology and Pharmacology. J. L. GORDON and B. L. HAZLEMAN (Eds). Elsevier/North-Holland, Amsterdam 1977, pp. 211–221
[18] OSSOWSKI, L., J. P. QUIGLEY, and E. REICH: J. biol. Chem. **249**, 4312–4320 (1974)
[19] CHRISTMAN, J. K., S. C. SILVERSTEIN, and G. ACS in: Proteinases in Mammalian Cells and Tissues. A. J. BARRETT (Ed.). North-Holland, Amsterdam 1977, pp. 90–149
[20] CHRISTMAN, J. K., and G. ACS: Biochim. biophys. Acta **340**, 339–347 (1974)

[21] CHRISTMAN, J. K., and G. ACS: Nature, Lond. **264**, 681 (only) (1976)
[22] KATUNUMA, N.: Rev. Physiol. Biochem. Pharmac. **72**, 83–104 (1975)
[23] KATUNUMA, N., and E. KOMINAMI in: Proteinases in Mammalian Cells and Tissues. A. J. BARRETT (Ed.). North-Holland, Amsterdam 1977, pp. 151–180
[24] HAAS, R., T. NAGASAWA, and P. C. HEINRICH: Biochem. biophys. Res. Commun. **74**, 1060–1065 (1977)
[25] KORANT, B. D.: Biochem. biophys. Res. Commun. **74**, 926–933 (1977)
[26] SAITO, M., T. YOSHIZAWA, T. AOYAGI, and Y. NAGAI: Biochem. biophys. Res. Commun. **52**, 569–575 (1973)
[27] UMEZAWA, H., and T. AOYAGI in: Proteinases in Mammalian Cells and Tissues. A. J. BARRETT (Ed.). North-Holland, Amsterdam 1977, pp. 637–662
[28] BHATTACHARYYA, A. K., L. J. D. ZANEVELD, B. M. DRAGOJE, G. F. B. SCHUMACHER, and J. TRAVIS: J. Reprod. Fert. **47**, 97–100 (1976)
[29] ARNON, R. in: Immunological Approaches to Fertility Control. E. DICZFALUSY (Ed.). Karolinska Institute, Stockholm 1974, pp. 133–153
[30] MORTON, D. B. in: Proteinases in Mammalian Cells and Tissues. A. J. BARRETT (Ed.). North-Holland, Amsterdam 1977, pp. 445–500
[31] BARRETT, A. J. in: Proteinases in Mammalian Cells and Tissues. A. J. BARRETT (Ed.). North-Holland, Amsterdam 1977, pp. 1–55 and 181–207
[32] OTTO, K. in: Tissue Proteinases. A. J. BARRETT and J. T. DINGLE (Eds). North-Holland, Amsterdam 1977, p. 1–28
[33] OTTO, K., H. AFROZ, R. MÜLLER, and P. FUHGE in: Intracellular Protein Catabolism II. V. TURK and N. MARKS (Eds). Plenum Press, New York 1977, pp. 282–289
[34] MCDONALD, J. K., and S. ELLIS: Life Sci. **17**, 1269–1276 (1975)
[35] KIRSCHKE, H., J. LANGNER, B. WIEDERANDERS, S. ANSORGE, P. BOHLEY, and U. BROGHAMMER: Acta biol. med. germ. **35**, 285–299 (1976)
[36] KIRSCHKE, H., J. LANGNER, B. WIEDERANDERS, S. ANSORGE, and P. BOHLEY: Eur. J. Biochem. **74**, 293 (1977)
[37] ETHERINGTON, D. J.: Biochem. J. **153**, 199–209 (1976)
[38] HUISMAN, W. L. LANTING, H. J. DODDEMA, J. M. W. BOUMA, and M. GRUBER: Biochim. biophys. Acta **370**, 297–307 (1974)
[39] BOHLEY, H. KIRSCHKE, J. LANGNER, B. WIEDERANDERS, and S. ANSORGE: Acta biol. med. germ. **35**, 301–307 (1976)
[40] DEAN, R. T.: Biochem. biophys. Res. Commun. **68**, 518–523 (1976)
[41] SAXENA, V. P., and D. B. WETLAUFER: Biochemistry **9**, 5015–5022 (1970)
[42] AURICCHIO, F., L. MOLLICA, and A. LIGUORI: Biochem. J. **129**, 1131–1138 (1972)
[43] NAKASHIMA, K., and K. OGINO: J. Biochem., Tokyo **75**, 355–365 (1974)
[44] FRIEDRICH, K., H. KIRSCHKE, and S. ANSORGE: Acta biol. med. germ. **36**, 1723 (1977)
[45] JUDAH, J. D., and P. S. QUINN: Personal communication (1977)
[46] BARRETT, A. J. in: Proteinases of Mammalian Cells and Tissues. A. J. BARRETT (Ed.). North-Holland, Amsterdam 1977, pp. 209–248
[47] DINGLE, J. T., A. R. POOLE, G. S. LAZARUS, and A. J. BARRETT: J. exp. Med. **137**, 1124–1141 (1973)
[48] DEAN, R. T.: Nature, Lond. **257**, 414–416 (1975)
[49] HARRIS, E. D. Jr., and E. CARTWRIGHT in: Proteinases of Mammalian Cells and Tissues. A. J. BARRETT (Ed.). North-Holland, Amsterdam 1977, pp. 249–283
[50] SELLERS, A., E. CARTWRIGHT, G. MURPHY, and J. J. REYNOLDS: Biochem. J. **163**, 303 to 307 (1977)
[51] KERR, M. A., and A. J. KENNY: Biochem. J. **137**, 477–488 (1974)
[52] KERR, M. A., and A. J. KENNY: Biochem. J. **137**, 489–495 (1974)
[53] KENNY, A. I. in: Proteinases of Mammalian Cells and Tissues. A. J. BARRETT (Ed.), North-Holland, Amsterdam 1977, pp. 393–443
[54] DUCKWORTH, W. C.: Biochim. biophys. Acta **437**, 531–542 (1976)
[55] HARTLEY, B. S.: A. Rev. Biochem. **29**, 45–72 (1960)
[56] BLOW, A. M. J., R. VAN HEYNINGEN, and A. J. BARRETT: Biochem. J. **145**, 591–599 (1975)

[57] Dayton, W. R., W. J. Reville, D. E. Goll, and M. H. Stromer: Biochemistry **15**, 2159 (1976)
[58] Guroff, G.: J. biol. Chem. **239**, 149–155 (1964)
[59] Aswanikumar, S., and A. N. Radhakrishnan: Biochim. biophys. Acta **384**, 194–202 (1975)
[60] McQuillan, M. T., and V. M. Trikojus in: Tissue Proteinases. A. J. Barrett and J. T. Dingle (Eds). North-Holland, Amsterdam 1971, pp. 157–166
[61] Marks, N. in: Intracellular Protein Catabolism II. V. Turk and N. Marks (Eds). Plenum Press, New York 1977, pp. 85–102
[62] McRorie, R. A., R. B. Turner, M. M. Bradford, and W. L. Williams: Biochem, biophys. Res. Commun. **71**, 492–498 (1976)
[63] Kohn, L. D., C. Isersky, J. Zupnik, A. Lenaers, G. Lee, and C. M. Lapière: Proc. natn. Acad. Sci. U.S.A. **71**, 40–44 (1974)
[64] Cleveland, D. W., S. G. Fischer, M. W. Kirschner, and U. K. Laemmli: J. biol. Chem. **252**, 1102–1106 (1977)
[65] Berman, M. B. in: Trace Components of Plasma: Isolation and Clinical Significance. G. A. Jamieson and T. J. Greenwalt (Eds). Alan R. Liss Inc., New York 1976, pp. 225–253
[66] Mittman, C. (Ed.): Pulmonary Emphysema and Proteolysis. Academic Press, New York 1972
[67] Ignarro, L. J.: Agents Actions **4**, 241–258 (1974)
[68] Barrett, A. J., C. B. Sledge, and J. T. Dingle: Nature, Lond. **211**, 83–84 (1966)
[69] Shaw, I. H., C. G. Knight, and J. T. Dingle: Biochem. J. **158**, 473–476 (1976)
[70] Schorlemmer, H.-U., P. Davies, and A. C. Allison: Nature, Lond. **261**, 48–49 (1976)
[71] Brostoff, S. W., W. Reutter, M. Hichens, and E. H. Eylar: J. biol. Chem. **249**, 559–567 (1974)
[72] Fehr, K., M. Velvart, A. Böni, H. Watanabe, M. A. Spycher, and J. R. Rüttner: Ann. Rheum. Dis. **35**, 85 (1976)
[73] Ferguson, R. K., G. A. Turini, H. R. Brunner, N. Gavras, and D. N. McKinstry: Lancet **1977**/I, 775–778
[74] Parsons, J. A. (National Institute for Medical Research, London): Personal communication (1977)
[75] Poole, A. R. in: Lysosomes in Biology and Pathology. Vol. **3**, pp. 303–337. J. T. Dingle (Ed.). North-Holland, Amsterdam 1973
[76] Rao, G. J. S., and H. L. Nadler: Pediat. Res. **9**, 739–741 (1975)
[77] Golde, D. W., M. Territo, T. N. Finley, and M. J. Cline: Ann. Int. Med. **85**, 304 to 309 (1976)
[78] McAdoo, M. H., A. M. Dannenberg, C. J. Hayes, S. P. James, and J. H. Sanner: Infec. Immun. **7**, 655–665 (1973)
[79] Barlow, G. H., A. Rueter, and I. Tribby: Proteases and Biological Control. E. Reich, D. B. Rifkin, and E. Shaw (Eds). Cold Spring Harbor Laboratory, New York 1975, pp. 325–331
[80] Egberg, N.: Thromb. Res. **4**, 35–53 (1974)
[81] IUPAC-IUB: Enzyme Nomenclature: Recommendations (1972) of the Internation. Union of Pure and Applied Chemistry and the International Union of Biochemistry. Elsevier Publ. Co., Amsterdam 1973
[82] Barrett, A. J., H. Keilova, H. Kirschke, K. Otto, G. Siebert, V. M. Stepanov, and V. Turk in: Proteases and Biological Control. E. Reich, D. B. Rifkin and E. Shaw (Eds). Cold Spring Harbor Laboratory, New York 1975, pp. 481–482. Also in Intracellular Protein Catabolism. H. Hanson and P. Bohley (Eds). Barth, Leipzig 1975, pp. 555–557
[83] McDonald, J. K., and C. Schwabe in: Proteinases in Mammalian Cells and Tissues. A. J. Barrett (Ed.). North-Holland, Publ. Co., Amsterdam 1977, pp. 311–391
[84] Barrett, A. J. in: Proteinases in Mammalian Cells and Tissues. A. J. Barrett (Ed.). North-Holland Publ. Co., Amsterdam 1977, pp. 181–208
[85] Kirschke, H., J. Langner, B. Wiederanders, S. Ansorge, P. Bohley, and H. Hanson: Acta biol. med. germ. **36**, 185 (1977)
[86] Dingle, J. T., A. M. J. Blow, A. J. Barrett, and P. E. N. Martin: Biochem. J. (in press)
[87] Turnsek, T., I. Kregar, and D. Lebez: Biochim. biophys. Acta **403**, 514–520 (1975)

CONTENTS

СОДЕРЖАНИЕ

Страница

INHALT

Bezugsmöglichkeiten

Bestellungen sind zu richten:

- **in der DDR** an eine Buchhandlung oder an den Akademie-Verlag DDR-108 Berlin, Leipziger Straße 3–4
- **im sozialistischen Ausland** an eine Buchhandlung für fremdsprachige Literatur oder an den zuständigen Postzeitungsvertrieb
- **in der BRD und Westberlin** an eine Buchhandlung oder an die Auslieferungsstelle KUNST UND WISSEN, Erich Bieber, 7 Stuttgart 1, Wilhelmstraße 4–6
- **in Österreich** an den Globus-Buchvertrieb, 1201 Wien, Höchstädtplatz 3

im übrigen Ausland an den Internationalen Buch- und Zeitschriftenhandel; den Buchexport, Volkseigener Außenhandelsbetrieb der Deutschen Demokratischen Republik, DDR-701, Leipzig, Postfach 160, oder an den Akademie-Verlag,
- DDR-108, Berlin, Leipziger Straße 3–4.